T0201447

EMERGENCY MEDICINE ORAL BOARD REVIEW ILLUSTRATED

Second Edition

EMERGENCY MEDICINE ORAL BOARD REVIEW ILLUSTRATED

Second Edition

Edited by

YASUHARU OKUDA, MD

Associate Professor of Emergency Medicine, University of Central Florida College of
Medicine; National Medical Director, SimLEARN, Veterans Health Administration,
Orlando, FL, USA.

BRET P. NELSON, MD

Director of Emergency Ultrasound, Department of Emergency Medicine,
Icahn School of Medicine at Mount Sinai, New York, NY, USA

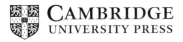

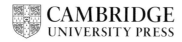

Shaftesbury Road, Cambridge CB2 8EA, United Kingdom

One Liberty Plaza, 20th Floor, New York, NY 10006, USA

477 Williamstown Road, Port Melbourne, VIC 3207, Australia

314–321, 3rd Floor, Plot 3, Splendor Forum, Jasola District Centre, New Delhi – 110025, India

103 Penang Road, #05–06/07, Visioncrest Commercial, Singapore 238467

Cambridge University Press is part of Cambridge University Press & Assessment,
a department of the University of Cambridge.

We share the University's mission to contribute to society through the pursuit of
education, learning and research at the highest international levels of excellence.

www.cambridge.org
Information on this title: www.cambridge.org/9781107627901

© Yasuharu Okuda and Bret P. Nelson (2010) 2015

This publication is in copyright. Subject to statutory exception
and to the provisions of relevant collective licensing agreements,
no reproduction of any part may take place without the written
permission of Cambridge University Press & Assessment.

First published 2010
Second edition 2015 (version 19, April 2024)

Printed in the United Kingdom by TJ Books Limited, Padstow Cornwall, April 2024

A catalogue record for this publication is available from the British Library

Library of Congress Cataloging-in-Publication data
Emergency medicine oral board review illustrated / edited by Yasuharu Okuda, Bret P. Nelson. – Second edition.
     p. ; cm.
Includes bibliographical references and index.
ISBN 978-1-107-62790-1 (Paperback : alk. paper)
I. Okuda, Yasuharu, editor.   II. Nelson, Bret, 1973– , editor.
[DNLM: 1. Emergency Medicine–methods–Case Reports.   2. Decision Making–Case Reports.   3. Emergency
Medical Services–Case Reports.   WB 105]
RC86.9
616.02´5076–dc23   2014050226

ISBN 978-1-107-62790-1 Paperback

Cambridge University Press & Assessment has no responsibility for the persistence or accuracy
of URLs for external or third-party internet websites referred to in this publication and does not
guarantee that any content on such websites is, or will remain, accurate or appropriate.

Every effort has been made in preparing this book to provide accurate and up-to-date information which
is in accord with accepted standards and practice at the time of publication. Although case histories are
drawn from actual cases, every effort has been made to disguise the identities of the individuals involved.
Nevertheless, the authors, editors and publishers can make no warranties that the information contained
herein is totally free from error, not least because clinical standards are constantly changing through
research and regulation. The authors, editors and publishers therefore disclaim all liability for direct
or consequential damages resulting from the use of material contained in this book. Readers are
strongly advised to pay careful attention to information provided by the manufacturer of any
drugs or equipment that they plan to use.

The authors dedicate this book to their shared mentor, Sheldon Jacobson, MD. Having spent decades perfecting the art of bedside teaching, he has been a role model and an advocate for generations of young faculty. With his support and guidance the authors have begun what they hope will be an equally long and rewarding journey in patient care, advocacy, and medical education.

YO: To my wife, who is my strength and best friend; my two daughters who show me how to enjoy life every day to its fullest; my parents who always allowed me to question; my family, friends, and colleagues for their timeless support; and my residents and students who teach me something new every day.

BPN: Throughout my career I have been fortunate to work with passionate, talented individuals who continually exceed my expectations. I am proud to have worked with so many of them in creating this book. I am humbled by the love and support of my family; they are responsible for all the great joys of my life.

Table of Contents

Color plate section can be found between pages xvi and 1.

Section Editors

Lars K. Beattie, MD, MS
Department of Emergency Medicine, University
   of Florida College of Medicine Gainesville, FL
(Cases 55 – 65, 118 and 119)

Kriti Bhatia, MD
Department of Emergency Medicine, Brigham &
   Women's Hospital, Boston, MA
(Cases 77 – 87, 122 and 123)

David Caro, MD
Department of Emergency Medicine, University of
   Florida College of Medicine, Jacksonville, FL
(Cases 88 – 98)

Michael Cassara, DO
Associate Professor of Emergency Medicine,
   Hofstra North Shore-LIJ School of Medicine,
   Associate Program Director, Residency in
   Emergency Medicine, North Shore University
   Hospital, Associate Medical Director, North
   Shore-LIJ Health System Patient Safety
   Institute / Emergency Medical Institute, NY
(Cases 1 – 11, and 126)

Bharath Chakravarthy, MD, MPH
Department of Emergency Medicine, University
   of California Irvine, Irvine, CA
(Cases 12 – 22, 116, and 117)

Anne Chipman, MS, MD
Department of Emergency Medicine, Alameda
   County Health System-Highland Hospital, San
   Francisco, CA
(Case 124)

Michael G. Gonzalez, MD
Baylor College of Medicine, Houston, TX
(Cases 44 – 54, 114, and 115)

Colleen Hickey
Baylor College of Medicine, Houston, TX
(Cases 33 – 43, 110, and 111)

Amy Leuthauser, MD, MS
Department of Emergency Medicine,
   Mount Sinai School of Medicine,
   New York, NY
(Cases 66 – 76, 112, and 113)

Jacqueline Nemer, MD
Associate Professor of Emergency Medicine,
   Department of Emergency Medicine,
   University of California, San Francisco,
   CA
(Cases 99 – 109, 124, and 125)

Thomas Nguyen, MD
Assistant Professor, Assistant Program Director,
   Department of Emergency Medicine, Beth
   Israel Medical Center, NY
(Cases 23 – 32, 120, and 121)

Peter S. Pang, MD
Associate Chief | Emergency Medicine
   Associate Professor | Medicine Center for
   Cardiovascular Innovation, Chicago, IL
(Cases 33 – 43, 110, and 111)

Contributors

Yuemi An-Grogan, MD
Fellow, Pediatric Emergency Medicine,
Department of Pediatrics, Northwestern
University Feinberg School of Medicine, Ann
and Robert H. Lurie Children's Hospital of
Chicago, Chicago, IL

Sunil Aradhya, MD
Resident, Department of Medicine, Emergency
Medicine Section, Baylor College of Medicine,
Houston, TX

Ani Aydin, MD
Clinical Instructor, Department of Emergency
Medicine, Yale School of Medicine, New
Haven, CT

Lars K. Beattie, MD, MS
Department of Emergency Medicine, University
of Florida College of Medicine, Gainesville,
FL, USA

Jessica Berrios, MD
Department of Emergency Medicine, Nassau
University Medical Center, East Meadow, NY

Michael Cassara, DO
Associate Professor of Emergency Medicine,
Hofstra North Shore-LIJ School of Medicine,
Associate Program Director, Residency in
Emergency Medicine, North Shore University
Hospital, Associate Medical Director, North
Shore-LIJ Health System Patient Safety
Institute / Emergency Medical Institute, NY

Bharath Chakravarthy, MD, MPH
Department of Emergency Medicine,
University of California Irvine, Irvine, CA

David Cherkas, MD
Department of Emergency Medicine, Icahn
School of Medicine at Mount Sinai, Elmhurst
Hospital Center, Elmhurst, NY

Joseph Chiang, MD
Medical Director, Department of Emergency
Medicine, Memorial Hospital Los Banos, Los
Banos, CA

Anne Chipman, MS, MD
Resident Physician, Department of Emergency
Medicine, Alameda County Health
System-Highland Hospital,
San Francisco CA

Evelyn Chow, MD
Department of Emergency Medicine, Kaiser
Permanente, Fremont, CA

Meka Close, MD
Department of Emergency Medicine, Jersey City
Medical Center, Jersey City, NJ

Michael A. Cole, MD
Associate Physician Department of Emergency
Medicine Brigham and Women's Hospital,
and Clinical Instructor in Medicine
(Emergency Medicine) Harvard Medical
School, Boston, MA

Matthew Constantine, MD
Assistant Professor, Department of Surgery,
   Division of Emergency Medicine, UT
   Southwestern Medical Center, Dallas, TX

Abiola Fasina, MD
The Memorial Hospital of Salem County,
   Salem, NJ

Desmond Fitzpatrick, MD
Department of Emergency Medicine, University
   of Florida College of Medicine, Gainesville, FL

Nicholas Genes, MD, PhD
Department of Emergency Medicine, Icahn School
   of Medicine at Mount Sinai, New York, NY

Daniel Goldstein, MD
Resident, Department of Emergency Medicine,
   Beth Israel Medical Center, New York, NY

Tarlan Hedayati, MD
Assistant Professor, Department of Emergency
   Medicine, Rush Medical College, Chicago, IL

Luke Hermann, MD
Department of Emergency Medicine, Icahn School
   of Medicine at Mount Sinai, New York, NY

Braden Hexom, MD
Department of Emergency Medicine, Icahn School
   of Medicine at Mount Sinai, New York, NY

Alan Huang, MD
Sutter Tracy Community Hospital, Tracy, CA

Bashar A. Ismail, MBBS
Resident, Department of Medicine, Emergency
   Medicine Section, Baylor College of Medicine,
   Houston, TX

Lisa Jacobson, MD
Assistant Professor of Emergency Medicine,
University of Florida College of Medicine,
   Jacksonville, FL

Maxwell Jen, MD
Resident, Department of Emergency Medicine,
   UC Irvine School of Medicine, Irvine, CA

Ravi Kapoor, MD, MPH
Instructor, Icahn School of Medicine at Mount
   Sinai, New York, NY

Raashee Kedia, MD
Assistant Professor, Department of Emergency
   Medicine, UT Southwestern Medical Center,
   Dallas, TX

Satjiv Kohli, MD, MBA
Department of Emergency Medicine, Icahn
   School of Medicine at Mount Sinai, Hospital of
   Queens, New York, NY

Bonnie Lau, MD
Medical Education Fellow,
Department of Emergency Medicine, University
   of California, San Francisco, Belmont, CA

Elisabeth Lessenich, MD, MPH
Harvard-Affiliated Emergency Medicine
   Residency, Brigham & Women's Hospital /
   Massachusetts General Hospital, and
   Department of Emergency Medicine, Boston,
   MA

Edward R. Melnick, MD, MHS
Assistant Professor, Department of Emergency
   Medicine, Yale School of Medicine, New
   Haven, CT

Denise Nassisi, MD FACEP
Associate Professor, Department of Emergency
   Medicine, Icahn School of Medicine at Mount
   Sinai, New York, NY

Bret P. Nelson, MD
Director of Emergency Ultrasound,
Department of Emergency Medicine, Icahn
   School of Medicine at Mount Sinai,
   New York, NY

Jacqueline Nemer, MD
Associate Professor of Emergency Medicine,
Department of Emergency Medicine, University
   of California, San Francisco, CA

Thomas Nguyen, MD
Assistant Professor Department of Emergency
   Medicine, Assistant Program Director, Beth
   Israel Medical Center, NY

Uyen Nguyen, MD
Resident, Department of Emergency Medicine,
   Beth Israel Medical Center, New York, NY

Yasuharu Okuda, MD
Associate Professor of Emergency Medicine,
University of Central Florida College of Medicine;
   National Medical Director, SimLEARN,
   Veterans Health Administration, Orlando, FL

Ruben Olmedo, MD
Department of Emergency Medicine, Icahn
   School of Medicine at Mount Sinai, New York,
   NY

Ram Parekh, MD
Assistant Clinical Professor, Department of
   Emergency Medicine, Icahn School of
   Medicine at Mount Sinai, New York, NY

Matthew Ryan, MD, PhD
Assistant Professor, Department of Emergency
   Medicine, University of Florida College of
   Medicine, Gainesville, FL

Sheler Sadati, MD
University of Rochester Medical Center School
   of Medicine and Dentistry, Rochester, NY

Raghu Seethala, MD
Department of Emergency Medicine, Surgical
   Intensive Care Unit, Brigham Women's
   Hospital, Instructor of Medicine, Harvard
   Medical School, Boston, MA

Amish Shah, MD
Department of Emergency Medicine, Icahn School
   of Medicine at Mount Sinai, New York, NY

Peter Shearer, MD
Department of Emergency Medicine, Icahn School
   of Medicine at Mount Sinai, New York, NY

Bing Shen, MD
Department of Emergency Medicine, Kaiser
   Permanente Medical Center, Hayward/
   Fremont, CA

Mason Shieh, MD, MBA
Resident, Department of Emergency Medicine,
   Beth Israel Medical Center, New York, NY

Benjamin H. Slovis, MD
Department of Emergency Medicine, Icahn School
   of Medicine at Mount Sinai, New York, NY

Natasha Spencer, MD, PhD
VA Connecticut Healthcare System – West
   Haven Campus, West Haven, CT

Reuben Strayer, MD
Assistant Clinical Professor, Department of
   Emergency Medicine, Icahn School of
   Medicine at Mount Sinai, New York, NY

Christopher Strother, MD
Assistant Professor, Department of Emergency
   Medicine, Icahn School of Medicine at Mount
   Sinai, New York, NY

Jeffrey R. Suchard, MD
Professor of Clinical Emergency Medicine and
   Clinical Pharmacology, UC Irvine School of
   Medicine, Irvine, CA

Shefali Trivedi, MD
Department of Emergency Medicine, Icahn School
   of Medicine at Mount Sinai, New York, NY

Tiffany Truong, MD, MPH
Medical Director, St. Mary's Medical Center, San
   Francisco, CA

Anita Vashi, MD
Robert Wood Johnson Foundation Clinical
   Scholars Program, Department of Internal
   Medicine, Yale School of Medicine,
   New Haven, CT

Scott Weingart, MD, FCCM
Associate Professor Director of ED Critical Care,
   Icahn School of Medicine at Mount Sinai,
   New York, NY

Alisa Wray, MD
Resident, Department of Emergency Medicine,
   UC Irvine School of Medicine, Irvine, CA

Lisa Zahn, MD
Attending Physician,
Emergency Department, Ocean Medical Center,
   Brick, NJ

Shawn Zhong, MD
Chief of Emergency Critical Care at Staten Island
   University Hospital, Staten Island, NY

Preface

The accreditation process for emergency medicine in the United States is considered to be one of the most difficult among all medical specialties, with residents required to pass both a written and oral examination to gain certification. This book allows the reader to apply a case-based interactive approach to studying for the oral board examination, while also providing an excellent introduction to the field. Featuring more than 100 cases derived from the *Model of Clinical Practice of Emergency Medicine*, with an emphasis on EKGs, CT scans, x-rays, and ultrasounds, this book is a model resource for the practicing emergency medicine resident. The reader can easily practice cases alone or with a partner and can follow up with key points of critical actions, clinical pearls, and references. The appendixes are loaded with high-yield information on subjects emphasized in the oral board examination, such as pediatric, cardiovascular, traumatic, and toxicological disorders. This book truly allows the reader to feel actively immersed in the case.

Some of the diagnoses featured in this book include: Iron overdose, congenital hyper-trophic pyloric stenosis, hemorrhagic stroke, tension pneumothorax, Boerhaave syndrome, necrotizing fasciitis, Henoch-Schönlein purpura, abdominal aortic aneurysm, thermal burn 30%, Steven-Johnson syndrome, febrile syndrome, ectopic pregnancy, inferior wall myocardial infarction, thrombotic thrombocytopenic purpura, Ludwig's angina, cavernous sinus thrombosis, Kawasaki syndrome, high altitude cerebral edema, Fournier gangrene, neck trauma, pancreatitis, alcohol withdrawal, pelvis fracture, childhood trauma—abuse, necrotizing enterocolitis, cold water immersion, congenital coarctation, isoniazid overdose, elder abuse, and carotid artery dissection.

Dr. Yasuharu Okuda is the Director of the Institute for Medical Simulation and Advanced Learning for the Health and Hospitals Corporation (HHC) of New York City and is responsible for training clinical providers across all 11 NYC HHC hospitals using case-based simulation. He holds dual appointments in Emergency Medicine (EM) and Medical Education at The Mount Sinai School of Medicine and has significant experience in residency education as a former associate program director of EM. He received his MD from New York Medical College and completed his training at Mount Sinai Emergency Medicine Residency. He holds appointments on multiple national committees including Co-Chair of the Emergency Medicine Special Interest Group for the Society for Simulation in Healthcare and Vice-Chair of the SAEM Simulation Academy. He has received numerous awards in education and is published in the areas of simulation and neurological emergencies. His research focus is in human factors in health care, using simulation to improve safety and quality of patient care.

Dr. Bret P. Nelson is an assistant professor of Emergency Medicine at the Mount Sinai School of Medicine. He is the Associate Residency Director and the Director of Emergency Ultrasound for the department. He received his MD from SUNY Stony Brook School of Medicine and completed his training at the Harvard Affiliated Emergency Medicine residency program at the Massachusetts General and Brigham & Women's Hospitals. He has lectured throughout the United States, Europe, and Asia and has earned awards for teaching from Harvard Medical School and Mount Sinai. His research interests include bedside ultrasound and medical education, and he is coauthor of the *Manual of Emergency and Critical Care Ultrasound* (Cambridge University Press).

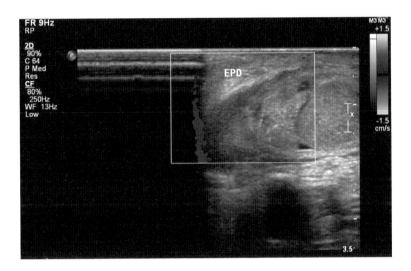

Figure 20.3

Figure 114.1

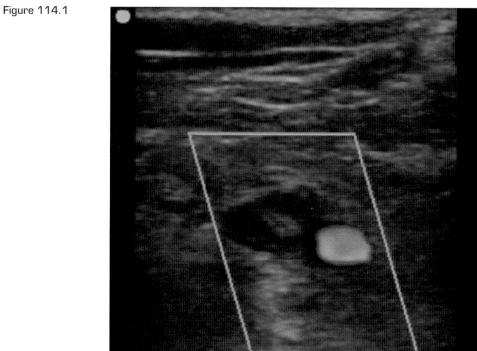

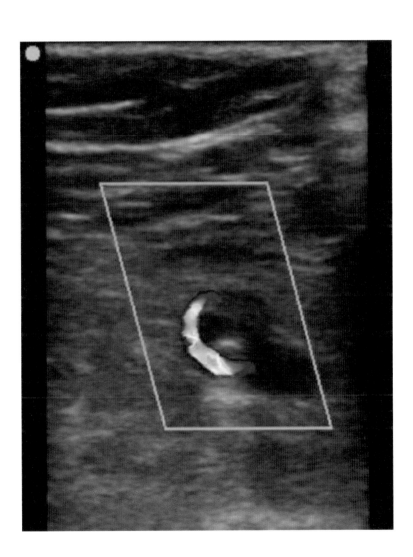

Figure 114.2

Figure 116.1

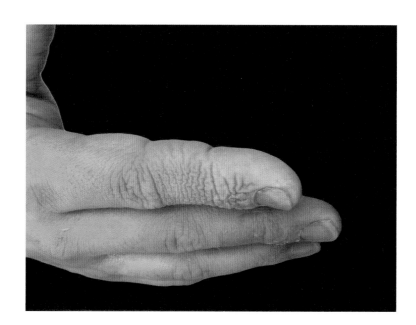

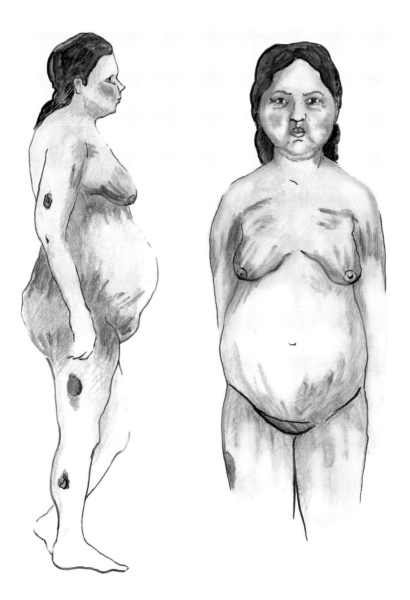

Figure 120.1

Figure 121.2

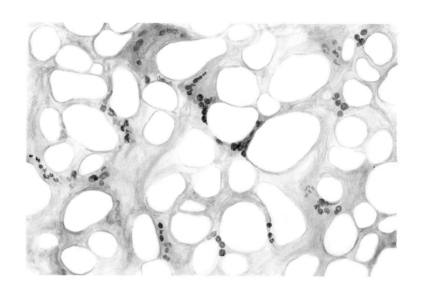

CHAPTER 1

How to use this book

Bret P. Nelson, MD

HOW TO USE THIS BOOK

The amount of information that must be transferred from books, patients, journals, mentors, and so on into the brain of an aspiring emergency physician is overwhelming. Many physicians create study plans, purchase books, fall behind schedule, and readjust timelines in an endless process akin to yo-yo dieting. Whatever the means we use to study while not actively caring for patients, inevitably we learn as our forebears did – one patient at a time.

Thus, this book was crafted as a case-based approach to the art and science of emergency medicine. Although the format stresses an approach useful in preparation for the emergency medicine oral boards, the cases serve as a review (or introduction) to the practice of emergency medicine. These pages contain heuristics on the general approach to patient management, pearls on the care of children, tips on performing common bedside procedures, and a litany of cases.

ORAL BOARD PREPARATION

Working with a Partner

As described in Chapter 3, during the oral boards you will be taken through a series of cases by an American Board of Emergency Medicine examiner. To mimic this process as closely as possible, you should review the cases in this book with a partner. Pairing with another emergency physician is ideal, as they will be familiar with the format of the boards and the medical decision making in the cases, and they will have more fun throwing curveballs at you to make the cases more interesting (or difficult)! If you cannot find a colleague with a medical background to take you through the cases, a friend, family member, or significant other will do. The "examiner instructions" for each case are written to help a nonphysician approach the case. It is quite likely that your family and friends already know a lot of the jargon in this book. Like most physicians, you have probably regaled them with enough stomach-turning stories over the dinner table to make them experts. If you are fortunate enough to have a partner (examiner), read through the introductory section and appendices and become familiar with the format for the boards, but do not look at the images or cases. The examiner will take you (the candidate, to use ABEM's term) through the cases. You should read through each case on your own after working through it with your examiner, and look up any areas you had difficulty with. References for standard emergency medicine texts; Tintinalli's *Emergency Medicine: A Comprehensive Study Guide*, 7th ed. by Tintinalli and colleagues, 2011; *Rosen's Emergency Medicine: Concepts and Clinical Practice*, 8th ed. by Marx and colleagues, 2014, are included for each case. Please ask your partner to read the next section (Examiner Instructions) and the sample case before you tackle the cases in the rest of the book.

Examiner Instructions

Thank you for helping your friend, family member, or colleague (the candidate) to review for the oral board exam. This is the final step in their quest to become a board-certified emergency physician. It is probably not the first (and certainly not the last) time you will ask yourself, "What have I gotten myself into?" when dealing with them. Your efforts will greatly exceed whatever reward you have been offered, especially if you were convinced by dinner in any restaurant they can afford on a resident's salary.

If you are a physician, nurse, emergency medical technician (EMT), or other medical provider, the case-based format should be familiar to you. Your goal is to provide the candidate with bits of information about the case and take the case in different directions based on their actions (or inaction). If you have no medical background, don't be intimidated! You already understand enough about medical care to appreciate the daily struggles the candidate faces in taking care of patients. Keep in mind that none of the actors on today's "doctor shows" ever attended medical school. Yet they can sound convincing, and you can appreciate the medical plot points, with a little coaching.

Each case focuses on a patient presenting with some acute manifestation of illness. Some will have subtle signs such as headache or nausea, and others will be quite obviously sick (vomiting blood, major motor vehicle accident, etc.). Many patients will have straightforward problems such as broken bones, and others will have diagnoses that are difficult to pin down (poisonings, drug reactions, or more rare illnesses). Start by reading the examiner instructions for each case; these will give you an overall picture of what the medical problem and major critical actions are. Within the description there will often be additional points on how to deal with situations that will arise in the course of the case – playing the part of a consultant, when to reveal certain key information, how to deal with common medical errors, and so on. Next, read the case from beginning to end to see the flow, starting with the "chief complaint" (reason for evaluation) to initial impressions (What do I see when I walk into the room?) to basic historical information about the patient and the physical examination, followed by ordering tests, giving medications, interpreting the test results, calling upon consultants, and establishing patient disposition (admitting to the hospital, going to the operating room, discharging them, etc.).

The cases are meant to be fun (in a nerdy sort of way). At first, you'll probably present the cases pretty "straight." You can state the patient's complaint and examination as written in the text, speak about consultants in the third person ("the cardiologist says they will see the patient in the morning"), and "stick to the script." As you become more comfortable with the oral boards' format, feel free to get into the character a bit more. Patients, consultants, nurses, and other "characters" in oral board cases are typically portrayed in the first person by examiners. Instead of saying, "the patient reports they are in pain," try, "Doctor, my arm still hurts" or "Why isn't my son getting anything for pain? Who's in charge here?" You probably know someone who thought karaoke was stupid but then would not give up the microphone after trying it. Taking a friend through these cases can be similarly entertaining, even without the aid of alcohol.

When you become fairly comfortable with the format (this is easier for medical professionals), you can deviate a bit from the cases to make them more interesting and challenging. Examples of how to do this are given in some cases with a "curveball" described. Some of these curveballs will involve reluctant consultants, patients who aren't forthcoming with the truth, or other factors which can make proper diagnosis and treatment difficult. Many of these types of curveballs can appear on the real oral boards, because the candidate is being tested partially on their ability to work effectively in the emergency medicine practice system. Some are so important that they should be expected in every case, even when not explicitly stated in the instructions. For example, if the candidate orders a medication before checking the patient's allergies, that patient should exhibit an allergic reaction to the medication. This is good practice for the boards (where points can be deducted for such mistakes) but more important in real life, where "points" are people.

Working Alone

Don't worry if you couldn't convince anyone to nurse you through all of the cases. You can still use this book effectively to engage in "active learning," which is much more effective for adult learners than flipping through pages and passively reading the text. You'll have to use a bit of discipline in approaching the cases and force yourself to think about your management for each case.

After reading the sample case, take each case one by one. Read through the chief complaint and think about what you would do with that patient immediately. Usually, the next question to ask is, "What do I see when I look at the patient?" After the text reveals the answer, stop and think of your next action. For example, if you saw an ashen, unresponsive patient, you will want to move immediately toward resuscitation. For a well-appearing patient in no distress, you will likely start with a primary survey, history, and physical examination.

Try to think ahead as much as possible, focusing on what specific historical or physical examination items you are especially interested in. You will get more out of asking yourself, "Does this patient have a carotid bruit?" than simply thinking, "Now I'll examine the patient." Remember that the real oral board examiners will not just give away the entire examination; they will often ask for what specific actions you would like to perform. There are no tricks in this book, and there should not be any on the boards either. When a test or physical examination is described as "normal," move on with the case as if it is.

By the end of each case, you will see a checklist of critical actions. These types of actions are the basis for scoring on the real oral boards. The examiner instructions are near the end. These will often provide insights into the case, confirming or revealing the diagnosis, and often elucidating why certain actions were or were not mandated, why that computed tomography (CT) scan was never available, or why the consultant gave you such a hard time. While the case is fresh in your mind, refer to the appropriate chapters in Rosen's or Tintinalli's to ensure you are comfortable with the material.

EMERGENCY MEDICINE STUDY GUIDE

Emergency Medicine Residents, Medical Students, Nurses, EMTs, PAS, and Other Providers

Sometimes it's more interesting and engaging to go through cases rather than to read textbook chapters. An individual case can be reviewed in a very short time, making it ideal for reading on public transportation or when you have only a few minutes. Ideally, use the "active" reading method described in the board review section. You can also give the cases a straight read-through, though it's not as effective as engaging your limbic system a bit by challenging yourself to think, "What should I do next?"

The cases should then be used as a springboard for further reading or discussion. Primary textbook references are given, but these should be supplemented by a search for more current literature (using PubMed, UptoDate, or other online research tool). Ask colleagues or mentors about similar cases they've encountered and how they managed them. The management decisions in this book are meant to represent "textbook" answers, but real-world management often differs significantly. By anchoring your supplemental reading in cases, you will have a greater retention of the management pearls and other facts discussed.

SAMPLE CASE

The following sample case is presented twice. First, the case is written in the standard format used throughout the book. Next, a sample dialogue describes the case as it would be presented by an examiner to a candidate. By looking back and forth between the case and the dialogue, you should get some sense of how the book can be used and how the oral boards are administered.

CASE A: Back Pain

A. Chief complaint
a. 55-year-old male with backache

B. Vital signs
a. Blood pressure (BP): 165/90, heart rate (HR): 90, respiratory rate (RR): 16, temperature (T): 36.8°C orally oxygen saturation (Sat): 98% on room air (RA)

C. What does the patient look like?
a. Patient lying on stretcher, appears stated age; appears in mild distress as he attempts to find a position of comfort

D. Primary survey
a. Airway: speaking in full sentences
b. Breathing: no respiratory distress, no cyanosis
c. Circulation: warm and moist skin, normal pulses, and capillary refill

E. History
a. History of present illness (HPI): the patient is a 55-year-old male with no significant past medical history who presents with a backache for several hours. He reports

walking to work when he noted a sharp, burning pain in his mid to lower back, worse on the left than the right side. The pain began rather abruptly and was severe. He felt that it radiated up to his posterior chest and down to his leg when it was most pronounced. It has since improved a bit. There is no position that makes the pain better or worse, and the patient is unable to localize the pain to an exact point on his back. He denies any difficulty urinating, blood in the urine, or trauma.

  b. Past medical history (PMHx): none
  c. Past surgical history (PSHx): none
  d. Allergies: none
  e. Medications: none
  f. Social: lives with wife; drinks alcohol socially, smokes one-half pack of cigarettes per day, denies the use of other drugs. Works as a manager at a box company
  g. Family history (FHx): no significant family history
  h. Primary medical doctor (PMD): Dr Underhill

F. Action
  a. Oxygen via nasal cannulae (NC) or nonrebreather mask
  b. Two large-bore peripheral intravenous (IV) lines
  c. Monitor: BP: 165/95 HR: 95 RR: 18 Sat: 100% on 2L NC

G. Secondary survey
  a. General: mild pain, discomfort
  b. Head: normocephalic, atraumatic
  c. Eyes: normal
  d. Ears: normal
  e. Nose: normal
  f. Neck: supple, nontender, normal range of motion, no carotid bruit
  g. Pharynx: normal dentition, no lesions, no swelling
  h. Chest: nontender, no lesions
  i. Lungs: normal air movement, clear breath sounds bilaterally
  j. Heart: normal rate, rhythm regular; no murmurs, rubs, or gallops
  k. Abdomen: normal bowel sounds, soft, nontender or distended
  l. Rectal: normal tone, brown stool, occult blood negative
  m. Urogenital: normal examination
  n. Extremities: full range of motion; no deformity; normal femoral, radial, and dorsalis pedis pulses
  o. Back: nontender, no costovertebral angle tenderness, no muscle spasm, no signs of trauma
  p. Neurologic: alert and oriented; cranial nerves intact; normal strength, sensation, gait
  q. Skin: warm to touch. No rash noted
  r. Lymphatic: no lymphadenopathy

H. Studies
  a. CBC, BMP, coagulation studies, blood type and cross-match
  b. Lactate, UA
  c. EKG (electrocardiogram, also known as ECG)

I. Nurse
  a. EKG (Figure 1.1)

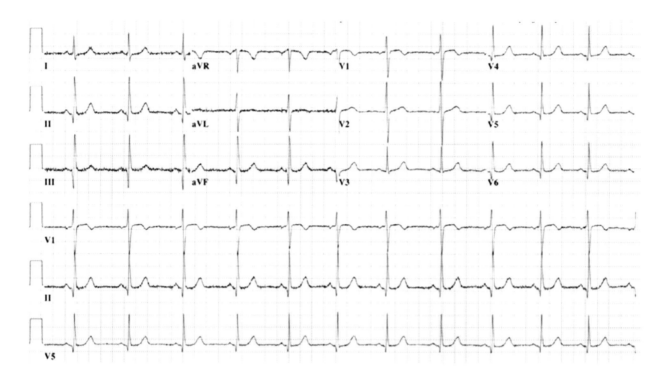

Figure 1.1

J. Action
a. Imaging
  i. Chest x-ray (CXR)
b. Medications
  i. Morphine IV
c. Reassess
  i. Pain improved with morphine

K. Results

Complete blood count (CBC):

White blood cells (WBC)	11.1×10^3/uL
Hematocrit (Hct)	40.3%
Platelets (Plt)	438×10^3/uL

Basic metabolic panel (BMP):

Sodium (Na)	134 mEq/L
Potassium (K)	3.9 mEq/L
Chloride (Cl)	101 mEq/L
Bicarbonate (CO_2)	29 mEq/L
Blood urea nitrogen (BUN)	20 mEq/dL
Creatinine (Cr)	1.2 mg/dL%
Glucose (Gluc)	113 mg/dL

Coagulation panel:

Prothrombin time (PT)	11.9 sec
Partial thromboplastin time (PTT)	24.0 sec
International normalized ratio (INR)	1.1

Liver function panel:

Aspartate aminotransferase (AST)	31 U/L
Alanine aminotransferase (ALT)	29 U/L
Alkaline phosphatase (Alk Phos)	52 U/L
Total bilirubin (T bili)	0.9 mg/dL
Direct bilirubin (D bili)	0.1 mg/dL
Amylase	42 U/L
Lipase	19 U/L
Albumin	4.1 g/dL

Urinalysis (UA):

Specific Gravity (SG)	1.019
pH	6
Protein (Prot)	Neg
Glucose (Gluc)	Neg
Ketones	Neg
Bilirubin (Bili)	Neg
Blood	Neg
Leukocyte esterase (LE)	Neg
Nitrite	Neg
Color	Yellow

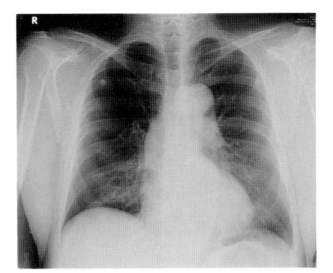

Figure 1.2

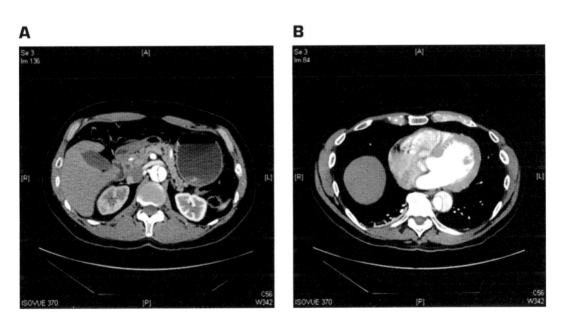

Figure 1.3
A and B

a. Lactate: 1.5
b. CXR (Figure 1.2)

L. Reassess
a. Patient describes worsening of pain, now with nausea and some chest discomfort as well

M. Action
a. Imaging
   i. Computed tomography (CT) scan of chest and abdomen (must describe differential diagnosis to radiologist protocoling study)

N. Nurse
a. CT scan (Figure 1.3) demonstrates dissection of the descending thoracic aorta extending to the abdominal aorta and the left iliac artery. There is no involvement of the aortic arch.

O. Action

a. Consultation

    i. Vascular surgery

    ii. Intensive care unit

    iii. Notify primary care doctor

b. Meds

    i. Esmolol, Labetalol, or other β-antagonist IV

    ii. Morphine IV

    iii. Sodium nitroprusside IV

P. Reassess

a. (β-antagonists given) Monitor: BP: 110/55 HR: 55 RR: 18 Sat: 100% on 2L NC; pain improved

b. (β-antagonists not given) Monitor: BP: 170/100 HR: 100 RR: 18 Sat: 100% on 2L NC; pain continues

Q. Diagnosis

a. Type B aortic dissection

R. Critical actions

▪ EKG

▪ CXR

▪ Analgesia

▪ Thorough neurologic and vascular examinations

▪ CT scan to assess for dissection

▪ Verbalize differential diagnosis (dissection, aneurysm, renal colic) with consultant (radiologist, ICU staff, etc)

▪ Blood pressure control

▪ ICU consultation and admission

S. Examiner instructions

a. This is a case of aortic dissection. The aorta is the largest artery in the body and carries blood from the heart to the chest and abdomen. Its wall is composed of several layers that can tear, causing blood to dissect in between the layers. High blood pressure, smoking, and chronic medical conditions can increase the risk of this disorder. The patient's back pain and shortness of breath were due to tearing of the layers of the aorta, and therefore will not be improved with moving to a different position. The aorta should be suspected because of the severity and radiation of pain, and taking into account the patient's risk factors (smoking) and abnormal vital signs (high blood pressure). If the patient is not placed on a cardiac monitor, they should complain of feeling "woozy." The patient's pain will continue to worsen in the ED until he is treated with a β-antagonist (such as Labetalol, Esmolol, Propranolol) and a pain medication such as morphine. If the patient does not undergo imaging or is discharged, he should lose consciousness. A CT scan should be readily available if requested, but ultrasound and MRI will "take a few hours."

T. Pearls

a. Dissections are often classified according to their anatomic involvement: Type A involves the ascending aorta; type B does not.

b. Up to 12% of patients with aortic dissection have a normal CXR; the test should not be used to exclude the diagnosis.

c. Magnetic resonance imaging (MRI) has the best sensitivity and specificity for the diagnosis of aortic dissection; however, this test is often not feasible as it requires a stable patient and more time than other modalities, such as transesophageal echo (TEE) or CT scan. Among these options, CT scan is most commonly employed as the test of choice in the ED.

d. When considering aortic dissection in a patient with chest pain or difficulty breathing, other diagnoses in the differential include myocardial ischemia, congestive heart failure, pericarditis, and pulmonary embolus (PE). The diagnosis should also be considered for atypical back pain where renal colic or musculoskeletal causes are being considered, especially in patients with risk factors, such as advanced age, smoking, or hypertension.

e. Goals of emergency department therapy for dissection include blood pressure reduction and decreasing shear forces acting on the dissection site. Thus, β-blockers such as Esmolol, Metoprolol, and Propranolol are considered first-line agents. Vasodilators such as sodium nitroprusside may be administered after these agents are used. Analgesia is important for patient comfort; it reduces sympathomimetic drive contributing to blood pressure and shear forces.

f. Surgical management reduces in-hospital mortality for type A dissections and is the standard of care. Initial treatment of type B acute aortic dissections is generally medical (blood pressure control and observation). Patients with persistent pain, uncontrolled hypertension, occlusion of a major arterial trunk, aortic leak or rupture, or development of a localized aneurysm may require surgical intervention.

U. References
a. Tintinalli's: Chapter 62. Aortic Dissection and Related Aortic Syndromes
b. Rosen: Chapter 85. Aortic Dissection

SAMPLE CASE SCRIPT

Here is one example of how the sample case could play out between an examiner and a candidate. Each case will run a very different course depending on the examiner and the choices the candidate makes. This example is intended to highlight a few common circumstances that will come up during the cases. This is **NOT** an example of a "perfectly run" case.

EXAMINER:
You are working an overnight shift at General Hospital, and the next patient is a 55-year-old man with back pain. *(If you are making up the case, you get to name the hospital! Most cases should take place in an emergency department associated with a large hospital, but you can alter the scenarios as you like. During the boards, "ABEM General" is the default location.)*

CANDIDATE:
What do I see when I walk into the room?

EXAMINER:
(From What does the patient look like?) The patient is lying on a stretcher, appears stated age; he is in mild distress as he attempts to find a position of comfort.

CANDIDATE:
May I have the vital signs?

EXAMINER:
(From Vital signs) Blood pressure: 165/90, heart rate: 90, respiratory rate: 16, temperature: 36.8°C orally, oxygen saturation: 98% on room air.

CANDIDATE:
I'd like to perform a primary survey. Is the patient able to speak?

EXAMINER:
(From the Primary survey) Yes, he is speaking in full sentences.

CANDIDATE:
How is his breathing? What does his skin look like?

EXAMINER:
(From the Primary survey) He is in no respiratory distress; there is no cyanosis. His skin is warm and moist, and he has normal capillary refill.

CANDIDATE:
The patient seems stable enough to obtain a further history. Sir, what brings you to the emergency department today?

EXAMINER:
(From the HPI) Well, Doc, my back's been hurting me for a few hours now. I got this sharp pain in my lower back while I was walking to work. It came out of nowhere. It seemed to go down my left leg and up to my chest. *(If you are just starting out, you can just read the HPI as written. Once you become comfortable with the cases, it will be more interesting and true to the oral board format to act out the case a bit and speak as the patient in the first person.)*

CANDIDATE:
Was there a particular position that makes the pain worse or better?

EXAMINER:
No, and I can't seem to get into a comfortable position now, either. I've never had anything like this before.

CANDIDATE:
Were you exerting yourself at all? Have you been working out recently, or have you had any injury to the area?

EXAMINER:
No, nothing I can think of.

CANDIDATE:

Are you having any chest pain, trouble breathing, or palpitations?

EXAMINER:

The back pain seemed to go toward the chest as well. No trouble breathing or palpitations. *(If a symptom isn't mentioned in the case, feel free to say it is negative.)*

CANDIDATE:

I'd like to put this patient on a cardiac monitor, place an intravenous line, and start him on oxygen. We should hold some blood tubes for laboratory testing as well.

EXAMINER:

All right. The nurse has established a cardiac monitor, IV access, and placed the patient on oxygen. *(If you are comfortable with the way cases typically run, you can ask the candidate what type of IV and how much oxygen. If all these words are like a foreign language for you, just play the cases straight. Also, note how the candidate has the nurse place a line and draw labs early in the case. Since it is not yet clear which labs will need to be sent, the candidate just requests the nurse "hold" the blood for now. The cases in the rest of the book list lab tests early on, but that doesn't mean the candidate needs to order them before examining the patient or obtaining a history first. They are listed early so the examiner has a rough idea of what might be requested or relevant. The examiner can have the nurse ask, "What labs would you like?" as the IV is placed, and the candidate should practice the reply, "Let's hold the samples for now until I have a bit more information.")*

CANDIDATE:

I'd like to examine the patient. How is the head and neck examination?

EXAMINER:

(Read Secondary survey section, but do not give it away yet because the candidate was too vague) What are you looking for?

CANDIDATE:

I'd like to examine the head for signs of injury. I'll check the pupils for reactivity, examine the retina for vascular abnormalities, check carotid pulses in the neck, listen for carotid bruits, ensure that the neck is supple and nontender...

EXAMINER:

(Now satisfied that the candidate knows how to examine the head and neck region) The head and neck examination is normal. The neck is nontender, and there are no bruits. *(Some specific findings are listed, both normal and abnormal, to help the candidate in the case. In this case, it will be useful to note the lack of carotid bruits. The retina examination can be described as normal, because the entire eye examination was normal according to the case.)*

CANDIDATE:

Now I'll look at the chest and abdomen for signs of injury or other visible abnormalities. I'll listen to the lungs and heart as well.

EXAMINER:

The chest, heart, and lung examination is normal. *(Let's skip ahead a bit – the remainder of the physical examination in this case was unremarkable. Just remember to have the candidate specify what they are examining before giving them the examination results from the case.)*

CANDIDATE:

Sir, are you a smoker? Do you have any other medical problems? Are you allergic to any medications?

EXAMINER:

(From History section) Yes, I smoke approximately three to four packs per week. I don't have any other medical problems or allergies. *(Note the candidate seems to be skipping around a bit. That's fine – you have all the answers in front of you and the examiner instructions tell you where the case should go. The candidate, however, may have an easier time if they follow a more algorithmic method of assessing the patient, as described in Chapter 3. This will significantly reduce the candidate's chances of missing something, and it should reduce anxiety on test day.)*

CANDIDATE:

I'd like to order some tests. May I have an EKG, chest x-ray, and labs including a CBC, chemistry panel, coagulation panel, UA, and type and hold?

EXAMINER:

(Checks Studies section and examiner instructions) No problem; the tests have been sent, and the patient will have an EKG and chest x-ray. Is there anything else you'd like?

CANDIDATE:

No, that's all for now.

EXAMINER:

(Following examiner instructions) The nurse informs you that the patient is still having quite a bit of pain.

CANDIDATE:

Thank you. I'd like to order 6 mg of morphine intravenously.

EXAMINER:

The patient's pain is improved after receiving the morphine. *(If you are familiar with drug dosing, ask the candidate to be more specific with drug dosages and routes. Dosages are not mentioned in this book for simplicity.)*

EXAMINER:

Results of the tests are back. *(Also show candidate laboratory results as printed in the case. Since the table can't be split up, show all the laboratory results in the table even if they weren't all requested. However, do not show images [EKG, CXR, etc] for tests that were not ordered. Note there is no reading for the CXR and EKG in the case – the candidate is expected to interpret these images on his or her own. The interpretations are discussed at the end of each case, and a brief interpretation for each figure in the book is given in Appendix H. For other types of tests which the candidate is not expected to interpret on their own [such as an MRI], results will be communicated to the candidate by the examiner.)*

CANDIDATE:

Sir, how is your pain now?

EXAMINER:

(Following case, Reassess section) It was better for a while, but now it's back as bad as ever. I'm starting to feel a little chest pain and nausea.

CANDIDATE:

Let's repeat the vital signs.

EXAMINER:

(There are some repeat vital signs listed – since the patient hasn't received a β-antagonist, we'll use the vitals in the "no β-antagonists" section of Reassess.) Blood pressure: 170/100, heart rate: 100, respiratory rate: 18, oxygen saturation: 100% on 2L NC.

CANDIDATE:

All right. I'd like to consult cardiology.

EXAMINER:

(This consultation was not described in the instructions! When this happens, the consultant will offer no useful information to the candidate, and the candidate will have to continue with the case as they would manage the case on their own. If the candidate is having trouble with some aspect of the case, the consultant can be used to give them a hint. For the purposes of the boards, consultants generally serve to perform some specific action that an emergency physician cannot, such as performing an operation, admitting a patient, or performing a specialized study. When asked to give their opinion on a case or provide a diagnosis, they will not be helpful.) We have Dr. Harmon from cardiology on the phone. *(In character)* This is Dr. Harmon, what's going on?

CANDIDATE:

I have a patient here with back pain radiating to the chest *(describes the case)*. I need a consult.

EXAMINER:

I'm not sure what you need me to do. What do you think is going on with the patient?

CANDIDATE:

Well, it could be a heart attack, renal colic, an aortic aneurysm or dissection, or some trauma we've missed. But I think he might be sick.

EXAMINER:

Why don't you figure it out a bit more and call me if you need me. *(Hangs up)*

CANDIDATE:

I'd like to order a CT scan of the abdomen.

EXAMINER:

All right. The radiologist wants to know what you're looking for so they can protocol the study appropriately.

CANDIDATE:

Renal colic, an aortic aneurysm or dissection; less likely to be some occult trauma.

EXAMINER:

The patient gets the CT scan. *(Show candidate Figure 1.3)*

CANDIDATE:

This looks like an aortic dissection. Do we have an official reading on this?

EXAMINER:

Yes. It is read as a dissection of the descending thoracic aorta extending to the abdominal aorta and left iliac artery. There is no involvement of the aortic arch. *(Candidates would not normally be expected to interpret this type of study. Thus, the results are given in the text of the case. These images are included in this book for their educational value.)*

CANDIDATE:

I'd like to move the patient to the critical care area of the ED. Place a second large-bore intravenous line, please. I'd like to start an esmolol drip.

EXAMINER:

Done. Would you like anything else?

CANDIDATE:

I'd like to repeat the vital signs and contact vascular surgery.

EXAMINER:

(Now we can use the vitals in the "β-antagonists" section of Reassess) Blood pressure: 110/55, heart rate: 55, respiratory rate: 18, oxygen saturation: 100% on 2L NC. Vascular surgery (Dr. Media) is on the phone for you.

CANDIDATE:

Dr. Media, this is Dr. Candidate in the ED. We have a type B aortic dissection in the ED who arrived with back pain radiating to his chest and leg. He was initially hypertensive but we've started him on an esmolol drip and his vital signs and symptoms have improved.

EXAMINER:

Thank you; can you admit him to the ICU and we'll see him there? *(The candidate has a similar discussion with the ICU staff and the patient's primary care physician, and the patient is admitted.)*

* * *

At this point, the candidate should read through the case him- or herself, focusing on the critical actions, examiner instructions, and pearls. References should be examined to solidify understanding of the disease processes from the case. Each case will contain a reference from "Rosen's" and "Tintinalli's," the formal references are detailed below.

REFERENCES

Marx A, Hockberger RS, Walls RM. *Rosen's Emergency Medicine: Concepts and Clinical Practice*. 8th ed. St. Louis, MO: Mosby; 2014.

Tintinalli JE, Cydulka RK, Meckler GD, The American College of Emergency Physicians, Stapczynski JF, Ma JO, Cline DM. *Tintinalli's Emergency Medicine: A Comprehensive Study Guide*. 7th ed. New York, NY: McGraw-Hill; 2011.

CHAPTER 2

EM medical decision making

Scott Weingart, MD, FCCM

This chapter discusses the cognitive processes of emergency medicine (EM). It is applicable to our approach in the department and to the more artificial environment of the board exam. Decision making in EM is quite different than most of the other fields in medicine. The novice may assume that we make most of our decisions using conscious contemplation, perhaps because this is the path the novice is forced to take. The reality is that if we had to think about every diagnosis and treatment during the course of a shift, we would be crushed under the cognitive load. Imagine for a moment how effortlessly you walk or speak; would these be as easy if you were consciously guiding each muscle contraction?

ILLNESS SCRIPTS

Thinking is the last resort; it is slow, and counterintuitively, predisposes us to error. Most of our decisions are made by pattern matching. Using only a few lines from the patient's history, a brief physical examination, some basic tests, like the glucose level, and most importantly a gestalt impression of how the patient looks, we can usually narrow the differential to one or perhaps a couple of possibilities. The process takes only seconds. We match the patient's presentation to an accumulation of all of the similar presentations we have seen or read about throughout our careers; this accumulation is referred to as an illness script. It is only when we do not have an illness script to match with the patient in front of us that we are forced to resort to other decision-making techniques.

All of the cases on the oral board exam should be approached by pattern matching. These patients should not be anomalies; they will be bread and butter presentations. If you cannot match the case, you are probably missing something, but do not give up hope. In this situation and in real life, we can fall back on three strategies: heuristics, analytic thinking, and shotgunning.

HEURISTICS

Heuristics are mental shortcuts; they are a pathway to rapid action without formal analysis. We use many heuristics in the practice of EM. Some of them can predispose us to error, for example, all reproducible chest pain is benign. However, there are

TABLE 2.1

Airway
Breathing
Circulation
Disability-pupillary reaction, GCS, and ability to move all four extremities
Exposure/Environment – see every inch of skin and then keep the patient warm
Finger stick (can also mean Finger-do Rectal if appropriate)
Girls and women get a pregnancy test
Hang antibiotics (early antibiotics for all of your sepsis patients and preprocedural antibiotics in your trauma patients)
Inject tetanus when appropriate (you may forget it later on)
GCS, Glasgow coma scale.

many heuristics that are indispensable and lead to good outcomes on both the exam and for our patients. Some examples of useful EM heuristics are described subsequently.

Sick/Not Sick Paradigm

The immediate dichotomization between sick/not sick is the most important heuristic in EM. Sometimes, we'll have no idea what is going on with a patient, but we have an intuition that they are unwell. That patient is going to be admitted and we are going to fix every vital-sign abnormality and address any positive diagnostic tests. If the patient looks well, but has a vague complaint, we may send them home with close follow-up even if we do not have a final diagnosis. Unfortunately, this heuristic can fail if the patient looks pristine, but has a life-threatening illness. For instance, an acute acetaminophen overdose can cause this heuristic to fail.

Age Heuristic

Another valuable heuristic relates to the elderly. Very few presentations should lead to the discharge of a patient older than 75 years old, similarly, a patient less than 40 needs to be pretty sick to get admitted. *If they're old we hold, if they're young they're sprung* will often lead to an appropriate decision.

The ABCs Heuristic

Fundamental to EM is falling back on the ABCs for our initial approach to any sick patient. Over the years, I have added to this alphabetical heuristic; Table 2.1 lists an approach to a sick patient for the boards or in the resuscitation room.

ANALYTIC THINKING

Careful use of deductive reasoning is the proper approach when the previous strategies have not yielded answers. Thinking is hard; we should reserve it for when it serves us best. As we gain experience, we need to think about fewer cases; most of our answers will come to us through subconscious pattern matching and the use of proven heuristics. If during the oral boards, you are forced to resort to analytic thinking, you are in a difficult situation. Thinking under enormous stress is difficult, but not insurmountable. It is acceptable to take a second, close your eyes, and reorganize your perceptions. By the same token, in the hectic, chaotic environment of the emergency department, finding a quiet corner for a moment can often improve our analytic processing.

SHOTGUNNING

This is a cognitively bereft heuristic, but every so often you are left with little else. Shotgunning involves sending every laboratory test and radiographic study that is vaguely applicable and hoping something comes back that reveals an answer. This is very low level cognitive reasoning. If you are resorting to shotgunning during your exam, it is doubtful that passing score will be the result. Using this technique in the department will lead to wasted money and unnecessary testing.

Cognitive Checkpoint

Before completing our care of any patient, we need to stop and consciously ask ourselves if we are missing anything. This is perhaps the most important error prevention strategy we can use in our field. During the board exam, it is just as important. Take a moment and review your performance; you may pick up errors that you initially missed. For example, after taking a history and completing a primary and secondary survey, it may be helpful to review the facts of the case thus far before ordering tests. This will give you an opportunity to fill in any gaps, allow yourself to see a pattern that you may have missed, and will better crystallize your thought processes for the examiner.

* * *

In conclusion, our approach to decisions in EM bears similarities to the fields of anesthesiology and critical care, but is different than the other fields in medicine. We arrive at thousands of decision nodes in the course of a shift. If we had to think about every one of them, we could not function at a high level. Most of our decisions are made by unconscious processes that can predispose us to error if our knowledge base is poor, our experience lacking, or our vision clouded by emotion or stress. However, when we are prepared and clear-minded, a shift can feel cognitively effortless; I hope your board exam experience is the same.

CHAPTER 3

About the Oral Boards: The approach and practical tips

Peter Shearer, MD and Yasuharu Okuda, MD

Emergency medicine (EM) is rich in what is known as narrative medicine. Stories are the foundation of our practice. Patients tell us their stories. We edit them and add in our own details (test results, radiography, etc). We often retell these stories: if we are students to attending physicians during clinical rotations; if we are attendings or residents to colleagues and consultants when we seek input into a complex case; and even back to patients when we have solved the case, or at least written the next chapter.

It is wholly appropriate that the American Board of Emergency Medicine (ABEM) incorporates an oral examination into its certification process. As a process the ABEM oral examination involves elements of an Observed Structured Clinical Encounter (OSCE) and simulation, though it does not incorporate high-fidelity simulation (yet). As with an OSCE the process must be organized and thorough because it is observed and scored. Like a simulated patient it evolves in a version of "real time" in which decisions and commitment to certain pathways must be made. You must interact with the examiner as if you are speaking to a real patient, a real family member, a real consultant, or other real staff.

The oral board examination "stories" actually unfold in hotel bedrooms. The exam is given at the Chicago Marriott O'Hare Airport Hotel. The cases are administered within the guest rooms along a long hallway. It is important to know this upfront so months of preparation are not undone by surprise at the setting. You will wait at the end of the hallway until your turn, then go to your assigned door and wait for the examiner inside to open it and invite you in. Sometimes there is a third person in the room to monitor the exam for quality.

An oral exam case differs from a conventional story in that you are very much a part of how the story unfolds, but you must always remember that it is already written. The authors have created a story for you with a beginning, a middle, and an ending. The beginning is handed to you: "It is Monday morning and you start your shift at ABEM General Hospital, a nurse approaches you with a worried look on her face." The middle of the story is a series of critical actions that you must take along the way. Many of these are similar from case to case: undress the patient; check a rapid blood glucose; ask EMS to stay to give further history. Others will be quite case specific: checking salicylate levels in an elderly patient with altered mental status. The ideal ending may be known, but it is flexible. Success on the test doesn't always mean that the patient walks away unharmed. Perhaps the patient is meant to die no matter what, and the goal of the case is to marshal the resources of your department (social worker, private family room) to deliver the news to the family and discuss organ donation?

The process is one of asking for more details, descriptions, and taking actions. After the scenario is given to you, often the best way to start is "I approach the patient and what do I see?" Though things may change rapidly as they do in real life, you should get a first impression of what intervention is needed. For example, ABCs for a patient in full arrest; lines and monitoring if the patient is critical; time for a further history if the patient is awake and talking to you. As you move through the case as with any good story, you must constantly ask, "And then? What happened next?" If you order tests, ask for the results. If you made an intervention, be sure you go back and reassess the patient and their vital signs afterward.

The examiner holds onto the details of the story until you ask for them. If you do not ask SPECIFICALLY for a blood urea nitrogen (BUN) or creatinine, do not expect to be given one. If you do not SPECIFICALLY say, "Nurse, please put the patient on a cardiac monitor with a continuous oxygenation saturation," it will not happen. You will need to ask "What is the oxygen saturation?" to learn the result. If you place a hypoxic patient on oxygen, reassess their saturation. If you fail to do so, you may miss methemoglobinemia, or a patient who will require intubation.

Over the course of 5 hours each participant goes through seven scenarios: four single case encounters, two multicase encounters managing three patients at once, and one single case that is a test case and is not scored. The single case encounters are 15 minutes and the triple case encounters are 30 minutes. You will not know which one is the test case. Though direct pathophysiology questions were dropped in 2002, the examiners still test knowledge base by asking for electrocardiogram (ECG/EKG) or radiography interpretations, or even in the information that you provide to a consultant or a family member in a scenario.

Your examiners are master storytellers. They are leaders in the field of emergency medicine. They have been well trained in the cases they are giving, and will probably only work with two or three cases over the days that the test is administered. They know the details of their stories inside out. Some will try more than others to act out the script: you might be expected to interact with them as if they were the pregnant teenager in their case. Others might just stick to narrating the case for you. Though the resources of the hospital are available to you, examiners will not let you use consultants for answers to questions or look up information in a textbook. If the question is one an emergency physician should know (such as common drugs, fracture patterns, ECG interpretation, etc) your examiner may tell you that the consultant is not available.

The key to preparation is practice. The knowledge content is similar to that of the written exam, which you will have already passed as a requisite to sit for the oral exam. There is a slight focus on cardiovascular topics, toxicology, and trauma; if these have been your weak areas in the past they definitely require review. It is best to sit down with this book and practice as many scenarios as possible, out loud, with a friend. The back and forth exchange is different from your typical conversations about patients at work though the content will be similar.

The ABEM oral certifying examination can be nerve-wracking. Remember though that you have been doing this through residency and every working day since finishing your residency – only in a different format. Instead of getting the story from a patient, you are getting it from your examiner. Your confidence will grow with repetition as you practice cases in this book. At the most basic level the examiner holds a story about one (or three) patients. Your challenge is to get the details of that story from the examiner in a smooth and rational manner. The subsequent text contains practical tips for the day as well as one approach to the oral board encounter.

PRACTICAL TIPS

- Arrive early the prior day. The last thing you want to do is get to the hotel late the night before because of a delayed flight.
- Stay at the hotel and reserve the room well in advance of the test. Again, you want to minimize stress. Avoid a long commute to the hotel the morning of the test. The hotel is adjacent to the airport and NOT in downtown Chicago.
- Sleep well and eat well. Nothing too heavy to eat the night before; make sure you eat and go to sleep at a reasonable time. You want to keep your mind sharp for the next day. Eat breakfast the following morning but don't stuff yourself so that you're uncomfortable during the exam. If you think you might get hungry, put a snack (like a granola bar) in your coat pocket just in case.
- Dress professionally but comfortably. Dress as you would for a job interview. You don't want to be distracted by feeling self-conscious for underdressing. Most candidates will be wearing suits.
- Smile and be polite. Once you are called into the room for your encounter by the examiner, introduce yourself and greet them with a smile and handshake if appropriate. Though these exams are standardized, it never hurts to be pleasant to the examiner. We are all human including the examiners. Never argue with the examiner, no matter what.
- Play the game. Don't think, "This is so artificial" or, "I'd get it if it were a real patient." The examination is what it is; an exam to test your skills. Be compassionate when you are talking to the family or patient. Try to pretend you are really there in the clinical environment.
- Wear a watch without a calculator to help with keeping track of time.
- You will be given a pencil and a blank piece of paper with a picture of a human body on the side to use during the encounter. Use them. This will be detailed in the next section.
- The examiner will ask you to let them know when you are ready to begin. This means you have a minute to prepare yourself. Use it.
- Once you have finished the encounter, the examiner will let you know that the time is up. Thank them and walk out. Don't read into what they say or don't say when the case is over. They are not supposed to give you any hints on how you did; just because you don't hear "great job" or see a smile on their face doesn't mean you didn't do well. Just clear your mind and go to the next case. It may be that they are hungry or need to go to the bathroom.

THE APPROACH

There are many ways to approach the oral boards cases. It is likely that you have done some mock oral boards exams during your residency and have learned a format that works for you. If it works, stick with it. As described in Chapter 2, EM physicians' brains work in ways that differ from many specialties. Because we work in a chaotic environment with multiple patients and typically high volumes, we rely on pattern matching and heuristics. The experienced EM physician knows when a patient is sick because of their "look," abnormal vital signs, or concerning trends in their appearance upon reassessment. Unfortunately, the oral boards are an artificial environment and we lose the edge that we've come to rely on, our senses. The smell of melena, cyanotic lips, the use of accessory muscles to breathe, and subtle hints of delirium in an older patient must be revealed through asking questions instead of automatically presenting themselves to the candidate. So the candidate theoretically starts at a slight disadvantage in the encounter compared to the true clinical environment. Fortunately there is one aspect of the oral boards that we can use to our advantage: the examiner cannot lie and they are not there to trick you. This means if you ask them about breath sounds on the left side of the chest, they have to say "yes" or "no." We do not have to second-guess ourselves and wait for the chest x-ray (CXR) to place a chest tube in a penetrating trauma.

To overcome the situational disadvantage of the artificial physician–patient encounter, we have to maximize our data collection in an efficient way. The following approach may seem overly detailed and time consuming. However, if done correctly and practiced it will likely save you time in the long run. This is so you don't have to go back to ask, "What was the rectal exam again?" or say, "Whoops, that patient had a penicillin allergy?"

■ When you walk into the room, you will find a pencil and paper on the desk. The paper will have the outline of a person, much in the shape of the gingerbread person, on the left side of the paper taking up one-sixth of the page (Figure 3.1). The rest of the paper will be blank. The examiner will allow you to take a moment to get yourself ready. Use that time and divide the paper into four quadrants, labeled as illustrated in Figure 3.2. Do this *before* starting the case. This should take you less than 1 minute.

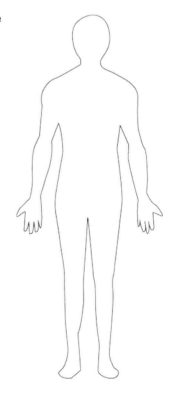

Figure 3.1 Sample Oral Boards Note Sheet.

  ▶ HISTORY BOX: The top left box will be where you record information relevant to the patient's chief complaint as well as history and review of systems (ROS).
  ▶ EXAM BOX: The bottom left box is the vitals and physical examination box. Memorize and write down all of the abbreviations before beginning so that you won't forget to ask about certain aspects of the examination. You might not end up asking for all of them (like a rectal examination in a patient with an ANKLE sprain). But some things may not be obvious unless you ask everything about it. For example, you may encounter a patient with left-sided sharp chest

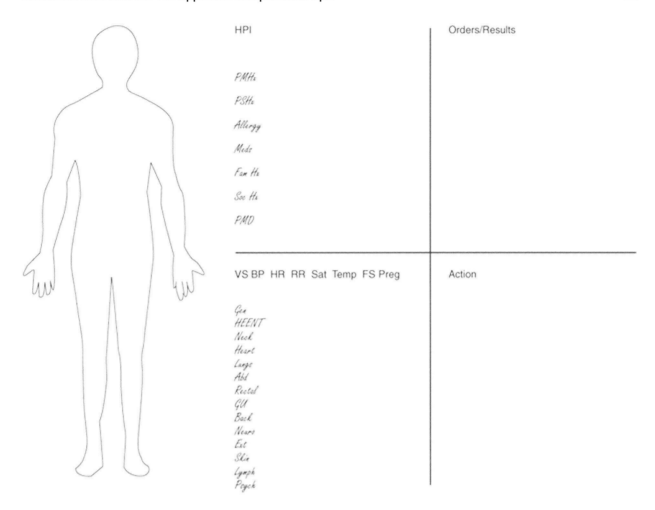

HPI		Orders/Results
PMHx		
PSHx		
Allergy		
Meds		
Fam Hx		
Soc Hx		
PMD		

VS BP HR RR Sat Temp FS Preg	Action
Gen	
HEENT	
Neck	
Heart	
Lungs	
Abd	
Rectal	
GU	
Back	
Neuro	
Ext	
Skin	
Lymph	
Psych	

Figure 3.2 Sample Oral Boards Note Sheet with Suggested Labels.

pain for 3 days, which is constant and not made worse with breathing. Unless you ask about the skin examination, you may miss the vesicular lesions along a dermatomal distribution seen in zoster. Be vague initially; if a portion of the examination is normal, the examiner will just say "normal" and you can move on. If it is especially relevant to the case or there are abnormalities to be discovered, they may ask you, "What are you looking for?" Then you would need to be more detailed by asking questions such as, "Are there equal breath sounds, crackles, wheezes, rubs, crepitus, etc."

▷ ORDERS AND RESULTS: The top right box is where you order tests and put the results. If you ask for a test such as a complete blood count (CBC) or basic metabolic panel (BMP), be sure to ask for the results later, they are not obligated to give it to you automatically. One technique is to say, "Nurse, can I have a CBC, BMP, PT/PTT, and type and cross and can you give the results to me as soon as they're available." The other way to keep track is to write it down in the box. Once you have the result, you can write it down or put a check next to it.

▷ ACTION: The bottom right box is your action box. Here you'll record what you've done: whether antibiotics or tetanus was administered, consults you've requested, and disposition (such as the OR or ICU).

▷ The picture on the left of the paper can be used to help visualize the patient. In a multitrauma patient, it may be helpful to circle areas affected, such as the right femur, head, left chest. Other uses include marking the procedures you've done, such as the rectal examination, nasogastric tube, intubation, chest tube.

▪ Now you're ready to start the case – it begins when you tell the examiner, "I'm ready."

▷ The examiner will give you the chief complaint as described earlier.

▷ "50-year-old male brought in by ambulance with severe substernal chest pain radiating to the left shoulder."

▪ At this point you need to assess if the patient is sick or not sick, get the vitals, and perform the ABCDEs, intervening when necessary.

▷ The first question should always be either "what does the patient look like" or "what do I see, hear, and smell as I walk into the room." Either will give you a gestalt of how sick the patient is. If the patient is critical you will need to act immediately to stabilize the patient.

▷ The next step is to obtain vital signs. Ask the nurse and/or EMS about key vital signs including blood pressure, heart rate, respiratory rate, oxygen saturation, temperature, and blood glucose when relevant. Vitals are extremely important and will tell you a lot about the status of the patient. Continue throughout the case to frequently repeat vitals signs *especially* after an intervention, such as medications, administration, or procedure.

▷ The third step is the *primary survey* – ABCDEs. This is also done when you want to ask the nurse to start an intravenous line (IV), O_2, and monitor if appropriate. Specifically, place two large bore (16- to 18-gauge) angiocatheters in the anticubital fossa, start oxygen either by nasal canula or nonrebreather mask, and place the patient on a monitor. Not all patients may warrant these steps (the patient with an ankle sprain, for example) but the majority of sick patients will need these as a minimum. If the patient has an abnormal ABCD or E, you may need to intervene before moving on.

▷ The patient with GCS < 8 in a trauma or respiratory distress may need to be intubated.

▷ With altered mental status, check a blood sugar and give the coma cocktail.

▷ Place a chest tube or needle decompression in a tension pneumothorax.

▷ Start blood or fluid boluses in a hypotensive patient.

▷ Apply pressure to large wounds that are bleeding.

▷ This is also when you may ask for stat items like EKG or CXR if the patient has severe chest pain or respiratory distress.

▪ Now the history

▷ EMS offers valuable information but if you wait too long, they will leave the ED. Ask them to stick around early in the case so you don't lose them if you need to stabilize the patient first. They can give you valuable information about mechanism of injury, pills at the bedside, or the condition of the patient's home, as well as what treatments were given in the field.

▷ Now use the History Box to record the history of present illness (HPI) and other history. Don't forget important things like drug, alcohol, smoking history, do not resuscitate (DNR) status, as well as allergies. Use all resources available, such as the patient, nursing home papers, family or friends, and primary medical doctor (PMD). Do NOT order a medication for a patient until you have checked their allergies.

- Once you have some idea of the history and have stabilized the patient, you can move on to the *secondary survey*. Refer to the Physical Examination box. As discussed earlier, ask general questions like "What is the lung exam like?" If the examiner wants to know what you're thinking, they will ask, "What are you looking for?" otherwise, they will say "Normal."
- Continue to repeat vitals signs throughout the case, especially after an intervention (such as oxygen or drug administration). Also, ask the patient how he or she is doing after each intervention (for example, asking, "How is the pain?," after giving morphine).
- **Orders and Results Box**: Once you have an idea of what's going on with the patient, you will usually order laboratory tests, radiology studies, and so on. You may have already sent basic laboratory work but you can add relevant data here. Avoid trying to shotgun lots of tests, as the examiner can deduct points if you are wasting resources. Mark down what you ordered because you may forget and the nurse does not have to voluntarily offer you the information once the results are available. Ask the nurse to give you the results when available.
- **Action Box**: Treat pain, give antibiotics for infections early, order tetanus for wounds, get appropriate consultants, and manage all of the issues relevant to the chief complaint. You may be asked to describe how you would perform a procedure, so be prepared (refer to Appendix G). Also, don't forget social workers or child protective services in abuse cases, calling primary care doctors to discuss the patient, talking to family and the patient to update them on their status, explain all procedures, and appropriate disposition.
- Upon completion of the case, the examiner will tell you that the time is up. Thank them and excuse yourself from the room. Clear your mind and move on to the next case.

CHAPTER 4

About the Oral Boards: Format and scoring

Michael Cassara, DO

INTRODUCTION

Oral Certification Examinations in Emergency Medicine are objective structured oral examinations (OSOE) constructed for the high-stakes assessment of clinical judgment of candidates seeking certification in emergency medicine. Successful completion of an OSOE is a mandatory component of the pathways for initial certification in emergency medicine as established by both the American Board of Emergency Medicine (ABEM) and the American Osteopathic Board of Emergency Medicine (AOBEM). Regardless of the board sponsoring the test, Oral Certification Examinations in Emergency Medicine are, at the base level, low-technology ("pencil-and-paper") constructs (games) in which candidates and examiners collaboratively role play the management of simulated patients in a virtual emergency department setting. As with other role-playing constructs, candidates are allowed (within predetermined rules and guidelines) to freely respond to the situations presented and to the characters (patients, family members, consultants, etc.) portrayed by examiners. Decisions made by candidates influence the turns and twists cases take and, ultimately, the outcomes of patients "treated." Candidates preparing for these simulation-based examinations benefit immensely from understanding the structure, content, procedures, technical characteristics, and scoring rubrics defining the "game." The aim of this chapter is to provide the critical information candidates need for optimal performance. Whenever possible, similarities and differences between the ABEM and AOBEM examinations will be presented.

STRUCTURE OF THE ABEM ORAL CERTIFICATION EXAMINATION[1-3]

The ABEM Oral Certification Examination in Emergency Medicine is provided biannually during a three-day testing period incorporating one weekend (Saturday through Monday) in the spring and fall of each calendar year. Each testing day is subdivided into a morning and an afternoon session; each session is approximately 5½ hours in duration. Candidates are assigned by ABEM to one of these sessions and notified by mail before the date of the examination. On the day of the examination, during the registration period, candidates receive an individualized itinerary for the session. The itinerary divides the session into multiple 15-minute and 30-minute blocks; blocks will be identified as test periods or breaks. During the 15-minute test periods, examiners administer **simulated patient encounters** (SPEs; "single case scenarios"). During SPEs, candidates manage one simulated patient. During the 30-minute test periods, examiners administer **simulated situation encounters** (SSEs; "triple case scenarios"). During SSEs, candidates must simultaneously manage three simulated patients. **All candidates must complete all critical actions and case-related tasks within 15 and 30 minutes for SPEs and SSEs, respectively.**

During the ABEM Oral Certification Examination, candidates participate in six scored standardized oral simulations and one field-test case[1-3]. Four of the scored simulations are SPEs, and two of the scored simulations are SSEs. The examiners assessment of the candidates is therefore based on the candidate's management of 10 simulated patients (four "single case scenarios" plus two "triple case scenarios"). Candidates should remember that their management for all simulated patients is assessed individually, regardless of whether the candidate meets the simulated patient within a SPE or SSE. ABEM provides no specific information describing how the field-test case is incorporated within the examination (e.g. whether it appears as a SPE or embedded within a SSE).

A description of the implementation of the ABEM Oral Certification Examination is provided in other chapters in this text. A video demonstration of a simulated SPE is available on the ABEM website[4].

STRUCTURE OF THE AOBEM ORAL EXAMINATION

The AOBEM Oral Examination in Emergency Medicine is provided biannually during a two-day testing period in the spring and fall of each calendar year. Candidates are assigned by AOBEM to one of these sessions and notified by mail before the date of the examination. During the examination, candidates move through three testing stations. Each testing station consists of two simulated patient encounters. **Candidates are provided 30 minutes to complete the pair of cases provided at each station.** Additional information regarding the Oral Examination may be found at the AOBEM website[5].

ORAL CERTIFICATION EXAMINATION CONTENT

All content for the ABEM Oral Certification Examinations in Emergency Medicine is derived from and described in the Model of the Clinical Practice of Emergency Medicine ("the Model")[5]. The Model defines the breadth and depth of Emergency Medicine. Key content areas are defined along a matrix of critical, urgent, and non-emergent presentations. Knowledge expected of candidates seeking ABEM certification in Emergency Medicine is presented along the framework of 16 physician tasks. Unlike the ABEM Qualifying Examination, the percentage breakdown of the content upon which the ABEM Oral Certification Examination is based is not explicitly described. ABEM states that the content of the Oral Certification Examination may originate from any content area within the Model, although the conditions, presentations, and diseases that are within the domains of cardiovascular, traumatic, and toxicologic disorders are routinely emphasized[1,3]. Variable acuity time frames, as well as modifying factors, are routinely represented in the case scenarios provided during the examination. The ratio of critically ill to emergent patient presentations portrayed on the ABEM Oral Board Examination is reported as 2:1[1]. In contrast to the

Qualifying Examination, where pediatric and geriatric content represents a minimum of 8% and 4% of the content, respectively, the Oral Certification Examination presents candidates with a significant, but undefined, percentage of pediatric patients.

In contrast, all content for the AOBEM Oral Examination is derived from the AOBEM Table of Specificity for Certification Examinations[7], which was adapted from the Core Content in Emergency Medicine[8], and last revised in 2008. No further delineation or breakdown of the content contained within the AOBEM Oral Examination is publicly available.

SCORING RUBRIC FOR THE ABEM ORAL CERTIFICATION EXAMINATION

Candidate performance on the ABEM Oral Certification Examination is assessed across eight domains ("performance criteria") on a scale from 1 (worst performance) to 8 (best performance). The eight performance criteria are: **Data Acquisition, Problem Solving, Patient Management, Resource Utilization, Health Care Provided (Outcome), Interpersonal Relations and Communication Skills, Comprehension of Pathophysiology,** and **Clinical Competence (Overall)**[1-3]. ABEM defines each performance criterion as follows:

- **Data Acquisition:** candidate demonstrates the ability to acquire the *appropriate data critical for correctly diagnosing and managing the patient in a timely, orderly, and efficient manner,* using a *data collection approach* that is *well-integrated into the overall management plan*
- **Problem solving:** candidate demonstrates an *organized approach* to the evaluation of the patient, and *collects data that differentiates between reasonable alternative diagnoses* while *contemporaneously stabilizing/managing the patient* and *anticipating complications*
- **Patient management:** candidate *appropriately sequences management actions* with data-acquisition activities and problem-solving strategies, *provides proper interventions* at the right times, *makes appropriate referrals,* and *manages multiple patients simultaneously*
- **Resource utilization:** candidate demonstrates a *logical, judicious, economical, efficient, and appropriate use of resources (e.g. laboratory, diagnostic tests, etc.)* in a simulated setting
- **Health care provided (outcome):** candidate *provides timely and appropriate medical care,* and *stabilizes and maximally improves* the patient's condition (*based on the actual patient outcome*)
- **Interpersonal relations and communication skills:** candidate demonstrates an ability to communicate clinical information (e.g. diagnosis, management, test results, procedures, options) clearly with patients, staff, and consultant, while simultaneously demonstrating respect, empathy, and concern
- **Comprehension of pathophysiology:** candidate demonstrates an understanding of *the scientific rationale and evidence-basis for treatments and procedures, interprets procedure and diagnostic tests* proficiently, and *avoids implementation of "routine" procedures* without considering underlying cause–effect relationships
- **Clinical competence (overall):** candidate demonstrates c*ompetency providing emergency care* based on the examiner's *overall assessment of the candidate's cognitive and procedural skills*

Along with these eight performance criteria, ABEM explicitly defines "critical actions" for each simulated case provided within a SPE or SSE. **Critical actions are behaviors deemed critical to the essential completion of a task and for successful outcomes**[2,3,9]. They are usually constructed as imperative sentences (e.g. "order chest x-ray," "treat pneumothorax," or "explain procedure to patient"). Critical actions are developed to differentiate among candidates with different levels of performance[9], and are part of the scoring of every case appearing on the Oral Certification Examination. They are "cornerstones" of performance which help guide examiners rating performances of candidates[2,9]. Each case typically has three to seven clearly defined critical actions[10]. SSEs may possess as many as 16 critical actions[3]. All critical actions are linked to one (and only one) of the aforementioned eight performance criteria. Possible critical action–performance criteria links, using the previous examples, could include the following: "order chest x-ray" linked with "data acquisition;" "treat pneumothorax" linked with "patient management;" and, "explain procedure to patient" linked with "interpersonal relations and communication skills." A review of the Sample Examiner Rating Sheet in Appendix D in ABEM's *Examination Information for Candidates* demonstrates these links explicitly[1]. The significance of linking critical actions to performance criteria is described in the section on **Scoring the ABEM Oral Certification Examination**.

As described above, each of the eight domains of performance are rated for each case using an 8-point ordinal scale. ABEM divides the scale into quartiles of performance using the following categories: **Very Acceptable (7,8); Acceptable (5,6); Unacceptable (3,4);** and **Very Unacceptable (1,2).** ABEM defines these categories using the following anchors:

Very Acceptable (7,8)
- Candidate performs <u>all</u> critical actions
- Examiner without significant objections or criticisms
- Candidate demonstrates efficient, confident, appropriate data acquisition skills
- Candidate uses current, evidence-based, generally accepted principles and guidelines to guide diagnostic and management decisions
- Candidate demonstrates a sophisticated and sound understanding of the pathophysiology inherent in the case
- Candidate anticipates and addresses psychological, social, and economic needs of patients and their families

Acceptable (5,6)
- Candidate performs <u>all</u> critical actions related to the domain (performance criteria) being rated, and avoids committing **dangerous actions**. Exceptions are possible (at the discretion of the examiner) if correctly documented (this is known as a **4/5 Exception**[§]).

[§] The **4/5 Exception** provides examiners with scoring flexibility, especially when judging critical actions. Credit for performing a critical action is likely given only when candidates perform the action as explicitly written. However, there are (uncommon) circumstances when candidates <u>may meet the intent of a critical action without performing the action as explicitly written</u>. Assume, for example, that the examiner presents the candidate with a patient with altered mental status. One likely critical action could be to *obtain an emergent serum glucose level (Problem Solving)*. The 4/5 Exception could be granted by the examiner if the candidate empirically orders the administration of 25 grams dextrose (50 mL of 50% dextrose water) in lieu of obtaining the serum glucose level. The rule is likely termed a 4/5 Exception because, under normal circumstances, missing a critical action would result in a score no greater than 4 in the performance criteria to which the critical

▓ Candidate demonstrates minor inefficiencies, error, or incomplete data acquisition and patient management, but performance remains within the range of generally accepted guidelines and practice standards; patient experiences additional time, expense, or (some) pain as a result

▓ Candidate successfully diagnoses and correctly manages the case, but with some difficulty

▓ Candidate performs an "adequate" history and physical examination

▓ Candidate avoids unnecessary life-threatening procedures or treatments

▓ Candidate demonstrates a sufficient "working knowledge" of pathophysiology

▓ Candidate demonstrates a reasonable concern about the patient's psychological, social, and economic issues

Unacceptable (3,4)

▓ Candidate misses <u>one or more</u> critical actions related to the domain (performance criteria) being rated, or commits **dangerous actions**. Exceptions are possible (at the discretion of the examiner) if correctly documented ("**4/5 Exception**").

▓ Candidate demonstrates significant gaps in data acquisition and management

▓ Candidate provides care that is incomplete, disorganized, and inefficient, but may recognize his/her limitations, and may demonstrate a concern for the patient's welfare by recruiting help from consultants and using other resources to overcome deficiencies

▓ Candidate demonstrates a partial, inadequate, or incomplete knowledge of pathophysiology, procedures, and generally accepted evidence-based management principles

▓ Candidate does not anticipate complications or problems

▓ Candidate demonstrates a lack of concern for the patient's psychological, social, and economic issues

Very Unacceptable (1,2)

▓ Candidate <u>misses two or more</u> critical actions

▓ Candidate selects inappropriate or dangerous actions

▓ Candidate demonstrates gross negligence or mismanagement without recognizing his/her own deficiencies and inadequacies

▓ Candidate demonstrates rudimentary history acquisition and patient stabilization/management skills along with a deficient fund of knowledge

▓ Candidate does not obtain appropriate consultation when indicated

▓ Candidate discharges the patient when hospitalization and emergent specialized care is necessary

Each category provides the examiner with two possible ratings (a high and low point within each quartile of level of performance) with which to score the candidate's performance. For example, an examiner assessing a candidate who functions at the "Very Acceptable" level for the performance criteria of **Data Acquisition** may apply (at his or her discretion) a rating of either 7 or 8. Unfortunately, ABEM does not publicly describe how examiners discriminate candidate performance between these two points on the scale within each category (quartile of level of performance).

---

action is keyed. In the example above, the 4/5 Exception would allow the examiner to upgrade the rating in the performance criterion Problem Solving from 4 to 5 even though the explicit critical action has not technically been met.

SCORING THE ABEM ORAL CERTIFICATION EXAMINATION[1,3]

Candidates who successfully pass the ABEM Oral Certification Examination fulfill one of two possible pass/fail criteria:

1. **Pass/Fail Criterion #1:** candidate achieves a minimum case rating of 5.75 across the eight performance criteria described above for each standardized oral simulation case faced during the examination session that is included for scoring (not a field-test case); OR,
2. **Pass/Fail Criterion #2:** candidate achieves an average minimum score of 5.00 across all scored cases, when:
   a. The candidate's scores for all eight performance criteria for every scored case are averaged to create six individual case scores; AND
   b. The highest individual case score and the lowest individual case score are averaged, and the high-low average is 5.00 or greater; AND
   c. All other remaining case scores total 5.00 or greater.

The examples below help provide clarity in deducing how examiners apply this complex set of rules for rating candidates' performances.

Sample Oral Certification Examination Case (SPE): The examiner presents the candidate with Mr. Red, a 63-year-old man with chest pain resulting from ST-segment-elevation myocardial infarction (STEMI). Initial vital signs are: pulse, 84/minute; respirations, 14/minute; blood pressure, 160/80 mmHg; temperature, 37C (98.6F); and oxygen saturation, 99% (FiO_2=0.21). The patient has a past medical history of hypertension, insulin-dependent diabetes mellitus, and hypercholesterolemia. He has no medication allergies. His medications include metformin, sildenafil (taken within the past 12 hours), and amlodipine. The candidate is presented with the initial case information, and then moves forward with the primary survey, initial diagnostic and stabilizing management interventions, history and data acquisition, and the secondary survey. ECG, if requested by the candidate, reveals an obvious anterior wall STEMI. Chest x-ray, if requested, reveals clear lung fields and a normal mediastinum. During the case play, the patient's condition suddenly deteriorates; he develops ventricular fibrillation and sudden cardiac arrest. The examiner and candidate role play "four minutes" of the resuscitation, including CPR, procedures (endotracheal intubation, defibrillation), medication administration (epinephrine), and post-resuscitation management (post-arrhythmia management, therapeutic hypothermia, discussion with consultants and the patient's family, admission to ICU). For the examples below, the critical actions (and performance criteria to which they are linked) for this sample case are:

1. **Order ECG (Data Acquisition)**
2. **Obtain chest x-ray (Problem Solving)**
3. **Administer aspirin (Patient Management)**
4. **Perform defibrillation (Patient Management)**
5. **Consult cardiologist (Resource Utilization)**

Scoring example 1 – Candidate Performs "Well" on SPE, Earns "Very Acceptable" Rating: Candidate performs all critical actions. Candidate performs a problem-focused history and primary survey as initial stabilization measures are implemented.

Candidate anticipates alternative diagnoses (e.g. aortic dissection) and obtains ECG and chest x-ray. Candidate recognizes anterior wall STEMI and orders aspirin. Candidate avoids nitroglycerin (dangerous action). Candidate anticipates complications, and applies defibrillator pads to patient. Candidate demonstrates knowledge of and applies evidence-based guidelines when sudden cardiac arrest occurs (initiates immediate CPR, defibrillation, and sequences medications and interventions appropriately). Candidate succinctly and accurately describes how to perform endotracheal intubation and defibrillation. Candidate requests consultation with a cardiologist, effectively explains the situation to the consultant and family members, and admits the patient to the ICU until cardiac catheterization can be arranged. The patient survives the event.

The examiner provides the following ratings for the eight performance criteria (using the scoring rubric and eight-point ordinal scale) as shown in **Table 1**:

TABLE 1. SAMPLE EXAMINER RATING FORM FOR EXAMPLE 1

Performance Criteria	Very Unacceptable		Unacceptable		Acceptable		Very Acceptable	
Data Acquisition	1	2	3	4	5	6	7	**8**
Problem Solving	1	2	3	4	5	6	**7**	8
Patient Management	1	2	3	4	5	6	7	**8**
Resource Utilization	1	2	3	4	5	6	**7**	8
Health Care Provided	1	2	3	4	5	6	7	**8**
Interpersonal Relations and Communication Skills	1	2	3	4	5	6	7	**8**
Comprehension of Pathophysiology	1	2	3	4	5	6	**7**	8
Clinical Competence	1	2	3	4	5	6	7	**8**

The examiner also marks the critical action checklist as follows:

☑ Order ECG (Data Acquisition)
☑ Obtain chest x-ray (Problem Solving)
☑ Administer aspirin (Patient Management)
☑ Perform defibrillation (Patient Management)
☑ Consult cardiologist (Resource Utilization)

Note that, because the candidate has performed each critical action for this case, the examiner must provide a minimum rating within the "Acceptable" category (rating no less than 5) for each performance criterion to which the critical action is linked.

The overall score for this case (7.63) is calculated by averaging the scores for each performance criterion. This candidate's performance has been rated "Very Acceptable" by the examiner using this rubric, and the candidate would **PASS** this SPE. If this candidate's performance on all scored cases on the entire Oral Certification Examination were similar, then this candidate would easily pass the examination by **Pass/Fail Criterion #1**.

<u>**Scoring example 2 – Candidate Misses Critical Action on SPE, Earns "Unacceptable" Rating:**</u> Candidate performs a problem-focused history and primary survey but is inefficient and disorganized with implementing initial stabilization measures. Candidate does not anticipate alternative diagnoses (e.g. aortic dissection) and only orders

an ECG (does not obtain a chest x-ray). Candidate recognizes anterior wall STEMI and orders aspirin. Candidate avoids nitroglycerin (dangerous action). Candidate does not anticipate sudden cardiac arrest as a potential complication, however, and does not apply defibrillator pads to patient before the sudden cardiac arrest. Candidate requests immediate defibrillation when sudden cardiac arrest occurs, but cannot describe the procedure appropriately. Candidate requests consultation with a cardiologist, but provides only a rudimentary explanation of the situation to the consultant, and does not engage family members. The candidate admits the patient to the ICU. The patient survives the event.

The examiner provides the following ratings for the eight performance criteria (using the scoring rubric and eight-point ordinal scale) as shown in **Table 2**:

TABLE 2. SAMPLE EXAMINER RATING FORM FOR EXAMPLE 2

Performance Criteria	Very Unacceptable		Unacceptable		Acceptable		Very Acceptable	
Data Acquisition	1	2	3	4	**5**	6	7	8
Problem Solving	1	2	3	**4**	5	6	7	8
Patient Management	1	2	3	4	**5**	6	7	8
Resource Utilization	1	2	3	4	**5**	6	7	8
Health Care Provided	1	2	3	4	**5**	6	7	8
Interpersonal Relations and Communication Skills	1	2	3	4	**5**	6	7	8
Comprehension of Pathophysiology	1	2	3	4	**5**	6	7	8
Clinical Competence	1	2	3	4	**5**	6	7	8

The examiner also marks the critical action checklist as follows:

☑ Order ECG (Data Acquisition)
☑ Obtain chest x-ray (Problem Solving)
☑ Administer aspirin (Patient Management)
☑ Perform defibrillation (Patient Management)
☑ Consult cardiologist (Resource Utilization)

Note that, because the candidate failed to perform the second critical action for this case (obtain chest x-ray), the examiner must provide a minimum rating within the "Unacceptable" category (rating no greater than 4) for Problem Solving (the performance criterion to which the critical action "obtain chest x-ray" is linked).

The overall case score is 4.88. This candidate's overall performance for this case is "Unacceptable" according to the rubric, and, because the candidate **fails** to earn a case rating of 5.75 or greater for this SPE, the candidate could possibly fail the entire Oral Certification Exam (by not meeting **Pass/Fail Criterion #1**).

It is important to remember that because each simulated oral encounter is scored independently, candidates who achieve a poor rating (less than 5.75) for one case may still pass the examination if they are able to meet **Pass/Fail Criterion #2**. In this circumstance, upon completion of the entire Oral Certification Examination, the candidate's entire performance is evaluated. Let's assume that the candidate for Scoring Example 2 recovers from the performance in the case above, and earns the following ratings for the remainder of the examination (see **Table 3**):

TABLE 3. SAMPLE CANDIDATE PERFORMANCE FOR AN ENTIRE ORAL CERTIFICATION EXAMINATION

	SPE1[*]	SPE2	SPE3	SPE4	SSE1[#]	SSE2[#]
Average of Ratings for the Eight Performance Criteria by Case ("Case Scores")	4.88	5.00	6.13	5.38	6.04	6.04

* *This score is from the* Scoring Example 2 – Candidate Misses Critical Action on SPE, Earns "Unacceptable" Rating *(above)*

This score is likely the average of all three cases within the SSE, although it is possible that one or more of these cases could be field-test cases.

Under **Pass/Fail Criterion #2**, the highest (blue) and lowest (red) case scores are averaged. This average (5.51), and all other remaining case scores, are greater than 5.00; this candidate would **PASS** the Oral Certification Examination.

ADDITIONAL NOTES

- Frederick et al. (2011)[11] demonstrated a predictive correlation between candidate scores on the ABEM In-Training Examination (taken as the PGY-3) and the ABEM Oral Certification Examination
- Lunz and Bashook (2008)[12] demonstrated that the candidate communication ability (cited by some as a source for construct-irrelevant variance) did not influence candidate outcomes on oral certification examinations in Orthopedic Surgery administered by trained examiners.
- Interexaminer agreement (interrater reliability) with scoring candidate performance using both critical actions and the eight performance criteria across all simulated cases on the ABEM Oral Certification Examination, has been demonstrated to be high[2].

CONCLUSIONS

To optimize performance on the Oral Certification Examination in Emergency Medicine, candidates should focus on:

- Demonstrating an organized approach to the emergent assessment and management of one or more critically ill or injured adult or pediatric patients
- Demonstrating an ability to appropriately sequence and perform data acquisition and problem-solving tasks while simultaneously initiating stabilizing interventions
- Meeting every critical action for every standardized oral simulation faced on the test
- Maximizing ratings within each of the eight performance criteria against which their performances are judged
- Avoiding dangerous actions

REFERENCES

1. American Board of Emergency Medicine. Examination Information for Candidates-Oral Certification Examination: October 5–7, 2013. http://www.abem.org/public/docs/default-source/publication-documents/fall2013_oralifc_final.pdf?3Fsfvrsn=6. Accessed: October 19, 2013.

2. Bianchi L, Gallagher EJ, Korte R, Ham HP. Interexaminer agreement on the American Board of Emergency Medicine Oral Certification Examination. *Ann Emerg Med.* 2003;41(6): 859–864.

3. Platts-Mills TF, Lewin MR, Ma S. The Oral Certification Exam. *Ann Emerg Med.* 2006; 47(3):278–282.

4. American Board of Emergency Medicine. Oral Examination Candidate Orientation Video. https://www.abem.org/public/emergency-medicine-(em)-initial-certification/oral-examination/oral-examination-information-for-candidates. Accessed October 19, 2013.

5. American Osteopathic Board of Emergency Medicine. Part 2 Oral Examination Certification Requirements. http://www.aobem.org/part2requirements.html. Accessed: October 19, 2013.

6. Perina DG, Brunett P, Caro DA, Char DM, Chisholm CD, Counselman FL, Heidt J, Keim SM, Ma OJ; for the 2011 EM Model Review Task Force, The 2011 Model of the Clinical Practice of Emergency Medicine. *Acad Emerg Med.* 2012; 19(7): e19–40. doi: 10.1111/j.1553–2712. 2012.01385.x.

7. American Osteopathic Board of Emergency Medicine. Table of Specificity for Certification/ Cognitive Assessment. http://www.aobem.org/tableofspecificity.html. Accessed: October 19, 2013.

8. Task Force on the Core Content for Emergency Medicine Revision: Core content for emergency medicine. *Ann Emerg Med.* 1997; 29:792–811.

9. Flanagan JC. The critical incident technique. *Psychol Bull.* 1954;51:327–358.

10. Reinhart M. Educational Measurement Issues for Oral Patient Simulations. In: *Society for Academic Emergency Medicine Annual Meeting. May 21*, 1999. (conference proceedings).

11. Frederick RC, Hafner JW, Schaefer TJ, Aldag JC. Outcome measures for emergency medicine residency graduates: do measures of academic and clinical performance during residency training correlate with American Board of Emergency Medicine test performance? *Acad Emerg Med* 2011; 18:S59–S64.

12. Lunz ME, Bashook PG. Relationship between candidate communication ability and oral certification examination scores. *Med Edu* 2008:42:1227–1233.

CASES

CASE 1: Overdose (Tiffany Truong, MD)

A. Chief complaint

a. 22-year-old female brought in by EMS for nausea, vomiting, and diarrhea after intentional overdose

B. Vital signs

a. BP: 119/71 HR: 96 RR: 22 T: 37.1°C Sat: 98% on RA FS: 170

C. What does the patient look like?

a. Young female, vomiting

D. Primary survey

a. Airway: speaking in full sentences
b. Breathing: no apparent respiratory distress, no cyanosis
c. Circulation: dry and cool skin, normal capillary refill

E. History

a. HPI: a 22-year-old female with a history of anemia took "half bottle" of her ferrous sulfate pills 4 to 5 hours before arrival. She had an argument with her boyfriend the night prior and took the pills as an intentional suicidal attempt. She reported no other ingestion. She stated that she had vomited twice with scant hematemesis and had one bout of non-bloody diarrhea before ED arrival. Patient denies fever, chills, shortness of breath, chest pain, recent travel, current antibiotic use, back pain, urinary symptoms, or vaginal discharge. Patient complains of mild epigastric pain in the ED. EMS brought the patient to the ED after being called by the patient. They reported finding an empty 30-tablet bottle of iron pills in her apartment.
b. PMHx: anemia, history of profuse vaginal bleeding
c. PSHx: none
d. Allergies: none
e. Meds: ferrous sulfate, 325 mg once a day
f. Social: lives alone, denies tobacco, alcohol, recreational drugs, or alternative medicines; sexually active with boyfriend
g. FHx: no family history of liver disease
h. PMD: none

F. Action

a. Oxygen via nasal cannula or nonrebreather mask
b. Two large-bore peripheral IV lines
c. Labs
   i. CBC, BMP, LFT, coagulation studies, blood type and cross-match
   ii. UA, urine pregnancy test, alcohol level, acetaminophen level, salicylate level, urine toxicology screen
d. 1 L NS bolus
e. Monitor: BP: 98/61 HR: 99 RR: 21 Sat: 100% on 2 L O_2
f. EKG
g. Urine pregnancy test

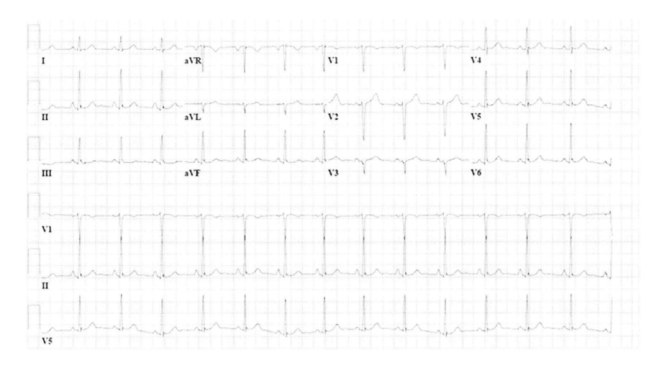

Figure 1.1

G. Nurse
 a. EKG (Figure 1.1)
 b. 1 L NS
    i. BP: 101/69 HR: 93 RR: 20 Sat: 100% on O_2
 c. Urine pregnancy test negative

H. Secondary survey
 a. General: alert, oriented × 3, vomited once at triage but comfortable
 b. Head: normocephalic, atraumatic
 c. Eyes: extraocular movement intact, pupils equal, reactive to light
 d. Ears: normal tympanic membranes
 e. Nose: no discharge
 f. Neck: full range of motion, no jugular vein distension, no stridor
 g. Pharynx: normal dentition, no lesions, no swelling
 h. Chest: nontender
 i. Lungs: clear bilaterally
 j. Heart: rate and rhythm regular, no murmurs, rubs, or gallops
 k. Abdomen: no distention, mild epigastric tenderness, bowel sounds normal, no
     masses, no hernias, nontender at McBurney's point, negative Murphy's sign, no
     rebound, no guarding, no rigidity
 l. Rectal: normal tone, dark stool, occult blood negative
 m. Extremities: full range of motion, no deformity, normal pulses
 n. Back: nontender
 o. Neuro: cranial nerves II to XII intact; normal sensation, strength; normal reflexes
     and gait

p. Skin: warm and dry

q. Lymph: no lymphadenopathy

I. Action

a. Reassess

    i. Patient vomited two more times since triage

b. NGT placement

c. Meds

    i. Metoclopramide for vomiting

    ii. Whole bowel irrigation with polyethylene glycol solution at 2 L/hr by nasogastric tube

    iii. Deferoxamine 5 mg/kg/hr IV infusion (can increase to 15 mg/kg/hr if no rate-related hypotension, not to exceed total daily dose of 6 g/d). Consults

        i. Poison Control Center notified

        ii. Psychiatry consulted and patient is placed on one-to-one observation

d. Imaging

    i. CXR

    ii. AXR

e. Labs

    i. Call labs to add serum iron levels

    ii. Calculate elemental iron dose: 325 mg per pill $\times$ 20% (ferrous sulfate contains 20% elemental iron) $\times$ ~15 pills = 975 mg ingested elemental iron

f. 2nd L NS bolus

J. Nurse

a. BP: 121/78 HR: 90 RR: 18 Sat: 98% on O_2 (after 2 L)

b. Patient: comfortable

K. Results

Complete blood count:

WBC	10.3×10^3/uL
Hct	35.7%
Plt	350×10^3/uL

Basic metabolic panel:

Na	138 mEq/L
K	4.3 mEq/L
Cl	105 mEq/L
CO_2	20 mEq/L
BUN	12 mEq/dL
Cr	1.1 mg/dL
Gluc	100 mg/dL

Coagulation panel:

PT	12.6 sec
PTT	26.0 sec
INR	1.0

Liver function panel:

AST	23 U/L
ALT	26 U/L
Alk Phos	42 U/L
T bili	1.0 mg/dL
D bili	0.3 mg/dL
Amylase	50 U/L
Lipase	25 U/L
Albumin	4.7 g/dL

Urinalysis:

SG	1.010–1.030
pH	5–8
Prot	Neg mg/dL
Gluc	Neg mg/dL
Ketones	Neg mg/dL
Bili	Neg
Blood	Neg
LE	Neg
Nitrite	Neg
Color	Yellow

Arterial blood gas:

pH	7.36	PCO$_2$	35 mmHg
PO$_2$	88 mmHg	HCO$_3$	20 mmol/L

a. Lactate 2.2 mmol/L
b. Serum iron 666 mcg/dL
c. Aspirin level negative
d. Acetaminophen level negative
e. CXR (Figure 1.2)
f. AXR (Figure 1.3A and 1.3B)

L. Action

a. Admit for observation and treatment

M. Diagnosis

a. Iron overdose

N. Critical actions

▥ Large-bore IV access and fluid bolus
▥ EKG
▥ Whole bowel irrigation
▥ Deferoxamine
▥ Aspirin and acetaminophen

O. Examiner instructions

a. This is a case of intentional iron overdose presenting within six hours of ingestion. Large iron overdoses can have significant consequences including liver failure,

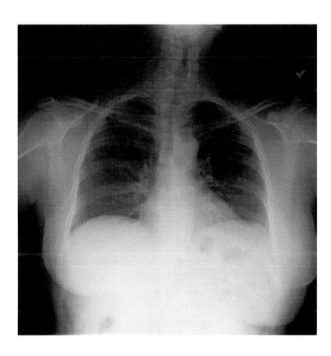

Figure 1.2

A

B

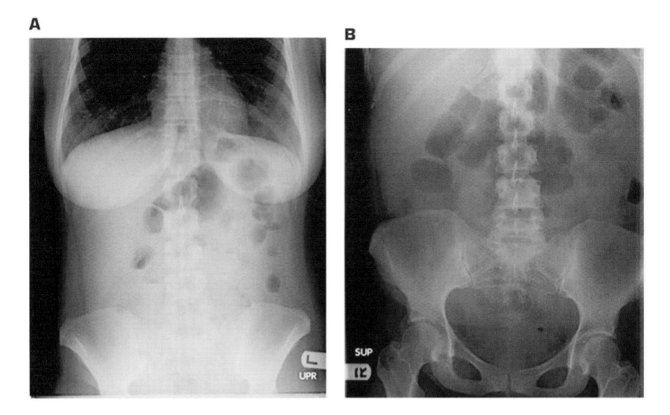

Figure 1.3 A and B

coma, and death. This patient has symptoms of nausea, vomiting, hematemesis, and diarrhea which are consistent with the first stage of iron poisoning. Important actions early in the case include obtaining an ECG (to exclude tricyclic anti-depressant overdose), a pregnancy test (required in any female of child-bearing age), and serum iron levels. The patient needs IV fluids for hypotension, whole bowel irrigation, and chelation therapy to reduce the amount of iron absorbed by the intestines.

P. Pearls

a. Toxic ingestions are determined by the amount of elemental iron contained in the tablet and the number of tablets ingested. In general, toxic overdoses are reported following overdoses as low as 10 to 20 mg/kg elemental iron.

b. Serum iron levels between 300 and 500 mcg/dL correlate with significant GI and mild systemic toxicity, and serum iron levels between 500 mcg/dL and 1000 mcg/dL correlate with moderate systemic toxicity.

c. Significant morbidity is associated with levels greater than 1000 mcg/dL. However, low levels of serum iron may be due to variable times to peak levels of different iron preparations and do not necessarily mean absence of toxicity.

   i. Iron preparations
      1. Ferrous fumarate (33% elemental iron)
      2. Ferrous sulfate (20% elemental iron)
      3. Ferrous gluconate (12% elemental iron)

   d. Clinical stages of iron poisoning

      i. Stage I (1/2–6 hours): vomiting, diarrhea, abdominal pain, hematemesis, hematochezia

      ii. Stage II (4–12 hours) or "Latent stage": GI symptoms may resolve: Despite improvement of GI symptoms, patient may have ongoing clinical illness and progressive systemic deterioration. Monitor for signs of early hypoperfusion and worsening metabolic acidosis

      iii. Stage III (6–72 hours) or "Systemic Toxicity": coma, lactic acidosis, coagulopathy, shock, seizures

      iv. Stage IV (12–96 hours) or "Hepatic Stage": hepatic failure with jaundice, hypoglycemia, coagulopathy

      v. Stage V (2–4 weeks) or "Delayed Sequelae": vomiting, abdominal pain, pyloric scarring, gastric outlet, and small bowel obstruction

   e. Total iron binding capacity (TIBC) has little value in assessment of iron-poisoned patients.

   f. Blood glucose and WBC, formerly thought to be predictive of serum iron levels >300 mcg/dL, are now known to be insensitive.

   g. Radiopaque iron tablets are visible on x-ray and can guide GI decontamination when visualized. This can be helpful if you see any radiopaque iron tablets but is not always reliable if you do not.

   h. Activated charcoal does not absorb significant amounts of iron, and its use is not recommended.

   i. Whole bowel irrigation is indicated for large ingestion. Administer 250 to 500 ml/hr of polyethylene glycol solution in children and 2 L/hr in adults.

   j. Deferoxamine therapy

      i. Indications

         1. Serum iron >350 mcg/dL in a symptomatic patient (including protracted vomiting)

         2. Shock

         3. Coma/seizures

         4. Acidosis

      ii. Administration: 5 mg/kg/hr IV infusion (can increase to 15mg/kg/hr if no rate-related hypotension, not to exceed total daily dose of 6 g)

      iii. Iron-deferoxamine complexes are excreted in the urine and turn it an orange-red color (classically described as "vin rose" urine). Compare urine to pre-deferoxamine baseline samples to judge color difference

Q. References

a. Tintinalli's: Chapter 192. Iron

b. Rosen's: Chapter 157. Heavy Metals

CASE 2: Vomiting infant (Abiola Fasina, MD)

A. Chief complaint

a. 3-week-old baby brought in with vomiting and poor feeding

B. Vital signs
a. HR: 170 BP: 50/palp RR: 60 T: 37.2°C wt: 2.8 kg

C. What does the patient look like?
a. Small pale baby that is sucking air hungrily. The baby has sunken eyes and is lethargic.

D. Primary survey
a. Airway: weak cry
b. Breathing: tachypneic, no cyanosis
c. Circulation: pale skin with decreased elasticity, slow capillary refill, and weak pulses

E. Action
a. Establish IV access
b. Labs
    i. BMP, CBC, ABG, and liver function tests
    ii. Bedside serum glucose (result: 85 mg/dL)
    iii. Serum lactate
    iv. Blood and urine cultures, if sepsis is suspected
c. 20 ml/kg saline bolus × 2, followed by D5 ¼ NS infusion
d. Nothing by mouth (NPO)

F. History
a. HPI: This is a 3-week-old male infant brought in by his mother with vomiting and poor feeding. The mother states that three days ago, the baby started to spit up food after several of his feedings. Symptoms have progressively worsened; he now vomits food forcibly after every feeding. The mother reports that the vomit appears clear with only occasional streaks of blood. She states the baby always appears hungry but is unable to keep food down. He has become progressively more lethargic and weak. She reports having to change a diminishing number of wet diapers over the past few days. The mother occasionally sees the baby's "stomach churning," and that the baby is starting to turn "yellow." She denies fever, chills, or night sweats. There are no sick contacts at home. She reports that the infant had an uncomplicated prenatal course and was born by normal spontaneous vaginal delivery. The baby has received all age-appropriate vaccinations.
b. PMHx: none, birth wt: 3 kg
c. PSHx: none
d. Allergies: none
e. Meds: none
f. FHx: only child
g. PMD: Dr Roberts

G. Nurse
a. NS bolus
b. Vital signs: HR: 160 BP: 60/p RR: 60 T: 99.8°F
c. Patient now NPO

H. Secondary survey
a. General: small pale lethargic baby with a weak cry, sucking air avidly
b. HEENT: depressed fontanelles and dry mucous membranes

   c. Neck: normal

   d. Chest: normal

   e. Heart: tachycardic, sinus rhythm, no murmurs, rubs, or gallops

   f. Abdomen: Firm, peristaltic waves noted passing from the left to the right across the upper abdomen

   g. Rectal: normal, no stool in the vault

   h. GU: normal

   i. Back: normal

   j. Extremities: decreased tone, moving all four extremities weakly

   k. Neuro: normal

   l. Skin: poor skin turgor; jaundice over torso

I. Action

a. Abdominal x-ray

b. Abdominal US

c. Meds/IV fluids: continue IV hydration with D5 ¼ NS at 1.5 to 2 times maintenance rate

d. Reassess

   i. Patient appears more comfortable following rehydration

e. Surgical consult

J. Nurse

a. Vital signs: HR: 160 BP: 70/30 RR: 50, afebrile (after two 20 ml/kg boluses)

K. Results

Complete blood count:

WBC	4.8×10^3/uL	D bili	0.1 mg/dL
Hct	38%	Amylase	260 U/L
Plt	165×10^3/uL	Lipase	250 U/L
		Albumin	3.6 g/dL

Basic metabolic panel:

Na	140 mEq/L	**Urinalysis:**	
K	2.9 mEq/L	SG	1.030
Cl	90 mEq/L	pH	6
CO_2	30 mEq/L	Prot	Neg
BUN	11 mEq/dL	Gluc	Neg
Cr	0.8 mg/dL	Ketones	Neg
Gluc	90 mg/dL	Bili	Neg
		Blood	Neg
Coagulation panel:		LE	Neg
PT	12.5 sec	Nitrite	Neg
PTT	26 sec	Color	Yellow
INR	1.0		
		Arterial blood gas:	
		pH	7.55
Liver function panel:		PO_2	85 mmHg
AST	20 U/L	PCO_2	40 mmHg
ALT	25 U/L	HCO_3	30 mmol/L
Alk Phos	40 U/L		
T bili	1.5 mg/dL		

a. US (Figure 2.1) significant for thickened pylorus with a diameter of 6 mm

Figure 2.1

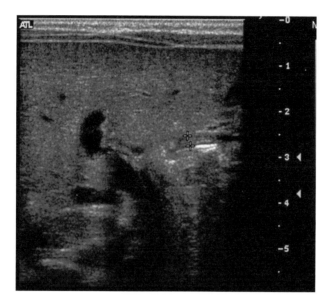

L. Action
a. Admit to pediatrics and continue to monitor fluid input and output, daily weights
b. Continue maintenance fluids including potassium supplementation
c. Pylorotomy in OR, not emergent in this case

M. Diagnosis
a. Congenital hypertrophic pyloric stenosis

N. Critical actions
▨ IV access and adequate rehydration
▨ Abdominal examination
▨ Nasogastric tube, nothing by mouth (NPO)
▨ Abdominal US

O. Examiner instructions
a. This is a case of congenital hypertrophic pyloric stenosis. In this illness, muscles at the stomach outlet become overgrown (hypertrophied) and obstruct normal food transit from the stomach to the small intestine. Digestion and absorption are consequently impaired. Initial vital signs demonstrate tachycardia and hypotension resulting from hypovolemia (normal neonatal vital signs include: HR between 120 and 160; systolic BP, greater than 70; RR, less than 60). These will correct only with fluid administration. If no fluids are given, have the nurse remind the doctor of the vital signs. Labs early in the course of the disease are generally normal; once significant vomiting and dehydration occurs, hypochloremic hypokalemic metabolic alkalosis is commonly seen. Ultrasound (US) is the preferred diagnostic study and demonstrates a hypertrophied pylorus (greater than 4 mm diameter is significant). To make this particular case more challenging, state that care providers cannot obtain venous access upon arrival. In this case, the neonate is ill enough to warrant intraosseus needle placement if IV access is not rapidly established.

P. Pearls
a. Abdominal US is the preferred diagnostic study.
b. Physical examination is the most important diagnostic tool.

    i. Peristaltic waves may be seen after a feeding.

    ii. Palpation of an "olive" is pathognomonic. When this is present, no further diagnostics are necessary.

c. Fluid resuscitation and nasogastric decompression in sick infants.

d. Occurs in infants typically present in the 2nd to 3rd week of life and are usually first-born males.

Q. References

a. Tintinalli's: Chapter 123. Vomiting, Diarrhea, and Dehydration in Children.

b. Rosen's: Chapter 172. Gastrointestinal Disorders.

CASE 3: Altered mental status (Abiola Fasina, MD)

A. Chief complaint

a. 81-year-old female brought in by EMS, unconscious

B. Vital signs

a. BP: 140/60 HR: 60 RR: 6 T: 37°C Sat: 80%

C. What does the patient look like?

a. The patient appears her stated age. Patient is unresponsive to all stimuli including pain.

D. Primary survey

a. Airway: agonal respirations, slight gurgling at back of throat

b. Breathing: being ventilated by EMS, good air movement bilaterally

c. Circulation: mottled cyanotic skin, normal pulses and capillary refill

E. Action

a. Endotracheal intubation

    i. Bag valve mask with good technique (oral airway, good mask seal, jaw thrust, etc.) to optimally preoxygenate

    ii. Rapid sequence intubation using medications to protect against possible brain injury:

        a. Premedication with lidocaine and fentanyl

        b. Induction with etomidate

        c. Paralysis with rocuronium or succinylcholine

b. Two large-bore peripheral IV lines

c. Labs

    i. CBC, BMP, PT/PTT/INR, type and cross-match, aspirin, acetaminophen level, lactate, ABG, cardiac enzymes, and UA

d. 1 L NS bolus

e. Monitor (after bolus): BP: 149/69 HR: 55 RR: 18 Sat: 100% on 100% FiO_2

f. EKG and portable CXR

g. Foley catheter

h. Finger stick glucose (Result=395)

i. Dextrose, thiamine, and naloxone

j. Head CT

k. Place patient on ventilator

F. History

a. HPI: An 81-year-old female with a history of bronchitis, non-insulin-dependent diabetes mellitus, hypertension, and chronic atrial fibrillation (on warfarin) brought in by EMS for respiratory failure. Witness states that while patient was being assisted to the bathroom, she collapsed on the floor. Some trembling of the arms was noted but the patient was still verbal. The patient subsequently complained of shortness of breath and became unresponsive. The family states the patient never complained of chest pain, fever, or cough. Patient has no history of seizure. Her baseline mental status is "normal." The patient ambulates without walkers, canes, or assistance at baseline, and is able to walk for 3-to-4 blocks before experiencing fatigue. The patient's other medications are unknown. EMS arrived at the scene and observed a mottled, cyanotic female, unresponsive to all stimuli with a weak, thready pulse

b. PMHx: bronchitis, non-insulin-dependent diabetes mellitus, hypertension, atrial fibrillation (chronic)

c. PSHx: unknown

d. Allergies: none

e. Meds: warfarin, metformin, metoprolol (these are not known to EMS)

f. Social: no history of smoking, drinking, or drugs; patient lives with family and is able to perform her usual daily activities without assistance at baseline

g. FHx: noncontributory

h. PMD: unknown

G. Nurse

a. EKG: (Figure 3.1)

b. 1 L fluid bolus given

c. CXR: (Figure 3.2)

Figure 3.1

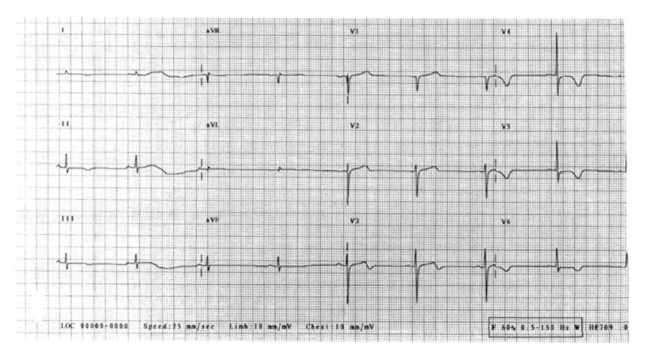

Figure 3.2

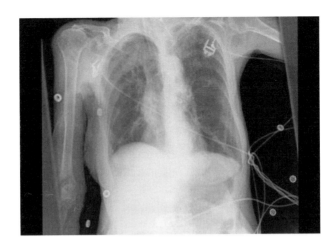

H. Secondary survey

a. General: elderly, frail, and pale female

b. HEENT: normocephalic, atraumatic, 1 mm pupils nonreactive to light, no gag, not triggering the ventilator, no tongue lacerations noted

c. Neck: normal

d. Chest: clear bilaterally, no crackles or rales

e. Heart: bradycardic with barely palpable peripheral pulses, prolonged capillary refill

f. Abdomen: normal

g. Rectal: normal tone, hemoccult negative, brown stool

h. GU: Foley catheter in place

i. Back: no abrasions, hematomas, or ecchymoses

j. Neuro: unresponsive to sternal rub or other noxious stimulation, Glasgow Coma Scale: Eye=1, Verbal=1, Motor=1, intubated. Could also be described as "3T."

k. Extremities: no peripheral edema noted; weak radial and dorsalis pedis pulses bilaterally

l. Skin: mottled appearance improved

m. Lymph: normal

I. Action

a. Meds: continue fluids

b. Reassess

   i. Patient still unresponsive; heart rate decreasing and blood pressure increasing

J. Nurse

a. BP: 199/104 HR: 45 RR: 16 RT: 99 Sat: 100%

K. Results

Complete blood count:

WBC	10.9 × 103/uL	BUN	16 mEq/dL
Hct	33%	Cr	0.8 mg/dL
Plt	261 × 103/uL	Gluc	405 mg/dL

Basic metabolic panel:

Na	134 mEq/L	**Coagulation panel:**	
K	3.9 mEq/L	PT	30 sec
Cl	102 mEq/L	PTT	26 sec
CO_2	24 mEq/L	INR	2.9

Liver function panel:

AST	25 U/L	Gluc	+
ALT	33 U/L	Ketones	Neg
Alk Phos	44 U/L	Bili	Neg
T bili	1.2 mg/dL	Blood	Neg
D bili	0.2 mg/dL	LE	Neg
Amylase	204 U/L	Nitrite	Neg
Lipase	223 U/L	Color	Yellow
Albumin	3.2 g/dL		

Urinalysis:

Arterial blood gas:

		pH	7.40
SG	1.028	PO_2	85 mmHg
pH	6.5	PCO_2	40 mmHg
Prot	Neg	HCO_3	25 mmol/L

a. Aspirin and acetaminophen levels: negative
b. Troponin: negative
c. Head CT (Figure 3.3)

L. Action

a. Neurosurgical consult for ventriculostomy placement and neurosurgical intensive care unit (ICU) admission
b. Central line and arterial line placement (optional for ED evaluation)
c. Vitamin K and fresh frozen plasma or prothrombin complex concentrate to reverse anticoagulation

M. Diagnosis

a. Non-traumatic intracranial hemorrhage (ICH)

N. Critical actions

▪ Manage airway upon arrival
▪ Large-bore IV access and fluids
▪ Bedside serum glucose level
▪ Laboratory evaluation (coagulation factors)
▪ Head CT for new onset coma
▪ Reversal of anticoagulation (with one or more of the following: FFP, vitamin K, PCC)
▪ Neurosurgical and ICU consult

Figure 3.3

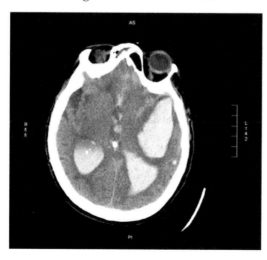

O. Examiner instructions

a. This is a case of nontraumatic intracranial hemorrhage (ICH) in a patient on anticoagulation for atrial fibrillation. Anticoagulation agents increase the risk of bleeding complications (gastrointestinal and intracranial bleeding are the most dangerous sites for hemorrhage to occur). Important early actions include: checking proper ETT placement on patient arrival and obtaining ABG, peripheral venous access with immediate fluid resuscitation; administering naloxone, thiamine, and dextrose (if the blood sugar is not known to be normal). In this case, the patient's bleeding will not improve with medical therapy and she will require emergent operative intervention. Head CT is necessary to make the diagnosis of ICH, initiate therapy, and to obtain the proper consults. It is also important to remember to reverse any anticoagulation that might be contributing to the ICH with vitamin K, fresh frozen plasma (FFP), or blood products once the diagnosis is made.

b. Curveball: In every patient, airway, breathing, and circulation should be addressed first. An alternate presentation for this case would be that the patient arrives intubated by EMS but experiences a rapid deterioration in vital signs on arrival suggesting improper placement of the tube in the esophagus (and not the trachea). The patient's oxygen saturation will drop, followed by the heart rate. When the ETT placement is investigated esophageal placement will be noted and the candidate can re-intubate appropriately. With proper ETT placement the vital signs will return to their previous values.

P. Pearls

a. Coma occurs with bilateral hemispheric pathology, such as hemorrhage or infarct or with damage to the reticular activating system.

b. Other dangerous causes of coma include trauma, infarction, or hemorrhage; central venous thrombosis, meningitis, hydrocephalus, malignancy, cerebral abscess, toxic overdose hepatic or renal failure, sepsis and metabolic derangements (such as hypoglycemia) or exposures to carbon monoxide.

c. The Cushing reflex (bradycardia and hypertension) is exhibited in this case. It is a common physiologic response to increased intracranial pressure.

d. After initial resuscitation, the most important diagnostic test in this patient is to obtain a head CT quickly.

Q. References

a. Tintinalli's: Chapter 160. Spontaneous Subarachnoid and Intracerebral Hemorrhage; Chapter 162. Altered Mental Status and Coma

b. Rosen's: Chapter 16: Depressed Consciousness and Coma

CASE 4: Chest trauma (Abiola Fasina, MD)

A. Chief complaint

a. 34-year-old male stabbed in the chest

B. Vital signs

a. BP: 88/42 HR: 110 RR: 28 T: 37.9°C Sat: 92% on nonrebreather mask

C. What does the patient look like?

a. Young disheveled-looking male, intoxicated. Patient is gasping and complaining of difficulty in breathing. Patient appears to be slightly somnolent but is following commands and answering questions.

D. Primary survey

a. Airway: speaking in short sentences, breathing fast, and gasping for air
b. Breathing: moderate respiratory distress with decreased breath sounds on the right. Mild tracheal deviation to the left (candidate must ask)
c. Circulation: patient has slightly cool extremities but capillary refill is normal, distended neck veins

E. Action

a. Needle or tube thoracostomy (describe procedure), hiss of air audible after insertion of needle or tube
b. Two large-bore peripheral IV lines
c. Labs
    i. CBC, BMP, PT/PTT, serum toxicology screen, blood type and cross-match
d. 2 L NS bolus
e. Monitor: BP: 98/72 HR: 110 RR: 28 T: 37.9°C Sat: 98% on nonrebreather mask (after thoracostomy)
f. EKG
g. Tetanus vaccine administered
h. Prepare for emergent intubation (if needed)

F. History

a. HPI: a 34-year-old male with no significant past medical or surgical history reports being stabbed in the right chest by a broken bottle. Patient admits to drinking several beers but denies additional drug use. There was no loss of consciousness. Patient denies any head or neck trauma.
b. PMHx: none
c. PSHx: none
d. Allergies: penicillin (rash)
e. Meds: none
f. Social: works in construction, lives with three friends; denies tobacco and illicit drug use, but admits recent alcohol use ("several beers")
g. FHx: noncontributory
h. PMD: none ("has not seen a physician in several years")

G. Nurse

a. NS bolus
b. EKG (sinus tachycardia)
c. Monitor and pulse oximetry
d. Repeat vital signs after needle/tube thoracostomy
    i. BP: 130/80 HR: 96 RR: 18 Sat: 98% on nonrebreather mask

H. Secondary survey

a. General: young disheveled male, somnolent, arousable, oriented, appears intoxicated
b. HEENT: normal except injected conjunctiva, no injury or bruising noted, pupils equal, reactive
c. Neck: trachea is now midline; neck veins appear normal, no stridor noted

d. Chest: needle or tube thoracostomy in right chest; breath sounds are still slightly diminished on the right; no crackles or rales, symmetric excursion; deep six-centimeter laceration present along the right anterior chest wall, near fourth to fifth rib space. No visible foreign body, no active bleeding

e. Heart: normal; no murmurs or rub

f. Abdomen: soft, nondistended; no peritoneal signs; bowel sounds normal

g. Rectal: normal, fecal occult blood (guaiac test) negative

h. GU: normal

i. Extremities: moving all four extremities well, normal pulses bilaterally, slightly pale, good tone and 5/5 strength

j. Back: normal

k. Neuro: patient is following commands easily, normal on examination

l. Skin: as stated earlier

m. Lymph: normal

I. Action

a. Tube thoracostomy (chest tube) if not placed earlier (describe procedure)

b. Portable upright CXR after chest tube

c. Foley catheter

d. Right-sided anterior chest wall laceration dressed

e. Surgical consult

f. Another 1 L bolus

J. Nurse

a. Vital signs stable after tube thoracostomy and 1 L crystalloid bolus
   i. BP: 128/80 HR: 96 RR: 18 Sat: 98% on 2 LPM oxygen by nasal cannula

b. Patient complaining of some chest pain

c. 1 L saline bolus × 2

K. Results

Complete blood count:

WBC	$14.2 \times 10^3/uL$
Hct	39%
Plt	$300 \times 10^3/uL$

Basic metabolic panel:

Na	140 mEq/L
K	3.8 mEq/L
Cl	107 mEq/L
CO_2	27 mEq/L
BUN	21 mEq/dL
Cr	0.9 mg/dL
Gluc	110 mg/dL

Coagulation panel:

PT	12.3 sec
PTT	31 sec
INR	1.0

Liver function panel:

AST	44 U/L
ALT	34 U/L
Alk Phos	55 U/L
T bili	0.8 mg/dL
D bili	0.1 mg/dL
Amylase	200 U/L
Lipase	23 U/L
Albumin	3.9 g/dL

Urinalysis:

SG	1.028
pH	6
Prot	Neg
Gluc	Neg
Ketones	Neg
Bili	Neg
Blood	Neg
LE	Neg
Nitrite	Neg
Color	Yellow

Arterial blood gas:

pH	7.40	PCO$_2$	40 mmHg
PO$_2$	90 mmHg	HCO$_3$	27 mmol/L

a. Blood type: AB$^+$

b. Serum toxicology: alcohol level – 190 mg/dL, no aspirin and acetaminophen negative

c. EKG (Figure 4.1)

L. Action

a. Imaging: CXR (Figure 4.2) no foreign body noted

b. Meds

    i. Morphine IV

    ii. Antibiotics

    iii. Tetanus toxoid IM

c. Reassess

    i. Patient is more comfortable, breathing easier, and saturating well, awaiting surgical consult to assess and repair chest laceration, will be admitted to SICU

M. Diagnosis

a. Tension pneumothorax

N. Critical actions

▨ Needle thoracostomy (If the candidate performed a tube thoracostomy first, no need for needle thoracostomy.)

▨ Tube thoracostomy

▨ Upright CXR

▨ Pain management

▨ Diligent search for other traumatic injuries

▨ Surgical consult

O. Examiner instructions

a. This is a case of tension pneumothorax resulting from penetrating trauma. Air has become trapped outside the lung within this patient's chest, impairing the normal mechanics of respiration and causing obstructive shock (preload decreases with increased intrathoracic pressure, as venous return to the heart by the inferior and superior vena cavae is diminished). It is a diagnosis that the candidate should make during the primary survey before ordering radiologic or laboratory tests based solely on the physical examination findings. Classic signs and symptoms include: labored breathing, hypotension, and diminished right ventricular preload, distended neck veins, tracheal deviation to the unaffected (contralateral) side, diminished or absent breath sounds, and ipsilateral hyperresonance. The most important early action is to perform immediate needle or tube thoracostomy to convert the tension pneumothorax to a simple pneumothorax. The patient's vital signs will deteriorate (oxygen saturation and blood pressure will drop, heart rate will rise, and the patient will lose consciousness) until needle or tube thoracostomy is performed. The patient should be kept on supplemental oxygen and monitored while a thoracostomy tube is placed. Ideally, only after these critical steps should a chest

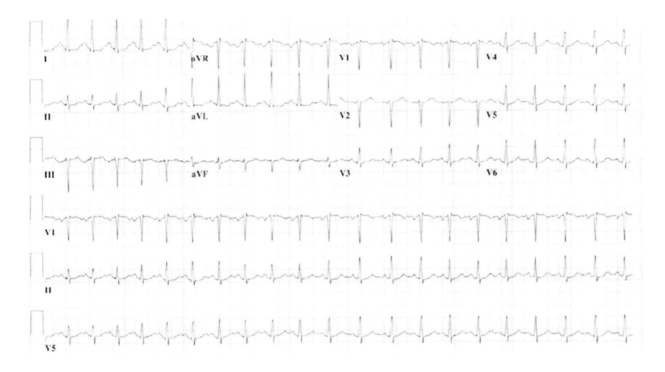

Figure 4.1

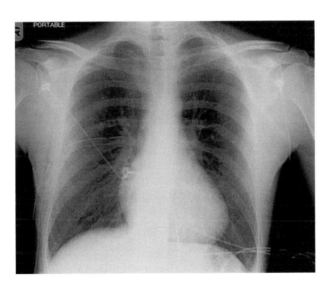

Figure 4.2

radiograph be ordered and obtained. Other important early actions include IV fluid administration, continuous cardiac monitoring and oximetry, diagnostic testing (serum, ultrasound, etc.) as part of a diligent search for other traumatic injuries, and early surgical consultation.

P. Pearls

a. Tension pneumothorax should be diagnosed clinically; no CXR needed initially.

b. Immediate needle thoracostomy and/or tube thoracostomy are critical actions.

c. Tracheal deviation is a rare and very late finding in tension pneumothorax. Although this finding is often used as a pathognomonic sign for tension pneumo-thorax, its absence certainly does not exclude the diagnosis.

    d. Monitor patients closely for signs of shock; adequate tissue perfusion should be maintained with crystalloids or blood products.

    e. Tension pneumothorax is a form of obstructive shock. Another cause of obstructive shock that has a high-likelihood of existing in this patient is pericardial tamponade. A rapid method for distinguishing these two etiologies on the oral board exam is with ultrasound. Other causes of obstructive shock (unlikely in this patient, but presented here to be complete) are acute large pulmonary embolism ("saddle embolism") and large diaphragmatic hernia with tension gastrothorax. Other forms of shock (hemorrhagic shock, distributive shock from traumatic cord injury) are also possible in the patient with multiple traumatic injuries.

Q. References
a. Tintinalli's: Chapter 250. Trauma in Adults.
b. Rosen's: Chapter 45. Thoracic Trauma.

CASE 5: Abdominal pain and vomiting (Shefali Trivedi, MD)

A. Chief complaint
a. 45-year-old female suffering from abdominal pain

B. Vital signs
a. BP: 145/85 HR: 93 RR: 16 T: 38.6°C Sat: 99% on RA

C. What does the patient look like?
a. Patient appears stated age, overweight, lying in stretcher holding abdomen, uncomfortable due to pain, in mild distress.

D. Primary survey
a. Airway: patent, speaking in full sentences
b. Breathing: no apparent respiratory distress, no cyanosis
c. Circulation: warm, dry skin, normal capillary refill

E. History
a. HPI: a 45-year-old female with a past medical history of hypertension, hypercholesterolemia, and gallstones presents with worsening abdominal pain for 1 day. She states that her pain is constant, sharp, and worst in the right upper quadrant, occasionally radiating to the right shoulder. She has had several similar episodes over the past 2 years that have either resolved spontaneously or with pain medications after about 1 to 2 hours. All episodes have begun after eating a "heavy" meal as did this episode. She complains of a subjective fever and chills for 1 day and nausea and three episodes of non-bilious, non-bloody vomiting. She denies diarrhea, constipation, chest pain, shortness of breath, sick contacts, recent travel history, unusual food intake, trauma, or urinary symptoms.
b. PMHx: hypertension, hypercholesterolemia
c. PSHx: none
d. Allergies: no known drug allergies
e. Meds: none

f. Social: lives with her husband and two children, denies smoking, alcohol, drug use, sexually active with her husband only

g. FHx: mother with hypertension, father with hypercholesterolemia and hypertension

h. PMD: none

F. Secondary survey

a. General: alert and oriented, overweight, mild distress due to pain

b. HEENT: normal

c. Neck: normal

d. Chest: normal

e. Heart: normal

f. Abdomen: normal bowel sounds, soft, severe tenderness in the right upper quadrant with voluntary guarding, positive Murphy's sign, nontender at McBurney's point, no pulsatile masses, no hepatosplenomegaly, no hernia, no rebound or guarding

g. Rectal: brown stool, fecal occult blood (guaiac test) negative, normal rectal tone

h. GU: normal

i. Extremities: normal

j. Back: normal, no costovertebral angle tenderness

k. Neuro: normal

l. Skin: normal

m. Lymph: normal

G. Action

a. Supplemental oxygen

b. Two large-bore peripheral IV lines

c. Labs
   i. CBC, BMP, liver function panel, PT/PTT, blood type and hold, urinalysis, blood culture, urine culture, qualitative or quantitative hCG (urine or serum)

d. 1 L NS bolus

e. Monitor: BP: 139/83 HR: 96 RR: 16 Sat: 100% on oxygen 2 LPM by nasal cannula

f. Imaging
   i. CXR
   ii. Right upper quadrant US
   iii. EKG

g. Meds
   i. Ampicillin sodium/sulbactam (or other appropriate antibiotic) IV
   ii. Morphine sulfate IV
   iii. Acetaminophen PO

h. Reassess
   i. Patient's pain has improved somewhat, but still complains of right-sided upper quadrant abdominal pain

H. Nurse

a. BP: 142/76 HR: 86 RR: 16 Sat: 100% on oxygen 2 LPM by nasal cannula

I. Results

Complete blood count:

WBC	15.6×10^3/uL	Alk Phos	325 U/L
Hct	41.7%	T bili	5.0 mg/dL
Plt	350×10^3/uL	D bili	3.5 mg/dL
		Amylase	56 U/L
Basic metabolic panel:		Lipase	24 U/L
Na	142 mEq/L	Albumin	4.0 g/dL
K	4.2 mEq/L		
Cl	105 mEq/L	**Urinalysis:**	
CO_2	24 mEq/L	SG	1.015
BUN	15 mEq/dL	pH	6
Cr	0.9 mg/dL	Prot	Neg
Gluc	110 mg/dL	Gluc	Neg
		Ketones	Neg
Coagulation panel:		Bili	Pos
PT	13.2 sec	Blood	Neg
PTT	27 sec	LE	Neg
INR	0.9	Nitrite	Neg
		Color	Yellow
Liver function panel:			
AST	22 U/L		
ALT	20 U/L		

a. Urine pregnancy test negative
b. EKG (Figure 5.1)
c. CXR (Figure 5.2)
d. RUQ US (Figure 5.3)

Figure 5.1

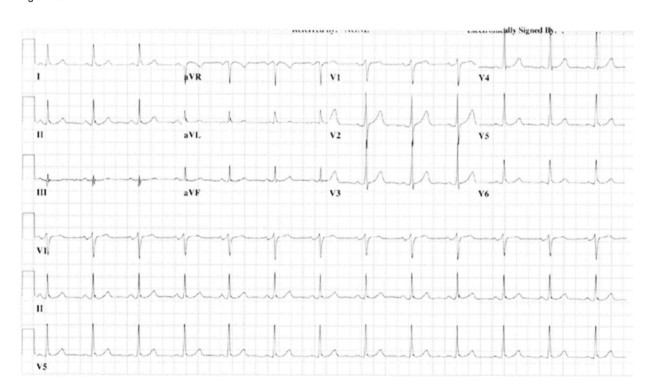

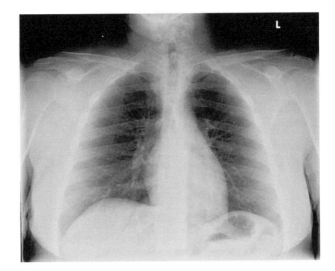

Figure 5.2

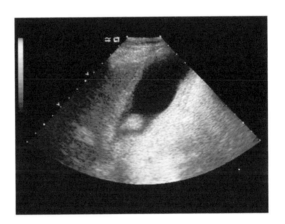

Figure 5.3

J. Action

a. Surgery consult
   i. Admit for IV antibiotics and possible OR for cholecystectomy
b. Discussion with patient regarding need for admission and possible cholecystectomy

K. Diagnosis

a. Cholecystitis

L. Critical actions

▨ Large-bore IV access
▨ Right upper quadrant US
▨ Pain management
▨ Surgery consultation
▨ Antibiotics

M. Examiner instructions

a. This is a case of acute cholecystitis. Symptoms are often worse after eating fatty meals. The patient continues to complain of fever until acetaminophen or other antipyretic is administered, and will continue to complain of pain until an analgesic is given. It is important that the candidate administers antibiotics early, and describes their concern for cholecystitis adequately to the surgical consultant (fever, Murphy's sign, elevated white blood cell count, vomiting, etc).

N. Pearls

a. Fever and tachycardia are often absent in cholecystitis. In these cases, the patient is often misdiagnosed as having "cholelithiasis" or "gastroenteritis."

b. Ultrasound is the preferred imaging modality in acute care settings. The presence of gallstones, a thickened gallbladder wall, and pericholecystic fluid have a positive predictive value exceeding 90%.

c. The differential diagnosis includes ascending cholangitis, choledocholithiasis, hepatitis, Mirizzi syndrome (obstruction of the common bile duct by gallstone obstruction of the cystic duct), hepatic abscess, Fitz-Hugh-Curtis syndrome (fibrinous perihepatitis as a consequence of pelvic inflammatory disease), pyelonephritis, right lower lobe pneumonia/pleurisy, pleural effusion, pancreatitis, peptic ulcer disease (of the duodenum with perforation), and appendicitis.

d. Consider atypical myocardial infarction, particularly in elderly or diabetic patients presenting with similar symptoms.

e. In pregnant patients and young women, elicit a sexual history and consider performing a pelvic examination to exclude Fitz-Hugh-Curtis syndrome (as described above).

f. Patients with diabetes have an increased risk for bacterial invasion into the gallbladder wall and emphysematous cholecystitis.

g. Treatment includes broad-spectrum antibiotics with coverage against Gram-positive and -negative aerobic and anaerobic bacteria.

h. Five percent of patients may not have gallstones.

i. Patients with acalculous and emphysematous cholecystitis are at increased risk for gangrene and perforation and require emergent cholecystectomy.

O. References

a. Tintinalli's: Chapter 82. Pancreatitis and Cholecystitis.

b. Rosen's: Chapter 90. Disorders of the Liver and Biliary Tract

CASE 6: Weak infant (Christopher Strother, MD)

A. Chief complaint

a. 4-week-old female with fever, lethargy, weakness worsening over the past two days

B. Vital signs

a. BP: 50/20 HR: 205 RR: 58 T: 39.2°C Sat: 94% on RA wt: 5 kg

C. What does the patient look like?

a. Patient appears stated age, lethargic, tachypneic, febrile, and flushed.

D. Primary survey

a. Airway: patent, weak cry

b. Breathing: tachypnea, no cyanosis, lungs clear

c. Circulation: warm flushed skin, capillary refill three seconds, tachycardia

E. Action

a. Oxygen supplementation (nonrebreather mask)

b. Largest possible peripheral IV $\times$ 2, likely anticubital fossa, interosseous (IO) line if difficulty with peripheral line

c. Labs

    i. CBC, BMP, LFT, PT/PTT, blood culture, UA, urine culture

    ii. Lumbar puncture and spinal fluid studies deferred until patient stabilized

    iii. Bedside serum glucose = 30 mg/dl

d. 20 ml/kg bolus NS

e. Monitor: BP: 50/25 HR: 200 RR: 58 Sat: 100% on O_2

f. Dextrose bolus 0.5 to 1 g/kg (Dosing: 10% dextrose = 5 ml/kg; 25% dextrose = 4 ml/kg)

F. History

a. HPI: a 4-week-old female, born full term by normal spontaneous vaginal delivery without complications, doing well until past two days, when she was noted by the parents with (initially) fussiness, sleepiness, and poor feeding. These symptoms and signs were followed by "really high" tactile fever and lethargy today. Fever, lethargy, poor feeding, irritability were noticed today and are present on initial examination. There is no history of vomiting, diarrhea, cough, travel, or recent exposure to other sick contacts.

b. PMHx: none

c. PSHx: none

d. Allergies: none

e. Social: lives with parents, two older siblings

f. FHx: not relevant

g. PMD: Dr Chris

G. Nurse

a. NS bolus 20 ml/kg (100 ml)

    i. BP: 60/40 HR: 190 RR: 50 Sat: 100% on O_2

b. If no fluids, then

    i. BP: 50/25 HR: 205 RR: 55 Sat: 100% on O_2

H. Secondary survey

a. General: lethargic, weak cry and motions, tachypnea, febrile

b. HEENT: anterior fontanelle open soft and flat, normal

c. Neck: normal

d. Chest: normal

e. Heart: mild vibratory murmur, tachycardia

f. Abdomen: normal

g. Rectal: normal

h. GU: normal

i. Extremities: normal

j. Back: normal

k. Neuro: normal

l. Skin: warm, flushed

m. Lymph: normal

Figure 6.1

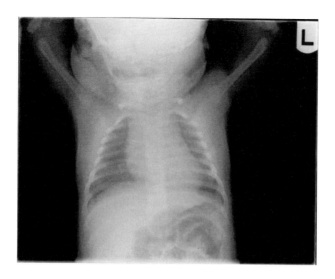

I. Action

a. Endotracheal intubation for airway protection in sepsis/lethargy
    i. Ventilator settings: volume 10 ml/kg, rate 30, O_2 100%
b. Meds
    i. Cefotaxime IV
    ii. Ampicillin IV
    iii. Multiple fluid boluses up to 80 ml/kg total (four standard doses)
    iv. Acetaminophen rectally
c. Reassess
    i. Patient with mild improvement in fever after 15 minutes so decreased warmth and flush, some decrease in HR and tachypnea, but only after multiple fluid boluses (as stated above)
d. Imaging
    i. CXR (Figure 6.1)

J. Nurse

a. BP: 65/45 HR: 170 RR: 50 (after NS boluses) Sat: 100% on O_2 (or vent)
b. Patient: mild global improvement

K. Results

Complete blood count:	
WBC	20.1×10^3/uL
Hct	45.5%
Plt	325×10^3/uL

Coagulation panel:	
PT	11.4 sec
PTT	29 sec
INR	1.0

Basic metabolic panel:	
Na	140 mEq/L
K	3.8 mEq/L
Cl	110 mEq/L
CO_2	13 mEq/L
BUN	3 mEq/dL
Cr	0.6 mg/dL
Gluc	35 mg/dL

Liver function panel:	
AST	90 U/L
ALT	75 U/L
Alk Phos	200 U/L
T bili	3.1 mg/dL
D bili	0.8 mg/dL
Amylase	40 U/L
Lipase	20 U/L
Albumin	3.5g/dL

Urinalysis:

SG	1.030	Nitrite	Neg
pH	7	Color	Yellow
Prot	Neg		
Gluc	Neg	**Arterial blood gas:**	
Ketones	Neg	pH	7.1
Bili	Neg	PO_2	160 mmHg
Blood	Neg	PCO_2	35 mmHg
LE	Neg	HCO_3	12 mmol/L

a. Lactate 3.6 mmol/L

b. LDH: 610

L. Action

a. Pediatric intensive care unit (PICU) consult

b. Discussion with family and PMD need for ICU admission and monitoring for likely sepsis

c. Meds

    i. Continued fluid support

M. Diagnosis

a. Sepsis

N. Critical actions

▨ IV or IO access

▨ Multiple fluid boluses

▨ Early antibiotics

▨ ICU consult

O. Examiner instructions

a. This is a case of an infant in septic shock from bacteremia. Early and generous fluid support is essential to maintain blood pressure and cardiac output. Antibiotics should be given early. If the infant is very lethargic, intubation should be performed to protect the airway and to decrease the metabolic demands (work) of breathing. In a stable child, a full work-up is required, including a lumbar puncture to obtain cerebrospinal fluid for culture and analysis. In an unstable child, blood and urinalysis are usually obtained quickly, but lumbar puncture may not; this procedure may be deferred, as it may delay emergent stabilizing interventions and could unnecessarily physiologically stress the critically ill neonate. This patient will need to be expeditiously moved to an intensive care setting as continuous hemodynamic monitoring and frequent serial reassessments will be needed.

P. Pearls

a. Septic shock is a form of distributive shock. Other forms of shock (e.g. hypovolemic shock) may be superimposed. The recommended initial management for septic shock is the rapid administration of crystalloid fluids (a minimum volume of 30 ml/kg up to 80 ml/kg, may be required). Vasopressor support may be required for patients with septic shock and hypotension refractory to fluid administration.

b. Broad-spectrum antibiotics should be given early in the management of an infant who may be septic.

c. Sepsis should be considered high on the differential diagnosis of any newborn presenting *in extremis*; empiric treatment should be initiated before diagnostic test can confirm the diagnosis.

Q. References

a. Tintinalli's: Chapter 113. Fever and Serious Bacterial Illness

b. Rosen's: Chapter 167. Pediatric Fever.

c. Camacho-Gonzalez, A, Spearman PW, Stoll BJ. Neonatal infectious diseases: evaluation of neonatal sepsis. *Pediatr Clin N Am* 60 (2013) 367–389.

CASE 7: Chest pain (Alan Huang, MD)

A. Chief complaint

a. 19-year-old male complaining of chest pain

B. Vital signs

a. BP: 115/65 HR: 100 RR: 18 T: 37.8°C Sat: 99% RA

C. What does the patient look like?

a. Patient is alert but appears uncomfortable, anxious, and diaphoretic.

D. Primary survey

a. Airway: speaking normally

b. Breathing: no respiratory distress

c. Circulation: skin diaphoretic, pulses are full in the peripheral extremities

E. Action

a. Oxygen via nasal cannula or nonrebreather mask

b. Two large-bore peripheral IV lines

c. Monitor: BP: 115/65 HR: 100 R: 18 T: 37.8°C Sat: 99% RA

d. 1 L NS bolus

e. Labs

    i. CBC, BMP, cardiac enzymes, D-dimer, coagulation studies, blood type and hold

f. EKG

g. CXR

F. History

a. HPI: a 19-year-old male with a history of psychiatric disease including depression and anxiety presents with sudden onset of burning chest pain while at rest this morning. The pain is rated a 10 out of 10, diffuse, radiating to the shoulders and back. He reports binging on alcohol last night, and had multiple episodes of non-bloody, non-bilious vomiting through the night. He denies having any shortness of breath, but he is diaphoretic. He denies tobacco, cocaine, or other illicit drug use. He denies taking extra doses of his psychiatric medicines. He denies any personal history of blood clots and any family history of cardiac disease. He reports no history of swelling in his legs.

b. PMHx: depression, anxiety

c. PSHx: none

d. Allergies: none

e. Meds: paroxetine, clonazepam

f. Social: no tobacco or illicit drug use; occasional alcohol "binges"

g. FHx: noncontributory

G. Nurse

a. EKG (Figure 7.1)

H. Secondary survey

a. General: alert, oriented, diaphoretic, remains uncomfortable

b. Head: normal

c. Eyes: normal

d. Neck: full range of motion, no jugular vein distension, palpable crepitus bilaterally (provide only if candidate asks)

e. Chest: nontender

f. Lungs: clear bilaterally

g. Heart: rate and rhythm regular, no murmurs, rubs, or gallops

h. Abdomen: normal bowel sounds, soft, non tender, or distended

i. Skin: warm and dry

I. Action

a. Review portable CXR (Figure 7.2)

b. Meds

   i. Morphine IV

   ii. Imipenem/cilastatin IV (or other broad-spectrum antibiotic regimen)

   iii. H_2 blocker IV

Figure 7.1

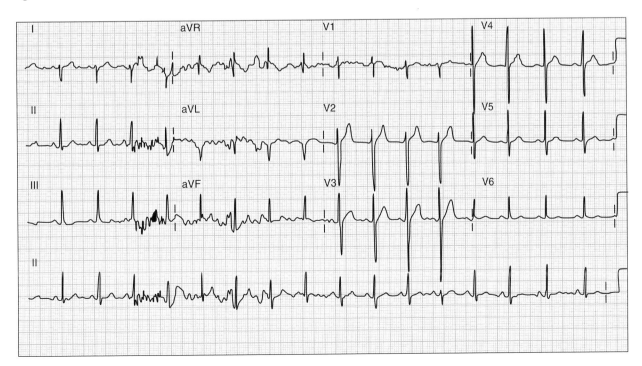

Figure 7.2

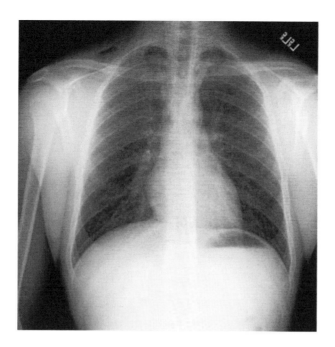

Figure 7.3

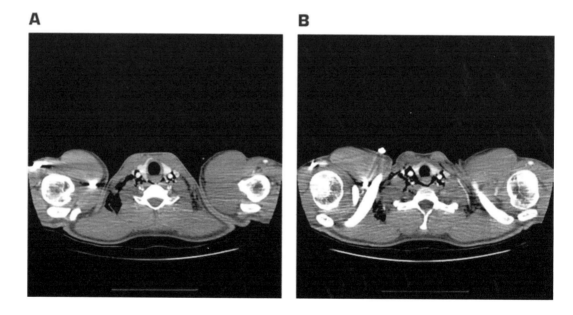

c. Gastroenterology (GI), cardiothoracic surgery, or otolaryngology (ENT) consult
d. Arrange CT neck/chest with contrast (Figure 7.3)

J. Results

Complete blood count:

WBC	15.8×10^3/uL	Cl	102 mEq/L
Hct	35.2%	CO_2	20 mEq/L
Plt	258×10^3/uL	BUN	15 mEq/dL
		Cr	0.8 mg/dL
Basic metabolic panel:		Gluc	85 mg/dL
Na	135 mEq/L		
K	4.5 mEq/L		

Coagulation panel:

PT	14.1 sec	Prot	Neg
PTT	28.4 sec	Gluc	Neg
INR	1.0	Ketones	Neg
		Bili	Neg
Liver function panel:		Blood	Neg
AST	33 U/L	LE	Neg
ALT	38 U/L	Nitrite	Neg
Alk Phos	45 U/L	Color	Yellow
T bili	0.5 mg/dL		
D bili	0.1 mg/dL	**Arterial blood gas:**	
Amylase	40 U/L	pH	7.37
Lipase	200 U/L	PO_2	80 mmHg
Albumin	3.8 g/dL	PCO_2	44 mmHg
		HCO_3	20 mmol/L

Urinalysis:

SG	1.018
pH	7

a. Cardiac enzymes negative

b. D-dimer negative

c. Alcohol negative

K. Diagnosis
a. Boerhaave's syndrome

L. Critical actions
▨ Note crepitus on physical examination

▨ Consider esophageal tear in differential of chest pain in this patient

▨ CXR to evaluate lungs and mediastinum

▨ Emergent GI, ENT, and/or CT surgery consultations (for endoscopy and operative intervention)

▨ Resuscitation with fluids and addition of broad-spectrum antibiotics to treat mediastinitis

M. Examiner instructions
a. This is a case of Boerhaave's syndrome (tear of the esophagus) due to episodes of vomiting. Keys include recognition of this etiology as an extremely deadly cause of chest pain, especially in the setting of vomiting and very uncomfortable-appearing patient. Aggressive fluid resuscitation should begin early, or the patient's vital signs will deteriorate (heart rate will rise, blood pressure will fall, skin will become more clammy and mental status will deteriorate).

b. Curveball: consultants should be reluctant to see a "vomiting psych patient." They will only become interested when the candidate describes concern for esophageal rupture given crepitus on physical examination and x-ray findings. At faculty discretion, CT scanning could be made unavailable while the candidate evaluates the case using other means (e.g. consultation with GI, etc.).

N. Pearls
a. A large proportion of esophageal tears are iatrogenic. However, spontaneous esophageal ruptures, or Boerhaave's syndrome, is associated with acts that increase intraluminal pressures, including vomiting, coughing, straining, seizures.

b. Most common location of distal esophageal tear is left posterolateral.
c. It can be associated with pleural effusion on CXR.
d. Severity of systemic toxicity dictates conservative versus operative management.
e. Mortality of full-thickness ruptures is very high.

O. References
a. Tintinalli's: Chapter 80. Esophageal Emergencies, Gastroesophageal Reflux Disease, and Swallowed Foreign Bodies.
b. Rosen's: Chapter 45. Thoracic Trauma.

CASE 8: Back pain (Alan Huang, MD)

A. Chief complaint
a. 27-year-old male with back pain

B. Vital signs
a. BP: 130/80 HR: 110 RR: 20 T: 36.1°C Sat: 100% RA

C. What does the patient look like?
a. Patient appears well, no sign of distress, alert, and oriented.

D. Primary survey
a. Airway: speaking normally in full sentences
b. Breathing: no respiratory distress, normal breath sounds
c. Circulation: skin dry, bounding pulses

E. History
a. HPI: a 27-year-old male with spinal cord injury three years ago presents with lower back pain for one week. He has been feeling feverish for two days and reports vomiting today. No cough, shortness of breath, headache or stiffness of neck, no diarrhea, no new weakness or numbness, and no recent trauma noted.
b. PMHx: spinal cord injury from motor vehicle collision three years ago; residual numbness of buttocks and thighs. Chronic urinary retention; patient self-catheterizes his bladder several times a day.
c. PSHx: none
d. Allergies: none
e. Meds: naproxen
f. Social: no tobacco or alcohol
g. FHx: noncontributory

F. Secondary survey
a. General: appearing well, no distress
b. HEENT: normal
c. Chest: normal
d. Heart: pulse regular, tachycardic; no murmurs, rubs, or gallops
e. Abdomen: normal bowel sounds, soft, nontender, nondistended, slight decrease in rectal tone
f. Back: tender to palpation in the lumbar spine

g. Neuro: cranial nerves II to XII intact, normal motor function, decreased sensation to thighs and buttocks posteriorly, normal cerebellar examination and gait, normal deep tendon reflexes; diminished sensation over perineum

h. Skin: warm and dry, no lesions

G. Action

a. Oxygen via nasal cannula or nonrebreather mask
b. Two large-bore peripheral IV lines
c. Labs
   i. CBC, BMP, PT/PTT, erythrocyte sedimentation rate (ESR), blood type and hold, urinalysis, blood and urine cultures
d. One liter 0.9% normal saline bolus
e. Monitor: BP: 130/80 HR: 110 R: 20 T: 39.0°C (rectal) Sat: 100% RA
f. Meds
   i. Morphine IV
   ii. Acetaminophen PO
g. CT or MRI of lumbosacral spine

H. Results

Complete blood count:

WBC	15.0×10^3/uL
Hct	36.2%
Plt	300×10^3/uL

Basic metabolic panel:

Na	138 mEq/L
K	4.3 mEq/L
Cl	97 mEq/L
CO_2	28 mEq/L
BUN	10 mEq/dL
Cr	1.0 mg/dL
Gluc	125 mg/dL

Coagulation panel:

PT	12.3 sec
PTT	30.5 sec
INR	1.1

Liver function panel:

AST	38 U/L
ALT	40 U/L
Alk Phos	55 U/L

T bili	1.1 mg/dL
D bili	0.1 mg/dL
Amylase	244 U/L
Lipase	200 U/L
Albumin	4.1 g/dL

Urinalysis:

SG	1.020
pH	6
Prot	+
Gluc	Neg
Ketones	Neg
Bili	Neg
Blood	Neg
LE	+
Nitrite	+
Color	Yellow

Arterial blood gas:

pH	7.38
PO_2	86 mmHg
PCO_2	41 mmHg
HCO_3	27 mmol/L

a. ESR: 75
b. MRI (Figures 8.1 and 8.2)

I. Action

a. Neurosurgery consult
b. IV antibiotics

J. Diagnosis
a. Epidural abscess

K. Critical actions
▪ Consider this diagnosis in an individual with back pain and fever
▪ Obtain a rectal temperature
▪ Obtain stat imaging
▪ Neurosurgery consult for possible operative intervention
▪ Determine cause – urinary tract infection

L. Examiner instructions
a. This is a case of spinal epidural abscess. Spinal epidural abscesses are infections that surround the spinal cord and often compress it, causing acute neurologic complications. The examiner should portray the radiologist and the neurosurgeon with a reluctance to evaluate this patient quickly, as fever and back pain are common complaints of ED patients. The candidate should note fever, spine tender-

Figure 8.1

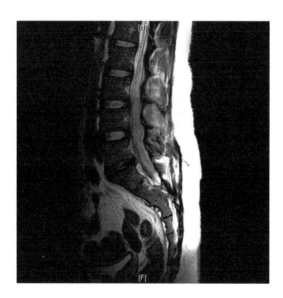

Figure 8.2

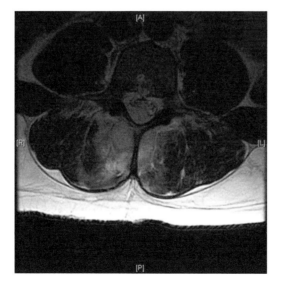

ness, and a baseline abnormal neurologic examination with consultants. If a urinalysis is not ordered, the patient could recall that the urine has looked cloudier recently. Note that the rectal temperature was elevated in this case; this method is more accurate than other types of triage temperature assessment.

M. Pearls

a. Epidural abscess is a rare entity, but associated with high morbidity if not diagnosed promptly.

b. Hematogenous spread is the most common cause, followed by contiguous spread. A small number are idiopathic.

c. IV drug use, diabetes, steroid use, trauma, recent procedures, and diminished immunity are risk factors.

d. ESR is universally elevated.

e. Treatment is usually surgical.

N. References

a. Tintinalli's: Chapter 276. Neck and Back Pain

b. Rosen's: Chapter 106. Spinal Cord Disorders

CASE 9: Leg swelling (Alan Huang, MD)

A. Chief complaint

a. 57-year-old male with left leg swelling

B. Vital signs

a. BP: 139/103 HR: 56 RR: 18 T: 36.4°C Sat: 98% RA

C. What does the patient look like?

a. Patient is lethargic, oriented to person and to place, but not to time

D. Primary survey

a. Airway: speaking normally in full sentences

b. Breathing: no respiratory distress

c. Circulation: skin moist, thready pulses

E. Action

a. Oxygen via nasal cannula or nonrebreather mask

b. Two large-bore peripheral IV lines

c. Labs
   i. CBC, BMP, LFTs, coagulation studies, blood type and hold, urinalysis, blood, and urine cultures

d. Monitor: BP: 139/103 HR: 56 R: 18 T: 36.4°C Sat: 98% RA

e. EKG

f. CXR

g. Finger stick glucose = 55

h. Administer dextrose IV (usually supplied as 50 ml ampule of 50% dextrose in water, for a dose of 25 g)

F. Nurse

a. If no finger stick obtained, patient becomes completely unresponsive

b. EKG (Figure 9.1)

c. CXR (Figure 9.2)

G. History

a. HPI: a 57-year-old male nursing home resident brought in for progressive left leg swelling over the past 24 hours. He rapidly developed blisters, skin weeping.

b. PMHx: congestive heart failure, hypertension, diabetes, venous stasis disease

c. PSHx: gastric bypass 3 years ago

d. Allergies: none

e. Meds: furosemide, isosorbide nitrate, omeprazole, carvedilol, aspirin, gabapentin

f. Social: former tobacco use, quit 10 years ago, former IV drug use, social alcohol use

g. FHx: noncontributory

H. Secondary survey

a. General: remains lethargic

b. Head: normal

c. Eyes: normal

d. Neck: normal

e. Chest: nontender, bilateral basilar rales

f. Heart: pulse is tachycardic, no murmurs, rubs, or gallops

g. Abdomen: normal

Figure 9.1

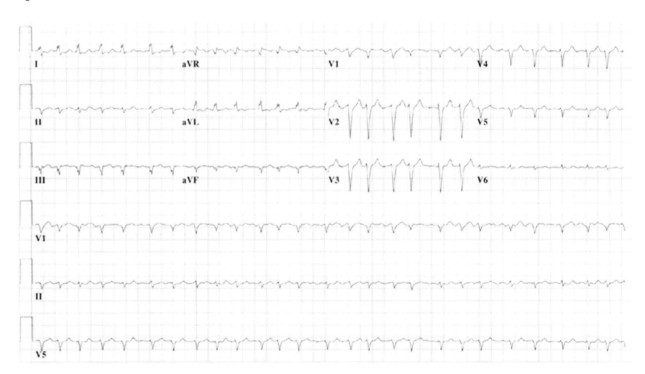

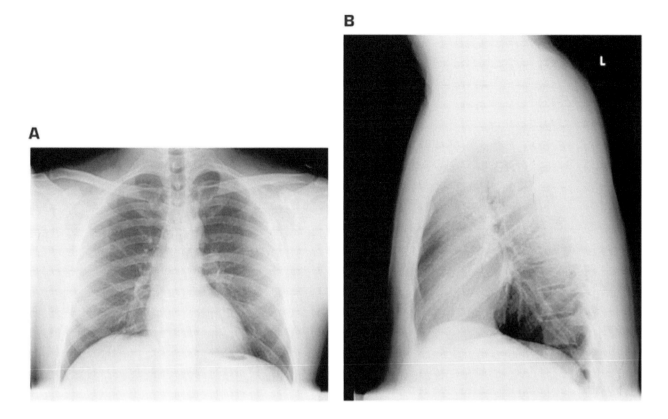

Figure 9.2 A and B

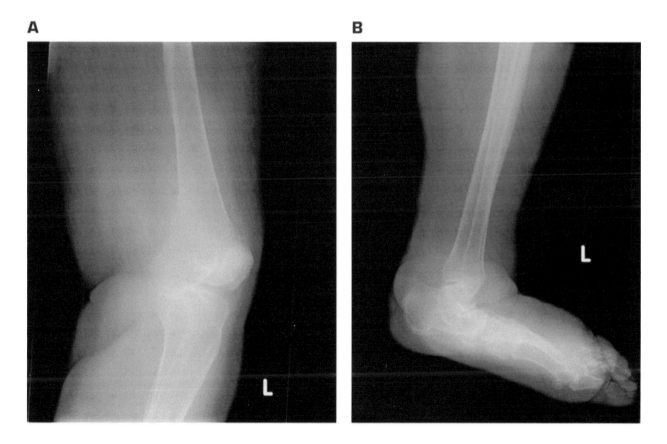

Figure 9.3 A and B

h. Skin
  i. Left leg: 2+ pitting edema to the knee is present, multiple hemorrhagic bullae are present, faint distal pulses
  ii. Right leg: chronic venous stasis, no ulcers, no warmth, redness, or erythema
i. Recheck vital signs: BP: 100/65 HR: 150 R: 25 Sat: 97% 2 L via NC

I. Action
a. IV antibiotics: imipenem/meropenem or vancomycin + clindamycin + ciprofloxacin
b. 1 L NS bolus
c. General surgery consult STAT
d. x-ray of left lower extremity (Figure 9.3A and 9.3B)

J. Results

Complete blood count:

WBC	13.9×10^3/uL	D bili	0.2 mg/dL
Hct	36.0%	Amylase	246 U/L
Plt	229×10^3/uL	Lipase	155 U/L
		Albumin	3.9 g/dL

Basic metabolic panel:

Na	136 mEq/L	**Urinalysis:**	
K	5.4 mEq/L	SG	1.030
Cl	104 mEq/L	pH	5
CO_2	17 mEq/L	Prot	Neg
BUN	95 mEq/dL	Gluc	Neg
Cr	4.8 mg/dL	Ketones	Neg
Gluc	70 mg/dL	Bili	Neg
		Blood	Neg
Coagulation panel:		LE	Neg
PT	15.0 sec	Nitrite	Neg
PTT	34.9 sec	Color	Yellow
INR	1.1		

Liver function panel:

AST	40 U/L	**Arterial blood gas:**	
ALT	44 U/L	pH	7.30
Alk Phos	100 U/L	PO_2	80 mmHg
T bili	1.1 mg/dL	PCO_2	30 mmHg
		HCO_3	16 mmol/L

a. Cardiac enzymes negative

K. Nurse
a. Surgery consult returns phone call
  i. Requests CT of leg; recommends fluids, continued antibiotics, and will follow as an inpatient, admit to medicine

L. Action
a. Candidate should decline request for CT
b. Candidate should insist on need for immediate operative intervention

M. Diagnosis
a. Necrotizing fasciitis

N. Critical actions
▧ Early recognition of condition based on appearance, rapidity of symptom development, amount of pain, and possible development of sepsis.
▧ Aggressive resuscitation with IVF.
▧ IV antibiotics
▧ Immediate surgical consult
▧ Do not delay operative intervention (definitive treatment is surgical debridement)

O. Examiner instructions
a. This is a case of necrotizing fasciitis. Necrotizing fasciitis is a rapidly progressive bacterial infection of the deep tissues of the body. It is associated with extremely high morbidity and mortality. Surgical consultants will delay evaluating the patient and the patient's condition will worsen (mental status will deteriorate, blood pressure will fall, and heart rate will rise) unless the candidate articulates the reasons for concern about necrotizing fasciitis.

P. Pearls
a. Necrotizing fasciitis is usually a polymicrobial infection of aerobes and anaerobes.
b. Mortality is high.
c. Diabetes is a risk factor for spontaneous disease (even without preexisting manipulation or trauma).
d. Surgical debridement is mandatory.
e. Avoid vasopressors if at all possible as they will only decrease blood flow to the dying limb (or body part).
f. Lower extremity is the most common site, followed by upper extremities.
g. Consider hyperbaric oxygen therapy.

Q. References
a. Tintinalli's: Chapter 147. Soft Tissue Infections.
b. Rosen's: Chapter 137. Skin and Soft Tissue Infections.

CASE 10: Weakness (Alan Huang, MD)

A. Chief complaint
a. 77-year-old male complaining of chest pain, shortness of breath, and weakness

B. Vital signs
a. BP: 137/64 HR: 66 RR: 18 T: 36.7°C Sat: 97% RA

C. What does the patient look like?
a. Patient is comfortable, alert, and oriented.

D. Primary survey
a. Airway: speaking normally in full sentences
b. Breathing: no respiratory distress
c. Circulation: skin warm and dry, pulses intact

E. Action

a. Oxygen via NC or nonrebreather mask

b. Two large-bore peripheral IV lines

c. Labs

    i. CBC, BMP, coagulation studies, blood type and cross-match, cardiac enzymes

d. Monitor: BP: 137/64 HR: 66 RR: 18 T: 36.7°C Sat: 97% RA

e. CXR

f. EKG

F. History

a. HPI: a 77-year-old male with a history of coronary artery disease, coronary artery bypass, congestive heart failure, hypertension, asthma presents with a 3-day history of what he thought was an asthma exacerbation. Patient additionally notes bilateral chest pain, non-radiating, improved with sitting up and worsened when lying down. He notes a fifty pack-year smoking history, no fever or cough. No swelling or pain in the leg.

b. PMHx: above, also hypothyroidism, asthma

c. PSHx: coronary artery bypass graft

d. Allergies: none

e. Meds: salmeterol-fluticasone, aspirin, levothyroxine, atorvastatin, lisnopril

f. Social: fifty pack per year tobacco history

g. FHx: noncontributory

G. Secondary survey

a. General: alert and oriented, comfortable

b. Head: normal

c. Eyes: normal

d. Neck: normal, no jugular vein distension

e. Chest: nontender

f. Lungs: clear to auscultation bilaterally

g. Heart: 2/6 systolic murmur, no rubs, or gallops

h. Abdomen: normal

i. Skin: normal

H. Nurse

a. If no EKG obtained, vital signs change: HR: 45 BP: 90/60 Sat: 90% NRB

b. EKG (Figure 10.1)

c. CXR (Figure 10.2)

I. Action

a. Calcium gluconate or calcium chloride IV

b. Dextrose and insulin IV

c. Albuterol nebulizer

d. Sodium bicarbonate IV

e. Kayexalate PO or PR

f. Furosemide IV

g. Consider bicarbonate and insulin continuous infusion

h. STAT electrolytes

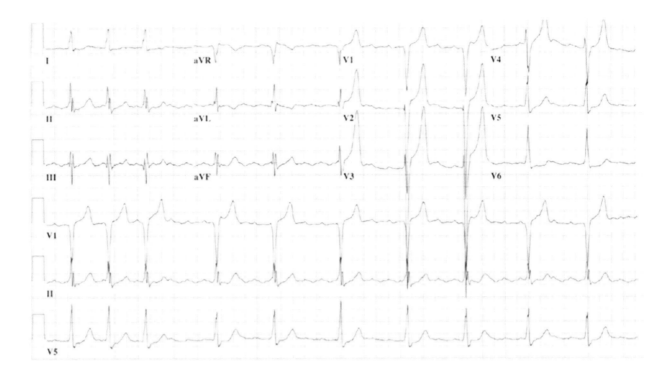

Figure 10.1

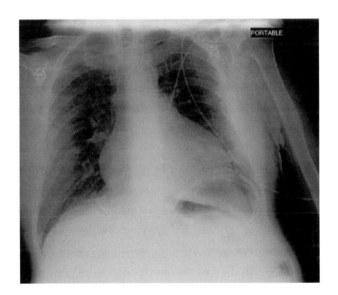

Figure 10.2

J. Results

Complete blood count:

WBC	10.1×10^3/uL
Hct	35.9%
Plt	466×10^3/uL

Basic metabolic panel:

Na	135 mEq/L
K	6.6 mEq/L
Cl	106 mEq/L
CO_2	18 mEq/L
BUN	56 mEq/dL
Cr	2.8 mg/dL
Gluc	74 mg/dL

Coagulation panel:		Urinalysis:	
PT	12.5 sec	SG	1.030
PTT	25.9 sec	pH	7
INR	1.1	Prot	Neg
		Gluc	Neg
Liver function panel:		Ketones	Neg
AST	30 U/L	Bili	Neg
ALT	34 U/L	Blood	Neg
Alk Phos	44 U/L	LE	Neg
T bili	1.2 mg/dL	Nitrite	Neg
D bili	0.2 mg/dL	Color	Yellow
Amylase	67 U/L		
Lipase	78 U/L	**Arterial blood gas:**	
Albumin	4.1 g/dL	pH	7.4
		PO_2	90 mmHg
		PCO_2	40 mmHg
		HCO_3	19 mmol/L

a. Cardiac enzymes negative

K. Diagnosis
a. Hyperkalemia

L. Critical actions
▪ Obtain EKG
▪ Note hyperkalemia (based on EKG and/or labs)
▪ Immediate stabilization of cardiac membranes with calcium
▪ Administration of medications that shift potassium into cells and also medications that decrease total body potassium
▪ Admission

M. Examiner instructions
a. This is a case of hyperkalemia (elevated potassium levels) due to acute renal insufficiency with possible contribution from angiotensin converting enzyme (ACE) inhibitors (lisinopril). Early treatment is imperative; the candidate should obtain an EKG and potassium level rapidly. The candidate should not wait for the results of the labs before treatment.

N. Pearls
a. Early EKG findings of hyperkalemia include peaked T waves and PR interval prolongation. With increased potassium levels, QRS widening can occur, and ultimately the sine waves of severe hyperkalemia.
b. Other EKG abnormalities include complete heart block, ventricular fibrillation, and asystole.
c. In slowly progressive hyperkalemia, EKG findings will be evident only with higher levels of serum potassium.
d. The most common cause of hyperkalemia is a hemolyzed sample (especially in the setting of a normal creatinine level); confirm with laboratory for presence of hemolysis or recheck value.
e. Causes of hyperkalemia include renal insufficiency, medications such as potassium-sparing diuretics or ACE inhibitors; β-blockers; digoxin, hypoaldosteronism including

adrenal insufficiency and type 4 renal tubular acidosis; increased intake or absorption; cellular injuries, such as rhabdomyolysis or tumor lysis syndrome; pseudo-hyperkalemia such as phlebotomy-induced hemolysis; severe thrombocytosis or leukocytosis; or laboratory error.

f. Medications which redistribute potassium most rapidly include bicarbonate followed by insulin.

g. Kayexelate and furosemide actually decrease total body potassium.

h. Consider nephrology consult for emergent hemodialysis, especially in patients on dialysis and patients with acute renal failure.

O. References

a. Tintinalli's: Chapter 21. Fluids and Electrolytes.

b. Rosen's: Chapter 125. Electrolyte Disorders.

CASE 11: Eye pain (Alan Huang, MD)

A. Chief complaint

a. 52-year-old female with pain in the left eye and blurry vision

B. Vital signs

a. BP: 142/91 HR: 95 RR: 16 T: 36°C Sat: 100% RA

C. What does the patient look like?

a. Patient appears uncomfortable due to pain, but is speaking normally, is alert and oriented.

D. Primary survey

a. Airway: speaking normally in full sentences

b. Breathing: no respiratory distress

c. Circulation: skin warm and dry, distal pulses intact

E. History

a. HPI: a 52-year-old female with a history of hypertension awoke today with significantly decreased vision of the left eye described as blurry vision. Right eye is unaffected. No headache or trauma. Patient notes nausea and one episode of vomiting.

b. PMHx: hypertension

c. PSHx: none

d. Allergies: none

e. Social: noncontributory

f. FHx: noncontributory

F. Secondary survey

a. General: alert and oriented, mild pain distress

b. Head: normal, temples nontender

c. Eyes: extraocular movements intact, no periorbital edema, conjunctiva normal. Left globe firm compared to right; left pupil mid-dilated, nonreactive, right eye visual acuity 20/30, left eye unable to visualize largest characters

      i. Slit lamp examination: left cornea "steamy," left eye intraocular pressure (IOP) is 60, right eye normal
- d. Lungs: normal
- e. Heart: normal
- f. Abdomen: normal
- g. Neuro: normal, except left eye vision as noted
- h. Skin: normal

G. Action
- a. Oxygen via NC or nonrebreather mask
- b. Two large-bore peripheral IV lines
- c. Labs
      i. CBC, BMP, PT/PTT, erythrocyte sedimentation rate or c-reactive protein
- d. Emergent ophthalmology consult
- e. Meds
      i. Brimonidine or other α-agonist to left eye
      ii. Timolol or other β-blocker to left eye
      iii. Acetazolamide or another carbonic anhydrase inhibitor PO or IV
      iv. Mannitol IV
      v. Prednisolone or other topical steroid in left eye
      vi. Pilocarpine or other muscarinic agonist in left eye every 6 hours once intraocular pressure <40

H. Results

Complete blood count:

WBC	4.9×10^3/uL	BUN	26 mEq/dL
Hct	40.2%	Cr	1.3 mg/dL%
Plt	405×10^3/uL	Gluc	110 mg/dL

Basic metabolic panel:

		Coagulation panel:	
Na	135 mEq/L	PT	15.0 sec
K	3.5 mEq/L	PTT	26.9 sec
Cl	96 mEq/L	INR	1.1
CO$_2$	24 mEq/L		

- a. ESR: 20

I. Action
- a. Arrange surgical intervention with ophthalmology (immediate surgery vs. medical management to stabilize ocular pressure and follow up within 24 hours)

J. Diagnosis
- a. Acute angle-closure glaucoma

K. Critical actions
- ▓ Thorough eye examination, including visual acuity, intraocular pressure (IOP), and slit lamp examination
- ▓ Early administration of glaucoma medications
- ▓ Frequent administration until normalization of IOP
- ▓ Emergent ophthalmology consult

L. Examiner instructions

a. This is a case of acute narrow angle or angle-closure glaucoma. In this disorder, the normal flow of fluid within the eye is interrupted, leading to pressure buildup, pain, decreased blood flow, and potential loss of vision. This is an ophthalmologic emergency. Critical actions include rapid identification of the diagnosis, brisk administration of a combination of medicines aimed at decreasing IOP via different mechanisms. Ophthalmology must be consulted emergently. Any delays in diagnosis or appropriate administration of medications increase the likelihood of permanent loss of vision. Laboratory evaluation is not necessary; if sent, results will be normal.

M. Pearls

a. Acute angle-closure glaucoma more likely to occur in patients without a history of chronic glaucoma.

b. In patients with sickle cell disease acetazolamide is contraindicated because it encourages sickling of red cells.

c. It is more common in patients of Asian descent who have narrower angles at baseline.

d. It is more common in older patients, who have larger lenses causing narrower angles.

e. In addition to pain in the eye and blurry vision, patients will often complain of "halos around lights," headache, nausea/vomiting, and even abdominal pain.

N. References

a. Tintinalli's: Chapter 238. Face and Jaw Emergencies.

b. Rosen's: Chapter 20. Headache and Chapter 22. Red and Painful Eye

CASE 12: Abdominal pain (Joseph Chiang, MD)

A. Chief complaint

a. 55-year-old male with severe abdominal pain, nausea, and vomiting

B. Vital signs

a. BP: 86/57 HR: 89 RR: 20 T: 37.1°C Sat: 99% on 2 L O_2

C. What does the patient look like?

a. Patient appears uncomfortable and in pain.

D. Primary survey

a. Airway: speaking in full sentences

b. Breathing: no apparent respiratory distress

c. Circulation: peripheral pulses equal, normal capillary refill

E. History

a. HPI: a 55-year-old male presents with 1 day of worsening abdominal distension, pain, and two episodes of vomiting. He reports swelling and tenderness in the right groin as well. He has had swelling in the groin before, but it has gotten worse, more painful, and has become "hard." He denies fever or chest pain.

   b. PMHx: hypertension, diabetes, asthma
   c. PSHx: cholecystectomy
   d. Allergies: penicillins
   e. Meds: metformin
   f. Social: lives with wife at home, denies alcohol, smoking, drugs, monogamous sex with wife
   g. FHx: hypertension, diabetes
   h. PMD: Dr Chang

F. Nurse
   a. EKG: normal sinus rhythm, left ventricular hypertrophy

G. Secondary survey
   a. General: alert and oriented, tachycardic, moderate distress due to pain
   b. HEENT: normal, oral mucosa dry
   c. Neck: normal
   d. Chest: normal
   e. Heart: tachycardic
   f. Abdomen: distended, diffusely tender, bowel sounds absent, no pulsatile masses, no masses, positive rebound, positive guarding
   g. Rectal: hemoccult negative, normal tone, no masses
   h. GU: large right inguinal hernia, not reducible, overlying skin is dusky, no testicular tenderness or swelling
   i. Extremities: normal
   j. Back: normal, no costovertebral angle tenderness
   k. Neuro: normal
   l. Skin: pale, no rashes, no edema
   m. Lymph: normal

H. Action
   a. Oxygen via NC or nonrebreather mask
   b. Two large-bore peripheral IV lines
   c. Labs
        i. CBC, BMP, LFT, PT/PTT, blood type and hold, lactate
   d. 1 L NS bolus
   e. Monitor: BP: 86/57 HR: 89 RR: 20 T: 37.1°C Sat: 99% on 2 L O_2
   f. EKG
   g. Consult
        i. Surgery
   h. Imaging
        i. Upright CXR
        ii. Obstructive series
   i. Meds
        i. NS 1L bolus
        ii. IV antiemetic
        iii. IV analgesia
        iv. IV antibiotics
   j. Nasogastric tube insertion (describe technique)

I. Results

Complete blood count:

WBC	18.4×10^3/uL	D bili	0.5 mg/dL
Hct	52.0%	Amylase	123 U/L
Plt	288×10^3/uL	Lipase	140 U/L
		Albumin	3.9 g/dL

Basic metabolic panel:

Na	139 mEq/L	**Urinalysis:**	
K	4.6 mEq/L	SG	1.030
Cl	92 mEq/L	pH	6
CO_2	31 mEq/L	Prot	Neg
BUN	18 mEq/dL	Gluc	Neg
Cr	1.2 mg/dL	Ketones	Neg
Gluc	160 mg/dL	Bili	Neg
		Blood	Neg
Coagulation panel:		LE	Neg
PT	12.9 sec	Nitrite	Neg
PTT	31.2 sec	Color	Yellow
INR	1.1		

Arterial blood gas:

Liver function panel:		pH	7.4
AST	40 U/L	PO_2	86 mmHg
ALT	23 U/L	PCO_2	40 mmHg
Alk Phos	107 U/L	HCO_3	27 mmol/L
T bili	1.6 mg/dL		

a. Lactate 1.9 mmol/L

b. EKG (Figure 12.1)

c. CXR (Figure 12.2A and 12.2B)

d. AXR (Figure 12.3A and 12.3B)

J. Action

a. Surgery consult

   i. Patient taken to OR for repair of incarcerated hernia

K. Diagnosis

a. Incarcerated hernia with bowel obstruction

L. Critical actions

▨ Recognition of hernia

▨ Large-bore IV access and fluid bolus

▨ Upright chest x-ray with obstructive series

▨ Nasogastric tube (NGT) placement

▨ Pain management

▨ Surgery consult

M. Examiner instructions

a. This is a case of an strangulated hernia. The patient's bowel has slipped from the abdominal cavity into a defect in the inguinal wall where it has become trapped. Trapped, irreducible bowel defines incarcerated hernia. The skin findings over the site of the hernia suggest strangulation (loss of blood supply). In the event of skin

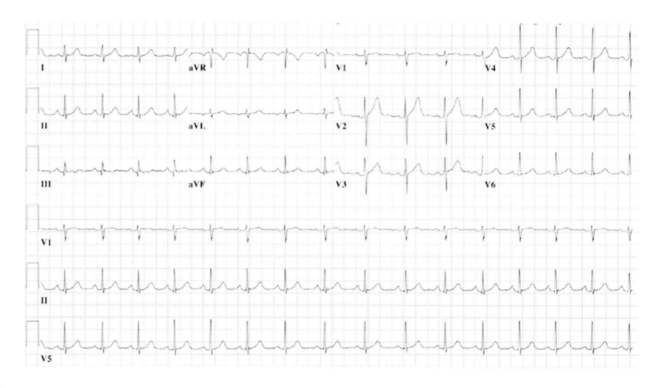

Figure 12.1

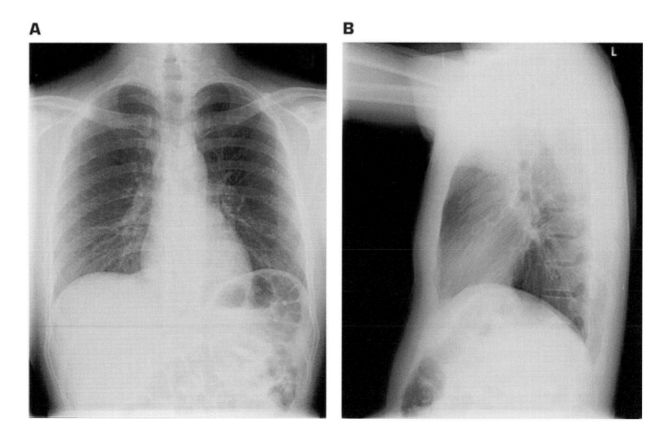

Figure 12.2 A and B

A   **B**

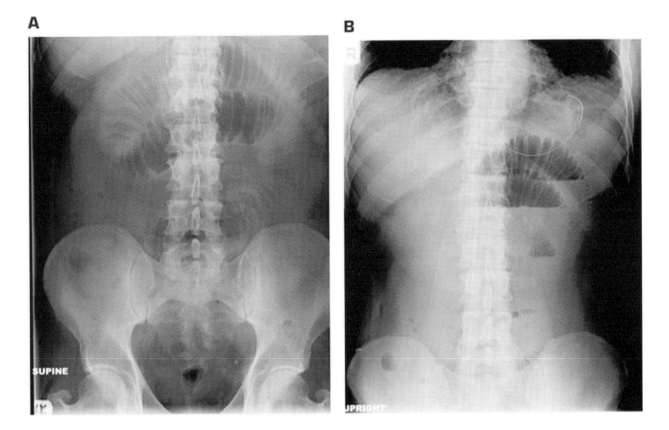

Figure 12.3 A and B

findings the physician should refrain from reducing the hernia as this may increase the likelihood of bowel perforation. Incarcerated or strangulated hernias lead to obstruction of normal digestion with pain, distension of the abdomen, and tissue damage. Dilated loops of bowel with air-fluid levels on abdominal x-ray confirm the diagnosis of obstruction. Nasogastric suction should be initiated to assist in deflation of the distended bowel. IV fluids are used to treat dehydration and correct electrolyte abnormalities caused by the continuous vomiting. IV antibiotics may be indicated as well, especially in patients who are febrile or have signs of peritonitis. Patients should be hospitalized for monitoring and treatment; surgery is often indicated.

N. Pearls
a. Upright chest x-ray is more sensitive than KUB for free air.
b. Peritoneal signs are ominous in cases of obstruction, and often suggest a surgical emergency. Consider NGT, fluids, and surgical consultation immediately. If bowel perforation is suspected, early antibiotics and surgery are indicated.
c. Note that the patient has a "relative" hypotension. Given the history of high blood pressure, a systolic blood pressure in the 90s is more ominous than in a patient with baseline normal blood pressure.
d. A high white blood cell count may be seen with bowel gangrene, abscess, or peritonitis.

O. References

a. Tintinalli's: Chapter 86. Bowel Obstruction and Volvulus; Chapter 87. Hernias in Adults

b. Rosen: Chapter 92. Disorders of the Small Intestine

CASE 13: Ringing in the ears (Joseph Chiang, MD)

A. Chief complaint

a. 17-year-old female with nausea, tremor, and ringing in the ears

B. Vital signs

a. BP: 107/56 HR: 117 RR: 22 T: 37.2°C

C. What does the patient look like?

a. Patient appears stated age, comfortable, in no acute distress while lying in stretcher, alert, and oriented.

D. Primary survey

a. Airway: speaking in full sentences

b. Breathing: no apparent respiratory distress, slightly tachypneic

c. Circulation: warm skin, good pulses bilaterally

E. History

a. HPI: a 17-year-old female notes headache last night for which she took aspirin. Headache improved, and she went to sleep soon after. Woke up in the morning and felt nauseated, tremulous and had ringing in her ears. No cough, fever, or chills. Reports a total dose of six 325 mg tablets of aspirin (only if asked).

b. PMHx: none

c. PSHx: none

d. Allergies: none

e. Meds: none

f. Social: lives with family, nonsmoker, occasional alcohol use

g. FHx: diabetes

F. Secondary survey

a. General: alert and oriented, afebrile, tachycardic, and tachypneic

b. HEENT: normal, tympanic membranes clear

c. Neck: normal

d. Chest: normal

e. Heart: normal

f. Abdomen: bowel sounds normal; no distension or peritoneal signs; mild tenderness in right upper and lower quadrants

g. Extremities: normal

h. Back: normal

i. Neuro: normal

j. Skin: warm, dry, normal color

k. Psychiatric: normal affect; judgment and insight normal; remote and recent memory normal; no suicidal or homicidal ideation

G. Action

a. Oxygen via NC or nonrebreather mask

b. Two large-bore peripheral IV lines

c. Monitor: BP: 107/56 HR: 117 RR: 22 T: 37.2°C

d. Labs

  i. CBC, BMP, LFT, lipase and amylase, PT/PTT, salicylate, acetaminophen, and alcohol levels

e. EKG

f. CXR

g. Urinalysis

h. Urine pregnancy test

H. Nurse

a. Patient: remains symptomatic

b. EKG (Figure 13.1)

c. CXR (Figure 13.2A and 13.2B)

I. Results

Complete blood count:

WBC	12.3×10^3/uL	D bili	0.1 mg/dL
Hct	36.6%	Amylase	153 U/L
Plt	300×10^3/uL	Lipase	35 U/L
		Albumin	4.4 g/dL

Basic metabolic panel:

Na	146 mEq/L	**Urinalysis:**	
K	3.1 mEq/L	SG	1.020
Cl	117 mEq/L	pH	6
CO_2	17 mEq/L	Prot	Neg
BUN	10 mEq/dL	Gluc	Neg
Cr	0.8 mg/dL	Ketones	Neg
Gluc	105 mg/dL	Bili	Neg
		Blood	Neg
		LE	Neg

Coagulation panel:

PT	12.7 sec	Nitrite	Neg
PTT	25.9 sec	Color	Yellow
INR	1.1		

Arterial blood gas:

Liver function panel:

		pH	7.54
AST	21 U/L	PO_2	90 mmHg
ALT	16 U/L	PCO_2	21 mmHg
Alk Phos	68 U/L	HCO_3	17 mmol/L
T bili	0.5 mg/dL		

a. Salicylate level: 60 mg/dL

b. Acetaminophen level negative

c. Alcohol level negative

d. Urine pregnancy: negative

e. UA (after initiation of medication)

  i. pH: 8.0

  ii. All other values: normal

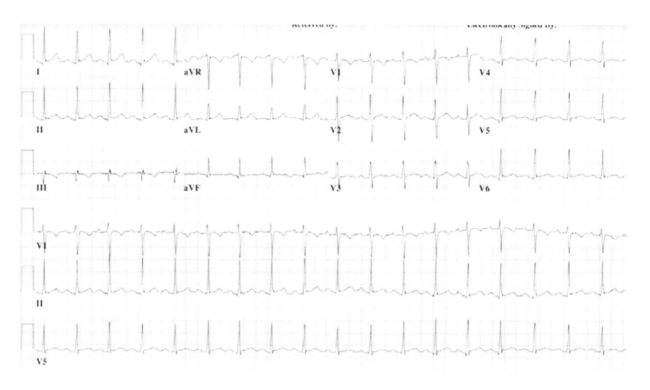

Figure 13.1

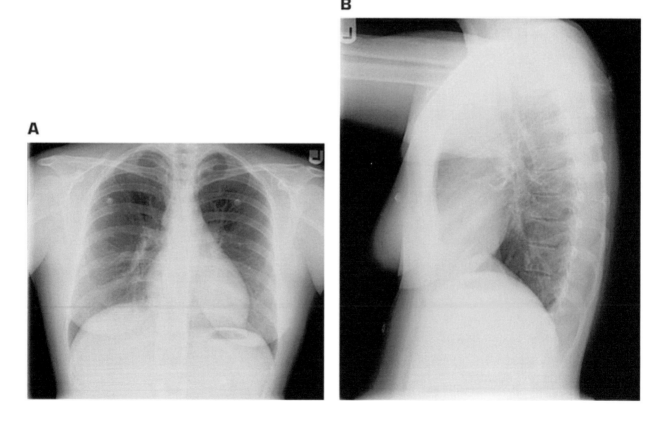

Figure 13.2 A and B

J. Action

a. ICU consult

    i. Admission for close monitoring

b. Discussion with patient and family regarding acute overdose of aspirin and its presentation and treatments

c. Meds

    i. Metoclopramide IV (for nausea)

    ii. Bicarbonate drip

d. Repeat salicylate levels 2 hours after bicarbonate was initiated

e. Continued monitoring of vital signs

f. Local Poison Control Center contacted – recommends frequent labs and continued treatment until salicylate level falls below 20

K. Diagnosis

a. Aspirin toxicity

L. Critical actions

▨ Large-bore IV access

▨ Pregnancy test

▨ Obtain history of salicylate use

▨ Alkalinization of urine with sodium bicarbonate

▨ Close monitoring of patient and salicylate levels

▨ ICU admission

M. Examiner instructions

a. This is a case of acute salicylate overdose. Her presentation is classic: nausea, tremor, tinnitus, tachycardia, and tachypnea. Cardiac and pulmonary causes of shortness of breath should be sought (through careful physical examination, EKG, CXR). The patient should not disclose the headache initially. She won't connect last night's headache with today's symptoms unless specifically asked about other recent illnesses or medications.

N. Pearls

a. Activated charcoal is usually only reserved for patients that present soon after a toxic ingestion.

b. Salicylate blood levels may peak in less than 1 hour or after more than 6 hours depending on the type of tablets ingested.

c. Urinary salicylate clearance can be increased by the administration of sodium bicarbonate bolus followed by maintenance doses until salicylate levels fall below 20 mg/dL and clinical improvement noted.

d. Patients present initially with respiratory alkalosis due to direct stimulation of the medulla leading to tachypnea and hyperpnea. Later, increased anion gap metabolic acidosis develops. Patients usually remain alkalemic with a pH >7.4.

e. Development of acidemia is an ominous sign. A decrease in pH is a poor prognostic marker and is often a preterminal event.

f. Early consultation with the ICU and a toxicologist is prudent.

g. Worsening of patient symptoms manifesting in end-organ damage will require emergent hemodialysis.

h. Hypokalemia interferes with urine alkalinization; potassium levels should be monitored, and hypokalemia corrected.

O. References
a. Tintinalli's: Chapter 183. Aspirin and Salicylates
b. Rosen: Chapter 149. Aspirin and Nonsteroidal Agents

CASE 14: Vomiting child (Joseph Chiang, MD)

A. Chief complaint
a. 6-year-old male with vomiting since yesterday

B. Vital signs
a. BP: 96/63 HR: 136 RR: 28 T: 36.1°C wt: 23 kg

C. What does the patient look like?
a. Patient appears uncomfortable; complaining of pain.

D. Primary survey
a. Airway: speaking in full sentences
b. Breathing: no apparent respiratory distress, no cyanosis
c. Circulation: peripheral pulses equal

E. History
a. HPI: a 6-year-old male presents with abdominal pain, hematemesis, diarrhea (one episode bloody), and decreased oral intake. Patient also has bilateral joint pain, and difficulty in walking. No sick contacts, travel history, unusual food, or raw meat and no fever noted in the patient.
b. PMHx: attention deficit hyperactivity disorder, strep throat 1 year ago
c. PSHx: none
d. Meds: none
e. Allergies: none
f. Social: lives with parents
g. FHx: no sick contacts

F. Secondary survey
a. General: awake, alert, appropriate for age
b. HEENT: pupils equal, round, reactive; sunken eyes, purplish hue around eyes, fundi sharp, no papilledema
c. Neck: tonsils enlarged; left ear erythematous
d. Chest: no rashes
e. Heart: tachycardic, no murmurs
f. Abdomen: no distension, positive epigastric tenderness, decreased bowel sounds, no rebound or guarding
g. Rectal: hemoccult positive
h. GU: minor rectal irritation due to diarrhea
i. Extremities: normal
j. Back: normal, no CVA tenderness

k. Neuro: normal
l. Skin: palpable purpura on bilateral elbows; purpura on lower extremity and buttocks
m. Lymph: normal

G. Action

a. Largest possible peripheral IV
b. Labs
   i. CBC, BMP, LFT, PT/PTT, blood type and cross-match
c. 20 mL per kg NS saline bolus intravenously
d. Monitor: BP: 96/63 HR: 136 RR: 28
e. Consult
   i. Pediatric surgery
f. Imaging
   i. Upright CXR with obstructive series
   ii. US abdomen
g. Meds
   i. NS 20 ml/kg IV bolus
   ii. Continue ½ NS at maintenance rate thereafter
   iii. Methylprednisolone IV
   iv. Ranitidine IV
h. Additional labs
   i. IgA, urinalysis

H. Results

Complete blood count:

WBC	15.3×10^3/uL
Hct	35.1%
Plt	595×10^3/uL

Basic metabolic panel:

Na	138 mEq/L
K	3.8 mEq/L
Cl	100 mEq/L
CO_2	21 mEq/L
BUN	15 mEq/dL
Cr	0.6 mg/dL
Gluc	71 mg/dL

Coagulation panel:

PT	12.3–15.5 sec
PTT	25.4–35.0 sec
INR	0.9–1.3

Liver function panel:

AST	21 U/L
ALT	43 U/L
Alk Phos	179 U/L
T bili	1.3 mg/dL
D bili	0.2 mg/dL
Amylase	61 U/L
Lipase	200 U/L
Albumin	3.9 g/dL

Urinalysis:

SG	1.025
pH	6
Prot	+
Gluc	Neg
Ketones	+
Bili	Neg
Blood	Neg
LE	Neg
Nitrite	Neg
Color	Yellow

a. IgA – 299
b. AXR (Figure 14.1)
c. US abdomen – limited examination demonstrates no evidence of intussusception

Figure 14.1

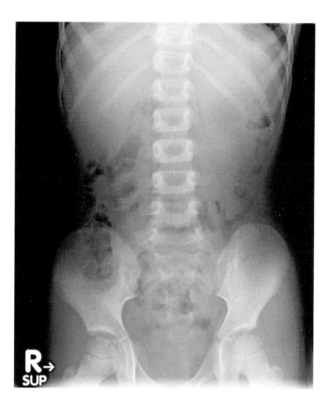

I. Action
a. Pediatric surgery consult – no intussusception or other surgical pathology; continue medical management
b. Admission to floor for hydration and steroids
c. Continue hydration, prednisone

J. Diagnosis
a. Henoch-Schönlein purpura

K. Critical actions
▓ Fluid resuscitation
▓ Abdominal x-ray
▓ Pain management
▓ Laboratory evaluation of liver and renal injury
▓ Surgery consult

L. Examiner instructions
a. This child is suffering from Henoch-Schönlein purpura, or HSP. HSP disease is a small-vessel vasculitis (inflammatory disease) characterized by purpura (rash), arthritis, abdominal pain, and hematuria. The cause is unknown, but often follows an upper respiratory infection and is immunologically mediated. When prompted, the mother will describe a rash on the lower extremity and buttocks for a few days.

M. Pearls
a. HSP is a clinical diagnosis.
b. The rash often begins as pink maculopapules that blanch on pressure and progresses to petechiae or purpura. It is often palpable (and henceforth the

pathognomonic findings of "palpable purpura"). The lesions favor the lower extremities and occur in crops lasting from 1 week to 10 days.

c. Severe, colicky abdominal pain may indicate possible intussusception, bowel obstruction, or gastrointestinal hemorrhage brought on by the damage to the GI vasculature. An abdominal radiograph or ultrasound may aid in the diagnosis of intussuception, but the gold standard is a barium enema test.

d. IgA level may aid in the recognition of the disease. However, imaging and labs should be ordered on the basis of the clinical picture, and to evaluate other abdominal pain causes (such as intussusception).

e. Major complications involve renal function and bowel perforation. However, the overall prognosis is excellent for the vast majority of children.

f. Admission to the hospital may be appropriate if the diagnosis is in doubt, in children with severe symptoms, or concern for renal and abdominal symptoms. Well-appearing children with classic HSP may be safely managed as outpatients.

N. References
a. Tintinalli's: Chapter 124. Acute Abdominal Pain in Children; Chapter 128. Renal Emergencies in Infants and Children.
b. Rosen: Chapter 172. Gastrointestinal Disorders

CASE 15: Snake bite (Joseph Chiang, MD)

A. Chief complaint
a. "My son was bitten by a snake!"

B. Vital signs
a. BP: 101/57 HR: 97 RR: 20 T: 36.0°C
b. No pain

C. What does the patient look like?
a. Patient appears comfortable.

D. Primary survey
a. Airway: speaking in full sentences; playful
b. Breathing: no apparent respiratory distress, no cyanosis
c. Circulation: peripheral pulses equal

E. History
a. HPI: a 10-year-old male was bitten on the right leg by a snake while on a hike with his family. They were on a trail and he felt a sharp pain in his leg before anyone realized there was a snake on the side of the trail. The family briefly saw a brown and white snake and heard it make a rattling noise after the incident. Rattlesnakes are known to be found in this area. A tourniquet was placed above the wound by the family, who drove immediately to the emergency department. The injury occurred 25 minutes ago. The patient is unable to give further description and currently complains only of pain at the site of the bite.
b. PMHx: none, immunizations up-to-date.
c. PSHx: none

d. Allergies: none

e. Meds: none

f. Social: lives with family

g. FHx: none

h. PMD: Dr Torres

F. Secondary survey

a. General: alert and oriented, no acute distress

b. HEENT: normal

c. Neck: normal

d. Chest: normal

e. Heart: normal

f. Abdomen: soft, nontender

g. Extremities: Right lateral lower leg with two puncture wounds, with no active bleeding or discharge. Tourniquet in place proximal to wound. Delayed capillary refill. Full range of motion, motor and sensory intact, no erythema, no edema, no induration; otherwise unremarkable examination

h. Back: normal, no marks

i. Neuro: normal; appropriate for age

j. Lymph: normal

G. Action

a. EKG

b. Labs

    i. CBC, BMP, PT/PTT, UA, fibrinogen, fibrin split products, blood type and cross-match

c. Normal saline bolus 20cc/kg

d. Remove tourniquet (constriction band may be placed instead)

e. Contact hospital pharmacy to ensure rattlesnake antivenom is available

H. Results

Complete blood count:

WBC	9.1×10^3/uL
Hct	36.2%
Plt	462×10^3/uL

Coagulation panel:

PT	12.3 sec
PTT	25.4 sec
INR	0.9

Basic metabolic panel:

Na	135 mEq/L
K	3.7 mEq/L
Cl	101 mEq/L
CO_2	22 mEq/L
BUN	14 mEq/dL
Cr	0.5 mg/dL
Gluc	93 mg/dL

Urinalysis:

SG	1.022
pH	6
Prot	Neg
Gluc	Neg
Ketones	Neg
Bili	Neg
Blood	Neg
LE	Neg
Nitrite	Neg
Color	Yellow

a. Fibrinogen, fibrin split products: Normal

I. Actions
a. Observe patient for 12 hours (symptoms will not progress during this time)

J. Diagnosis
a. Pit viper bite without envenomation ("dry bite")

K. Critical actions
▦ Assess ABCs

▦ Assess wound

▦ Identify snake, risk for venom exposure

▦ Evaluate for laboratory signs of envenomation

▦ Observe for physical signs of envenomation

▦ Thorough history and examination, including total exposure

▦ Contact nearby Poison Control Center

L. Examiner instructions
a. This is a case of a snake bite. The most important intervention is to assess the patient's respiratory and cardiovascular status. The candidate should determine if airway management or cardiovascular resuscitation with fluids or pressors is needed. Identification of the snake is paramount. The local Poison Control Center can provide invaluable assistance. If possible, collect the snake in question (local animal control authorities may be contacted). Meanwhile, assess bite marks for local progression and expose the patient to visualize any other possible bites. Luckily for the child in this case, the snake did not envenomate the wound.

M. Pearls
a. Antivenin is specific for each group of snakes; the local Poison Control Center may be helpful in determining the need. The majority of snakes are nonpoisonous but two major groups do pose a threat: crotalids (pit vipers including rattlesnakes, cotton mouths) and elapids (coral snakes, cobras). Venom effects may not develop in up to 25% of cases; these are referred to as "dry bites."

b. Crotalid venom is predominantly cytolytic and may cause edema, hemorrhage, and necrosis close to and far away from the bite. Systemic signs and symptoms may include hemolysis, thrombocytopenia, disseminated intravascular coagulopathy, vomiting, and cardiovascular and respiratory failure.

c. Elapids tend to have neurotoxic venom producing neurological symptoms (diplopia, ptosis, respiratory depression, parasthesia). These symptoms tend to be delayed.

d. Surgery consult is warranted if compartment syndrome is suspected.

e. Tetanus should be updated and antibiotics administered in severe bites.

f. Patients requiring antivenin therapy should be admitted to an ICU for monitoring.

g. Note that first-aid treatments such as suction and incision along with tourniquets are contraindicated. Application of a constriction band with an elastic bandage or penrose drain, rope, or clothing wrapped proximal to the bite may retard venom absorption without compromising arterial flow.

N. References
a. Tintinalli's: Chapter 206. Reptile Bites

b. Rosen: Chapter 62. Venomous Animal Injuries

CASE 16: Visual impairment (Joseph Chiang, MD)

A. Chief complaint
a. 70-year-old female with decreased vision in right eye

B. Vital signs
a. BP: 146/74 HR: 84 RR: 20 T: 36.9°C Sat: 98% on RA

C. What does the patient look like?
a. Patient appears well and is in no acute distress.

D. Primary survey
a. Airway: speaking in full sentences
b. Breathing: no apparent respiratory distress, no cyanosis
c. Circulation: peripheral pulses equal

E. History
a. HPI: a 70-year-old female presents with loss of vision in the right eye for the past 4 days. She also complains of mild dizziness. No fever, chills, nausea, vomiting, chest pain, shortness of breath, trauma, numbness, tingling, and weakness noted. No eye pain, tearing, or sensation of a curtain coming down over eyes.
b. PMHx: hypertension, diabetes, asthma, hypercholesterolemia
c. PSHx: cataract extraction
d. Allergies: none
e. Meds: metformin, hydrochlorothiazide, albuterol, simvastatin
f. Social: denies smoking, alcohol, drugs
g. FHx: not relevant

F. Secondary survey
a. General: alert and oriented, well appearing, has mild pain
b. HEENT: [Proctor: Make sure the candidate asks for specific portions of the eye exam including the visual acuity]. Head is atraumatic, normal cephalic; visual acuity: 20/30 left eye, absent vision in right eye; no nystagmus; right pupil dilates in response to light, constricts when light is directed into unaffected eye. Fundoscopic examination demonstrates intraretinal blood and macular edema, intraocular pressures normal
c. Neck: normal
d. Chest: normal
e. Heart: regular rate rhythm, normal s1, s2.
f. Abdomen: normal
g. Extremities: normal
h. Neuro: alert and oriented, no focal motor, sensory deficits; no neglect with left eye; no facial asymmetry; normal memory; gait normal
i. Skin: pale, no rashes, no edema
j. Lymph: normal

G. Action
a. Oxygen via NC or nonrebreather mask
b. Two large-bore peripheral IV lines

   c. Labs

      i. CBC, BMP, PT/PTT

   d. Monitor: BP: 146/74 HR: 84 RR: 20 Sat: 98% on RA

   e. EKG

   f. Consult

      i. Ophthalmology consult

   g. Imaging

      i. Head CT

H. Results

Complete blood count:

WBC	5.3×10^3/uL
Hct	35.1%
Plt	265×10^3/uL

Basic metabolic panel:

Na	136 mEq/L
K	3.9 mEq/L
Cl	99 mEq/L
CO_2	33 mEq/L
BUN	26 mEq/dL
Cr	1.3 mg/dL
Gluc	146 mg/dL

Coagulation panel:

PT	14 sec
PTT	26 sec
INR	1.1

Urinalysis:

SG	1.030
pH	6
Prot	Neg
Gluc	Neg
Ketones	Neg
Bili	Neg
Blood	Neg
LE	Neg
Nitrite	Neg
Color	Yellow

   a. Lactate 0.8 mmol/L

   b. EKG (Figure 16.1)

   c. Head CT without contrast (Figure 16.2)

I. Action

   a. Ophthalmology consult

      i. Examination demonstrates unremarkable sclera, conjunctiva, and anterior chamber in both eyes. Right eye has intraretinal blood and macular edema. Findings consistent with retinal vascular occlusion.

   b. Discharge home with follow-up

J. Diagnosis

   a. Retinal vascular occlusion

K. Critical actions

▓ Ocular examination

▓ Ophthalmology consult

L. Examiner instructions

   a. This is a case of central retinal vein occlusion or blockage of blood flow to the eye. This causes unilateral painless loss of vision. This pathology occurs most commonly in the elderly with glaucoma or hypertension. Careful history and ocular examination is important to establish the diagnosis. CT scan is unnecessary, but

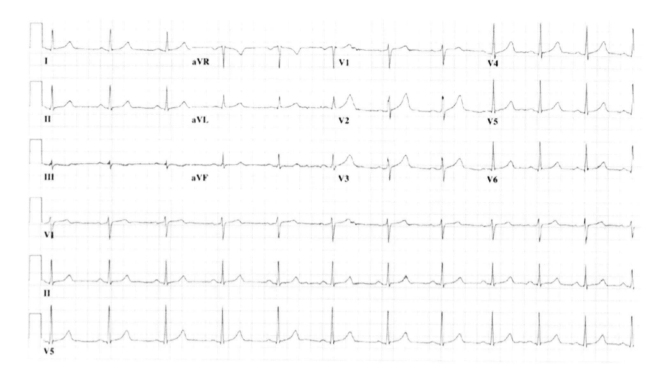

Figure 16.1

Figure 16.2
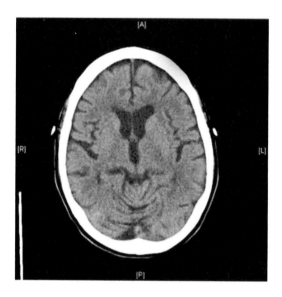

should be normal if obtained. If neurology consultation is attempted, the consultant will defer to the ophthalmologist's recommendations. No specific therapy is indicated. Patients should be referred to ophthalmologist within 24 hours for assessment of possible glaucoma or other pathologies.

M. Pearls

a. Optic disc edema and diffuse retinal hemorrhages in all quadrants are pathognomonic for central retinal vein occlusion.

b. Ophthalmoscopic examination reveals dilated and tortuous veins, retinal and macular edema, diffuse retinal hemorrhages and attenuated arterioles. An afferent pupillary defect may be noted in the affected eye – loss of vision in that eye prevents light information from being relayed to the brain. Thus, light shone in the affected eye will not be perceived, and the pupils dilate. When light is directed into the unaffected eye, the information is transmitted to the brain normally, and both pupils receive a signal to constrict.

c. Optic neuritis, though often presenting with similar symptoms as retinal vein occlusion, can be excluded as it is devoid of peripheral hemorrhage on examination.

N. References

a. Tintinalli's: Chapter 235. Eye Emergencies

b. Rosen: Chapter 71. Opthalmology

CASE 17: Syncope (Christopher Strother, MD)

A. Chief complaint

a. 11-year-old female brought in by EMS from school with the complaint of "passing out" twice today

B. Vital signs

a. BP: 100/70 HR: 96 RR: 18 T: 37.2°C Sat: 99% on RA FS: 115

C. What does the patient look like?

a. Patient appears stated age, no distress, sitting in stretcher.

D. Primary survey

a. Airway: speaking in full sentences

b. Breathing: no apparent respiratory distress, no cyanosis

c. Circulation: warm pink skin, normal capillary refill

E. Action

a. Labs
   i. UA, pregnancy test

b. Monitor: orthostatic vital signs (normal)

c. EKG

F. History

a. HPI: an 11-year-old female with no past medical history in usual state of health until physical education class today. During exercise she developed palpitations and shortness of breath followed by fainting. Initially recovered, briefly followed by a second episode about 2 minutes later. Symptoms now resolved except some residual fatigue and "weakness." Last meal taken by the patient was breakfast.

b. PMHx: none, premenarchal

c. PSHx: none

d. Allergies: none

e. Social: lives with parents at home, denies alcohol use, smoking, drugs, or sexual activity

f. FHx: no cardiac or sudden death history but mother "faints sometimes"

g. PMD: Dr Godwin

G. Nurse

a. BP: 100/75 HR: 90 RR: 18 Sat: 99% on RA

b. EKG (Figure 17.1)

H. Secondary survey

a. General: alert and oriented, fatigued but nontoxic

b. HEENT: mildly dry mucous membranes, otherwise normal

c. Neck: normal

d. Chest: normal

e. Heart: normal, no murmur, rub, or gallops

f. Abdomen: normal

g. GU: normal

h. Extremities: normal

i. Back: normal

j. Neuro: normal

k. Skin: normal

l. Lymph: normal

I. Status change

a. Patient now swoons and lapses into unconsciousness

J. Primary survey

a. Airway: clear, normal

b. Breathing: apneic

c. Circulation: pulseless

Figure 17.1

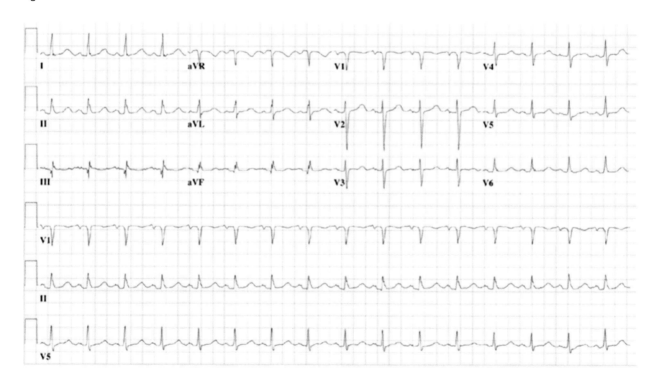

K. Action

a. Bag valve mask ventilation followed by intubation

b. Chest compressions

c. Monitor (Figure 17.2)

d. Defibrillate

    i. 4 joules/kg (effective on 2nd attempt)

e. Meds

    i. Epinephrine (no effect clinically)

    ii. Magnesium sulfate (no effect clinically)

f. Reassess

    i. Patient remains in ventricular fibrillation/torsades until two shocks and magnesium are administered.

    ii. Postresuscitation care includes antiarrhythmic drip, labs, endotracheal tube/ventilator set-up, and ICU consult, transfer

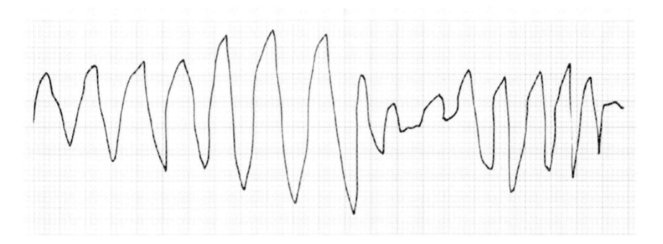

Figure 17.2

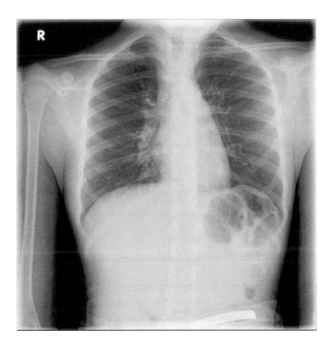

Figure 17.3

g. Imaging
    i. CXR (Figure 17.3)
h. Access
    i. IV access if not previously obtained

L. Results

Complete blood count:

WBC	10.7×10^3/uL	D bili	0.1 mg/dL
Hct	37.1%	Amylase	42 U/L
Plt	300×10^3/uL	Lipase	30 U/L
		Albumin	4.0 g/dL

Basic metabolic panel:

Na	140 mEq/L	**Urinalysis:**	
K	4.1 mEq/L	SG	1.018
Cl	108 mEq/L	pH	6
CO_2	22 mEq/L	Prot	Neg
BUN	3 mEq/dL	Gluc	Neg
Cr	0.6 mg/dL%	Ketones	Neg
Gluc	120 mg/dL	Bili	Neg
		Blood	Neg
Coagulation panel:		LE	Neg
PT	11.1 sec	Nitrite	Neg
PTT	35.2 sec	Color	Yellow
INR	1.0		
		Arterial blood gas:	
Liver function panel:		pH	7.4
AST	15 U/L	PO_2	100 mmHg
ALT	12 U/L	PCO_2	40 mmHg
Alk Phos	260 U/L	HCO_3	22 mmol/L
T bili	0.6 mg/dL		

a. Lactate 0.9 mmol/L

M. Action
a. ICU consult
b. Cardiology consult
c. Discussion with family and PMD need for ICU and cardiology evaluation
d. Discussion of prolonged QT syndrome with cardiology or ICU staff
e. Meds
    i. Lidocaine drip

N. Diagnosis
a. Prolonged QT syndrome
b. Torsades de pointes

O. Critical actions
▪ EKG ordered, look for prolonged QT syndrome
▪ Recognition of torsades after decompensation
▪ Resuscitation per pediatric advanced life support (PALS) guidelines
▪ Cardiology consultation

P. Examiner instructions

a. This is a case of a prolonged QT syndrome (an abnormal electrical conduction within the heart) leading to intermittent Torsades de pointes arrhythmia. Prolonged QT can be associated with syncope and sudden death from ventricular arrhythmias. Torsades de pointes ("twisting of the points") is classically associated with prolonged QT syndrome; the QRS complex alternates between low and high amplitude, as if it were twisting around the baseline. Any child with unexplained syncope should have an EKG checked for prolonged QT syndrome. In children of reproductive age, a urine pregnancy test is also useful. Once torsades occurs as in this patient, magnesium sulfate is the drug of choice for conversion, but unstable patients need defibrillation. Post-arrest care includes an antiarrhythmic such as lidocaine.

Q. Pearls

a. Prolonged QT is one of the more dangerous diagnoses that need to be excluded in a young patient with syncope.

b. Prolonged QT syndrome has the potential to decompensate into fatal ventricular arrhythmias, classically torsades de pointes.

c. Treatment of choice for torsades is magnesium and defibrillation.

R. References

a. Tintinalli's: Chapter 22. Cardiac Rhythm Disturbances

b. Rosen: Chapter 79. Dysrhythmias.

CASE 18: Sore throat (Lisa Zahn, MD)

A. Chief complaint

a. 3-year-old boy brought in for drooling and fever

B. Vital signs

a. BP: 114/80 HR: 150 RR: 28 T: 39.1°C Sat: 98% on RA Wt: 15 kg

C. What does the patient look like?

a. Comfortable-appearing male, slightly drooling and sitting upright, holding head and neck still.

D. Primary survey

a. Airway: speaking in full sentences, drooling slightly

b. Breathing: no apparent respiratory distress, no cyanosis

c. Circulation: moves all extremities, skin color within normal limits

E. Action

a. Oxygen supplementation (blow-by oxygen or nonrebreather mask)

b. Two large-bore peripheral IV lines

c. Labs

   i. CBC, BMP, coagulation studies, blood type and cross-match

d. 20 ml/kg (300 ml) NS bolus

e. Monitor: BP: 114/80 HR: 140 RR: 28 T: 39.1°C Sat; 100% on O_2

  f. Consult
   i. Otolaryngology consult
  g. Meds
   i. Ibuprofen

F. History

 a. HPI: a 3-year-old male with no past medical history, presents with three days of sore throat, now with drooling and increasing reluctance to move neck. Patient accompanied by grandmother. No fever, no cough, no photophobia, no nausea, no vomiting, no abdominal pain noted and no prior episodes noted.

 b. PMHx: immunizations up-to-date, no past medical history, normal spontaneous vaginal delivery at 40 weeks, uncomplicated pregnancy

 c. PSHx: none

 d. Allergies: none

 e. Meds: none

 f. Social: lives with grandmother

 g. FHx: noncontributory

 h. PMD: Dr Tsai

G. Nurse

 a. BP: 114/80 HR: 150 RR: 28 T: 39.1°C Sat: 98% on O_2

H. Secondary survey

 a. General: alert, oriented × 3, sitting upright in stretcher, holding head and neck in a fixed position, slightly drooling

 b. Head: normocephalic, atraumatic

 c. Eyes: extraocular movement intact, pupils equal, reactive to light

 d. Ears: normal tympanic membranes

 e. Nose: no discharge

 f. Neck: no stridor, no anterior cervical lymphadenopathy, pain with extension of neck

 g. Pharynx: normal dentition, no lesions, no tonsillar exudates, or edema

 h. Chest: nontender

 i. Lungs: clear bilaterally

 j. Heart: tachycardic rate, rhythm regular, no murmurs, rubs, or gallops

 k. Abdomen: normal bowel sounds, soft, nontender or distended

 l. Extremities: full range of motion, no deformity, normal pulses

 m. Back: nontender

 n. Neuro: cranial nerves II to XII intact; normal sensation, strength; normal reflexes and gait

 o. Skin: warm and dry

 p. Lymph: no lymphadenopathy

I. Action

 a. Prepare intubation equipment (no cricothyrotomy because of age)

 b. Meds
  i. Amplicillin/sulbactam
  ii. Ibuprofen

c. Reassess
    i. Patient condition is same as at presentation, repeat vitals within normal limits.
d. Consult
    i. Otolaryngology assessment shows swelling in soft tissue around the posterior pharynx, normal vocal cords without edema, patent airway. Recommends admission and observation with IV antibiotics.
e. Imaging
    i. Lateral neck soft tissue x-ray
    ii. CT neck with contrast if above is equivocal

J. Nurse

a. Antipyretic
    i. BP: 114/80 HR: 140 RR: 28 T: 38.2°C Sat: 98%
b. No antipyretic
    i. BP: 114/80 HR: 160 RR: 28 T: 39.6 Sat: 98%

K. Results

Complete blood count:

WBC	10.0×10^3/uL	Alk Phos	42 U/L
Hct	33.3%	T bili	1.0 mg/dL
Plt	191×10^3/uL	D bili	0.3 mg/dL
		Amylase	50 U/L
Basic metabolic panel:		Lipase	25 U/L
Na	138 mEq/L	Albumin	4.7 g/dL
K	4.3 mEq/L		
Cl	105 mEq/L	**Urinalysis:**	
CO_2	25 mEq/L	SG	1.020
BUN	18 mEq/dL	pH	7
Cr	0.6 mg/dL%	Prot	Neg mg/dL
Gluc	100 mg/dL	Gluc	Neg mg/dL
		Ketones	Neg mg/dL
Coagulation panel:		Bili	Neg
PT	12.6 sec	Blood	Neg
PTT	26.0 sec	LE	Neg
INR	1.0	Nitrite	Neg
		Color	Yellow
Liver function panel:			
AST	23 U/L		
ALT	26 U/L		

a. Lateral soft tissue neck radiograph (Figure 18.1)
    i. 1.5 cm prevertebral widening
b. CT of neck with contrast

L. Action

a. Surgery – otolaryngology consult
    i. Admit to PICU
    ii. Possible surgery in the morning
b. Discussion with family for admission and possible OR

Figure 18.1

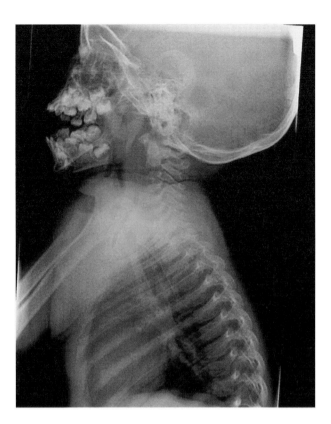

M. Diagnosis
a. Retropharyngeal abscess

N. Critical actions
▨ Preparation for intubation
▨ Antibiotics
▨ Soft tissue neck radiograph
▨ Otolaryngology consult
▨ ICU admission

O. Examiner instructions
a. This is a case of retropharyngeal abscess, a serious infection of the soft tissue behind the pharynx, which can in severe circumstances lead to a closing of the airway and inability to breath. The patient's symptoms of drooling, fever, sore throat, and neck stiffness are key findings. Important early actions include airway evaluation, obtaining IV access, administering antibiotics and IVF, obtaining radiographs, or CT scan, consulting otolaryngology and admitting the patient to an ICU setting. If the candidate does not order antibiotics, the patient will become more short of breath. If surgery or otolaryngology is not consulted, the patient will have increased difficulty in breathing and agitation. In unstable patients, CT should be deferred until the patient is stabilized or the airway is protected with intubation.

P. Pearls
a. In the setting of an acutely toxic-appearing child with airway compromise, rapid evaluation and airway assessment by an experienced intubator is critical. As much as possible an ill-appearing child who is maintaining their airway should be manipulated as little as possible until this can be arranged.

b. Retropharyngeal abscess most commonly affects children between the ages of 2 and 4 years.

c. History and physical examination are crucial for diagnosis. On physical examination, note the resistance to neck movement (with extension greater than flexion in the midline). Some patients are mistakenly worked up for meningitis because of the neck stiffness. Visual inspection of the oropharynx is frequently unremarkable. Presence of drooling is worrisome. Alternative diagnoses, such as epiglottitis and peritonsillar abscess, must be considered as well. In this case the gradual progression, nontoxic appearance, and full immunization status made epiglottitis less likely.

d. Although a lateral soft tissue neck radiograph is a good initial imaging study, it requires patient cooperation, which can be difficult in pediatric patients. The film must be taken as a perfect lateral, with the patient in inspiration. Otherwise, you may obtain a falsely positive study in which you see widening of the prevertebral space as an artifact. Crying can also cause a false positive. The prevertebral space is widened if it is greater than 7 mm at C2 or 14 mm at C6. For these technical reasons, further imaging studies of the neck such as a CT with contrast may be necessary.

e. Broad-spectrum antibiotics must be administered early. Retropharyngeal abscesses are polymicrobial. The most common organisms are gram positives, specifically group A *Streptococcus* and *Staphylococcus aureus*. Respiratory anaerobic species have been implicated as well.

f. Early surgical consultation by ENT should be obtained, because surgical drainage of the abscess may be necessary.

g. Late findings include extension into the mediastinum, airway compromise from abscess rupture, or direct pressure.

Q. References
a. Tintinalli's: Chapter 119. Stridor and Drooling, Chapter 241. Infections and Disorders of the Neck and Upper Airway
b. Rosen: Chapter 168. Pediatric Respiratory Emergencies

CASE 19: Knee pain (Edward R. Melnick, MD, MHS)

A. Chief complaint
a. 15-year-old male presents with left knee pain

B. Vital signs
a. BP: 118/77 HR: 84 RR: 16 T: 36.8°C Sat: 99% on RA

C. What does the patient look like?
a. Patient appears stated age, obese, limps into the examination room from the waiting room.

D. Primary survey
a. Airway: speaking in full sentences
b. Breathing: no apparent respiratory distress, no cyanosis
c. Circulation: warm and well-perfused, normal capillary refill

E. History

a. HPI: A 15-year-old obese male is brought in by his mother with the complaint of pain in the left knee and a limp since playing basketball in gym class yesterday. The pain has been a dull ache for the past 3 months but became more severe after gym class yesterday. He reports pain with bearing weight on his left lower extremity. He denies trauma, fever, recent respiratory infection, or decreased range of motion to the affected knee.

b. PMHx: none, immunizations up-to-date

c. PSHx: none

d. Allergies: none

e. Meds: none

f. Social: lives with parents and two younger sisters, denies alcohol, smoking, drugs, not sexually active

g. FHx: not relevant

h. PMD: Dr Smith

F. Secondary survey

a. General: alert and oriented, comfortable sitting on stretcher, pleasant, cooperative

b. HEENT: normal

c. Neck: normal

d. Chest: normal

e. Heart: normal

f. Abdomen: normal

g. Back: normal

h. Extremities

   i. Normal knee and ankle examination bilaterally, nontender, no effusion, full range of motion, knees stable to anterior drawer and Lachman test, 2+ dorsalis pedis and posterior tibial pulses bilaterally, normal capillary refill

   ii. Right hip examination normal, left hip externally rotated; range of motion limited in internal rotation

i. Neuro: antalgic gait but otherwise intact motor, sensory, and deep tendon reflexes in lower extremities bilaterally

j. Skin: warm and dry, no rashes, no edema, no cellulitis

k. Lymph: normal

G. Action

a. Meds

   i. Ibuprofen PO

b. Reassess

   i. Patient still with left knee pain and limp.

c. Imaging

   i. Bilateral hip x-ray

   ii. Consider knee x-ray

H. Nurse

a. Bilateral hip x-ray including lateral view (Figures 19.1 to 19.3)

I. Action
a. Strict non-weight-bearing on left lower extremity
b. Orthopedic consult
    i. To OR for percutaneous pinning
c. Discussion with family and PMD explaining slipped capital femoral epiphysis; need for prompt surgical management

J. Diagnosis
a. Slipped capital femoral epiphysis (SCFE)

K. Critical actions
▨ Physical examination of hips bilaterally
▨ Bilateral hip x-ray with lateral views
▨ Ortho consult for SCFE
▨ Pain medication

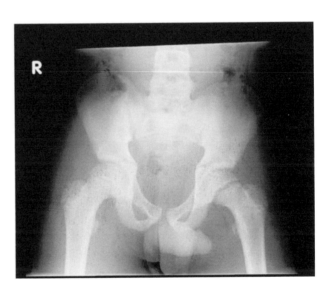

Figure 19.1

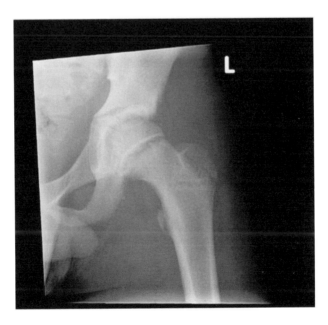

Figure 19.2

Figure 19.3

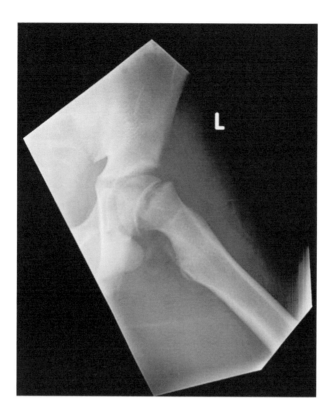

L. Examiner instructions

a. This is a case of slipped capital femoral epiphysis, the most common cause of hip disability in adolescents. In this injury, the growth plate near the end of the femur becomes disrupted, and the end of the bone "slips" out of place. Important early actions include physical examination of the hips and x-ray imaging of the hips bilaterally including lateral views. If the hips are not examined, the left knee pain and limp will persist. If the patient is discharged without a hip examination or x-ray, the patient will return 2 days later unable to walk.

M. Pearls

a. Slipped capital femoral epiphysis most commonly occurs in obese adolescents since the hips are exposed to repetitive minor trauma.

b. It may be acute, chronic, or acute on chronic. SCFE may manifest as pain in the hip or referred to the knee or thigh. One should examine the hip in any obese child complaining of knee pain.

c. It is three times more common in males, with an average age of 14 to 16 years old in males and 11 to 13 years old in females.

d. X-ray findings may only be apparent on lateral radiographic view. A line drawn along the superior aspect of the femoral neck (Klein's line) should transect the lateral quarter of the femoral head. In SCFE, no part of the femoral head is above Klein's line.

e. Delay in diagnosis can lead to significant disability due to avascular necrosis of the femoral head.

f. Inability to ambulate is ominous, and is a sign of unstable SCFE. These cases are at much higher risk of developing avascular necrosis than their stable (ambulatory) counterparts.

N. References
a. Tintinalli's: Chapter 133. Musculoskeletal Disorders in Children
b. Rosen: Chapter 176. Musculoskeletal Disorders

CASE 20: Abdominal pain (Edward R. Melnick, MD, MHS)

A. Chief complaint
a. 3-year-old male with abdominal pain

B. Vital signs
a. BP: 89/61 HR: 126 RR: 24 T: 36.9°C Sat: 100% on RA

C. What does the patient look like?
a. Patient appears stated age, carried in his mother's arms, crying and inconsolable despite verbal soothing by both parents.

D. Primary survey
a. Airway: crying and yelling, "Owie in my tummy"
b. Breathing: increased respiratory rate associated with pain, no cyanosis
c. Circulation: warm and well-perfused, normal capillary refill

E. History
a. HPI: a 3-year-old male brought in by parents with complaint of abdominal pain for 3 hours. The child has been colicky for 12 hours with decreased feeding, then began crying 3 hours ago and has not stopped since then. He vomited once 2 hours ago, nonbloody, nonbilious; denies fevers. Mother reports normal number of wet diapers and normal stool with no diarrhea, blood, or mucus. Mother also reports she noticed a new "diaper rash" when she changed the patient's diaper before trying to put him to bed that evening.
b. PMHx: full-term pregnancy with no complications, immunizations up-to-date
c. PSHx: none
d. Allergies: none
e. Meds: none
f. Social: lives with parents and 8-year-old brother
g. FHx: noncontributory
h. PMD: Dr Mehta

F. Nurse
a. Obtain largest IV access possible

G. Action
a. Labs
   i. CBC and BMP
b. Meds
   i. NS 20 mL/kg bolus × 2
   ii. Morphine IV

H. Secondary survey
a. General: crying, inconsolable, moderate distress due to pain
b. HEENT: normal, making tears, moist mucous membranes

   c. Neck: normal

   d. Chest: normal

   e. Heart: normal

   f. Abdomen: normal active bowel sounds, soft, nontender, nondistended, no rebound, no guarding

   g. Rectal: hemoccult negative brown stool, no mucus, no fissure

   h. GU: normal circumcised penis, no hernias, normal right testicle, left hemiscrotum mildly erythematous and edematous, left testicle enlarged and exquisitely tender, riding higher in the scrotum than the right testicle with a transverse lie, cremasteric reflex present on right but absent on left

   i. Extremities: normal

   j. Back: normal

   k. Neuro: normal

   l. Skin: warm and dry, rash-erythema noted to left hemiscrotum as per GU examination

   m. Lymph: normal

I. Action

   a. Consult

      i. Urology (or pediatric surgery depending on institutional availability) paged for emergency consult

   b. Imaging

      i. Testicular color-flow duplex Doppler US ordered – but sono tech must come in from home

   c. NPO

J. Nurse

   a. Vital signs

      i. IV fluids do not affect vital signs

      ii. If no pain medication given: BP: 87/63 HR: 148 RR: 24 T: 36.9°C Sat: 100% on RA

      iii. If pain medication given: BP: 87/63 HR: 116 RR: 24 T: 36.9°C Sat: 100% on RA

   b. Patient: still crying and inconsolable

   c. Still no response from page placed for urology/pediatric surgery consult and sono tech

K. Results

Complete blood count:

WBC	11.0×10^3/uL	BUN	14 mEq/dL
Hct	38.1%	Cr	0.4 mg/dL
Plt	350×10^3/uL	Gluc	70 mg/dL

Basic metabolic panel:

Na	135 mEq/L	PT	13.1 sec
K	4.6 mEq/L	PTT	27.5 sec
Cl	98 mEq/L	INR	0.9
CO_2	25 mEq/L		

Coagulation panel:

Urinalysis:

SG	1.020	Bili	Neg
pH	6	Blood	Neg
Prot	Neg	LE	Neg
Gluc	Neg	Nitrite	Neg
Ketones	Neg	Color	Yellow

L. Action
a. Discussion with family and PMD possibility of testicular torsion and need to attempt manual detorsion pending sono and urology consult
b. Meds
   i. Morphine IV
c. Attempt manual detorsion of left testicle (describe procedure)

M. Nurse
a. Vital signs
   i. BP: 85/63 HR: 106 RR: 20 T: 36.6°C Sat: 98% on RA
b. Patient: pain distress decreased, uncomfortable but consolable, patient states "my tummy is a little better"
c. Sono tech and surgical consult arrive 50 minutes later at which point the patient has started crying again and tachycardia has resumed
d. Testicular color-flow duplex Doppler US (Figures 20.1 to 20.3)
e. Patient taken directly to OR from sono by urologist for scrotal exploration and detorsion of left testicle

N. Diagnosis
a. Testicular torsion

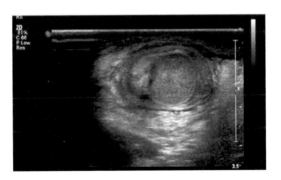

Figure 20.1

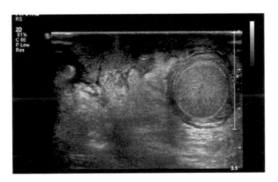

Figure 20.2

Figure 20.3
See color plate
section (in
some formats
this figure will
only appear in
black and
white).

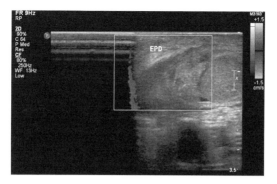

O. Critical actions

▨ Testicular examination
▨ Immediate, emergency urology/pediatric surgery consult
▨ Testicular color-flow duplex Doppler US
▨ Pain management
▨ Manual detorsion if prompt surgical consult not available
▨ OR for surgical exploration and detorsion
▨ Nothing by mouth

P. Examiner instructions

a. This is a case of testicular torsion, or twisting of the testicle around its attached
blood supply, causing decreased blood flow to the testicle and pain. The pain is
initially colicky indicating spontaneous torsion and detorsion. The sudden onset
of severe, constant pain and findings on physical examination indicate sustained
torsion and impending testicular infarction. Important early actions include
testicular examination, consulting urology or pediatric surgery, pain management, and ordering Doppler US of the testicles. His pain and tachycardia will
continue to increase until an opioid medication (such as morphine) is administered. Owing to slow response from the sono technician and surgical consult,
manual detorsion should be attempted by the ED physician to try to salvage the
patient's testicle.

Q. Pearls

a. Testicular torsion is the twisting of the spermatic cord causing decreased blood
flow to the testicle. Onset of testicular pain is usually sudden and severe. Pain is
often referred to the lower abdomen or inguinal canal.
b. Always include a GU examination in patients complaining of abdominal pain.
Conversely, always include abdominal examination in patients with GU
complaints.
c. Testicular salvage is usually possible with surgery after less than 12 hours of
symptoms but almost impossible after 24 hours of symptoms.
d. For adolescents and adults, the differential diagnosis includes epididymitis, and
work-up should include urinalysis and urethral swab for GC/chlamydia.
e. Manually detorse the testicle by elevating the affected testicle toward the inguinal
ring and rotate one and one half rotations (540°) in a medial to lateral motion in a
manner similar to opening a book. Procedural sedation will improve the patient's
tolerance of the procedure but will make it difficult to assess the efficacy of the
procedure. Relief of pain indicates successful detorsion but emergent urology

consultation is still necessary. However, this maneuver is usually unsuccessful and should be abandoned if the patient has worsening pain.

R. References
a. Tintinalli's: Chapter 127. Urologic and Gynecologic Problems and Procedures in Children.
b. Rosen: Chapter 99. Selected Urologic Problems

CASE 21: Abdominal pain (Yasuharu Okuda, MD)

A. Chief complaint
a. 79-year-old female brought in by husband with the complaint of worsening abdominal pain for the past 4 hours

B. Vital signs
a. BP: 85/63 HR: 96 RR: 18 T: 36.2°C Sat: 98% on RA FS: 110

C. What does the patient look like?
a. Patient appears stated age, uncomfortable secondary to pain in mild distress, lying still in stretcher.

D. Primary survey
a. Airway: speaking in full sentences
b. Breathing: no apparent respiratory distress, no cyanosis
c. Circulation: pale and cool skin, normal capillary refill

E. Action
a. Oxygen via NC or nonrebreather mask
b. Two large-bore peripheral IV lines
c. Labs
   i. CBC, Chem 7, LFT, PT/PTT, type and cross-match 2 units, lactate
d. 1 L NS bolus
e. Monitor: BP: 92/68 HR: 96 RR: 18 Sat: 100% on O_2
f. EKG

F. History
a. HPI: a 79-year-old female with a history of hypertension and hypercholesterolemia states that she has been constipated for the past few days. Today she was finally able to have a large "explosive" bowel movement which was brown and nonbloody. Since then over the past 4 hours she has developed progressive abdominal pain. The pain started in the epigastrum but now has become diffuse. The patient thought it might be indigestion. She rode a taxi to the hospital and the pain was exacerbated with shaking of taxi. Pain also worsened with shaking of the stretcher. The patient notes nausea, but denies vomiting, fever, chills, chest pain, shortness of breath, headache, back pain, urinary symptoms, or vaginal discharge; last meal was breakfast.
b. PMHx: hypertension and hypercholesterolemia
c. PSHx: none
d. Allergies: none

   e. Meds: simvastatin, aspirin, metoprolol

   f. Social: lives with husband at home, denies alcohol, smoking, drugs, not sexually active

   g. FHx: not relevant

   h. PMD: Dr Richardson

G. Nurse

   a. EKG (Figure 21.1)

   b. 1 L NS

      i. BP: 98/59 HR: 90 RR: 18 Sat: 98% on O_2

   c. No fluids

      i. BP: 70/45 HR: 118 RR: 20 Sat: 98% on O_2

H. Secondary survey

   a. General: alert, oriented × 3, moderate distress secondary to pain

   b. Head: normocephalic, atraumatic

   c. Eyes: mildly pale conjunctiva, extraocular movement intact, pupils equal, reactive to light

   d. Ears: normal tympanic membranes

   e. Nose: no discharge

   f. Neck: full range of motion, no jugular vein distension, no stridor

   g. Pharynx: normal dentition, no lesions, no swelling

   h. Chest: nontender

   i. Lungs: clear bilaterally

   j. Heart: rate and rhythm regular, no murmurs, rubs, or gallops

   k. Abdomen: distended, diffusely tender, bowel sounds absent, no masses, no hernias, nontender at McBurney's point, negative Murphy's sign, + rebound, + guarding, no rigidity

Figure 21.1

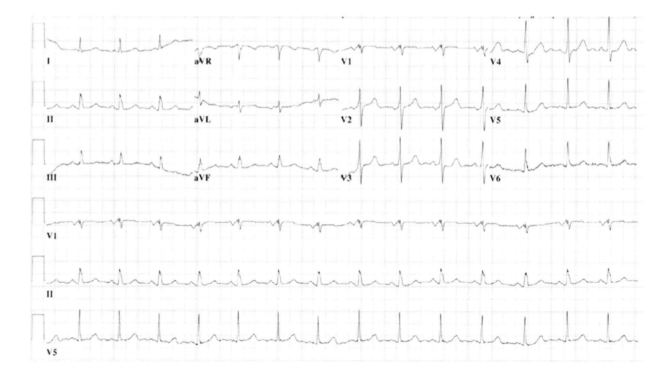

l. Rectal: normal tone, brown stool, occult blood positive
m. Urogenital: normal external genitalia
    i. Female: no blood or discharge, cervical os closed, no cervical motion tenderness, no adnexal tenderness.
n. Extremities: full range of motion, no deformity, normal pulses
o. Back: nontender
p. Neuro: cranial nerves II to XII intact; normal sensation, strength; normal reflexes and gait
q. Skin: warm and dry
r. Lymph: no lymphadenopathy

I. Action

a. Meds
    i. Ciprofloxacin
    ii. Flagyl
b. Reassess
    i. Patient still reports significant discomfort, worsening pain
c. Consult
    i. Surgery
d. Imaging
    i. Upright CXR (if supine CXR, inconclusive results)
    ii. Obstructive series
    iii. Morphine

J. Nurse

a. BP: 98/59 HR: 90 RR: 18 Sat: 98% on O_2 (after 1 L)
b. Patient: still with significant pain

K. Results

Complete blood count:

WBC	12.1×10^3/uL	Alk Phos	42 U/L
Hct	41.5%	T bili	1.0 mg/dL
Plt	253×10^3/uL	D bili	0.3 mg/dL
		Amylase	50 U/L
Basic metabolic panel:		Lipase	25 U/L
Na	138 mEq/L	Albumin	4.7 g/dL
K	4.3 mEq/L		
Cl	105 mEq/L	**Urinalysis:**	
CO2	30 mEq/L	SG	1.0.20
BUN	52 mEq/dL	pH	7
Cr	1.2 mg/dL%	Prot	Neg
Gluc	110 mg/dL	Gluc	Neg
		Ketones	Neg
Coagulation panel:		Bili	Neg
PT	12.6 sec	Blood	Neg
PTT	26.0 sec	LE	Neg
INR	1.0	Nitrite	Neg
		Color	Yellow
Liver function panel:			
AST	23 U/L		
ALT	26 U/L		

a. Lactate 2.2 mmol/L
b. Upright CXR (Figure 21.2)
c. Obstructive series (Figures 21.3 and 21.4)

Figure 21.2

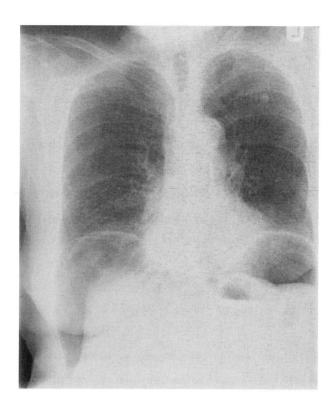

Figure 21.3

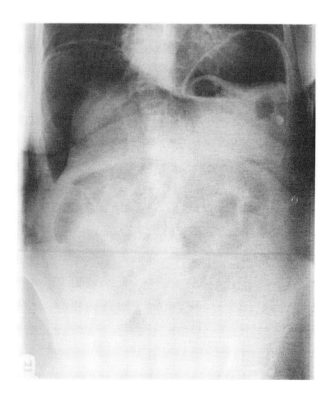

Figure 21.4

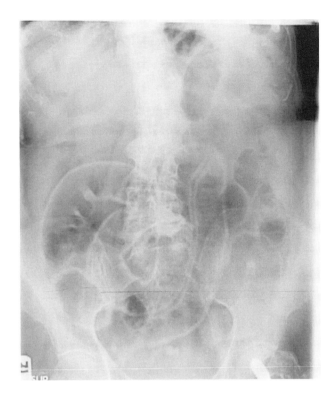

L. Action
a. Surgery consult
  i. To OR for laparotomy
b. Discussion with family and PMD need for emergent OR and suspicion for perforated viscus
c. Meds
  i. Morphine

M. Diagnosis
a. Gastric perforation

N. Critical actions
▓ Large-bore IV access and fluid bolus
▓ Upright chest x-ray
▓ Pain management
▓ Surgery consult

O. Examiner instructions
a. This is a case of a perforated viscus, likely from a small bowel obstruction. In this patient, an obstruction within the intestinal system caused a backup of pressure leading to rupturing of the stomach wall. The patient's symptoms of abdominal pain began fairly abruptly and her symptoms are significantly worsened with movement of any kind due to peritoneal irritation. Important early actions include administering IV fluids, consulting surgery, starting antibiotics, and advocating for the patient to go to the OR. If fluids are not administered, the patient's blood pressure will begin to drop. Her pain will continue to increase until an opioid medication (such as morphine) is administered. An obstructive series with upright

chest x-ray can be readily obtained; if a CT scan is ordered, note that the scanner is busy, and it will "be a while" before the test can be performed.

P. Pearls
a. Upright CXR is more sensitive than KUB for free air.
b. Peritoneal signs are ominous, and often suggest a surgical emergency. Consider early antibiotics, fluids, and surgical consultation.
c. Elderly patients with epigastric pain should be evaluated for coronary ischemia. Non-chest pain presentations are common in this age group, especially upper abdominal pain and/or shortness of breath.
d. Note that the patient has a "relative" hypotension. Given the history of high blood pressure, a systolic blood pressure in the 90s is more ominous than in a patient with baseline normal blood pressure.

Q. References
a. Tintinalli's: Chapter 86. Bowel Obstruction and Volulus
b. Rosen: Chapter 92. Disorders of the Small Intestine

CASE 22: Cough (Raghu Seethala, MD)

A. Chief complaint
a. 1-year-old male brought in with cough

B. Vital signs
a. BP: 100/60 HR: 170 RR: 24 T: 36.8°C Sat: 98% on room air

C. What does the patient look like?
a. Patient appears stated age, slightly underweight.

D. Primary survey
a. Airway: patient crying
b. Breathing: no apparent respiratory distress, no cyanosis
c. Circulation: normal pulses, normal capillary refill

E. History
a. HPI: a 1-year-old male with no significant medical history presents with nonproductive cough for the past 3 weeks. The patient had rhinorrhea and injected conjuctivae for 1 week and then developed a dry hacking cough. Coughing occurs in paroxysms, greater than 40 bouts per day, is worse at night, and is occasionally followed by vomiting and episodes of cyanosis. Patient gets extremely tired after coughing spells. Mother reports that the patient has been having decreased feeding. Mother denies any fevers, or hemoptysis.
b. PMHx: none, unclear immunization status
c. PSHx: none
d. Allergies: none
e. Meds: none
f. Social: lives with family at home, no recent sick contacts, patient and family are recent immigrants from Honduras

g. FHx: not relevant
h. PMD: pediatric clinic

F. Secondary survey

a. General: well-appearing, playful
b. HEENT: small subconjunctival hemorrhage in left eye, mucous membranes slightly dry
c. Neck: supple, no lymphadenopathy
d. Chest: scattered ronchi, no rales
e. Heart: regular rate and rhythm, no murmurs, rubs, or gallops
f. Abdomen: soft, nontender, normal bowel sounds
g. Urogenital: normal
h. Extremities: normal
i. Back: normal
j. Neuro: normal
k. Skin: pale, no rashes, no edema
l. Lymph: normal

G. Action

a. Oxygen supplementation (NC)
b. Labs
  i. CBC, BMP
c. Monitor
d. Imaging
  i. CXR
e. 20 ml/kg NS bolus

H. Nurse

a. BP: 100/60 HR: 120 RR: 18, Sat; 100% on O_2 (after 20 cc/kg NS bolus); if no bolus was administered, vitals remain unchanged from triage

I. Results

Complete blood count:			
WBC	40.6×10^3/uL	BUN	25 mEq/dL
Hct	41.5%	Cr	0.5 mg/dL%
Plt	253×10^3/uL	Gluc	102 mg/dL

Basic metabolic panel:		Coagulation panel:	
Na	139 mEq/L	PT	12.9 sec
K	3.8 mEq/L	PTT	25.4 sec
Cl	101 mEq/L	INR	0.9
CO_2	23 mEq/L		

a. CXR (Figure 22.1A and 22.1B)

J. Action

a. Admission to pediatric ward
  i. Respiratory isolation
b. Discussion with family and treatment of close contacts

A

B

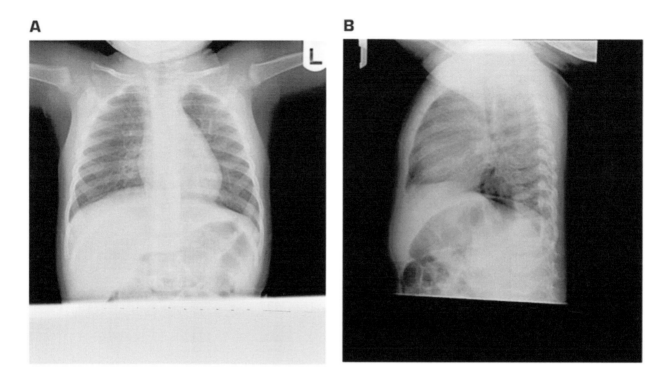

Figure 22.1 A and B

    c. Meds
      i. Erythromycin PO
   d. Further diagnostic testing
      i. Culture
      ii. Polymerase chain reaction (PCR) test for pertussis
      iii. Pertussis direct fluorescent antibody (DFA) stain

K. Diagnosis
a. Pertussis

L. Critical actions
▨ Oxygen
▨ Recognize tachycardia, give saline
▨ CXR
▨ Antibiotics for patient and close contacts
▨ Admission to respiratory isolation

M. Examiner instructions
a. This is a case of pertussis, a respiratory infection due to *Bordetella pertussis*. The patient presented in the paroxysmal phase of pertussis. Important early actions include oxygen administration if hypoxic, CXR, identifying the diagnosis, starting antibiotics for patient and close contacts. Correct antibiotics are macrolides (or sulfamethoxazole and trimethoprim if allergic). Once the diagnosis of pertussis is considered confirmatory diagnostic testing should be sent (culture, DFA, or PCR).

N. Pearls

a. The CXR is usually normal but look for complications such as super-infection, pneumonia, or pneumothorax from forceful coughing.

b. Look for atypical presentations in previously vaccinated adolescents, adults, and children who have completed vaccination series. Infants younger than 6 months (especially those younger than 4 weeks) may present with apnea, bradycardia, prolonged cough, poor feeding, and no paroxysms.

c. Note this patient's leukocytosis and lymphocytosis. Leukocytosis may reach up to 50×10^3/uL during paroxysmal phase.

d. Antibiotics have not been shown to reduce disease duration after the paroxysmal stage begins, but they can decrease transmission risk. Close contacts should receive antibiotic prophylaxis.

e. Patients who appear well, with stable vital signs and close follow-up can be discharged home with antibiotics.

O. References

a. Tintinalli's: Chapter 67. Acute Bronchitis and Upper Respiratory Tract Infections.

b. Rosen: Chapter 129. Bacteria.

CASE 23: Flank pain (Raghu Seethala, MD)

A. Chief complaint

a. 77-year-old male with flank pain

B. Vital signs

a. BP: 100/63 HR: 94 RR: 18 T: 36.9°C Sat: 99% on RA

C. What does the patient look like?

a. Patient appears stated age, appears uncomfortable due to pain, in mild distress; lying supine in stretcher.

D. Primary survey

a. Airway: speaking in full sentences

b. Breathing: no apparent respiratory distress, no cyanosis

c. Circulation: pale and cool skin, normal capillary refill

E. Action

a. Oxygen via peripheral NC or nonrebreather mask

b. Two large-bore lines IV

c. Labs
   i. CBC, BMP, LFT, PT/PTT, type and hold, lactate, UA

d. 1 L NS bolus

e. Monitor: BP: 95/64 HR: 93 RR: 18 Sat: 100% on O_2

f. EKG

F. History

a. HPI: a 77-year-old male with a history of hypertension, diabetes, and hypercholesterolemia states that a few hours after he woke up today he developed left-sided flank pain radiating to the groin. The pain is described as sharp, ripping and constant. Over the past few hours the pain has intensified. The patient also states he might have seen some blood in his urine. He denies any syncope, nausea, vomiting, diarrhea, melena, fever, headache, shortness of breath, or dysuria.

b. PMHx: hypertension, hypercholesterolemia, diabetes
c. PSHx: none
d. Allergies: none
e. Meds: simvastatin, metoprolol
f. Social: lives with wife at home, smokes one pack a day for 50 years, social drinker, denies drug use, not sexually active
g. FHx: not relevant
h. PMD: switched doctors, hasn't seen one in over a year

G. Nurse
a. EKG (Figure 23.1)
b. If 1 L NS given:
    i. BP: 98/62 HR: 91 RR: 18 Sat: 98% on O_2
c. If no fluids given:
    i. BP: 73/42 HR: 115 RR: 20 Sat 98% on O_2

H. Secondary survey
a. General: alert, oriented, moderate distress due to pain
b. HEENT: mildly pale conjunctivae, otherwise normal
c. Neck: normal
d. Chest: normal
e. Heart: normal

Figure 23.1

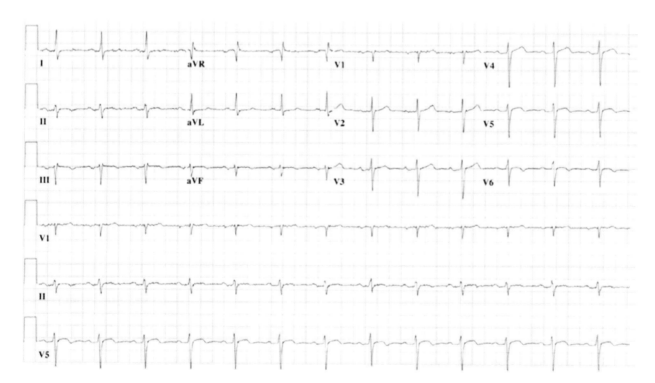

f. Abdomen: obese, non tender, bowel sounds present, no masses, no hernias, no rebound, no guarding, no rigidity, pulsatile mass palpated (must ask)

g. Rectal: hemoccult negative brown stool, normal rectal tone

h. Urogenital: normal

i. Extremities: normal

j. Back: normal, left costovertebral angle tenderness

k. Neuro: normal

l. Skin: pale, faint bilateral flank ecchymoses, no rashes, no edema, no cellulitis

m. Lymph: normal

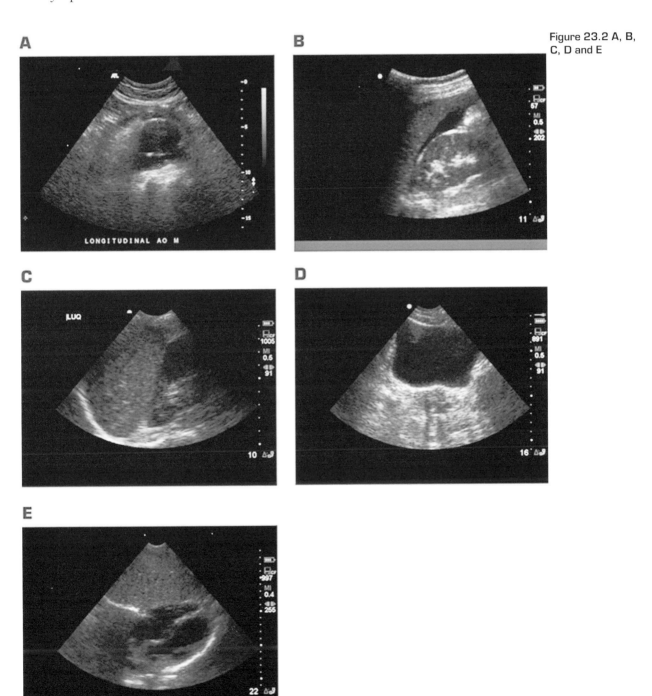

Figure 23.2 A, B, C, D and E

I. Action

a. Meds: morphine IV

b. Reassess

    i. Patient still with significant discomfort, worsening pain

c. Consult

    i. Surgery

d. Imaging

    i. Bedside US (Figure 23.2)

J. Nurse

a. BP: 98/59 HR: 90 RR: 18 Sat: 98% on O_2 (after 1 L)

b. Patient: still with significant pain

K. Results

Complete blood count:

WBC	9.1×10^3/uL	D bili	0.1 mg/dL
Hct	22.9%	Amylase	240 U/L
Plt	213×10^3/uL	Lipase	220 U/L
		Albumin	4.1 g/dL

Basic metabolic panel:

Na	139 mEq/L	**Urinalysis:**	
K	4.1 mEq/L	SG	1.020
Cl	101 mEq/L	pH	6
CO_2	19 mEq/L	Prot	Neg
BUN	40 mEq/dL	Gluc	Neg
Cr	1.4 mg/dL	Ketones	Neg
Gluc	202 mg/dL	Bili	Neg
		Blood	+
Coagulation panel:		LE	Neg
PT	13.1 sec	Nitrite	Neg
PTT	26 sec	Color	Yellow
INR	1.0		
		Arterial blood gas:	
		pH	7.33
Liver function panel:		PO_2	92 mmHg
AST	23 U/L	PCO_2	25 mmHg
ALT	19 U/L	HCO_3	19 mmol/L
Alk Phos	87 U/L		
T bili	0.7 mg/dL		

a. Lactate 2.9 mmol/L

b. CXR (Figure 23.3)

L. Action

a. Surgery consult

    i. To operating room for emergent surgical repair

b. Discussion with family and PMD regarding need for emergent surgical repair and diagnosis of aortic aneurysm

c. Meds

    i. Two units of uncross-matched blood

    ii. Call blood blank to make sure 10 to 16 units of blood and fresh frozen plasma will be available

Figure 23.3

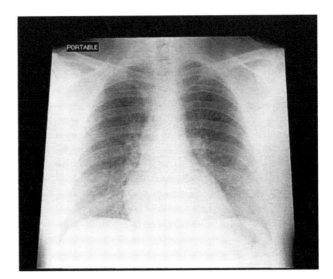

M. Diagnosis
a. Abdominal aortic aneurysm (AAA)

N. Critical actions
- Large-bore IV access and fluid bolus
- Bedside US
- Surgery consult
- Blood transfusion

O. Examiner instructions
a. This is a case of a leaking AAA. Weakness in the wall of the aorta causes dilation of the vessel, which causes increased pressure at the wall, increasing the rate of stretch until a leak occurs. This condition tends to progress slowly (over years) and the risk of rupture increases with the diameter of the vessel. Important early actions include administering IV fluids if hypotensive, obtaining a bedside US, consulting surgery, and advocating for the patient to go to the operating room (OR). If fluids are not administered, the patient's blood pressure will begin to drop. If the patient is still hypotensive then 2 units of uncrossed blood should be administered while multiple units of cross-matched blood are readied. A bedside US can readily be obtained; if a CT scan is ordered, note that the scanner is busy, and it will "be a while" before the test can be performed.

P. Pearls
a. Bedside US that is technically adequate has close to 100% sensitivity for demonstrating an AAA.
b. Once a ruptured AAA is suspected, all efforts should be concentrated on stabilizing the patient and transferring the patient to the OR.
c. Elderly patients with back or flank pain should be evaluated for AAA. Hematuria is also common in patients with ruptured AAA, which can lead to the incorrect diagnosis of nephrolithiasis.
d. Flank ecchymosis (Grey-Turner's sign) is a sign of retroperitoneal hematoma.

Q. References
a. Tintinalli's: Chapter 63. Aneurysms of the Aorta and Major Arteries
b. Rosen: Chapter 86. Abdominal Aortic Aneurysm

CASE 24: Weakness (Raghu Seethala, MD)

A. Chief complaint

a. 68-year-old female with lethargy

B. Vital signs

a. BP: 136/89 HR: 79 RR: 18 T: 36.5°C Sat: 98% on RA

C. What does the patient look like?

a. Patient appears stated age, lethargic, lying supine on stretcher.

D. Primary survey

a. Airway: speaking in full sentences

b. Breathing: no apparent respiratory distress, no cyanosis

c. Circulation: warm skin, normal capillary refill

E. Action

a. Oxygen via nonrebreather mask

b. Two large-bore peripheral IV lines

c. Labs

    i. CBC, BMP, LFT, PT/PTT, lactate, aspirin and acetaminophen levels

d. EKG

e. Monitor – unchanged from triage

f. Finger stick glucose (200; must ask)

F. History

a. HPI: a 68-year-old female with a history of hypertension and hypercholesterolemia presents after calling son and complaining of feeling extremely weak and lethargic. She reported feeling very depressed after her cat died last night, and "hasn't felt right" since. Son found patient lying on couch feeling too weak to get up. EMS administered O_2 and brought the patient to ED. Patient currently complaining of mild headache, generalized weakness, and malaise. She denies any chest pain, shortness of breath, syncope, seizure, nausea, or vomiting.

b. PMHx: hypertension and hypercholesterolemia

c. PSHx: none

d. Allergies: none

e. Meds: hydrochlorothiazide, simvastatin

f. Social: lives alone at home, denies alcohol, smoking, drugs, not sexually active

g. FHx: not relevant

h. PMD: Dr Weingart

G. Nurse

a. EKG (Figure 24.1)

H. Secondary survey

a. General: alert, oriented to self and place, moderately lethargic

b. HEENT: normal

c. Neck: supple neck, no nuchal rigidity

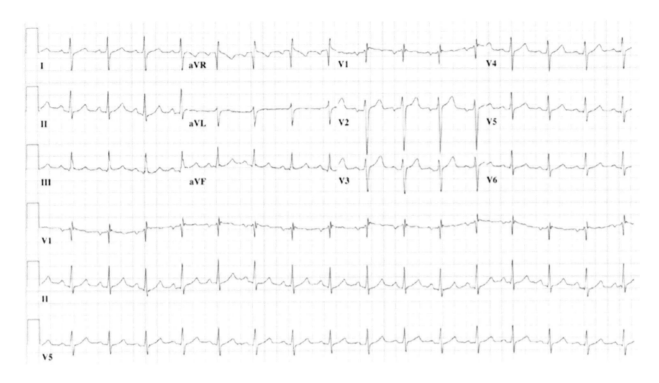

Figure 24.1

d. Chest: normal
e. Heart: normal
f. Abdomen: normal
g. Urogenital: normal
h. Extremities: normal
i. Back: normal
j. Neuro: alert, oriented to self and place, follows commands, generalized weakness, no focal motor deficits, normal sensory examination, normal reflexes, unsteady gait, + dysmetria
k. Skin: pale, no rashes, no edema
l. Lymph: normal
m. Psych: poor concentration

I. Further history
a. Son reports patient seems very out of sorts; when he arrived to her apartment today, he had to turn off the stove which she had left on

J. Action
a. Additional labs: carboxyhemoglobin (COHb), arterial blood gas
b. Reassess
  i. Patient feeling slightly better with O_2
c. Imaging
  i. CT head
  ii. CXR

K. Results

Complete blood count:

WBC	10.1×10^3/uL	D bili	0.3 mg/dL
Hct	39.5%	Amylase	200 U/L
Plt	253×10^3/uL	Lipase	47 U/L
		Albumin	4.1 g/dL

Basic metabolic panel:

Na	135 mEq/L	**Urinalysis:**	
K	3.5 mEq/L	SG	1.019
Cl	101 mEq/L	pH	7
CO_2	21 mEq/L	Prot	Neg
BUN	19 mEq/dL	Gluc	Neg
Cr	1.1 mg/dL	Ketones	Neg
Gluc	202 mg/dL	Bili	Neg
		Blood	Neg
Coagulation panel:		LE	Neg
PT	15.1 sec	Nitrite	Neg
PTT	30 sec	Color	Yellow
INR	1.0		

Arterial blood gas:

Liver function panel:		pH	7.31
AST	30 U/L	PO_2	399 mmHg
ALT	25 U/L	PCO_2	40 mmHg
Alk Phos	88 U/L	HCO_3	20 mmol/L
T bili	0.9 mg/dL	O_2 Sat	72%

a. Lactate 2.2 mmol/L

b. COHb: 23%

c. Portable CXR (Figure 24.2)

d. Head CT (Figure 24.3)

L. Action

a. Call nearest hyperbaric center

b. Transfer patient
  i. To hyperbaric chamber for hyperbaric oxygen (HBO) treatment

c. Discussion with family and PMD regarding need for emergent transfer for HBO treatment

M. Diagnosis

a. Carbon monoxide poisoning

N. Critical actions

▨ 100% nonrebreather mask

▨ Obtain finger stick blood glucose

▨ Obtain history consistent with carbon monoxide poisoning

▨ Obtain COHb level

▨ Transfer to hyperbaric treatment facility

O. Examiner instructions

a. This is a case of a carbon monoxide (CO) poisoning. Carbon monoxide is a colorless, odorless gas, which is commonly produced by combustion, and interferes

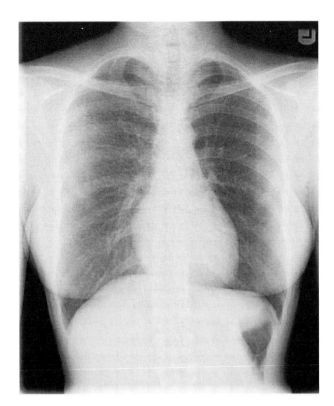

Figure 24.2

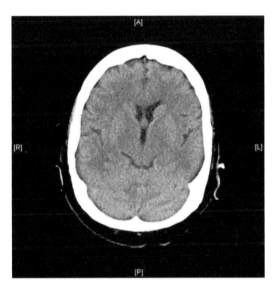

Figure 24.3

with the normal transport of oxygen in the cells. The patient had a significant exposure by leaving her stove on and falling asleep on the couch. The history of a stove being left on (or in many cases, space heaters or other combustion devices being used with poor ventilation) is the key to an otherwise nonspecific presentation. The death of her cat is not a red herring; the animal succumbed to the poisoning sooner than the patient did. These two components of the case can be made more or less accessible to the candidate depending on how difficult the examiner would like to make the case. Important early actions include placing the patient on 100% oxygen, ordering a COHb level, and identifying that the patient needed to be transferred to a hyperbaric treatment center. The decision to transfer to a hyperbaric treatment center is made because of the patient's neurologic deficits, not because of the COHb level. Once the diagnosis has been made and the critical actions completed, further testing should be done on a case by case basis such as an EKG to evaluate for cardiac ischemia from CO, or head CT/MRI to evaluate for cerebral edema.

P. Pearls
a. As with any case of altered mental status or weakness, early EKG and finger stick glucose are important.
b. Pulse oximetry cannot be used to determine arterial oxygenation because these devices mistake COHb for oxyhemoglobin and give falsely elevated levels.
c. COHb can be performed on venous blood drawn in a heparinized tube.
d. COHb levels do not correlate with symptoms or prognosis.
e. Definite indications for hyperbaric oxygen treatment are abnormal neurologic examination, altered mental status, coma, syncope, or seizure. Relative indications are persistent neurologic symptoms after 4 hours of 100% NRB treatment, myocardial ischemia, pregnancy with a history of CO exposure, persistent acidosis, and concurrent thermal or chemical burns.
f. Symptoms of CO poisoning are often subtle and insidious; when multiple family members become simultaneously ill, or when even pets seem affected, environmental exposures (such as CO poisoning) should be strongly considered. There is a higher incidence in the winter months.

Q. References
a. Tintinalli's: Chapter 217. Carbon Monoxide
b. Rosen: Chapter 159. Inhaled Toxins

CASE 25: Assault to face (Raghu Seethala, MD)

A. Chief complaint
a. 24-year-old male brought in by EMS after being assaulted to the face with a baseball bat

B. Vital signs
a. BP: 143/83 HR: 106 RR: 20 T: 36.2°C Sat: 95% on RA FS: 110

C. What does the patient look like?
a. Patient appears stated age, uncomfortable appearing in mild distress, lying still on backboard with c-collar in place. He has obvious facial deformities and a significant amount of facial bleeding.

D. Primary survey
a. Airway: patient is making gurgling noises
b. Breathing: some respiratory distress, no cyanosis
c. Circulation: warm skin, normal pulses, moderate epistaxis

E. Action
a. Chin lift, jaw thrust, oropharyngeal suctioning, pull tongue forward

b. Reassess
- i. No improvement in airway

c. Intubate using awake technique (describe procedure)
- i. If candidate attempts basic rapid sequence intubation (RSI), patient will desaturate and code
- ii. Have cricothyrotomy set up also
- iii. Post intubation management

d. Two 16- or 18-gauge IVs in antecubital fossa

e. Direct pressure to nares if unsuccessful, anterior and posterior packing

f. Labs
- i. CBC, Chem 7, PT/PTT, type and cross-match 2 units, lactate, EtOH level

g. 1 L NS bolus

h. Trauma team activation

i. Monitor: BP: 132/78 HR: 110 RR: 18 Sat: 100% on O_2

F. History

a. HPI: a 24-year-old male with no significant medical history presents after assault to the face with baseball bat. Patient was at a bar drinking that night. After the bar closed he was involved in an altercation with another individual in the parking lot. The assailant took out a wooden baseball bat from the back of his truck and hit the patient in the face multiple times. The patient fell to the ground with questionable LOC. When EMS arrived at scene the patient was moaning in pain, and cursing out loudly. He was intoxicated but able to answer EMS questions.

b. PMHx: none

c. PSHx: appendectomy

d. Allergies: none

e. Social: lives alone, binge drinker, denies tobacco use, + marijuana, denies IVDA

f. FHx: not relevant

g. PMD: none

G. Nurse

a. 1 L NS
- i. BP: 128/79 HR: 99 RR: 18 Sat: 100% on vent

H. Secondary survey

a. General: patient is intubated

b. HEENT: laceration under right zygoma, moderate epistaxis, depressed midface on examination, craniofacial dislocation present when rocking the maxillary arch, swelling, and deformity of nose, copious amount of blood in the oropharynx.

c. Neck: normal

d. Chest: normal

e. Heart: normal

f. Abdomen: normal

g. Rectal: brown stool, normal tone

h. Urogenital: normal

i. Extremities: no deformities, no ecchymosis

j. Back: normal

k. Neuro: normal

l. Skin: pale, no rashes, no edema

m. Lymph: normal

n. FAST examination: normal

I. Action

a. Meds

    i. Tetanus toxoid IM

b. Imaging

    i. CT head

    ii. CT C-spine

    iii. CT facial bones

    iv. CXR, pelvis AP

J. Nurse

a. BP: 123/79 HR: 90 RR: 18 Sat: 100% on vent

K. Results

Complete blood count:

WBC	5.3×10^3/uL	D bili	0.3 mg/dL
Hct	41.5%	Amylase	50 U/L
Plt	350×10^3/uL	Lipase	25 U/L
		Albumin	4.7 g/dL

Basic metabolic panel:

Na	138 mEq/L	**Urinalysis:**	
K	4.3 mEq/L	SG	1.0.20
Cl	105 mEq/L	pH	7
CO_2	30 mEq/L	Prot	Neg
BUN	12 mEq/dL	Gluc	Neg
Cr	1.1 mg/dL	Ketones	Neg
Gluc	100 mg/dL	Bili	Neg
		Blood	Neg
Coagulation panel:		LE	Neg
PT	12.6 sec	Nitrite	Neg
PTT	26.0 sec	Color	Yellow
INR	1.0		

Arterial blood gas:

pH	7.4
PO_2	95 mmHg
PCO_2	41 mmHg
HCO_3	24 mmol/L

Liver function panel:

AST	23 U/L
ALT	26 U/L
Alk Phos	42 U/L
T bili	1.0 mg/dL

a. Lactate 0.8 mmol/L

b. EtOH 340

c. CXR (Figure 25.1)

d. Pelvis x-ray (Figure 25.2)

e. CT head (Figure 25.3)

f. CT face Le Fort II fracture

g. CT C-spine normal CT Spine

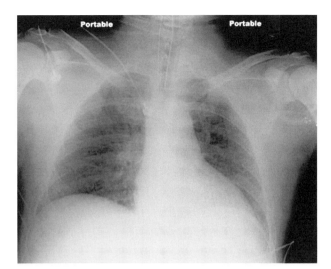

Figure 25.1

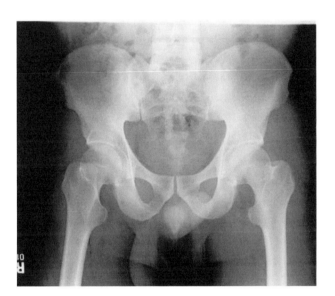

Figure 25.2

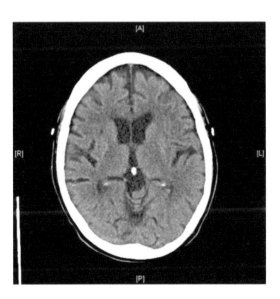

Figure 25.3

L. Action
a. Consult oral/maxillofacial surgery (OMFS)
b. Trauma consult
    i. Admission to trauma service

M. Diagnosis
a. Maxillofacial trauma

N. Critical actions
▇ Early airway control using an advanced airway technique, with cricothyrotomy set up simultaneously
▇ Hemorrhage control
▇ C-spine immobilization
▇ CT head, C-spine, facial bones

O. Examiner instructions
a. This is a case of a midface fracture. Important early actions include prompt and aggressive airway management. Simple airway maneuvers like chin lift, jaw thrust, oropharyngeal suctioning, or pulling tongue forward should be attempted first. If unsuccessful, intubation is required. Evaluation of degree of difficulty for mask ventilation should be undertaken before patient is paralyzed. If it is felt patient cannot be bagged or that intubation will be very difficult, awake intubation should be performed. Simultaneous cricothyrotomy setup should occur during intubation in severe maxillofacial trauma. Typical trauma protocol should be observed and appropriate imaging should be obtained including CTs of head, C-spine, and facial bones.

P. Pearls
a. Maintain C-spine precautions in patients with maxillofacial trauma. Patients with blunt facial injury have a higher incidence of C-spine injury.
b. If teeth are missing, a CXR can be obtained to visualize any teeth that may have been aspirated.
c. Assess for CSF rhinorrhea.
d. When controlling facial bleeding, direct pressure should be applied first. Try to avoid clamping vessels which could cause inadvertent injuries to the facial nerve, parotid duct, and other important such structures.
e. If there is copious amount of blood in oropharynx and unable to see vocal cords, may need to suction and/or perform cricothyrotomy.

Q. References
a. Tintinalli's: Chapter 256. Trauma to the Face
b. Rosen: Chapter 42. Facial Trauma

CASE 26: Burn (Raghu Seethala, MD)

A. Chief complaint
a. 24-year-old male brought in with burn

B. Vital signs
a. BP: 135/73 HR: 126 RR: 20 T: 37.2°C Sat: 98% on RA

C. What does the patient look like?

a. Patient appears stated age. Burns, soot, and blistering are present on face, neck, and chest. Patient suffers moderate distress due to pain and lying supine in stretcher.

D. Primary survey

a. Airway: speaking in full sentences; soot in nares and mouth; burns and blistering over face and mouth
b. Breathing: no apparent respiratory distress, no cyanosis
c. Circulation: normal pulses, normal capillary refill

E. Action

a. Oxygen via nonrebreather mask
b. Two large-bore peripheral IVs
c. Labs
   i. CBC, BMP, LFT, PT/PTT, carboxyhemoglobin, lactate
d. 1 L NS bolus
e. Monitor: BP: 139/79 HR: 116 RR: 20 Sat: 100% on O_2
f. EKG
g. Meds
   i. Morphine 6 mg IV (be sure to enquire about allergies before giving medications, even in emergent cases)

F. History

a. HPI: a 24-year-old male with no past medical history states he was out camping with friends. They were drinking beer and he lost his balance and fell face first into the campfire. Friends were able to pull the patient out. He currently complains of intense pain all over face, neck, arms, and torso.
b. PMHx: none
c. PSHx: none
d. Allergies: none
e. Meds: none
f. Social: social use of alcohol, smoker, denies drug use
g. FHx: not relevant
h. PMD: none

G. Nurse

a. EKG (Figure 26.1)
b. 1 L NS
   i. BP: 130/79 HR: 90 RR: 18 Sat: 98% on O_2

H. Secondary survey

a. General: alert and oriented, moderate distress due to pain
b. HEENT: painful, blistered burns to face, lips, soot on face, in nares, and mouth
c. Neck: painful, blistered burn to anterior neck, significant soft tissue swelling of neck, no stridor
d. Chest: painful, blistered burn involving entire anterior chest, breath sounds clear bilaterally
e. Heart: tachycardic, no murmur
f. Abdomen: painful, blistered burn to anterior abdomen, no guarding, no rebound

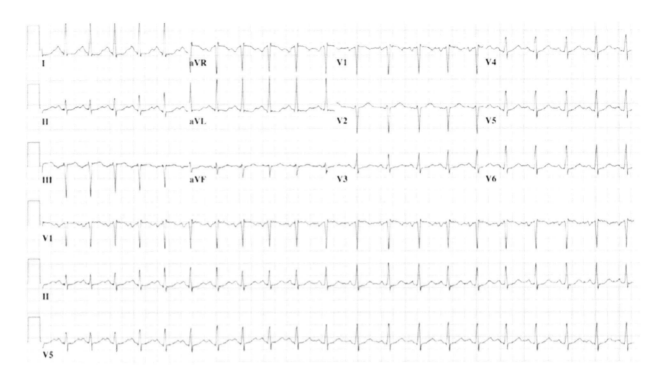

Figure 26.1

g. Urogenital: normal

h. Extremities: circumferential burn to left forearm, skin thickened, white with superficial charring, with minimal sensation, decreased distal pulses

i. Back: normal

j. Neuro: normal

k. Skin: burns as described earlier

l. Lymph: normal

I. Action

a. Intubate

   i. Rapid sequence intubation

b. Fluid administration

   i. Use Parkland formula (Appendix F) to calculate fluid requirements for the first 24 hours; one-half of total fluids should be administered within 8 hours of the burn and other half over the next 16 hours.

c. Nursing

   i. Place Foley catheter

d. Perform escharotomy

e. Imaging

   i. CXR

f. Meds

   i. Tetanus toxoid IM

g. Reassess

   i. Patient intubated requires ongoing sedation and analgesia

J. Nurse

a. BP: 107/80 HR: 99 RR: 18 Sat: 98% on O_2

K. Results

Complete blood count:

WBC	14.1×10^3/uL
Hct	44.5%
Plt	295×10^3/uL

Basic metabolic panel:

Na	138 mEq/L
K	4.2 mEq/L
Cl	101 mEq/L
CO_2	18 mEq/L
BUN	38 mEq/dL
Cr	1.6 mg/dL
Gluc	102 mg/dL

Coagulation panel:

PT	13.1 sec
PTT	26.0 sec
INR	1.0

Liver function panel:

AST	32 U/L
ALT	20 U/L
Alk Phos	89 U/L
T bili	1.5 mg/dL
D bili	0.6 mg/dL
Amylase	25 U/L
Lipase	34 U/L
Albumin	4.0 g/dL

Urinalysis:

SG	1.030
pH	6
Prot	Neg
Gluc	Neg
Ketones	Neg
Bili	Neg
Blood	Neg
LE	Neg
Nitrite	Neg
Color	Yellow

a. Lactate 4.2 mmol/L
b. Carboxyhemoglobin: 5.5
c. Portable CXR (Figure 26.2)

L. Action

a. Contact burn unit
  i. Transfer patient to burn unit
b. Discussion with family regarding need for emergent transfer of the patient to the burn unit
c. Meds
  i. Morphine (or other opioid) boluses or infusion

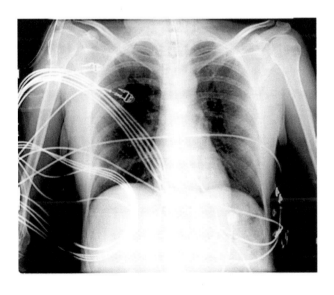

Figure 26.2

M. Diagnosis
a. Thermal burn

N. Critical actions
▪ Large-bore IV access and fluid resuscitation (following Parkland formula)
▪ Analgesia
▪ Intubation
▪ Escharotomy for circumferential third-degree burn to extremity
▪ Tetanus administration
▪ Transfer to burn unit

O. Examiner instructions
a. Important early actions in this case include obtaining large-bore IV access, initiating fluid resuscitation, intubating the patient, and transferring the patent to a burn center. Although the patient did not exhibit stridor or any respiratory distress upon arrival to the ED, it is critical to intubate burn patients presenting with significant swelling of the neck or lower face. If the patient is not intubated before ICU transfer, he will develop significant difficulty breathing due to throat swelling, and intubation will become very difficult. If this occurs, advanced airway techniques (such as fiberoptic intubation or cricothyroidotomy) will be required for successful intubation. If anesthesia or ENT consultants are called to manage the airway early in the case, they will argue that the patient appears well and does not require intubation. If consulted once the patient becomes symptomatic, they will be out of the hospital and unavailable for 20 minutes (necessitating the candidate must manage the airway themselves).

P. Pearls
a. Early intubation is warranted if impending airway compromise is suspected. Stridor, hoarseness, hypoxia, blood gas abnormalities, are often late signs of airway compromise, and signify that airway edema has already become critical.
b. Appropriate fluid resuscitation (following the Parkland formula) requires administration of half the total fluid requirement within 8 hours of the injury, not presentation to the ED. For example, if the patient presents 2 hours after injury the fluids need to be adjusted to administer half within the next 6 hours.
c. Assess for carbon monoxide and cyanide poisoning in all burn patients.
d. Note that this patient had deep circumferential burns to the extremities and required escharotomy. Loss of distal pulses is a late finding and patients with deep circumferential burns require escharotomy to prevent compartment syndrome.

Q. References
a. Tintinalli's: Chapter 210. Thermal Burns
b. Rosen: Chapter 63. Thermal Burns

CASE 27: Vomiting blood (Jessica Berrios, MD)

A. Chief complaint
a. 37-year-old female vomiting blood

B. Vital signs
a. BP: 76/45 HR: 126 RR: 18 T: 36.6°C O$_2$ Sat: 100% on RA

C. What does the patient look like?

a. Patient appears pale, lethargic, and in mild distress.

D. Primary survey

a. Airway: patent, able to speak

b. Breathing: clear lungs, equal breath sounds

c. Circulation: weak pulses, prolonged capillary refill time

E. Action

a. Oxygen via NC

b. Two large-bore peripheral IV lines

c. Place on monitor

d. Labs

    i. CBC, BMP, LFTs, PT/PTT, blood type and cross-match 6 units

e. EKG

f. CXR

g. Urine pregnancy

F. History

a. HPI: a 37-year-old female presents via EMS with three episodes of vomiting bright red blood. Initially the patient was nauseated, and notes epigastric abdominal pain and distension. She denies fevers, no known history of gastrointestinal bleeding.

b. PMHx: alcohol abuse, hepatitis C, cirrhosis

c. PSHx: none; alcohol use daily, denies smoking, drug use

d. Allergies: no known drug or food allergies

e. Meds: none

f. PMD: none

G. Nurse

a. EKG (Figure 27.1)

b. After 1 L saline: BP: 90/55 HR: 120

c. If no saline given: BP: 70/40 HR: 135

H. Secondary survey

a. General: alert and oriented, moderate distress

b. HEENT: pale mucous membranes, icteric sclera, oropharynx clear, no masses, no blood in nares or mouth

c. Neck: no lymphadenopathy, supple

d. Chest: clear, equal air movement bilaterally, no rales

e. Heart: regular rate, no murmurs, capillary refill time >2 seconds

f. Abdomen: tender epigastric area, distended, + fluid wave

g. Rectal: hemoccult negative brown stool

h. Extremities: no edema

i. Back: normal

j. Neuro: normal

k. Skin: cool, clammy skin of extremities, spider angiomas

I. Action

a. NS IV bolus

b. Octreotide drip

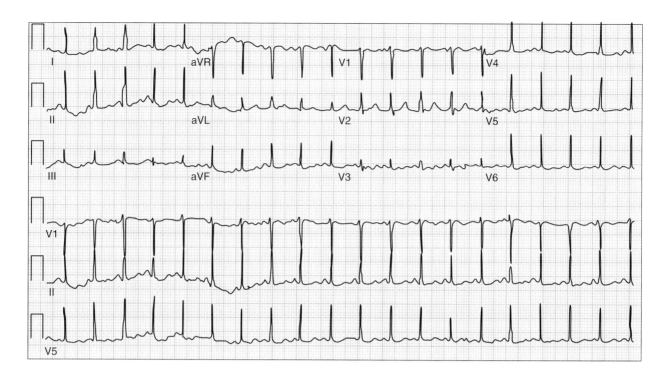

Figure 27.1

   c. Esomeprazole drip
   d. Transfuse 2 units packed red blood cells
   e. Place nasogastric tube
   f. Consult gastroenterologist (GI) for emergent esophagogastroduodenoscopy (EGD)

J. Results

Complete blood count:

WBC	4.5×10^3/uL	D bili	0.6 mg/dL
Hct	18.1%	Amylase	50 U/L
Plt	44×10^3/uL	Lipase	180 U/L
		Albumin	2.8 g/dL

Basic metabolic panel:

Na	130 mEq/L
K	4.6 mEq/L
Cl	101 mEq/L
CO_2	20 mEq/L
BUN	40 mEq/dL
Cr	1.0 mg/dL
Gluc	188 mg/dL

Urinalysis:

SG	1.030
pH	6.5
Prot	Neg
Gluc	Neg
Ketones	Neg
Bili	Neg
Blood	Trace
LE	Neg
Nitrite	Neg
Color	Yellow

Coagulation panel:

PT	12 sec
PTT	38 sec
INR	2.3

Arterial blood gas:

pH	7.4
PO_2	88 mmHg
PCO_2	40 mmHg
HCO_3	20 mmol/L

Liver function panel:

AST	47 U/L
ALT	26 U/L
Alk Phos	269 U/L
T bili	4.6 mg/dL

Figure 27.2

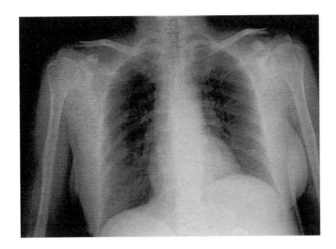

a. Urine pregnancy test: negative
b. CXR (Figure 27.2)

K. Action
a. Continue IV fluids
b. Fresh frozen plasma (FFP) transfusion
c. Platelet transfusion
d. Prophylactic antibiotics (such as ciprofloxacin)
e. Admission to ICU

L. Diagnosis
a. Variceal bleeding (upper GI bleeding)

M. Critical actions
▨ Large-bore IV access
▨ Hemodynamic monitoring
▨ Blood transfusion
▨ Platelet/FFP transfusion
▨ GI consultation
▨ ICU admission

N. Examiner instructions
a. This is a case of variceal bleeding in a cirrhotic patient. Patients with advanced liver disease due to long-term alcohol abuse often develop dilated veins (varices) in the esophagus which can rupture and bleed profusely. Red blood in vomitus is most likely variceal or due to gastric ulcers. Adequate IV access, early fluid resuscitation, blood transfusions, and emergent GI evaluation are critical steps in the management. If fluids and blood are not transfused rapidly, the patient's blood pressure will drop and she will become obtunded. The gastroenterologist should at first plan to manage the patient without EGD ("Keep giving her fluids, and I'll see her in the morning."); the candidate should advocate for emergent EGD, noting a strong suspicion for bleeding varices which would require banding or sclerotherapy. When the EGD is performed (in the ED or once the patient arrives in the ICU), it will reveal bleeding varices which were successfully banded.

O. Pearls

a. Three primary goals of emergent therapy for brisk upper GI bleeding are as follows:
   i. Hemodynamic resuscitation – two large-bore IV lines or central line, blood with clotting factors and platelets as needed;
   ii. Prevention and treatment of complications – prophylactic antibiotics in cirrhotic patients before endoscopy (ciprofloxacin or ceftriaxone);
   iii. Treatment of bleeding with medications and endoscopy.

b. Early endoscopy confirms the diagnosis and allows for definitive management in most cases.

c. If bleeding is not effectively controlled, balloon tamponade with a Sengstaken-Blakemore tube (for less than 24 hours) as a bridge to further therapy may be initiated. Severe cases failing medical management and EGD may be candidates for transjugular intrahepatic portosystemic shunt (TIPS). A trial of IV vasopressin could also be considered, especially when EGD is not readily available.

d. No need for aggressive fluids; permissive hypotension may result in a better outcome.

P. References

a. Tintinalli's: Chapter 78. Upper Gastrointestinal Bleeding
b. Rosen : Chapter 30. Gastrointestinal Bleeding
c. NICE Clinical Guideline 141. Acute Upper GI Bleeding. June 2012. Guidance.nice. org.uk/cg141

CASE 28: Light-headedness (Jessica Berrios, MD)

A. Chief complaint

a. 87-year-old female brought in with the complaint of light-headedness

B. Vital signs

a. BP: 116/65 HR: 36 RR: 18 T: 36.6°C O_2 Sat: 96% on RA

C. What does the patient look like?

a. Patient appears stated age, in mild respiratory distress.

D. Primary survey

a. Airway: patent, speaking in full sentences
b. Breathing: mild respiratory distress
c. Circulation: pale, cool skin, delayed capillary refill

E. Action

a. Oxygen via NC or nonrebreather mask
b. Finger stick blood glucose (235; must ask)
c. Two large-bore peripheral IV lines
d. Cardiac monitor
e. Labs
   i. CBC, BMP, cardiac enzymes, PT/PTT, blood type and hold
f. Obtain EKG
g. CXR

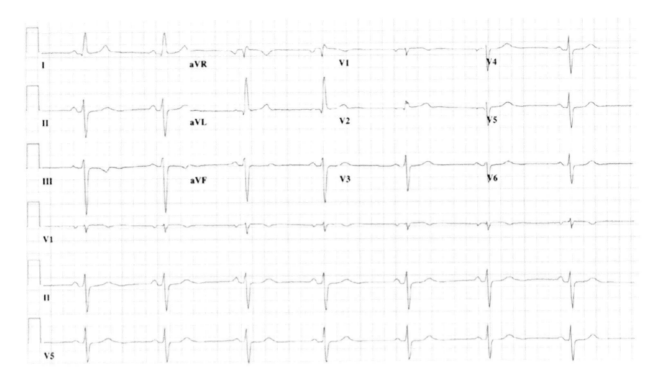

Figure 28.1

F. History

a. HPI: a 87-year-old female with substernal chest pain described as pressure different than previous chest pain. Also notes shortness of breath, nausea, and one episode of vomiting. Patient denies cough or fever, no neurological complaints, no recent travel or surgery; no known drug ingestions/overdose history.

b. PMHx: coronary artery disease, hypertension, type 2 diabetes, atrial fibrillation

c. PSHx: hysterectomy 40 years ago

d. Allergies: none

e. Meds: warfarin, metoprolol, insulin

f. Social: nonsmoker, denies alcohol use, lives alone

g. FHx: hypertension, diabetes

h. PMD: Dr Sharma

G. Nurse

a. EKG (Figure 28.1)

b. Place transcutaneous pacing pads on patient's chest

H. Secondary survey

a. General: alert and oriented, mild distress

b. HEENT: normal

c. Neck: no jugular venous distension, supple

d. Chest: clear, equal air movement bilaterally, no rales

e. Heart: regular rate, no murmurs, capillary refill time >2 seconds

f. Abdomen: normal

g. Rectal: hemoccult negative brown stool

h. Extremities: no edema, normal pulses

    i. Back: normal

    j. Neuro: normal

    k. Skin: cool, delayed capillary refill

I. Action

a. Atropine 0.5 mg IV can be given, up to 3 mg total, every 5 minutes

b. Cardiology consultation

c. Glucagon IV

J. Nurse

a. No response to atropine; heart rate remains in low 40s, patient complains of more shortness of breath, becoming hypotensive, lethargic

K. Action

a. NS bolus IV

b. Begin transcutaneous pacing

L. Results

Complete blood count:

WBC	10×10^3/uL	BUN	24 mEq/dL
Hct	36.0%	Cr	0.7 mg/dL
Plt	399×10^3/uL	Gluc	248 mg/dL

Basic metabolic panel :   **Coagulation panel :**

Na	133 mEq/L	PT	12 sec
K	4.4 mEq/L	PTT	38 sec
Cl	97 mEq/L	INR	2.2
CO_2	24 mEq/L		

a. CK: 77

b. Troponin: negative

c. Magnesium: 2.2 mg/dL

d. CXR: Figure 28.2

e. EKG: now paced at 70

Figure 28.2

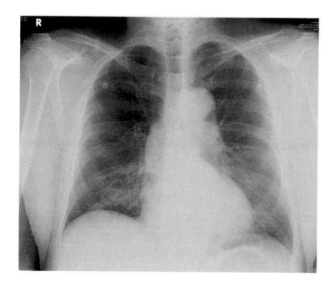

M. Action
a. Prepare for transvenous pacing (in ED or cardiac catheterization laboratory)
b. Admission to ICU

N. Diagnosis
a. Bradycardia

O. Critical actions
▓ EKG
▓ Obtain oxygen saturation
▓ Atropine 0.5 mg IV (may repeat up to total 3 mg) or Glucagon 5–10 mg IV
▓ Pacing (transcutaneous or transvenous)
▓ Cardiology consultation
▓ Admission to ICU

P. Examiner instructions
a. This is a case of symptomatic bradycardia. This patient's heart rate has become very low (likely due to rate-controlling medications like metoprolol), which is decreasing her blood flow and causing symptoms of dizziness and chest pain. Important management steps include immediate cardiac monitoring, electrocardiogram, transcutaneous pacing, and cardiology consultation. Assessing immediate response is important for further workup or need for transvenous pacing. If the candidate attempts to treat a possible β-blocker overdose with glucagon, this strategy will be ineffective and pacing will still be necessary.
b. Curveball: transcutaneous pacing could fail, forcing the candidate to place a transvenous pacemaker themselves; have them describe the procedure.

Q. Pearls
a. For patients who are symptomatic, transcutaneous pacing should be initiated immediately. If the external pacer fails to capture, a transvenous pacer should be inserted emergently.
b. Unstable patients (or any patient with signs of decreased perfusion due to bradycardia) may be treated with atropine.
c. Consider β-blocker toxicity in patients with significant bradycardia; a glucagon bolus and drip can be administered to diagnose and treat this condition.
d. Atropine is ineffective in patients with a deinnervated heart (eg, those patients who are postcardiac transplant).
e. In severe β-blocker toxicity, may consider vasopressors (epinephrine or norepinephrine). Intralipid therapy for lipid-soluble drugs may be effective in decreasing its bioavailability.

R. References
a. Tintinalli's: Chapter 22. Cardiac Rhythm Disturbances, Chapter 188. Beta Blockers
b. Rosen: Chapter 79. Dysrhythmias

CASE 29: Shortness of breath (Jessica Berrios, MD)

A. Chief complaint
a. 37-year-old male with shortness of breath

B. Vital signs

a. BP: 156/60 HR: 116 RR: 28 T: 36.8°C O_2 Sat: 90% on RA

C. What does the patient look like?

a. Patient appears stated age, in moderate respiratory distress.

D. Primary survey

a. Airway: patent

b. Breathing: moderate respiratory distress, using accessory muscles, wheezing bilaterally with prolonged expiration

c. Circulation: warm, normal capillary refill and pulses

E. Action

a. Oxygen via nonrebreather mask

b. Two large-bore peripheral IV lines

c. Labs

    i. CBC, BMP, cardiac enzymes, PT/PTT, blood type and hold

d. Cardiac monitor

e. Obtain EKG

f. CXR

g. Obtain peak flow reading

F. History

a. HPI: a 37-year-old obese male presents with complaint of progressive shortness of breath associated with dry cough for 2 hours, also states he has been having upper respiratory symptoms this week. He used his albuterol inhaler several times before coming to the ED. Patient denies fevers, nausea, vomiting, diarrhea, recent travel, or surgery.

b. PMHx: asthma (two previous intubations, two ICU visits in the last 5 years), hypertension, type 2 diabetes

c. PSHx: inguinal hernia repair

d. Allergies: none

e. Meds: albuterol and fluticasone inhalers, prednisone

f. Social: denies tobacco, drug, or alcohol use

g. FHx: asthma, hypertension, diabetes

h. PMD: Dr Franklin

G. Action

a. Albuterol nebulizers, continuous

b. Ipratropium nebulizer every 20 minutes x 3 doses

c. Methylprednisolone 125 mg IV

d. Magnesium 1–2 grams IV

H. Secondary survey

a. General: alert and oriented, moderate respiratory distress

b. HEENT: lips cyanotic, no stridor; oropharynx clear, no lesions, no lymphadenopathy, or masses

c. Neck: no jugular venous distension, supple

Figure 29.1

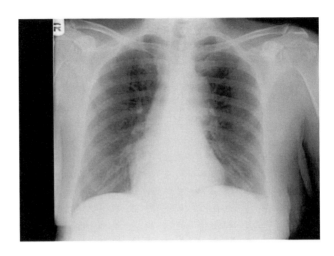

d. Chest: diffuse inspiratory and expiratory wheezing, poor air movement, no rales; peak flow: 180 L/minute

e. Heart: tachycardic, no murmurs

f. Abdomen: normal

g. Extremities: no edema, normal pulses

h. Back: normal

i. Neuro: normal

j. Skin: normal

I. Nurse

a. Patient is not responding to therapy: O$_2$ sat 90% on oxygen, and patient remains tachypneic

b. CXR (Figure 29.1)

J. Action

a. Administer terbutaline 0.25 mg SC or epinephrine 0.3 mg SC

b. Trial of bilevel positive airway pressure (BiPAP) with in-line continuous nebulized albuterol

c. ICU admission

K. Results

Complete blood count:			Coagulation panel :	
WBC	12.0 × 10³/uL		PT	12.3–15.5 sec
Hct	36.0%		PTT	25.4–35.0 sec
Plt	288 × 10³/uL		INR	0.9–1.3

Basic metabolic panel :			Arterial blood gas:	
Na	134 mEq/L		pH	7.45
K	4.2 mEq/L		PO$_2$	62 mmHg
Cl	102 mEq/L		PCO$_2$	24 mmHg
CO$_2$	21 mEq/L		HCO$_3$	20 mmol/L
BUN	11 mEq/dL			
Cr	1.0 mg/dL			
Gluc	210 mg/dL			

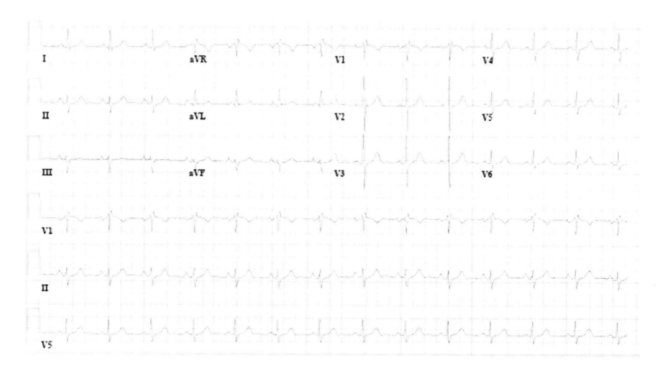

Figure 29.2

a. EKG (Figure 29.2)

L. Nurse

a. Patient has less accessory muscle use, more comfortable; RR: 24 O$_2$ sat: 96% on BiPAP

M. Diagnosis

a. Acute asthma exacerbation (status asthmaticus)

N. Critical actions

▨ Pulse oximetry

▨ Cardiac monitoring

▨ Supplemental oxygen

▨ Administration of albuterol, ipratropium, and steroids

▨ Frequent reassessment for clinical improvement

▨ Adjunctive therapies for severe asthma (such as magnesium, epinephrine or terbutaline, BiPAP)

▨ Admission to ICU

O. Examiner instructions

a. This is a case of a severe asthma exacerbation. A combination of bronchospasm (smooth muscle spasms in the lungs) and inflammation causes difficulty in breathing and cough. First-line therapies (nebulized β-agonists and anticholinergics in addition to steroids) were insufficient to provide rapid relief in this case; the candidate should recognize this and move to adjunctive therapeutic options (such as terbutaline or epinephrine, magnesium, BiPAP). If the patient is intubated, blood pressure should drop and heart rate increase unless a fluid bolus (at least 1L NS) is administered.

P. Pearls

a. Magnesium sulfate has shown benefit in severe asthma exacerbations; it is less useful in mild to moderate cases.

b. Helium-oxygen mixtures (Heliox) have not been shown to improve outcomes in acute asthma.

c. Empiric use of antibiotics is not recommended.

d. In patients who deteriorate despite usual therapeutic efforts, evidence supports a trial of positive-pressure mask ventilation before intubation.

e. Arterial blood gas (ABG) parameters are often used to guide treatment in patients with severe asthma and may aid in decision making by providing quantitative information on pulmonary gas exchange.

f. Hypercapnia is usually a late finding that reflects increasing airflow obstruction and fatigue because of the increased work of breathing. The decision to intubate should be based on clinical grounds, rather than on ABG determinations alone.

g. Indications for intubation include cardiac or respiratory arrest, severe hypoxia, exhaustion, or deterioration of mental status. Note that intubation alone does not correct the underlying pathology of the exacerbation (airflow obstruction). Ventilator settings on intubated asthmatic patients are very difficult to manage, and hypotension after intubation commonly occurs. This is due to decreased preload from high intrathoracic pressures in these patients. Vent settings should include low tidal volumes and prolonged expiratory times (1:3 I:E ratio) to avoid barotrauma.

Q. References

a. Tintinalli's: Chapter 72. Acute Asthma in Adults

b. Rosen: Chapter 73. Asthma

CASE 30: Rash and fever (Jessica Berrios, MD)

A. Chief complaint

a. 27-year-old female with rash and fever

B. Vital signs

a. BP: 106/65 HR: 86 RR: 20 T: 38.6°C O_2 Sat: 99% on RA

C. What does the patient look like?

a. Patient appears stated age, alert, in mild distress from pain.

D. Primary survey

a. Airway: patent, speaking full sentences

b. Breathing: clear bilaterally, no wheezing

c. Circulation: good radial pulses, capillary refill time normal

E. History

a. HPI: a 27-year-old female presents with fever, chills, and malaise that started 3 days ago. She noted a red rash last night to upper chest and neck area, now spreading to abdomen and arms. The rash is mildly tender, not pruritic. She also developed ulcers in her mouth and suffered pain with urination. HIV status unknown and no previous similar rash noted. Last menstrual period was 2 weeks ago, denies use of tampons.

b. PMHx: urinary tract infection (UTI)

c. PSHx: none

d. Allergies: no known drug or food allergies

e. Meds: started on sulfamethoxazole and trimethoprim for UTI 5 days ago

f. Social: smoker (1 pack per day for 10 years), occasional alcohol use, denies drugs, monogamous with husband

g. PMD: none

F. Action

a. IV access

b. Labs

i. CBC, BMP, UA, urine pregnancy test, blood and urine cultures, CXR

c. Monitor

d. EKG

e. CXR

f. Administer acetaminophen or ibuprofen for fever

G. Secondary survey

a. General: alert and oriented, comfortable after antipyretic administered

b. HEENT: small oral erosions to bilateral buccal mucosa, palate, and lips with crusting; injected sclera bilaterally; tympanic membranes normal, nares clear

c. Neck: supple, no lymphadenopathy

d. Chest: normal

e. Heart: normal

f. Abdomen: normal

g. Urogenital: small red erosions near introitus of vagina, no crusting or vesicles noted

h. Extremities: no edema, normal pulses

i. Back: normal

j. Neuro: normal

k. Skin: symmetric red, purpuric mildly tender macules and plaques over neck and chest, extensor surfaces of arms (~10%) with vesicles and bullae, some with sloughing and necrosis of larger plaques, bullae spread with pressure, some appear like target lesions

H. Nurse

a. EKG (Figure 30.1)

b. CXR (Figure 30.2)

I. Results

Complete blood count:

WBC	11.0×10^3/uL	BUN	14 mEq/dL
Hct	32.0%	Cr	0.7 mg/dL
Plt	332×10^3/uL	Gluc	121 mg/dL

Basic metabolic panel: | **Coagulation panel:**

Na	142 mEq/L	PT	15 sec
K	4 mEq/L	PTT	28.0 sec
Cl	101 mEq/L	INR	0.9
CO_2	22 mEq/L		

Liver function panel:

AST	22 U/L	Gluc	Neg
ALT	23 U/L	Ketones	Neg
Alk Phos	55 U/L	Bili	Neg
T bili	0.7 mg/dL	Blood	Trace
D bili	0.1 mg/dL	LE	Trace
Amylase	30 U/L	Nitrite	Neg
Lipase	100 U/L	Color	Yellow
Albumin	3.8 g/dL		

Arterial blood gas:

Urinalysis:

		pH	7.35
SG	1.015	PO_2	88 mmHg
pH	6	PCO_2	44 mmHg
Prot	Neg	HCO_3	25 mmol/L

J. Action

a. Dermatology consultation

b. ICU admission

c. NS bolus

K. Diagnosis

a. Stevens–Johnson Syndrome

L. Critical actions

▓ Obtain history of recent antibiotic use

▓ Skin examination

▓ Establish diagnosis of Stevens–Johnson Syndrome

Figure 30.1

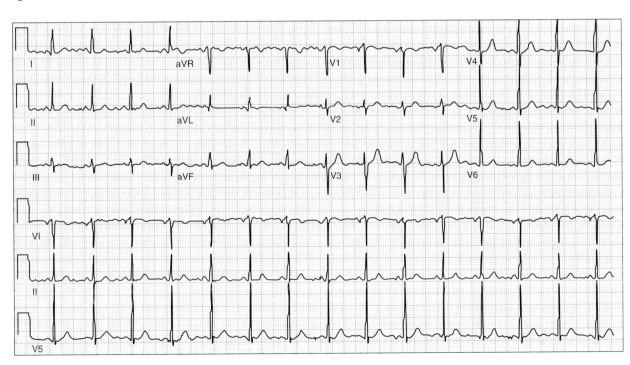

A

B

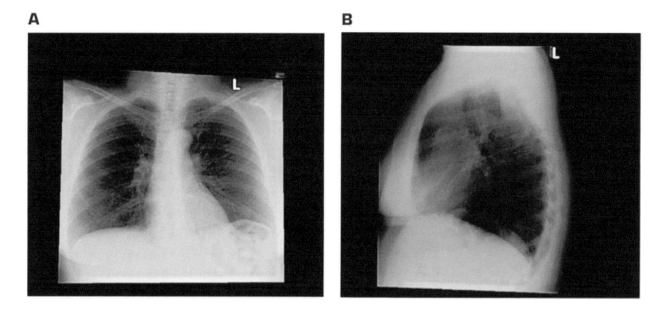

Figure 30.2 A and B

- Stop the offending agent
- Dermatology and ophthalmology consultation
- ICU admission

M. Examiner instructions

a. This is a case of Stevens–Johnson syndrome, a vesiculobullous disease with acute inflammatory reaction in the skin and mucosa. Although the exact pathophysiology is not well known, this syndrome is often associated with medication reactions and infections. This patient is taking a sulfur-containing antibiotic for her UTI, which is likely the culprit. Important actions include making the diagnosis on the basis of history and physical examination, contacting dermatology, and admitting the patient to a burn unit. When consulted, the dermatologist will not be able to provide any additional assistance beyond agreeing with the candidate's plan for admission and IV fluids. They will not be able to help make the diagnosis for the candidate. Early ophthalmology consult will prevent/treat involvement of the eyes.

N. Pearls

a. Medications are the most common trigger. Among those implicated include antibiotics (penicillins, sulfonamides, and cephalosporins), antiepileptics, nonsteroidal antiinflammatory agents, antipsychotics, and antigout medications.

b. Patients with HIV who take sulfamethoxazole and trimethoprim are at 40 times greater risk of developing Stevens–Johnson syndrome.

c. Ocular involvement is very common (70%)

d. The syndrome carries a 1% to 3% mortality. Sepsis is the major cause of death.

e. Prophylactic IV antibiotics are not routinely recommended – treatment includes removing the causative agent and supportive care.

f. Intravenous immunoglobulins (IVIGs), steroids, and plasmapharesis have been studied, but insufficient evidence exists to recommend their use in all patients.

O. References
a. Tintinalli's: Chapter 245. Serious Generalized Skin Disorders
b. Rosen: Chapter 120. Dermatologic Presentations

CASE 31: Weakness (Jessica Berrios, MD)

A. Chief complaint
a. 67-year-old male with weakness and difficulty walking

B. Vital signs
a. BP: 146/65 HR: 106 RR: 18 T: 37.6°C O$_2$ Sat: 95% on RA

C. What does the patient look like?
a. Patient appears comfortable, lying supine in stretcher.

D. Primary survey
a. Airway: patent, no secretions
b. Breathing: clear and unlabored
c. Circulation: strong pulses, normal capillary refill

E. History:
a. HPI: a 67-year-old male presents with weakness of both legs and difficulty walking. His symptoms have been progressively worsening over several days. He also complains of progressive shortness of breath, dry cough, dyspnea on exertion, dizziness, and parasthesias of his hands and feet. He notes recent diarrhea, now improving; denies fever, headache, vision changes, difficulty speaking or swallowing, denies pain, no known tick bites, no recent travel.
b. PMHx: hypertension
c. PSHx: none
d. Allergies: no known drug or food allergies
e. Meds: amlodipine
f. Social: smoker for 20 years, 1.5 packs per week, drinks two glasses wine daily, denies drug use
g. FHx: hypertension
h. PMD: none

F. Action
a. Oxygen via NC
b. Two large-bore peripheral IV lines
c. Labs
    i. CBC, BMP, erythrocyte sedimentation rate (ESR), UA, ABG
d. Cardiac monitor
e. Finger stick blood glucose (120)
f. EKG
g. CXR

G. Secondary survey

a. General: alert and oriented, comfortable

b. HEENT: normal cephalic, atraumatic, extraocular movements intact, pupils equal and reactive to light, 3 mm, oropharynx clear, no exudates

c. Neck: weakness of neck muscles; neck supple, no lymphadenopathy

d. Chest: clear, poor effort, no wheezing or rales

e. Heart: normal

f. Abdomen: soft, distended suprapubic area with associated mild pain with palpation, normal bowel sounds

g. Urogenital: normal

h. Extremities: no edema, normal pulses

i. Back: normal

j. Neuro: normal cranial nerves II to XII; 2/5 strength in lower extremities, 4/5 in upper extremities, no deep tendon reflexes of lower extremities; sensation intact, normal sphincter tone; unable to walk, appears ataxic in the upper extremities

k. Skin: normal, no lesions

H. Action

a. Lumbar puncture

I. Results

Complete blood count:

WBC	5.2×10^3/uL	D bili	0.1 mg/dL
Hct	32.8%	Amylase	50 U/L
Plt	232×10^3/uL	Lipase	78 U/L
		Albumin	3.8 g/dL

Basic metabolic panel:

Na	142 mEq/L	**Urinalysis:**	
K	4.0 mEq/L	SG	1.020
Cl	101 mEq/L	pH	5
CO_2	22 mEq/L	Prot	Neg
BUN	14 mEq/dL	Gluc	Neg
Cr	0.7 mg/dL	Ketones	Neg
Gluc	121 mg/dL	Bili	Neg
		Blood	Neg
Coagulation panel:		LE	Neg
PT	12.8 sec	Nitrite	Neg
PTT	25.0 sec	Color	Yellow
INR	1.0		
		Arterial blood gas:	
		pH	7.42
Liver function panel:		PO_2	80 mmHg
AST	24 U/L	PCO_2	48 mmHg
ALT	17 U/L	HCO_3	25 mmol/L
Alk Phos	77 U/L		
T bili	0.4 mg/dL		

a. ESR: 30

b. LP: Protein 400, normal cell count and glucose, Gram stain negative

c. EKG (Figure 31.1)

d. CXR (Figure 31.2)

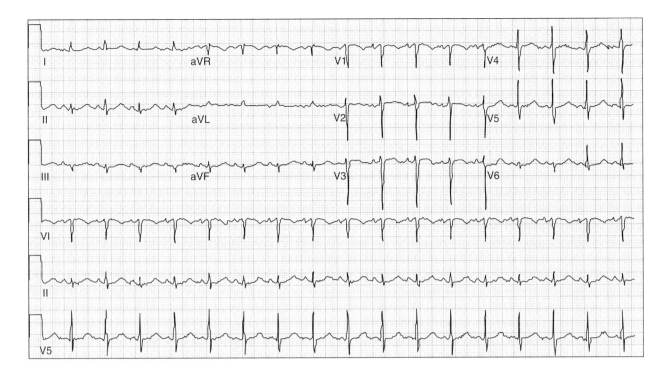

Figure 31.1

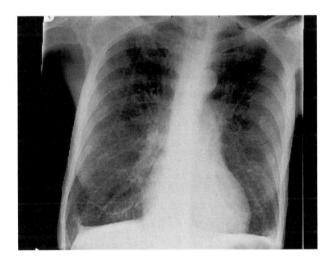

Figure 31.2

J. Nurse

a. Patient appears lethargic, more tachypneic, shallow breaths; O_2 sat 92% on 2 L via NC, complaining of increasing heaviness to head and arms

K. Action

a. Call respiratory therapist for forced vital capacity (FVC) and negative inspiratory force (NIF)
   i. FVC below normal
   ii. NIF below normal
b. Place non rebreather mask, prepare equipment for intubation

c. After discussion with patient and family, perform intubation for declining respiratory status, airway protection

d. Consult neurology

e. Admission to ICU

f. Administer IV immunoglobulin or plasma exchange

L. Diagnosis

a. Guillain–Barre syndrome (GBS)

M. Critical actions

▨ Obtain finger stick blood glucose

▨ Complete neurologic examination including motor, sensory and reflexes

▨ Establish diagnosis of GBS

▨ Neurology consultation

▨ Recognize worsening respiratory status, electively intubate

▨ Admission to ICU

▨ Begin plasma exchange or IV immunoglobulin

N. Examiner instructions

a. This is a case of Guillain–Barre syndrome (GBS), a demyelinating peripheral nerve disease characterized by progressive ascending symmetrical weakness/paralysis with loss of deep tendon reflexes. The diaphragmatic muscles may be affected, causing respiratory compromise and may require intubation. GBS is usually preceded by a viral illness or *Campylobacter jejuni* diarrhea infection. It is important to distinguish the GBS symptoms from stroke, metabolic disorders, or other causes of weakness. The candidate must recognize that the patient's symptoms have worsened, and intubation based on clinical assessment (worsening respiratory status) or pulmonary function (respiratory testing) should be initiated. A neurologist should be consulted, and the patient should be admitted to the ICU.

b. If the patient is intubated using succinylcholine as a paralytic, he will lose his pulse and demonstrate a wide-complex tachycardia (consistent with severe hyperkalemia) on the monitor. Standard ACLS protocols will be unsuccessful, unless calcium and other acute therapy for hyperkalemia are rapidly initiated.

O. Pearls

a. Up to 30% of patients with GBS will require ventilatory support. Predictors of respiratory failure include inability to cough, stand, lift the elbows or head, and elevated liver enzymes.

b. Indications for intubation are largely clinical; however, some quantitative measures include a forced vital capacity less than 20 cc/kg, NIF less than 30 cm H_2O, aspiration, rapid progression of weakness, and autonomic instability.

c. Succinylcholine should not be used when intubating patients with GBS. As with any demyelinating disorder, acetyl cholinesterase receptors are up-regulated. This can cause severe, prolonged hyperkalemia when a depolarizing neuromuscular blocker is used.

d. A lumbar puncture and/or nerve conduction studies may help to diagnose GBS.

P. References

a. Tintinalli's: Chapter 166. Acute Peripheral Neurologic Lesions

b. Rosen: Chapter 108. Neuromuscular Disorders

CASE 32: Abdominal pain and vomiting (Natasha Spencer, MD, PhD)

A. Chief complaint

a. 51-year-old female with abdominal pain and vomiting

B. Vital signs

a. BP: 136/78 HR: 64 RR: 20 T: 35.9°C Sat: 100% on RA

C. What does the patient look like?

a. Patient appears to be in severe pain.

D. Primary survey

a. Airway: speaking in full sentences
b. Breathing: no apparent respiratory distress, no cyanosis
c. Circulation: pale and cool skin, normal capillary refill

E. Action

a. IV access
b. Labs
    i. CBC, BMP, LFT, lipase, PT/PTT, HCG, blood type and cross-match, lactate
c. 1 L NS bolus
d. EKG
e. Morphine IV
f. Nothing by mouth (NPO)

F. History

a. HPI: a 51-year-old female with hypertension and asthma presents with lower abdominal pain for the past 2 days. The pain is intermittent, feels tight and squeezing and has been increasing in severity. She notes nausea and vomiting food for the past day. She denies diarrhea, fever, dysuria, chest pain, vaginal bleeding, or shortness of breath. Her last bowel movement was yesterday and normal in quality.
b. PMHx: hypertension, asthma
c. PSHx: appendectomy, tubal ligation, bladder surgery
d. Allergies: none
e. Meds: esomeprazole, loratadine, gabapentin, rofecoxib, fluticasone, zolpidem
f. Social: lives with family at home, denies alcohol, smoking, drugs
g. FHx: not relevant

G. Nurse

a. EKG (Figure 32.1)
    i. BP: 136/78 HR: 64 RR: 20 T: 35.9°C Sat: 100% on RA

H. Secondary survey

a. General: alert and oriented, severe distress due to pain
b. HEENT: normal
c. Neck: normal
d. Chest: normal

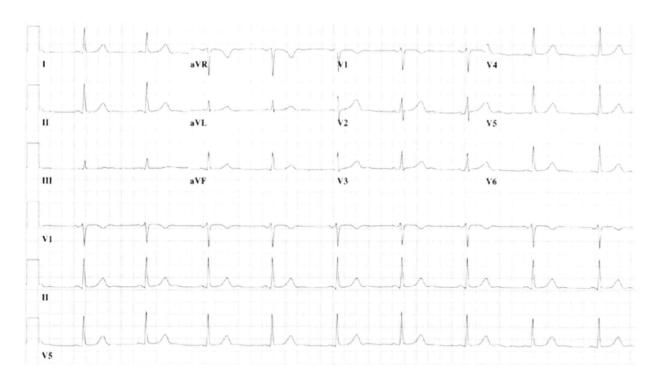

Figure 32.1

   e. Heart: normal
   f. Abdomen: bilateral lower quadrant tenderness with guarding; bowel sounds normal, mild distension, no masses, no hernias, nontender at McBurney's point, negative Murphy's sign
   g. Rectal: hemoccult negative
   h. Pelvic: normal
   i. Extremities: normal
   j. Back: normal
   k. Neuro: normal
   l. Skin: warm and dry; no rash or induration
   m. Lymph: normal

I. Action
  a. Meds
    i. Morphine IV
  b. Reassess
    i. Patient continues to have significant discomfort
  c. Consult
    i. Surgery
  d. Imaging
    i. Obstructive series
    ii. Abdominal CT with contrast

J. Nurse
  a. BP: 113/65 HR: 60 RR: 18 Sat: 100% on O_2 RA
  b. Patient: continues to have significant pain (until a total of 6 mg of morphine or equivalent is administered)

H. Results

Complete blood count:

WBC	12.6×10^3/uL	Alk Phos	181 U/L
Hct	37.4%	T bili	0.4 mg/dL
Plt	253×10^3/uL	D bili	0.2 mg/dL
		Amylase	71 U/L
Basic metabolic panel:		Lipase	77 U/L
Na	143 mEq/L	Albumin	4.1 g/dL
K	4.1 mEq/L		
Cl	105 mEq/L	**Urinalysis:**	
CO_2	25 mEq/L	SG	1.022
BUN	12 mEq/dL	pH	6
Cr	0.8 mg/dL	Prot	Neg
Gluc	96 mg/dL	Gluc	Neg
		Ketones	Neg
Coagulation panel:		Bili	Neg
PT	11.9 sec	Blood	Neg
PTT	28 sec	LE	Neg
INR	0.9	Nitrite	Neg
		Color	Yellow
Liver function panel:			
AST	24 U/L		
ALT	22 U/L		

a. CXR (Figure 32.2)

b. Obstructive series (Figures 32.3 and 32.4)

c. Abdominal CT with IV, oral, and rectal contrast (radiology report)

K. Action

a. Surgery consult

    i. Advocate for patient admission

b. Discussion with patient about need for admission

c. Meds

    i. Morphine IV (if patient remains in significant pain)

    ii. Antibiotics IV

d. Nasogastric tube for decompression

L. Diagnosis

a. Small bowel obstruction (SBO)

M. Critical actions

▓ IV access and fluid bolus

▓ Obstructive series with upright chest x-ray

▓ Pain management

▓ Surgery consult

▓ NG tube

N. Examiner instructions

a. This is a case of small bowel obstruction. The patient is at increased risk of obstruction because of her prior abdominal surgeries, which can lead to scarring

Figure 32.2

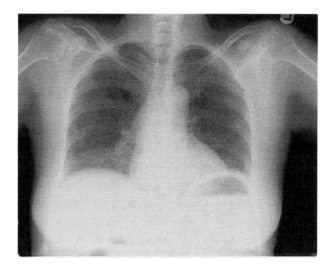

Figure 32.3

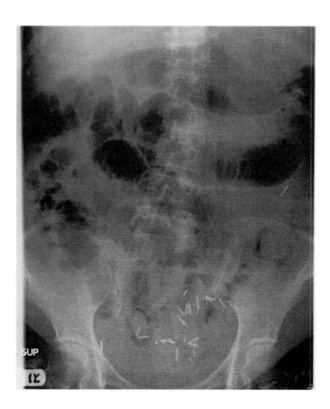

and adhesions that may block proper flow of intestinal contents. Important early actions include administering IV fluids, consulting surgery, decompressing the stomach, and pain control. If fluids are not administered, the patient may become tachycardic and hypotensive. Her pain will continue to increase until an opioid medication (such as morphine) is administered. An obstructive series (patient supine and then upright) and an upright chest x-ray can be readily obtained; if a CT scan is ordered, note that the scanner is busy, and it will "be a while" before the test can be performed. If a nasogastric tube is not placed after diagnosis, the patient may continue vomiting and aspirate. If the patient is sent home, the patient should return to the ED in 2 hours with peritonitis.

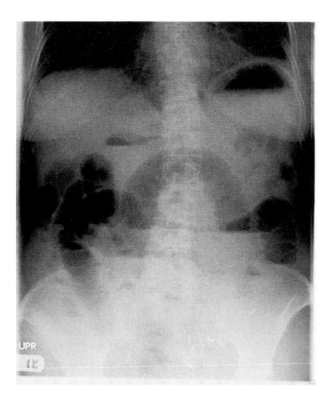

Figure 32.4

O. Pearls

a. Obstructive series (plain abdominal films with the patient supine and then upright) with upright CXR are useful for ruling out free air, and may help localize causes and sites of obstruction. The x-rays may reveal distended loops of small bowel and the upright abdominal film may show a pattern of intestinal air-fluid arranged similarly to a stepladder proximal to the obstruction.

b. Abdominal CT with contrast is not always necessary, but is often useful for differentiating a dynamic ileus from mechanical SBO, diagnosing bowel strangulation (which can occur with incarcerated hernia), and determining a specific transition point (such as a tumor) amenable to surgical intervention.

c. Middle-aged and elderly patients with epigastric pain should be evaluated for coronary ischemia. Non-chest pain presentations are common in this age group, especially upper abdominal pain and/or shortness of breath.

d. Patients should be hydrated with IV fluid to replace fluid loss (vomiting and intestinal third-spacing and lack of oral intake).

e. If an immediate operation is advocated or if the patient has signs of peritonitis or ischemia, the patient should be given broad-spectrum antibiotics.

f. Place NG tube for gastric decompression.

g. Surgical intervention is often needed to correct obstruction although a trial of medical management initially can be pursued for obstruction that has not been complicated by ischemia, peritonitis, or bowel perforation.

P. References

a. Tintinalli's: Chapter 86. Bowel Obstruction and Volvulus

b. Rosen: Chapter 92. Disorders of the Small Intestine

CASE 33: Chest pain (Natasha Spencer, MD, PhD)

A. Chief complaint

a. 37-year-old male with chest pain

B. Vital signs

a. BP: 143/69 HR: 100 RR: 20 T: 35.7°C Sat: 99% on RA

C. What does the patient look like?

a. Patient is agitated and uncomfortable.

D. Primary survey

a. Airway: speaking in full sentences
b. Breathing: clear to auscultation bilaterally, no apparent respiratory distress, no cyanosis
c. Circulation: tachycardic, radial pulses 2+ bilaterally, fingertips warm, pink

E. Action

a. Oxygen via NC or nonrebreather mask
b. Two large-bore peripheral IV lines
c. Labs
    i. CBC, BMP, PT/PTT, troponin, type and cross
d. Monitor
e. EKG
f. CXR – portable

F. History

a. HPI: a 37-year-old male, past medical history smoking, crack-cocaine abuse, alcohol abuse, and hypertension, presents with chest pain which began two hours ago after smoking cocaine. The pain is in the left chest and is accompanied by left arm tingling but no radiation of pain to the back, arm, or jaw. The pain is also accompanied by shortness of breath and sweating.
b. PMHx: hypertension
c. PSHx: none
d. Allergies: none
e. Meds: none
f. Social: smoking, crack-cocaine abuse, alcohol abuse
g. FHx: noncontributory

G. Nurse

a. Vital signs
    i. BP: 151/95 HR: 79 RR: 20 Sat: 95% on RA
b. EKG (Figure 33.1)

H. Secondary survey

a. General: alert and oriented, slightly agitated and uncomfortable due to chest pain
b. HEENT: pupils dilated bilaterally

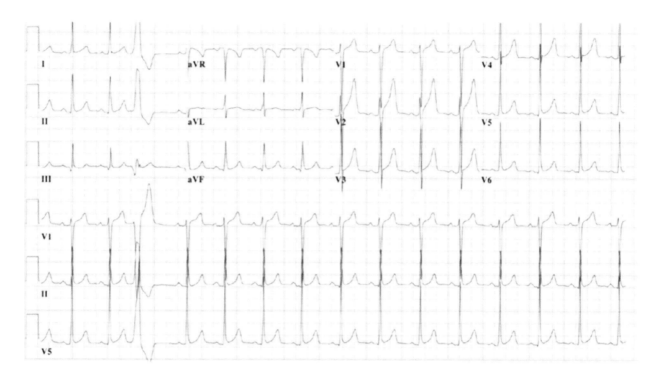

Figure 33.1

c. Neck: supple, symmetric, no LAD, no JVD
d. Chest: breath sounds equal; no respiratory distress; no chest tenderness
e. Heart: regular, tachycardic, no murmurs
f. Abdomen: soft, nontender; no masses, bowel sounds normal, no distension. No guarding, no rebound.
g. Extremities: no cyanosis, clubbing, or edema
h. Back: no gross abnormalities, no bruising, no tenderness to palpation to entire spine, no step offs
i. Neuro: no focal deficits, no pronator drift, normal gait, sensation intact to light touch
j. Skin: warm, diaphoretic
k. Vascular: equal pulses to carotid, radials, femorals, and DP

I. Action
a. Meds
  i. Lorazepam IV
  ii. Aspirin PO
  iii. Nitroglycerin sublingual
b. Reassess
  i. Patient less agitated; chest pain improved but still present
  ii. Repeat EKG – unchanged
c. Imaging
  i. Portable CXR (Figure 33.2)

J. Nurse
a. BP: 128/81 HR: 85 RR: 16 Sat: 98% on NC O_2

A

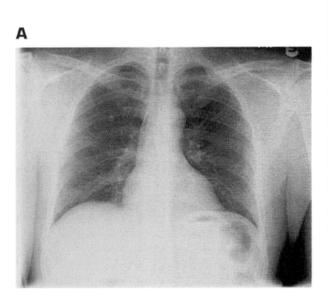

B

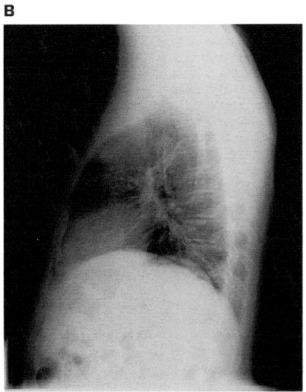

Figure 33.2 A and B

K. Results

Complete blood count:

WBC	12.1×10^3/uL
Hct	46.1%
Plt	389×10^3/uL

Basic metabolic panel:

Na	138 mEq/L
K	3.8 mEq/L
Cl	97 mEq/L
CO_2	20 mEq/L
BUN	14 mEq/dL
Cr	1.1 mg/dL
Gluc	74 mg/dL

Coagulation panel:

PT	13.0 sec
PTT	31.2 sec
INR	0.9

Urinalysis:

SG	1.030
pH	6
Prot	Neg
Gluc	Neg
Ketones	Neg
Bili	Neg
Blood	Neg
LE	Neg
Nitrite	Neg
Color	Yellow

a. Troponin normal

L. Action

a. Patient admitted to observation unit for monitoring and serial troponins, given cocaine chest pain

M. Diagnosis
a. Cocaine-induced chest pain

N. Critical actions
▨ EKG and vital signs monitor
▨ Oxygen administration
▨ Benzodiazepines
▨ Nitrates
▨ Troponin
▨ CXR
▨ Observation admission to monitor due to cocaine-induced chest pain

O. Examiner instructions
a. This is a case of chest pain in the setting of cocaine abuse. The patient's symptoms may be due to cocaine-induced vasoconstriction of the coronary arteries. Early critical actions include obtaining an EKG, administering nitrates for coronary vasodilation, and giving aspirin and benzodiazepines to control tachycardia and hypertension. Benzodiazepines are the recommended first-line agent for cocaine chest pain. If benzodiazapines are not administered, the patient will become more tachycardic and hypertensive. A CXR is important to rule out pulmonary etiologies that may result from cocaine-induced barotrauma. If the patient is sent home before standard acute coronary syndrome workup, the patient should return to the ED in 2 hours with signs/symptoms of acute coronary syndrome.

P. Pearls
a. Chest pain in the context of cocaine use may be caused by etiologies that are cardiovascular (such as myocardial ischemia/infarction, aortic dissection, or endocarditis with septic pulmonary emboli) or noncardiac (such as those from inhalation-related barotraumas including pneumomediastinum, pneumothorax, pneumopericardium, pulmonary hemorrhage/infarction).
b. Benzodiazapines (eg, lorazepam or diazepam) are useful to treat hypertension and tachycardia and thus reduce myocardial oxygen demand. Avoid haloperidol, droperidol, and chlorpromazine, as they may contribute to hyperthermia and may lower the seizure threshold.
c. Treat potential ischemia or acute coronary syndrome according to standard protocol, including nitrates, morphine, oxygen, aspirin and possible heparin and stress test and/or cardiac catheterization. Traditionally, β-adrenergic antagonists have been avoided because of concern that unopposed α-adrenergic stimulation may exacerbate symptoms. Consider IV phentolamine for patients with ischemic EKG changes and persistant hypertension and chest pain that have not responded to first-line medications.
d. Tachydysrhythmias or QRS-complex prolongation can be treated with sodium bicarbonate in order to alkalinize the serum to a target pH of 7.45 to 7.5.

Q. References
a. Tintinalli's: Chapter 181. Cocaine, Methamphetamine, and Other Amphetamines
b. Rosen's: Chapter 154. Cocaine and Other Sympathomimetics

CASE 34: Seizure (Natasha Spencer, MD, PhD)

A. Chief complaint
a. 34-month-old male with generalized shaking

B. Vital signs
a. HR: 140 RR: 30 T: 38.0°C Sat: 96% on RA

C. What does the patient look like?
a. Patient appears well, but is crying.

D. Primary survey
a. Airway: crying
b. Breathing: no apparent respiratory distress, clear lungs bilaterally, no cyanosis
c. Circulation: normal capillary refill, radial pulses 2+ bilaterally

E. History
a. HPI: a 34-month-old male with no past medical history, developmentally normal, presents after generalized shaking episode 45 minutes ago. An hour ago, the patient was noted by his mother to feel warm and was given ibuprofen. Patient's mother was rechecking his temperature when he had generalized, rhythmic shaking with eyes rolling back. The episode lasted for 5 minutes, after which the patient was sleepy. No incontinence was noted. The patient has had rhinorrhea for the past 2 days, but no cough, vomiting, or diarrhea and no fever before today. The patient had a well-child check in his pediatrician's office today.
b. PMHx: none. Born at term. Immunizations up-to-date.
c. PSHx: none
d. Allergies: none
e. Meds: ibuprofen
f. Social: lives with family at home
g. FHx: none

F. Action
a. Acetaminophen PO

G. Nurse
a. Vital signs
   i. HR: 140 RR: 30 T: 38.0°C Sat: 96% on RA wt: 24.5 kg
b. Finger stick glucose: 100 (must ask)

H. Secondary survey
a. General: well appearing, alert, active, in no apparent distress
b. HEENT: NC/AT. Normal
c. Neck: shoddy LAD, supple
d. Chest: normal
e. Heart: normal
f. Abdomen: normal
g. Extremities: normal
h. Back: normal

i. Neuro: awake, alert, appropriate for age; gait normal for age; can reach, grab, and hold onto objects with each hand

j. Skin: warm and dry, no rash or induration

k. Lymph: normal

I. Action

a. Reassess

    i. Patient in no apparent distress, playing with blocks

b. Discussion with patient's parents about diagnosis, prevention, precautions, and follow-up

c. Discharge patient home with outpatient pediatrician follow-up.

J. Results

Complete blood count:		Urinalysis:	
WBC	11.5×10^3/uL	SG	1.010
Hct	33.9%	pH	5.5
Plt	350×10^3/uL	Prot	Neg
		Gluc	Neg
Basic metabolic panel:		Ketones	Neg
Na	138 mEq/L	Bili	Neg
K	4.2 mEq/L	Blood	Neg
Cl	101 mEq/L	LE	Neg
CO_2	24 mEq/L	Nitrite	Neg
BUN	13 mEq/dL	Color	Yellow
Cr	0.4 mg/dL%		
Gluc	90 mg/dL		

K. Diagnosis

a. Simple febrile seizure

L. Critical actions

▪ Detailed history and physical examination to assess for meningitis or other obvious bacterial infection

▪ Acetaminophen administered every 4 hours and/or ibuprofen every 6 hours to reduce fever

▪ Counsel parents about simple febrile seizures and follow-up

M. Examiner instructions

a. This is a case of a simple febrile seizure. The patient's seizure is not likely due to central nervous system (CNS) infection or other dangerous cause. Important early actions include a careful history and physical examination. If acetaminophen or ibuprofen has not been given, the fever will persist and the patient will seize. If labs are drawn, the WBC count will be slightly elevated. If a lumbar puncture (LP) is performed, it will be normal. If a neurological consult is called, they will suggest sending the child home without blood work or an LP.

N. Pearls

a. Any child who is actively seizing in the ED should be presumed to be in status epilepticus and treated accordingly (oxygen, monitor, medication to stop seizure, identification and treatment of triggers, and further evaluation/treatment of etiology).

b. Febrile seizures by definition are seizures not caused by CNS infection or other defined etiologies in children aged 6 months to 5 years. A simple febrile seizure can be presumed in children with a normal neurological examination after a generalized seizure lasting less then 15 minutes in the setting of fever.

c. Laboratory evaluation (other than perhaps a glucose finger stick), lumbar puncture, and hospitalization are almost never needed for children with a simple febrile seizure. Any workup or treatment should be aimed at identifying the infectious etiology.

d. An LP, however, is strongly suggested for children under 6 months with a first-time seizure. LP should be considered in patients between 6 and 12 months of age who have not received *Haemophilus influenzae* type b (Hib) or *Streptococcus pneumoniae* immunizations appropriate for their age or if immunization status cannot be confirmed. An LP also should be considered for children 12 months and older with a first-time seizure if: the seizure is focal; the patient appears toxic and not playful after the postictal period; follow-up is a concern; or if the patient had already been receiving antibiotic treatment.

e. Treatment of simple febrile seizure is aimed at its etiology; acetaminophen or ibuprofen should be given to treat fevers.

f. Hospitalization for children with a simple febrile seizure is not needed unless the seizure recurs within several hours to 1 day and/or if the fever has a complicated etiology not easily treated at home.

O. References
a. Tintinalli's: Chapter 129. Seizures and Status Epilepticus in Children
b. Rosen: Chapter 175. Neurologic Disorders.

CASE 35: Chest pain (Natasha Spencer, MD, PhD)

A. Chief complaint
a. 45-year-old female with chest pain

B. Vital signs
a. BP: 125/79 HR: 102 RR: 18 T: 37.3°C Sat: 98% on RA

C. What does the patient look like?
a. Patient appears comfortable, alert, and oriented.

D. Primary survey
a. Airway: speaking in full sentences
b. Breathing: no apparent respiratory distress, no cyanosis, clear lungs bilaterally
c. Circulation: RRR, radial pulses 2+ bilaterally, normal capillary refill

E. Action
a. Oxygen via NC or nonrebreather mask
b. EKG

F. History
a. HPI: a 45-year-old female presents with chest pain for 1 day. The pain is located in the right chest under the breast, is stabbing, radiates to her back, and is worse with

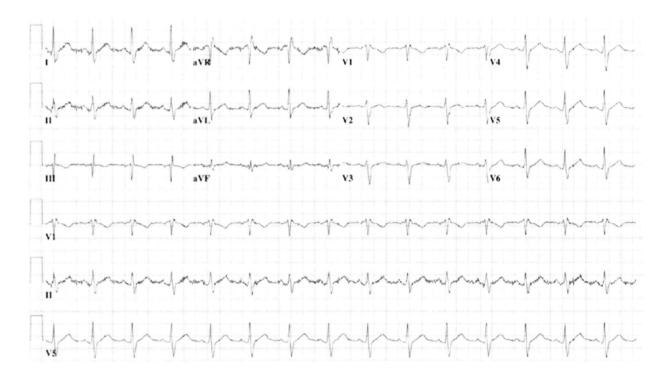

Figure 35.1

breathing. The pain is accompanied by shortness of breath. She denies cough, fever, or trauma.
b. PSHx: left ankle surgery 2 weeks ago
c. Allergies: none
d. Meds: none
e. Social: denies alcohol, smoking, drugs
f. FHx: hypertension, high cholesterol

G. Nurse
a. EKG (Figure 35.1)

H. Secondary survey
a. General: alert and oriented, no apparent distress
b. HEENT: normal
c. Neck: normal
d. Chest: chest is nontender; breath sounds normal; no respiratory distress
e. Heart: regular rate and rhythm; heart sounds normal; no extremity edema
f. Abdomen: nontender; bowel sounds normal, no distension, no masses
g. Rectal examination: hemoccult negative
h. Extremities: pitting edema in left leg; normal capillary refill; no calf tenderness, Dorsalis Pedis pulses 2+ bilaterally
i. Back: normal
j. Neuro: normal
k. Skin: warm and dry; no rash, erythema, or induration
l. Lymph: normal

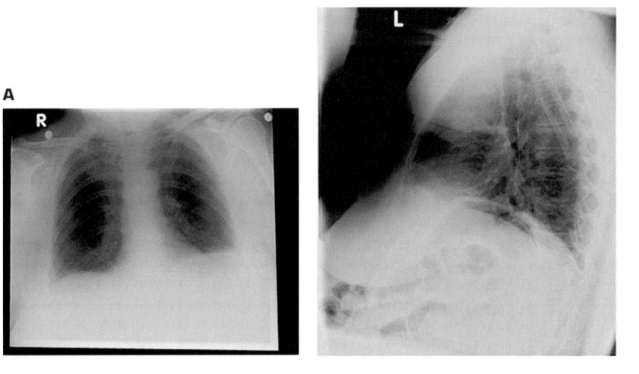

Figure 35.2 A and B

I. Action
a. Two large-bore peripheral IV lines
b. Labs
   i. CBC, BMP, PT/PTT, urine hCG
c. Monitor
d. Analgesia (acetaminophen PO or morphine IV)

J. Action
a. Monitor: BP: 116/78 HR: 103 RR: 18 Sat: 98% on RA
b. Reassess
   i. Patient still without pain; comfortable
c. Imaging
   i. CXR (Figure 35.2)
   ii. US of left lower extremity (unavailable until morning)

K. Nurse
a. BP: 114/55 HR: 99 RR: 20 Sat: 99% on RA

L. Results

Complete blood count:

WBC	12.5×10^3/uL
Hct	35.7%
Plt	339×10^3/uL

Basic metabolic panel:

Na	142 mEq/L
K	4.1 mEq/L
Cl	104 mEq/L
CO_2	25 mEq/L

Basic metabolic panel (continued):		Urinalysis:	
BUN	10 mEq/dL	SG	1.018
Cr	0.7 mg/dL%	pH	6
Gluc	84 mg/dL	Prot	Neg
		Gluc	Neg
Coagulation panel:		Ketones	Neg
PT	13.5 sec	Bili	Neg
PTT	30 sec	Blood	Neg
INR	1.1	LE	Neg
		Nitrite	Neg
		Color	Yellow

a. Urine pregnancy test negative

b. D-dimer positive

M. Action

a. Chest CT angiogram with IV contrast – multiple small emboli in distal right pulmonary vasculature

N. Action

a. Discussion with patient regarding need for treatment and admission

b. Admit patient to medicine service for continued anticoagulation

c. Meds

    i. Heparin sodium bolus and drip or low molecular weight heparin or novel oral anticoagulant

    ii. Acetaminophen PRN or morphine IV as needed for pain

O. Diagnosis

a. Pulmonary embolism

P. Critical actions

▨ EKG

▨ CXR

▨ Ventilation-perfusion (VQ) scan or chest CT angiogram

▨ Heparin treatment (low molecular weight heparin IM or unfractionated heparin IV) or novel oral anti coagulant may be chosen instead of heparin

▨ Admit patient for anticoagulation

Q. Examiner instructions

a. This is a case of pulmonary embolism (PE), or blood clot in the lung vasculature. Early EKG (to evaluate for cardiac ischemia or other obvious cause) is important in patients with chest pain. CXR is most commonly normal, but may demonstrate pleural effusion, atelectasis, or other nonspecific findings. If an US is requested of the extremities, US will not be available until morning (6 hours from now). If a D-dimer is ordered, it is positive and a CT scan should be ordered. If the patient is not admitted into the hospital and is discharged home, the patient will return to the ED the next day in cardiopulmonary arrest.

R. Pearls

a. Estimating the pretest probability for PE is useful to guide workup of chest pain. The PERC (Pulmonary Embolism Rule-out Criteria) are often used. When the clinician's pre-test probability of pulmonary embolism is less than 15% and all clinical criteria are present, there is less than a 2% chance of pulmonary embolism.

b. Low-risk criteria for PE include the following
    i. Age < 50 years
    ii. Pulse rate < 100 beats/min
    iii. O_2 sat > 94%
    iv. No history of hemoptysis, unilateral leg swelling, recent major surgery or trauma, prior PE or DVT, or exogenous estrogen use

c. D-dimer is most useful among patients with a low level of suspicion for PE, as PE can be ruled out with a negative quantitative D-dimer assay. If the D-dimer is positive in such patients, however, either a negative CT or a normal VQ scan can rule out the diagnosis.

d. Arterial blood gas and CXR are nonspecific for pulmonary embolism, but may show hypoxemia or basilar atelectasis, respectively. The studies may also be helpful when evaluating alternative diagnoses. A normal EKG is also nonspecific for PE, but may show a pattern consistent with right heart strain (tachycardia, T-wave inversion in V1–4, S1Q3T3 pattern and/or right bundle branch block).

e. PE is treated with anti coagulation. Traditionally, unfractioned heparin or LMWH have been used. If a major contraindication to heparin is present (eg, recent large cerebral infarction or major trauma), consider emergent inferior vena cava filter placement. Consider thrombolysis (e.g., with alteplase) for patients with cardiorespiratory collapse due to PE. Newer oral anti coagulants have been introduced which may also be used in lieu of "bridging" heparin to warfarin.

S. References
a. Tintinalli's: Chapter 60. Thromboembolism
b. Rosen: Chapter 88. Pulmonary Embolism and Deep Vein Thrombosis

CASE 36: Throat swelling (Natasha Spencer, MD, PhD)

A. Chief complaint
a. 5-year-old male with funny feeling in his throat

B. Vital signs
a. HR: 170 RR: 30, crying T: 36.5°C Sat: 93% on RA wt: 16.3 kg

C. What does the patient look like?
a. Patient is crying, uncomfortable

D. Primary survey
a. Airway: crying.
b. Breathing: some stridor, coughing noted; breath sounds otherwise clear and equal bilaterally, no accessory muscle use or retractions
c. Circulation: tachycardic; normal capillary refill

E. Action
a. Oxygen via NC
b. Two large-bore peripheral IV lines
c. Monitor

F. History

a. HPI: a 5-year-old male, no past medical history, presenting with coughing and anxiety after ingesting chocolate with peanuts 30 minutes ago. After eating the snack, he complained of itching, abdominal pain, and vomited. He was noted to be coughing and anxious and so was brought to the ED. He is now complaining he has "something weird on his throat."

b. PMHx: none

c. PSHx: none

d. Allergies: peanuts

e. Meds: none

f. Social: Lives at home with family

g. FHx: not relevant

G. Action

a. Epinephrine IM

b. NS 320 ml (20 mg/kg) IV bolus

c. Diphenhydramine IV

d. Ranitidine 25 mg IV

e. Albuterol nebulizer

f. Methylprednisolone IV

H. Nurse

a. Reassess vital signs

   i. BP: 85/50 HR: 130 RR: 28 Sat: 98% on RA

I. Secondary survey

a. General: cranky, crying, uncomfortable, interactive, alert

b. HEENT: mild erythema around mouth and mild lip swelling; trachea midline, no masses, no lymphadenopathy

c. Neck: normal

d. Pharynx: nonproductive cough, some stridor; diffuse bilateral wheezing; breath sounds equal bilaterally; no accessory muscle use or retractions

e. Heart: tachycardia

f. Abdomen: nontender, no masses, bowel sounds normal, no distension, no peritoneal signs.

g. Pelvic: deferred

h. Extremities: normal

i. Back: normal

j. Neuro: awake, alert, appropriate for age

k. Skin: mild erythema around mouth

l. Lymph: normal

J. Action

a. Reassess after medications administered

   i. Patient able to speak in full sentences.

   ii. HR: 80 RR: 24 Temp: 36.0 Sat: 97% on RA

K. Action

a. Observation for 6 hours in the ED

   i. Patient not coughing; is speaking in full sentences, and is without pruritis

   ii. BP: 96/52 HR: 87 Sat: 98% on RA

b. Counsel parents about avoiding allergen

c. Give parents epinephrine autoinjector as well as prescription for diphenhydramine, ranitidine, and steroids

d. Discharge patient home with pediatrician and allergist outpatient follow-up

L. Diagnosis

a. Anaphylaxis

M. Critical actions

▧ Airway assessment

▧ Oxygen

▧ Epinephrine IM

▧ NS (20 mg/kg) IV bolus

▧ Diphenhydramine or hydroxyzine

   ▶ Albuterol nebulizer

   ▶ Corticosteroids (PO or IV)

▧ Observation for at least 6 hours

▧ If discharged, should be given a prescription for an epinephrine autoinjector, antihistamine, and told to avoid the allergic trigger

N. Examiner instructions

a. This is a case of anaphlylaxis, a severe, multiorgan system allergic reaction. If epinephrine and diphenhydramine are not given, respiratory distress should continue and worsen. If ENT or anesthesia are consulted, they should say they are at another emergency and will be down after about 30 minutes. If the patient is monitored for less than 4 hours, the patient will have a relapse of respiratory distress. Any labs requested will be normal.

O. Pearls

a. Most fatalities from anaphylaxis happen within 30 minutes of antigen exposure. Fatalities occur from bronchospasm, laryngeoedema, and/or cardiovascular collapse.

b. Fluid resuscitation is critical in anaphylaxis. Multiple fluid boluses may be required, as patients often lose vascular tone with multisystem involvement.

c. Epinephrine is mainstay of initial therapy. IM injection into the thigh is more preferable than into the deltoid. If hemodynamically unstable, the drug should be administered intravenously via drip. Hypotensive patients not responding to IV fluids and epinephrine can be given additional vasopressors (such as dopamine or dobutamine).

d. Second-line therapy for anaphylaxis includes diphenhydramine, corticosteroids, and inhaled β-agonists. Consider use of an H_2 receptor blocker as well.

e. Racemic epinephrine, albuterol, ipratropium, and possibly magnesium may be used to treat signs of bronchospasm. Consider early endotracheal intubation for severe bronchospasm or laryngeal edema.

f. Patients who remain without symptoms after treatment can be discharged home after 4 to 6 hours of observation. Patients who remain hypotensive and symptomatic despite treatment should be admitted to an ICU.

P. References
a. Tintinalli's: Chapter 27. Anaphylaxis, Acute Allergic Reactions, and Angioedema
b. Rosen: Chapter 119. Allergy, Hypersensitivity, Angioedema, and Anaphylaxis

CASE 37: Abdominal pain (Ani Aydin, MD)

A. Chief complaint
a. 24-year-old female with nausea, vomiting, and abdominal pain

B. Vital signs
a. BP: 120/80 HR: 90 RR: 12 T: 38.2°C Sat: 98% on RA

C What does the patient look like?
a. Patient appears stated age, appears uncomfortable due to pain, lying supine and still on stretcher.

D. Primary survey
a. Airway: speaking in full sentences
b. Breathing: no apparent respiratory distress, no cyanosis, clear lungs
c. Circulation: RRR, pale and cool skin, radial pulses 2+, normal capillary refill

E. History
a. HPI: a 24-year-old female presents with abdominal pain, nausea, vomiting, and decreased oral intake for 1 day, with worsening abdominal pain for 3 hours. The pain started acutely yesterday. It began as a dull ache in the lower belly but has now moved to the right lower quadrant, and become more severe. She notes nausea and nonbloody vomitus today, but no diarrhea. She feels warm, but did not take her temperature at home. Her last menstrual period was 2 weeks ago, and she is on a regular menstrual cycle with periods occurring every 28 days. The patient denies any chest pain, shortness of breath, dysuria, hematuria, rectal bleeding, history of sexually transmitted diseases, or other history of gynecologic problems.
b. PMHx: none, no prior pregnancies, no history of ovarian cysts
c. PSHx: none
d. Allergies: none
e. Meds: none
f. Social: lives with husband at home; denies alcohol, smoking, or drugs; sexually active only with her husband
g. FHx: not relevant
h. PMD: Dr Miller

F. Action
a. Two large-bore peripheral IV lines
b. 1 L NS bolus

   c. Labs

     i. CBC, BMP, urine pregnancy test, UA

   d. Monitor

   e. Nothing by mouth (NPO)

   f. IV analgesia (such as opioid)

   g. Antiemetic

G. Nurse

   a. Pain assessment after opioids: 6/10

H. Secondary survey

   a. General: alert and oriented, moderate distress due to pain

   b. HEENT: normal

   c. Neck: normal

   d. Chest: normal

   e. Heart: normal

   f. Abdomen: tender to palpation greatest in right lower quadrant, with voluntary guarding, slight rigidity, and no rebound, bowel sounds present, no pulsatile masses, no masses, no hernia, negative Murphy's sign, + tenderness at McBurney's point, positive Rovsing sign, negative Psoas and Obturator signs

   g. Rectal: no rectal mass, no gross blood, hemoccult negative brown stool

   h. Pelvic: external vaginal normal, no blood or lesions in vaginal vault, no cervical motion tenderness, no ovarian masses

   i. Extremities: normal

   j. Back: normal

   k. Neuro: normal

   l. Skin: normal

   m. Lymph: normal

I. Action

   a. Meds

     i. Opioids (ie, morphine IV)

   b. Reassess

     i. Serial abdominal examination – unchanged from before

   c. Consult

     i. Surgery

   d. Imaging

     i. CT abdomen/pelvis with enteric (rectal) contrast. Some institutions may do oral or even noncontrast depending on the generation of CT scanner and expertise of the radiologist

J. Nurse

   a. BP: 120/80 HR: 90 RR: 12 T: 38.2°C Sat: 100% on RA

   b. Patient: still with significant pain

K. Results

Complete blood count:

WBC	12.1×10^3/uL
Hct	40.5%
Plt	253×10^3/uL

Basic metabolic panel:

Na	139 mEq/L
K	4.2 mEq/L
Cl	101 mEq/L
CO_2	23 mEq/L
BUN	10 mEq/dL
Cr	1.0 mg/dL
Gluc	90 mg/dL

Coagulation panel:

PT	14 sec
PTT	31 sec
INR	1.0

Urinalysis:

SG	1.022
pH	6
Prot	Neg
Gluc	Neg
Ketones	Neg
Bili	Neg
Blood	Neg
LE	Neg
Nitrite	Neg
Color	Yellow

a. Urine pregnancy test negative

b. CT abdomen/pelvis – acute appendicitis

L. Action

a. Surgery consult

    i. To OR for appendectomy

b. Discussion with family and PMD need for emergent OR and diagnosis of appendicitis

c. Meds

    i. Morphine IV

    ii. Antibiotics IV

M. Diagnosis

a. Appendicitis

N. Critical actions

▧ Urine pregnancy test

▧ UA

▧ Pelvic examination in woman of child-bearing age

▧ Pain management

▧ Antibiotics preoperatively

▧ Serial abdominal examination

▧ CT abdomen/pelvis with enteric contrast

▧ Surgery consult

O. Examiner instructions

a. This is a case of appendicitis in a young woman. Important early actions include administration of IV fluids and the patient should be made NPO. Pain medication should be administered early, especially if the surgical consult is delayed. A urine pregnancy test and pelvic and rectal examination must be performed on this patient. A CT abdomen/pelvis with enteric contrast should be obtained, but an ultrasound can be done if pregnancy is considered and the urine pregnancy test results are delayed.

P. Pearls

a. Appendicitis is a clinical diagnosis – early actions (such as surgical consultation) should be undertaken before CT scan when suspicion for the disease is high. If perforation is suspected, early antibiotics should be given.

b. Vital signs are often normal, especially early in appendicitis; the patient may have a low-grade fever.

c. CT abdomen/pelvis with enteric contrast should be performed in males and women of nonchild-bearing age with equivocal signs.

d. US can be used in thin children, pregnant women, and women of child-bearing age with a possible pelvic etiology of pain. However, this is often operator and institution dependent.

e. Pregnant women have the same risk of appendicitis as the general population; appendicitis most often presents in the 2nd trimester.

f. Perforation is more likely at the extremes of age.

g. It is unlikely that pain medication will mask the abdominal findings of appendicitis.

h. Peritoneal signs are ominous, and often suggest a surgical emergency; rebound tenderness is a late finding.

i. Uncomplicated appendicitis has a 0.1% mortality; this rate rises to 3% to 4% with perforation.

Q. References

a. Tintinalli's: Chapter 84. Acute Appendicitis

b. Rosen: Chapter 93. Acute Appendicitis

CASE 38: Altered mental status (Ani Aydin, MD)

A. Chief complaint

a. 85-year-old male with disorientation

B. Vital signs

a. BP: 135/70 HR: 88 RR: 13 T: 36°C Sat: 98% on RA

C. What does the patient look like?

a. Patient appears stated age, sleeping on stretcher but arousable and cooperative.

D. Primary survey

a. Airway: Speaking in full sentences

b. Breathing: No apparent respiratory distress, no cyanosis, clear lungs

c. Circulation: Pale and cool skin, RRR, radial pulses 2+, normal capillary refill

E. Action

a. Oxygen via NC or nonrebreather mask

b. Two large-bore peripheral IV lines

c. Finger stick blood glucose (107; must ask)

    d. Labs
      i. CBC, Chem 7, LFT, UA, PT, PTT, cardiac markers
    e. Cardiac monitor
    f. EKG
    g. CXR

F. History
a. HPI: a 85-year-old male was brought in by an ambulance after his wife noted that he was becoming more disoriented over the last 2 days. According to his wife, the patient was more forgetful. For example, he did not know his address or phone number today. Of note, the patient tripped and fell in the bathroom 3 days ago and complained of a slight headache at that time, but did not seek any medical attention. There was no loss of consciousness. He complains of midfrontal headache for 2 days without radiation. He denies neck pain, photophobia or phonophobia, reports no changes in vision or blurry vision, no nausea, or vomiting. This headache is worse than most of his prior headaches, and was not associated with aura at onset. He denies any shortness of breath, chest pain, abdominal pain, dysuria, hematuria, blood per rectum, or fever. There have been no changes in his appetite.
b. PMHx: hypertension, hypercholesterolemia
c. PSHx: umbilical hernia repair 20 years ago
d. Allergies: none
e. Meds: metoprolol, simvastatin, aspirin
f. Social: lives with wife (80 years old with multiple medical problems); drinks beer one to two times per month, denies any cigarette or drug use; at baseline able to perform all activities of daily living well
g. FHx: not relevant
h. PMD: Dr Stern

G. Nurse
a. EKG (Figure 38.1)
b. CXR (Figure 38.2)

H. Secondary survey
a. General: alert, oriented to person and place; unsure of date, appears comfortable on stretcher
b. HEENT: no ecchymoses or lacerations noted, tympanic membranes normal bilaterally; extraocular movements intact, pupils equal, round, reactive, conjunctiva normal, fundoscopic examination normal, no septal deviation, palate normal, uvula midline
c. Neck: normal
d. Chest: normal
e. Heart: normal
f. Abdomen: normal
g. Rectal: hemoccult negative brown stool, normal tone
h. Extremities: normal
i. Back: normal
j. Neuro: alert, oriented to self and place only (does not know the date), cooperative, 5/5 strength bilateral upper and lower extremities, sensation grossly intact, cranial nerves II to XII intact, reflexes 2/2 and symmetric bilaterally, no focal deficits, normal gait

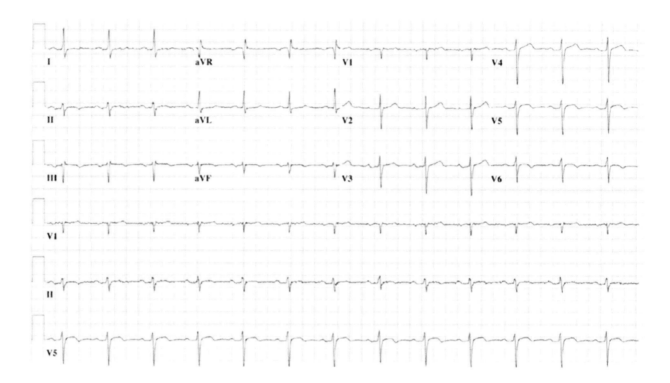

Figure 38.1

Figure 38.2

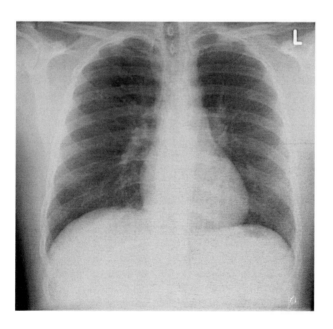

    k. Skin: no ecchymoses, lacerations, or abrasions noted
    l. Lymph: normal

I. Action
  a. Meds
     i. Acetaminophen PO for pain
  b. Imaging
     ii. Noncontrast head CT

J. Nurse

a. BP: 135/70 HR: 88 RR: 13 T: 36°C Sat: 98% on RA

b. Patient: no change in neurological examination, no apparent distress

K. Results

Complete blood count:

WBC	9.2×10^3/uL
Hct	41.5%
Plt	223×10^3/uL

Basic metabolic panel:

Na	137 mEq/L
K	4.2 mEq/L
Cl	108 mEq/L
CO_2	23 mEq/L
BUN	20 mEq/dL
Cr	0.6 mg/dL
Gluc	110 mg/dL

Coagulation panel:

PT	13.0 sec
PTT	29 sec
INR	1.1

Liver function panel:

AST	24 U/L
ALT	33 U/L
Alk Phos	120 U/L
T bili	0.9 mg/dL
D bili	0.1 mg/dL
Amylase	60 U/L
Lipase	104 U/L
Albumin	3.1 g/dL

Urinalysis:

SG	1.020
pH	7
Prot	Neg
Gluc	Neg
Ketones	Neg
Bili	Neg
Blood	Neg
LE	Neg
Nitrite	Neg
Color	Yellow

a. CT scan head (Figure 38.3)

L. Action

a. Consult neurosurgery (for drainage)

b. Discussion with family and PMD regarding need for admission to neurosurgical service for drainage of his subdural hematoma

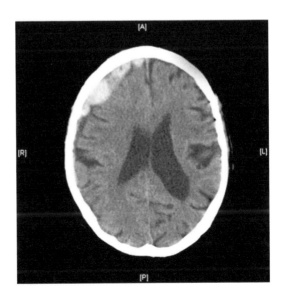

Figure 38.3

M. Diagnosis

a. Subdural hematoma with midline shift

N. Critical actions

▦ Early finger stick blood glucose

▦ Obtain history of recent fall

▦ Noncontrast head CT

▦ Laboratory evaluation

▦ Pain management; avoid nonsteroidal antiinflammatory (NSAID) medications which could make bleeding worse

▦ Neurosurgery consultation

▦ Admission to ICU

O. Examiner instructions

a. This is a case of a subacute subdural hemotoma (bleeding around the brain). This can occur after relatively minor head trauma in elderly patients, and leads to worsening mental status or even focal neurologic complaints. There are many processes that can cause confusion in the elderly; a rapid assessment of blood glucose levels, EKG, and a thorough history and physical examination are key steps in the patient's early management.

P. Pearls

a. Patients with moderate head trauma or high clinical suspicion for bleeding require observation, as the initial noncontrast head CT can be normal. Risk is increased if the patient is on antiplatelet or anticoagulant medications.

b. The noncontrast head CT can differentiate between acute intracranial and extracranial bleeding, subarachnoid hemorrhage, brain swelling, and large stroke.

c. The most common complaint after head trauma is a headache. A careful history and physical examination will reveal more subtle findings, including neurologic and mental status changes.

d. Patients at the extremes of age (greater than 60 or less than 2) should be considered high risk for intracranial injury, despite only having sustained minor head trauma.

e. Subdural hematomas (SDHs) occur as a blood clot forms between the dura and brain. In elderly patients and those with a history of alcoholism, brain atrophy causes stretching of the superficial bridging veins between the dura and brain. Thus, these patients are at increased risk for SDH. Since this venous bleeding is slow, signs and symptoms do not develop rapidly and extensive damage may have occurred by the time patients become symptomatic.

f. In epidural hematomas, the blood clot occurs outside the dura. The majority are associated with skull fractures. Since the bleeding is arterial, signs and symptoms usually develop earlier than in subdural hematomas. However, these patients can develop a "lucid interval" after an initial episode of loss of consciousness.

g. Traumatic subarachnoid hemorrhages (SAHs) result in blood within the meninges and spinal fluid. Up to two-thirds of patients with subarachnoid hemorrhage may have no bleeding noted on their initial noncontrast head CT, though this is time dependent. The sooner the head CT is performed in relation to the onset of symptoms, the more likely SAH will be observed on CT brain imaging. One of the most severe complications of SAH is the resulting vasospasm, which can result in significant ischemia.

Q. References

a. Tintinalli's: Chapter 254. Head Trauma in Adults and Children

b. Rosen: Chapter 41 Head Injury

CASE 39: Rectal pain (Ani Aydin, MD)

A. Chief complaint

a. 28-year-old male with pain in anal region

B. Vital signs

a. BP: 120/80 HR: 80 RR: 12 T: 37°C Sat: 100% on RA

C. What does the patient look like?

a. Patient lying prone on the stretcher due to pain in his anal region.

D. Primary survey

a. Airway: speaking in full sentences

b. Breathing: no apparent respiratory distress, no cyanosis

c. Circulation: pale and cool skin, normal capillary refill

E. History

a. HPI: a 28-year-old male with a history of Crohn's disease presents with pain in the anal region for 1 week. The pain is severe and located in the anal area without radiation. It has been progressive, dull, constant, worse with defecation and sitting, better with warm baths. The patient also noted some stains on his boxers this morning, but denies any rectal bleeding. He had a prior similar episode as a teenager, and required a "surgery" in the ED. He denies any fever, decreased appetite, nausea, vomiting, or blood per rectum.

b. PMHx: Crohn's disease

c. PSHx: "surgery" in ED 10 years ago

d. Allergies: none

e. Meds: mesalamine; no steroids at this time

f. Social: lives alone, single. Denies alcohol use, smoking, drugs. Sexually active with women, compliant with condom use

g. FHx: brother with Crohn's disease

h. PMD: Dr Langan

F. Action

a. Oxygen via NC

b. Two large-bore peripheral IV lines

c. Pain medication

d. Labs
   i. CBC, BMP, PT/PTT

e. Monitor: BP: 120/80 HR: 80 RR: 12 T: 37°C Sat: 100% on RA

G. Nurse

a. Reassess pain score

H. Secondary survey

  a. General: alert and oriented, moderate distress secondary to pain
  b. HEENT: normal
  c. Neck: normal
  d. Chest: normal
  e. Heart: normal
  f. Abdomen: normal
  g. Rectal: 2 cm × 2 cm fluctuant, indurated mass with some serous drainage near anal verge. No purulence; no surrounding erythema, no edema, no warmth; no hemorrhoids or lesions noted on anoscopy. No lesions and no palpable mass on rectal examination, no gross blood, hemoccult negative brown stool
  h. Urogenital: normal
  i. Extremities: normal
  j. Back: normal
  k. Neuro: normal
  l. Skin: normal
  m. Lymph: normal

I. Action

  a. Meds
      i. Morphine
      ii. Antibiotics not necessary (no systemic symptoms, no signs of overlying cellulitis)
  b. Reassess
      i. Patient with some improvements in pain symptoms after analgesia, but continues to complain of anal pain
  c. Consult
      i. None at this time
  d. Imaging
      i. None

J. Nurse

  a. BP: 120/80 HR: 80 RR: 12 T: 37°C Sat: 100% on RA
  b. Patient: lying prone with pain in anal region, somewhat improved with pain medication

K. Results

Complete blood count:

WBC	8.2×10^3/uL	BUN	19 mEq/dL
Hct	41.5%	Cr	0.9 mg/dL%
Plt	253×10^3/uL	Gluc	100 mg/dL

Basic metabolic panel:

		Coagulation panel:	
Na	137 mEq/L	PT	14.1 sec
K	3.9 mEq/L	PTT	31.5 sec
Cl	102 mEq/L	INR	1.0
CO_2	28 mEq/L		

L. Action

a. Incision and drainage, packing

b. Discussion with patient and PMD regarding the need for follow-up and wound checks, patient to return with any signs of infection or worsening symptoms

c. Meds

    i. Systemic pain medication (i.e., morphine IV)

    ii. Local anesthesia (i.e., local infiltration with lidocaine)

M. Diagnosis

a. Uncomplicated perianal abscess

N. Critical actions

▨ Pain medications

▨ Thorough examination to rule out signs of fistula formation and systemic involvement

▨ Incision and drainage (I & D)

▨ Discuss post-incision and drainage management – sitz baths, stool softeners, frequent dressing changes until incision is healed

▨ Arrange follow-up

O. Examiner instructions

a. This is a case of uncomplicated perianal abscess, or collection of pus. This is likely due to Crohn's disease. The prior "surgery" in the ED was an incision and drainage (I & D) of a similar lesion conducted 10 years prior. There are no signs of deeper involvement, fistula formation, or systemic signs on this examination. If a surgical consultation is requested, they should reply that they are in an emergency operative case and will follow up with the patient in the morning.

P. Pearls

a. There are four types of perirectal abscesses: perianal, ischiorectal, pelvirectal, and intersphincteric. Uncomplicated perianal abscesses may be incised and drained in the ED; however, for other types of perirectal abscesses and fistulas, treatment should be operative.

b. They are more common in adult males, but can also be found in the pediatric population.

c. They are associated with malignancies, Crohn's disease, tuberculosis, an immuno-compromised host, anal fissures, foreign bodies, anorectal trauma, and actinomycosis.

d. Most cases involve mixed anaerobic and aerobic flora.

e. Antibiotics are not necessary in patients unless the patient exhibits systemic involvement.

Q. References

a. Tintinalli's: Chapter 88. Anorectal Disorders

b. Rosen: Chapter 137. Skin and Soft Tissue Infections

CASE 40: Vaginal bleeding (Ani Aydin, MD)

A. Chief complaint
a. 25-year-old female with abdominal pain and vaginal bleeding

B. Vital signs
a. BP: 95/63 HR: 96 RR: 12 T: 37°C Sat: 100% on RA

C. What does the patient look like?
a. Patient appears stated age, scared, uncomfortable due to pain, lying still, supine in stretcher.

D. Primary survey
a. Airway: speaking in full sentences
b. Breathing: no apparent respiratory distress, no cyanosis
c. Circulation: pale and cool skin, normal capillary refill

E. History
a. HPI: a 25-year-old female, G2P2, with a history of bilateral tubal ligation after her last pregnancy 2 years prior, presents with abdominal pain and vaginal bleeding since this morning. Her last menstrual period was about 1 month ago. She soaked though five pads since this morning, which is unusually heavy for her periods. The patient did not note any clots. She has been sexually active with her husband, but has not been using any protection since her tubal ligation. She complains of some lightheadedness and dizziness. She denies any shortness of breath, chest pain, nausea, vomiting, fever, decreased appetite. She denies any history of sexually transmitted infections, including gonorrhea, chlamydia, HIV, or herpes.
b. PMHx: G2P2
c. PSHx: two prior caesarean sections (2 and 3 years ago); bilateral tubal ligation after her most recent pregnancy
d. Allergies: none
e. Social: lives with husband and two children at home; denies alcohol, smoking, drugs; sexually active with husband only, not using any protection
f. FHx: not relevant
g. PMD: Dr Johansen

F. Action
a. Two large-bore peripheral IV lines
b. Labs
   i. Urine pregnancy test, CBC, BMP, PT/PTT, blood type and cross-match 2 units, UA
c. 1 L NS bolus
d. Monitor: BP: 95/63 HR: 96 RR: 12 T: 37°C Sat: 100% on RA

G. Nurse
a. After 1 L NS: BP: 105/70 HR: 85 RR: 12 Sat: 100% on RA
b. If no fluids given: BP: 85/60 HR: 118 RR: 15 Sat: 98% on RA
c. Urine pregnancy test positive

H. Secondary survey

a. General: alert and oriented, moderate distress due to abdominal pain, nervous

b. HEENT: mildly pale conjunctiva, otherwise normal

c. Neck: normal

d. Chest: normal

e. Heart: normal

f. Abdomen: soft, nondistended, normal bowel sounds; mild tenderness in the hypogastrium; some voluntary guarding, no rebound, no rigidity; no palpable masses

g. Pelvic: external vagina normal; blood in vaginal vault, no clots; no vaginal lesions, lacerations, abrasions noted; no discharge; cervical os closed; mild tenderness on bimanual examination, no cervical motion tenderness

h. Rectal: hemoccult positive brown stool

i. Urogenital: normal

j. Extremities: normal

k. Back: normal

l. Neuro: normal

m. Skin: normal

n. Lymph: normal

I. Action

a. Meds

   i. Pain medication

b. Reassess

   i. Patient anxious about bleeding, continues to complain about abdominal pain.

c. Consult

   i. Obstetrics and gynecology

d. Imaging

   i. Pelvic US

e. Serum hCG

J. Nurse

a. Vitals signs: BP: 105/70 HR: 85 RR: 12 Sat: 100% on RA (after 1 L of fluid)

b. Patient: still with significant pain

K. Results

Complete blood count:		Coagulation panel:	
WBC	12.1×10^3/uL	PT	13.1 sec
Hct	29.8%	PTT	26 sec
Plt	253×10^3/uL	INR	1.0

Basic metabolic panel:	
Na	139 mEq/L
K	4.2 mEq/L
Cl	111 mEq/L
CO_2	23 mEq/L
BUN	10 mEq/dL
Cr	0.8 mg/dL
Gluc	92 mg/dL

Urinalysis:

SG	1.030	Bili	Neg
pH	6	Blood	Neg
Prot	Neg	LE	Neg
Gluc	Neg	Nitrite	Neg
Ketones	Neg	Color	Yellow

    a. Serum hCG: 10,500

       i. Blood Type O⁻

    b. Transvaginal US (Figure 40.1)

    c. FAST US (Figure 40.2)

L. Action

a. Meds

    i. Pain medication (such as morphine)

    ii. Rho (D) immune globulin IM

b. Obstetrics and gynecology consult

    i. To OR for laparotomy

c. Discuss with patient, family, and PMD need for emergent OR and diagnosis of ectopic pregnancy

M. Diagnosis

a. Ectopic pregnancy

Figure 40.1

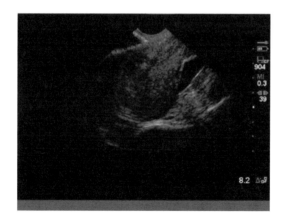

Figure 40.2

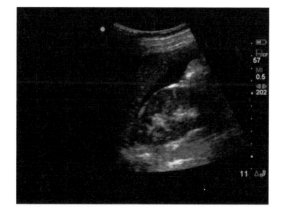

N. Critical actions
- Large-bore IV access and fluid bolus
- Blood type and cross-match
- Rho (D) immune globulin IM
- hCG
- Pelvic examination
- Pelvic US
- Pain management
- Obstetrics and gynecology consult

O. Examiner instructions
a. This is a case of an ectopic pregnancy, which is an abnormal implantation of the embryo outside of the uterus. Prior tubal ligations likely increased this patient's risk for ectopic pregnancy. Scarring from surgery, trauma, or pelvic infections can increase the risk as well. The patient presents with the classic triad: abdominal pain, vaginal bleeding, and amenorrhea. Important early actions include administering IV fluids, blood type and cross-match, hCG, US to confirm the absence of an intrauterine pregnancy, and consulting obstetrics and gynecology. If fluids are not administered, the patient's blood pressure will begin to drop. Her pain will continue to increase until addressed. While awaiting the quantitative hCG level, a US can be obtained in the ED which confirms the lack of an intrauterine pregnancy.

P. Pearls
a. Ectopic pregnancies are the leading cause of first-trimester pregnancy-related maternal deaths.
b. The incidence is higher in nonwhite women and teenagers.
c. There is an increased incidence in patient with prior sexually transmitted diseases, unsuccessful tubal ligations, assisted reproduction, intrauterine devices, prior ectopic pregnancies, previous pelvic surgeries, and exposure to diethylstilbestrol.
d. Most ectopic pregnancies occur in the fallopian tubes. Other sites include abdominal cavity, cervix, and ovary.
e. It is critical to administer Rho (D) immune globulin IM to Rh negative mothers to reduce the risk of maternal antibody formation against fetal hemoglobin. This sensitization can lead to neonatal hemolytic anemia and fetal hydrops in future pregnancies.
f. Peritoneal signs are ominous, and suggest an obstetrical emergency.

Q. References
a. Tintinalli's: Chapter 101. Ectopic Pregnancy and Emergencies in the First 20 Weeks of Pregnancy
b. Rosen's: Chapter 178. Acute Complications of Pregnancy

CASE 41: Agitation (Ani Aydin, MD)

A. Chief complaint
a. 49-year-old male with agitation

B. Vital signs
a. BP: 110/75 HR: 96 RR: 16 T: 37°C Sat: 98% on RA

C. What does the patient look like?

a. Patient appears older than stated age; slurring speech, eyelids drooping, disheveled, urine stains on clothing; attempting to get off the stretcher; small laceration noted on forehead

D. Primary survey

a. Airway: slurred speech, protecting airway and saturating well on RA
b. Breathing: no apparent respiratory distress, no cyanosis
c. Circulation: pale and cool skin, normal capillary refill

E. Action

a. Oxygen via NC or nonrebreather mask
b. Two large-bore peripheral IV lines
c. Labs
    i. UA, urine toxicology panel, alcohol level, BMP, CBC, LFTs, PT, PTT
d. Monitor: BP: 110/75 HR: 96 RR: 16 T: 37°C Sat: 98% on RA
e. 1 L D5 NS
f. Finger stick glucose (130; must ask)

F. History

a. HPI: a 49-year-old undomiciled male with a history of alcohol intoxication and hepatitis is brought in by ambulance for public intoxication and agitation. Upon presentation to the ED, the patient insists that he is fine and wants to be discharged immediately. He denies any headache, dizziness, lightheadedness, chest pain, shortness of breath, abdominal pain, nausea, vomiting, changes in vision, blurry vision, or fever. He states that he drinks approximately one pint of vodka per day, and his last drink was just before being picked up by the ambulance. He denies any other ingestion. The patient requests a sandwich and a change of clothing.
b. PMHx: alcohol abuse, hepatitis. Tetanus up-to-date
c. PSHx: none
d. Allergies: none
e. Social: undomiciled, unemployed, lives on the streets; drinks one pint of vodka per day; he has smoked one pack of cigarettes per day for the past 35 years. He denies any cocaine, crack, heroin, marijuana, or IV drug use; he is not currently sexually active
f. FHx: unknown
g. PMD: none

G. Nurse

a. 1 L NS
    i. BP: 120/75 HR: 96 RR: 16 T: 37°C Sat: 98% on RA

H. Secondary survey

a. General: thin with large abdomen, awake, oriented × 2 (knows his name, knows that he is in hospital), disheveled, agitated, slurred speech
b. HEENT: erythematous conjunctiva, eyelids drooping, 1.5 cm linear laceration located on left forehead with some ecchymosis
c. Neck: normal

d. Chest: clear to auscultation bilaterally; spider angiomas noted

e. Heart: normal

f. Abdomen: soft, nontender, distended, + bowel sounds; + fluid wave; hepatomegaly; no guarding, no rebound; small umbilical hernia, reducible

g. Rectal: hemoccult negative brown stool

h. Urogenital: normal

i. Extremities: asterixis

j. Back: normal

k. Neuro: normal

l. Skin: forehead laceration as above

m. Lymph: normal

I. Action

a. Meds

   i. Thiamine

   ii. Folate

   iii. D5 NS

b. Reassess

   i. Patient is belligerent at times, but able to be calmed by talking to him, awake and oriented × 2, unable to ambulate unassisted, hungry.

c. Imaging

   i. Noncontrast head CT

J. Nurse

a. BP: 120/75 HR: 96 RR: 16 T: 37°C Sat: 98% on RA

b. Patient: agitated but able to be calmed with talking, awake, slurred speech

K. Results

Complete blood count:

WBC	5.5×10^3/uL
Hct	31.4%
Plt	99×10^3/uL

Basic metabolic panel:

Na	138 mEq/L
K	4.2 mEq/L
Cl	107 mEq/L
CO_2	17 mEq/L
BUN	17 mEq/dL
Cr	1.2 mg/dL
Gluc	130 mg/dL

Coagulation panel:

PT	13.1 sec
PTT	31 sec
INR	1.5

Liver function panel:

AST	65 U/L
ALT	30 U/L
Alk Phos	100 U/L
T bili	0.5 mg/dL
D bili	0.2 mg/dL
Amylase	30 U/L
Lipase	23 U/L
Albumin	3.5 g/dL

Urinalysis:

SG	1.010
pH	6
Prot	Neg
Gluc	Neg
Ketones	Neg
Bili	Neg
Blood	Neg
LE	Neg
Nitrite	Neg
Color	Yellow

Figure 41.1

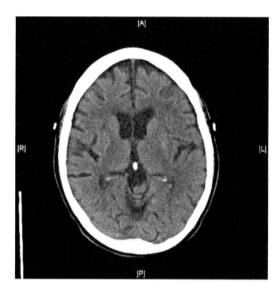

a. Osmolar gap = 9
b. Urine toxicology panel negative
c. Alcohol 350
d. Noncontrast head CT (Figure 41.1)

L. Action
a. Feed patient
b. Repair laceration

M. Diagnosis
a. Alcohol intoxication

N. Critical actions
- Finger stick glucose
- Noncontrast head CT
- Anion gap, osmolar gap
- Laceration repair

O. Examiner instructions
a. This is a case of alcohol intoxication. The patient is belligerent and has a head laceration. Since he is not fully oriented and unable to give an accurate history, a noncontrast head CT is appropriate. Should the patient become very agitated, chemical sedatives may be used, but the patient should be calmed by talking when appropriate.
b. Curveball: Although acute alcohol intoxication is a common ED presentation, patients often have other illnesses which may easily be missed. If the candidate does not request a finger stick glucose quickly, have the patient lose consciousness. The glucose in this scenario will be 35, and the patient will remain unresponsive until dextrose is administered intravenously.

P. Pearls
a. Alcohol intoxication contributes to 100,000 deaths per year.
b. About 2.5% of ED visits are related to alcohol use/abuse.

c. Screenings can be conducted in the ED using the "CAGE" questions and the Michigan Alcohol Screening Test.

d. In agitated patients, coingestants must be considered.

e. A noncontrast head CT is appropriate in an intoxicated patient with obvious head injury.

Q. References
a. Tintinalli's: Chapter 179. Alcohols
b. Rosen: Chapter 155. Toxic Alcohols

CASE 42: Abdominal pain (Nicholas Genes, MD, PhD)

A. Chief complaint
a. 45-year-old female with abdominal pain and fever

B. Vital signs
a. BP: 99/62 HR: 122 RR: 24 T: 38.4°C Sat: 97% on RA

C. What does the patient look like?
a. Patient appears stated age, uncomfortable due to pain in moderate distress, slowly writhing on stretcher.

D. Primary survey
a. Airway: speaking in full sentences
b. Breathing: no apparent respiratory distress, no cyanosis, increased respiratory rate
c. Circulation: warm and flushed skin, normal capillary refill

E. History
a. HPI: a 45-year-old female with severe diffuse abdominal pain for a day, fevers on and off since yesterday; persistent nausea with two episodes of vomiting today (yellowish material and food contents); no diarrhea; last menstrual period was one year ago.

b. PMHx: type I diabetes

c. PSHx: none

d. Allergies: none

e. Social: lives with husband at home, denies alcohol, smoking, drugs, sexually active

f. FHx: aunt had type I diabetes, father has hypertension, mother has hyperthyroidism

g. PMD: Dr Pomerleau

F. Action
a. Oxygen via NC or nonrebreather mask

b. Two large-bore peripheral IV lines

c. Labs
   i. CBC, BMP, LFT, arterial or venous blood gas, PT/PTT, blood type and cross-match two units, lactate, blood culture, urine culture, urinalysis, urine pregnancy test

d. Monitor: BP: 99/62 HR: 122 RR: 24 T: 38.4°C Sat: 97% on RA

e. Cardiac monitoring

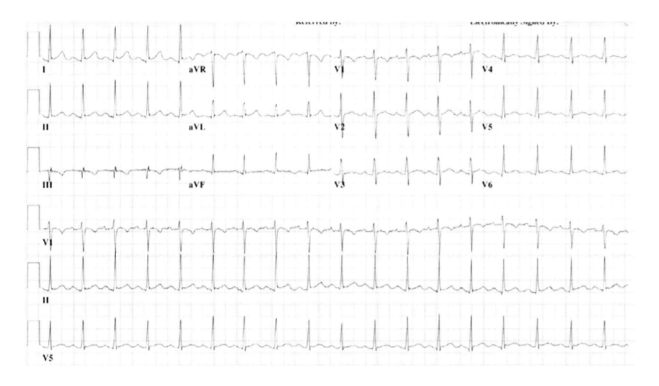

Figure 42.1

    f. 1 L NS bolus
    g. Finger stick glucose
    h. EKG

G. Nurse
    a. EKG (Figure 42.1)
    b. Glucose 335
    c. BP: 98/59 HR: 95 RR: 22 Sat: 98% on O_2

H. Secondary survey
    a. General: appears dry on examination, tachycardic; alert and oriented, moderate distress due to pain
    b. HEENT: mildly pale conjunctivae, otherwise normal
    c. Neck: normal
    d. Chest: lungs clear to auscultation bilaterally, tachypneic, no wheezes or rales
    e. Heart: tachycardic, regular rate and rhythm, no murmurs or rubs
    f. Abdomen: mildly distended, diffusely tender, bowel sounds decreased, no pulsatile masses, no masses, no hernias, nontender at McBurney's point, negative Murphy sign. Rebound and guarding are noted, no rigidity
    g. Rectal: hemoccult negative brown stool
    h. Urogenital: normal
    i. Extremities: normal
    j. Back: normal, no costovertebral angle tenderness
    k. Neuro: normal
    l. Skin: dry, poor turgor, no rashes, no edema, no cellulitis
    m. Lymph: normal

I. Action

a. Second liter IV fluid bolus

b. Recheck blood glucose

c. Start insulin drip; follow labs

J. Imaging

a. Upright CXR

b. Obstructive series

c. Meds

   i. Morphine IV

   ii. Reglan IV

d. Reassess

   i. Patient's heart rate returning to normal, pain subsiding (if analgesia given; if not, no change).

K. Nurse

a. BP: 112/69 HR: 90 RR: 18 Sat: 98% on O_2 (after 1 L)

b. Patient: still complains of some abdominal pain

L. Results

Complete blood count:

WBC	12.1×10^3/uL	T bili	0.5 mg/dL
Hct	41.5%	D bili	0.2 mg/dL
Plt	253×10^3/uL	Amylase	84 U/L
		Lipase	50 U/L
Basic metabolic panel:		Albumin	4.2 g/dL
Na	135 mEq/L		
K	4.0 mEq/L	**Urinalysis:**	
Cl	100 mEq/L	SG	1.035
CO_2	10 mEq/L	pH	8
BUN	34 mEq/dL	Prot	Neg
Cr	1.4 mg/dL	Gluc	+
Gluc	301 mg/dL	Ketones	+
		Bili	Neg
Coagulation panel:		Blood	+
PT	13.1 sec	Nitrite	+
PTT	26 sec	Color	Yellow
INR	1.0		
		Arterial blood gas:	
Liver function panel:		pH	7.1
AST	22 U/L	PO_2	80 mmHg
ALT	20 U/L	PCO_2	25 mmHg
Alk Phos	100 U/L	HCO_3	10 mmol/L

a. Lactate 2.2 mmol/L

b. Upright CXR (Figure 42.2)

c. AXR (Figures 42.3A and 42.3B)

M. Action

a. IVF bolus, insulin drip, replete K, follow labs, EKG, ICU admit, antibiotics for UTI (likely cause).

Figure 42.2

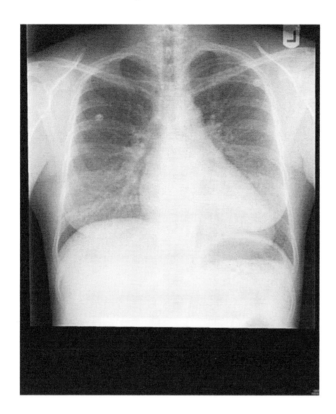

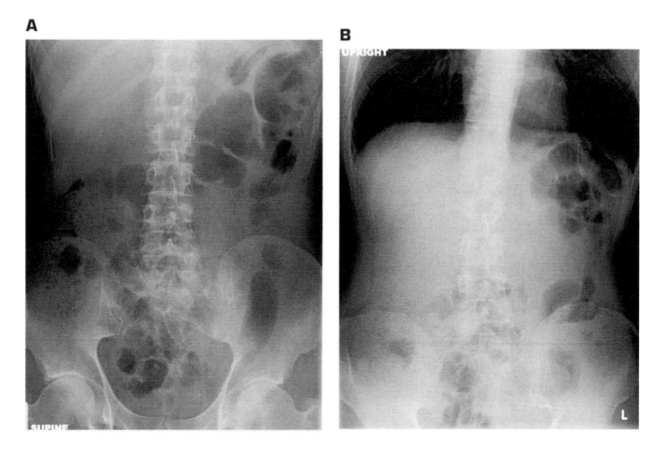

Figure 42.3 A and B

b. Meds

    i. Antibiotics (such as fluoroquinolone or cephalosporin)

    ii. Morphine IV if pain persists

c. Discussion with family and PMD regarding need for admission, hydration, insulin drip

d. EKG: normal sinus rhythm, no U waves

N. Diagnosis

a. Diabetic ketoacidosis

b. Urinary tract infection

O. Critical actions

▨ Early blood glucose assessment

▨ Fluid replacement (normal saline during the first hour, followed by ½ normal saline)

▨ Insulin drip

▨ Replete potassium

▨ EKG

▨ ICU admission

▨ Antibiotics for UTI

P. Examiner instructions

a. This is a case of diabetic ketoacidosis (DKA). DKA can be a presentation of new diabetes, a result of noncompliance with insulin therapy, or due to stressors, inflammation, or infection. If a blood glucose is assessed early (finger stick or venous sample), therapy for DKA may be started much earlier. Do not reveal the patient's blood glucose level unless it is specifically requested. The most important initial therapy in adults is IV fluids, not insulin. The patient's symptoms will worsen (blood pressure will fall and heart rate will rise), until fluid is administered. As fluid and insulin are administered, the symptoms of abdominal pain will resolve. Any evaluation for surgical cause of abdominal pain (surgical consultation, CT scan, etc) will reveal no pathology.

Q. Pearls

a. Diagnosis depends on a blood glucose of 250 mg/dL or higher, a bicarbonate level of 15 mEq/L or lower, and a pH (by arterial or venous blood gas) of 7.3 or lower with ketonuria.

b. Let the anion gap guide insulin therapy, not serum glucose or ketones.

c. Insulin should be continued until the anion gap resolves, not until the glucose normalizes. When glucose levels fall below 250 mg/dL, dextrose should be added to the IV fluid infusion to avoid hypoglycemia.

d. Be wary of potassium levels, they will drop as acidemia is corrected – begin repleting early.

e. Abdominal pain is a frequent complaint in DKA. It may be related to the precipitating cause, or it may be idiopathic. Peritoneal signs are ominous, and often suggest a surgical emergency. Consider early antibiotics, fluids, and surgical consultation.

f. There is little evidence that bicarbonate or phosphate repletion is of benefit. Giving insulin and fluids is usually ample therapy for treating the acidosis. The insulin given in DKA is not really for sugar reabsorption (insulin sometimes isn't given in mild DKA). Instead, the insulin is for ketogenesis and to overcome the acidosis.

R. References

a. Tintinalli's: Chapter 220. Diabetic Ketoacidosis

b. Rosen: Chapter 126. Diabetes Mellitus and Disorders of Glucose Homeostasis

CASE 43: Abdominal pain (Nicholas Genes, MD, PhD)

A. Chief complaint

a. 61-year-old man with epigastric pain and nausea

B. Vital signs

a. BP: 122/77 HR: 62 RR: 18 T: 36.3°C Sat: 97% on RA FS: 133

C. What does the patient look like?

a. Patient appears stated age, appearing uncomfortable due to pain, in moderate distress, looking pale and complaining of nausea.

D. Primary survey

a. Airway: speaking in full sentences

b. Breathing: no apparent respiratory distress, no cyanosis, increased respiratory rate

c. Circulation: cool and clammy skin, normal capillary refill

E. Action

a. Oxygen via NC or nonrebreather mask

b. Two large-bore peripheral IV lines

c. Labs

i. CBC, BMP, LFT, cardiac enzymes, PT/PTT, type and cross-match 2 units

d. 500 ml NS bolus

e. Cardiac monitor

f. Monitor: BP: 109/62 HR: 55 RR: 20 T: 37.3°C Sat: 97% on 2 L NC

i. If no fluids given: BP: 98/50 HR: 50 RR: 20 T: 37.3°C Sat: 97% on 2 L NC

ii. If nitroglycerin given: BP: 82/42 HR: 60 RR: 22 T: 37.3°C Sat: 95% on 2 L NC, distended neck veins

g. EKG

F. History

a. HPI: a 61-year-old male with history of type 2 diabetes and hypertension who felt weak and nauseous several times yesterday, unrelated to exertion. Today his stomach felt upset when walking into garage, he felt lightheaded and vomited once. The upset stomach settled into a heavy epigastric dullness; he felt weak and called 911.

b. PMHx: type 2 diabetes, hypertension, believes he has been told his cholesterol is high

c. PSHx: appendectomy, age 18

d. Allergies: none

e. Social: lives with wife, quit smoking 2 years ago, no alcohol, no drugs

f. FHx: father died of heart attack at age 50; mother has type 2 diabetes

g. PMD: Dr Brown

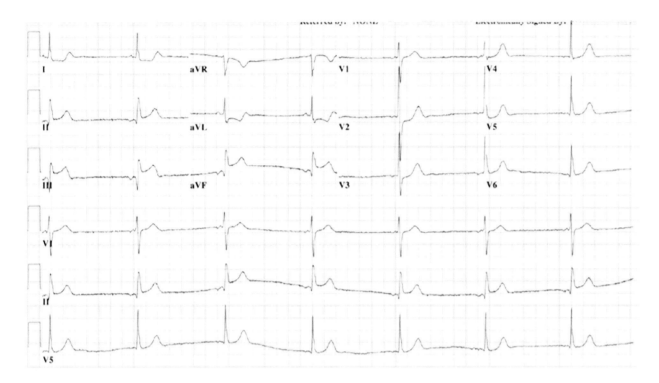

Figure 43.1

G. Nurse
  a. EKG (Figure 43.1)
  b. Patient still has epigastric sensation described in HPI

H. Actions
  a. EKG with right-sided leads
  b. CXR
  c. Aspirin chewable

I. Secondary survey
  a. General: alert and oriented, moderate distress due to pain, appears pale, clammy
  b. HEENT: normal
  c. Neck: normal
  d. Chest: lungs clear to auscultation, no wheezes, no rales
  e. Heart: bradycardic, no murmurs, rubs
  f. Abdomen: soft, nontender, no distension, no hepatosplenomegaly
  g. Rectal: hemoccult negative brown stool
  h. Urogenital: normal
  i. Extremities: normal
  j. Back: normal
  k. Neuro: normal
  l. Skin: pale, clammy, no rashes, no edema, no clubbing
  m. Lymph: normal

J. Action
  a. Consult cardiology/activate cardiac cathetenzation lab
  b. Repeat EKG (Figure 43.1)

Figure 43.2

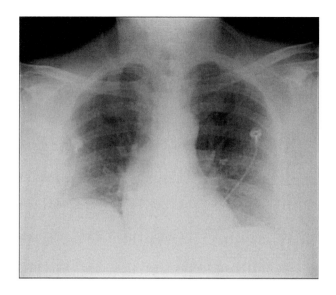

c. If 500 ml NS given: BP: 108/59 HR: 60 RR: 18 Sat: 98% on O_2

d. If no fluids given: BP: 80/45 HR: 52 RR: 20 Sat: 95% on O_2

e. If repeated nitroglycerin given, patient will go into shock which will require IV fluids and dobutamine to correct; dobutamine is started at 5 μg/kg/min and titrated up to 20 μg/kg/min. If these steps are not taken promptly, the patient will expire

K. Nurse

a. CXR (Figure 43.2)

L. Results

Complete blood count:

WBC	11.5×10^3/uL
Hct	40.0%
Plt	206×10^3/uL

Basic metabolic panel:

Na	138 mEq/L
K	3.8 mEq/L
Cl	103 mEq/L
CO_2	25 mEq/L
BUN	28 mEq/dL
Cr	1.2 mg/dL
Gluc	144 mg/dL

Coagulation panel:

PT	14 sec
PTT	30 sec
INR	1.1

Liver function panel:

AST	44 U/L
ALT	35 U/L
Alk Phos	67 U/L
T bili	0.9 mg/dL
D bili	0.2 mg/dL
Amylase	250 U/L
Lipase	66 U/L
Albumin	4.1 g/dL

Urinalysis:

SG	1.022
pH	7.1
Prot	Neg
Gluc	Neg
Ketones	Neg
Bili	Neg
Blood	Neg
LE	Neg
Nitrite	Neg
Color	Yellow

Arterial blood gas:

pH	7.4
PO_2	90 mmHg
PCO_2	44 mmHg
HCO_3	24 mmol/L

a. Troponin I: 1.2

M. Diagnosis
a. Inferior wall myocardial infarction with right ventricular involvement

N. Critical actions
▦ EKG
▦ Right-sided EKG
▦ IV access and fluid bolus
▦ Aspirin administration
▦ Avoid nitroglycerin administration
▦ Cardiology consultation
▦ Activating cardiac catheterization lab

O. Examiner instructions
a. This is a case of inferior wall myocardial infarction (MI) or heart attack. The patient's symptoms are vague and can suggest an abdominal process. This occurs frequently in diabetic patients with occluded coronary arteries overlying the diaphragm. Any delay in obtaining an EKG and diagnosing MI will worsen the patient's symptoms. Treating this patient with antiemetics, antacids, and pain medications might provide temporary relief, but the astute clinician should be concerned with cardiac pathology in any diabetic patient with nausea and vomiting. Note that nitroglycerin administration will cause the patient's blood pressure to drop and their symptoms to worsen.

P. Pearls
a. About one-third of inferior wall MIs involve the right ventricle, which has been associated with higher mortality and complications, especially in the setting of arrhythmias (though prognosis is good with prompt and appropriate therapy).
b. All EKGs with inferior ST elevations should have a right-sided lead V4–6 obtained – elevation in these leads is highly suggestive of right coronary artery occlusion and right ventricular infarction.
c. Any drugs that decrease preload – such as nitroglycerin but also diuretics – should be avoided. Even Foley catheter placement may cause vagal stimulation sufficient to worsen right ventricular function.
d. Several liters of IV fluids may be safely administered. If central venous pressure monitoring is in effect, a pressure of 15 mmHg is the target. Fluids above that limit are unlikely to improve hemodynamics; pressors may be of benefit at that point.
e. β-blockers and calcium channel blockers will slow heart rate and AV nodal conduction, and decrease contractility. Their use should be avoided in the hemodynamically unstable patient, and attempted only with careful monitoring in stable patients.
f. Reperfusion therapy, either through cardiac catheterization or thrombolysis, reduces morbidity and mortality for both inferior and right ventricular MI, just as it does for anterior MI.

Q. References
a. Tintinalli's: Chapter 53. Acute Coronary Syndromes
b. Rosen: Chapter 78. Acute Coronary Syndrome

CASE 44: Abdominal pain (Nicholas Genes, MD, PhD)

A. Chief complaint

a. 25-year-old female with abdominal pain

B. Vital signs

a. BP: 115/73 HR: 96 RR: 18 T: 37.2°C Sat: 98% on RA

C. What does the patient look like?

a. Patient appears stated age, sitting upright, clutching abdomen and grimacing in pain.

D. Primary survey

a. Airway: speaking in short sentences, phonating well

b. Breathing: no apparent respiratory distress, no cyanosis

c. Circulation: warm, flushed skin, good capillary refill

E. Action

a. Large-bore peripheral IV lines

b. Labs

    i. CBC, BMP, LFTs, urine pregnancy test, urinalysis, blood bank sample

F. History

a. HPI: a 25-year-old female with no significant past medical history states she experienced abrupt onset of right lower quadrant aching at work, several hours prior. She describes feeling "fine" beforehand, with normal bowel movements, no urinary burning or frequency, no fevers or chills, no cough or cold symptoms. States she had been out with friends the night prior. She had a similar pain once before, she thinks on the same side, but it resolved within minutes and was not this intense. She has vomited twice since the onset of pain.

b. PMHx: none

c. PSHx: none

d. Allergies: none

e. Meds: none

f. Social: nonsmoker, drinks alcohol socially, several male sexual partners in the past year. No prior pregnancies, no history of birth control; last menstrual period was 3 weeks ago, some menses are irregular with heavy bleeding and spotting in between periods

g. FHx: father has hypertension; mother has diabetes

h. PMD: none

G. Nurse

a. Urine pregnancy test negative

H. Action

a. Infuse 1 L NS IV

b. Reassess vital signs

    i. BP: 110/65 HR: 90 RR: 18 Sat: 98% on RA

I. Secondary survey

a. General: mildly obese, hirsute woman, alert and oriented, significant distress due to pain

b. HEENT: normal

c. Neck: normal

d. Chest: normal

e. Heart: normal

f. Abdomen: no distension, exquisitely tender over right lower quadrant, bowel sounds present, no masses, no hernias; negative Murphy sign, + guarding, no rigidity

g. Rectal: hemoccult negative brown stool

h. Urogenital: no external lesions; pelvic speculum examination shows no discharge, no blood at cervix; bimanual examination shows no cervical motion tenderness, but significant tenderness is noted at right adnexa

i. Extremities: normal

j. Back: normal

k. Neuro: normal

l. Skin: normal

m. Lymph: normal

J. Action

a. Meds

   i. IV pain and nausea medication such as morphine and metoclopromide

b. Reassess

   i. Patient's discomfort improving but still present

c. Imaging

   i. Doppler US of pelvis

   ii. If CT scan of abdomen/pelvis is ordered, inform candidate test will take time

K. Nurse

a. BP: 112/69 HR: 85 RR: 18 Sat: 98% on RA

L. Results

Complete blood count:

WBC	11.1×10^3/uL
Hct	38.5%
Plt	253×10^3/uL

Basic metabolic panel:

Na	137 mEq/L
K	4.1 mEq/L
Cl	101 mEq/L
CO_2	24 mEq/L
BUN	13 mEq/dL
Cr	0.9 mg/dL
Gluc	122 mg/dL

Coagulation panel:

PT	13.1 sec
PTT	26.2 sec
INR	1.0

Liver function panel:

AST	22 U/L
ALT	20 U/L
Alk Phos	55 U/L
T bili	0.5 mg/dL
D bili	0.2 mg/dL
Amylase	34 U/L
Lipase	30 U/L
Albumin	4.0 g/dL

Urinalysis:

SG	1.020
pH	6
Prot	Neg
Gluc	Neg
Ketones	Neg
Bili	Neg
Blood	Neg
LE	Neg
Nitrite	Neg
Color	Yellow

   a. Lactate 1.2 mmol/L (if ordered)

   b. Pelvic US (Figures 44.1, 44.2, and 44.3) shows edematous polycystic right ovary with decreased blood flow on Doppler imaging

M. Action

   a. Preop labs

      i. Blood type and cross, PT/PTT

   b. Meds

      i. IV pain medication (Morphine or Dilaudid)

   c. Gyn consult

      i. Emergent laparoscopy for detorsion

Figure 44.1

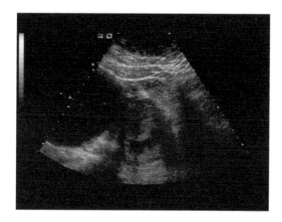

Figure 44.2

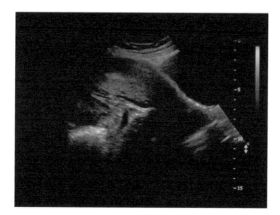

Figure 44.3

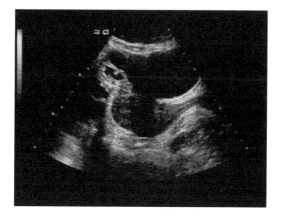

   d. Discussion with patient regarding need for emergent surgery for ovarian torsion, risk losing ovary, and infertility

   e. If US is not ordered and a course of observation is selected, patient will start to experience worsening symptoms.

N. Diagnosis
a. Ovarian torsion

O. Critical actions
▥ Pregnancy test

▥ Pelvic examination

▥ Pelvic US

▥ Ob/Gyn consultation for laparoscopy and detorsion

▥ Analgesia and re-assessment

P. Examiner instructions
a. This is a case of ovarian (adnexal) torsion. The ovary has twisted around its blood supply, causing lack of blood flow, pain, and threatening the viability of the organ. The patient's symptoms are severe, abrupt in onset, with occasional respites from a nonspecific but intense pain. Important early actions include ruling out pregnancy, identifying an enlarged ovary, and evaluating blood flow to the ovaries by Doppler US. A CT scan would show a large ovary but nothing explicitly pathological. Her pain will be partially relieved by pain medication, and her laboratory results will not aid in diagnosis. Treatment of ovarian torsion is extremely time-sensitive; the risk of losing the ovary increases with total ischemic time. If Gyn is consulted prior to obtaining Doppler US: The Gyn consultant should be reluctant to see the patient rapidly; candidate should explicitly describe a concern for ovarian torsion and understand the emergent need for operative intervention.

Q. Pearls
a. Adnexal torsion, a twisting of the ovary on its vascular pedicle, is a surgical emergency, responsible for approximately 3% of gynecologic emergencies. The duration of ischemia necessary to cause irreversible tissue necrosis is unknown, but a delay in diagnosis may result in the loss of the ovary and fallopian tube.

b. Torsion of a normal-sized ovary is rare; ovarian cysts greater than 5 cm and poly-cystic ovaries are more prone to torsion. Previous history of ovarian mass or infertility treatments have been reported as risk factors. Prior ectopic pregnancies, pelvic inflammatory disease, or endometriosis are not risk factors.

c. Laboratory findings are nonspecific in ovarian torsion, and cannot be used to assess tissue necrosis or ischemia.

d. Massive ovarian edema on imaging is suggestive of intermittently impaired blood flow.

R. References
a. Tintinalli's: Chapter 100. Abdominal and Pelvic Pain in the Nonpregnant Female

b. Rosen: Chapter 100. Selected Gynecologic Disorders

CASE 45: Altered mental status (Nicholas Genes, MD, PhD)

A. Chief complaint

a. 33-year old male found unconscious

B. Vital signs

a. BP: 95/63 HR: 66 RR: 11 T: 37.2°C SpO$_2$: 96% on RA

C. What does the patient look like?

a. Patient appears stated age, unconscious on stretcher.

D. Primary survey

a. Airway: not speaking; no apparent obstruction or trauma

b. Breathing: no respiratory distress, no cyanosis

c. Circulation: warm skin, normal capillary refill

E. Action

a. Oxygen via non-rebreather mask

b. Two large-bore peripheral IV lines

c. Labs

   i. CBC, BMP, serum acetaminophen, salicylates, alcohol, creatine phosphokinase (CPK), urine toxicology screen, +/- carboxyhemoglobin level

d. Monitor: BP: 96/68 HR: 71 RR: 10 Sat: 100% on O$_2$

e. EKG

f. Finger stick glucose (result is 98 mg/dL; must ask)

F. History

a. HPI: a 33-year-old male recently began working as home health aide for client with advanced cancer. EMS reports the patient voiced no complaints, behaved normally until he went to the bathroom about 2 hours ago. Client discovered the patient collapsed by the toilet.

b. PMHx: unknown

c. PSHx: unknown

d. Allergies: unknown

e. Social: unknown

f. FHx: unknown

g. PMD: unknown

G. Nurse

a. EKG (Figure 45.1)

H. Secondary survey

a. General: obtunded, minimally arousable, no apparent distress

b. HEENT: pupils equal, round and reactive to light, 2 mm to 1 mm

c. Neck: normal

d. Chest: lungs clear, normal breath sounds with no wheezes, rhonchi, or rales

e. Heart: normal, no murmurs, rubs, or gallops

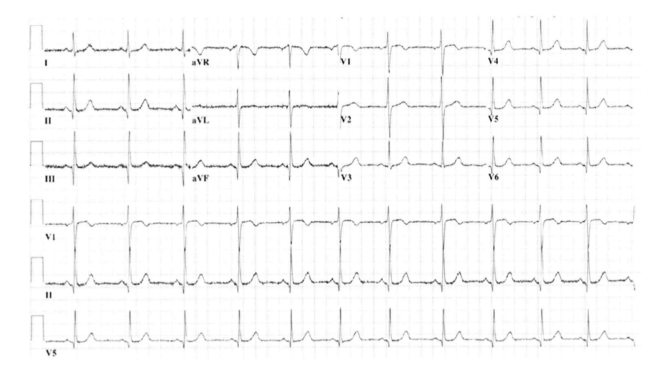

Figure 45.1

f. Abdomen: soft, nontender, nondistended
g. Rectal: hemoccult negative, good rectal tone
h. Urogenital: normal
i. Extremities: normal
j. Back: normal
k. Neuro: obtunded, barely arousable; moves all extremities, uncooperative with examination
l. Skin: pale, no rashes, edema, or cellulitis
m. Lymph: normal

I. Action
a. Meds
  i. Administer naloxone, dose 0.1–0.4 mg IV; thiamine and folate IV
b. Reassess
  i. Patient more easily aroused with noxious stimuli (e.g. sternal rub)
c. Imaging
  i. Portable CXR (evaluate for aspiration, radio-opaque pill fragments)
  ii. Consider head CT (not necessary if no signs of trauma, appreciable neuro deficit, and patient improves with antidote.)

J. Nurse
a. If naloxone given: BP: 98/59 HR: 80 RR: 13 Sat: 98% on O_2
b. If naloxone not given: BP: 98/59 HR: 80 RR: 8 Sat: 93% on O_2

K. Results

Complete blood count:

WBC	$6.1 \times 10^3/uL$
Hct	41.5%
Plt	$253 \times 10^3/uL$

Basic metabolic panel:

Na	137 mEq/L
K	4.1 mEq/L
Cl	103 mEq/L
CO_2	25 mEq/L
BUN	12 mEq/dL
Cr	0.8 mg/dL
Gluc	102 mg/dL

Liver function panel:

AST	45 U/L
ALT	40 U/L
Alk Phos	100 U/L
T bili	0.8 mg/dL
D bili	0.1 mg/dL
Amylase	40 U/L

Lipase	53 U/L
Albumin	4.1 g/dL

Urinalysis:

SG	1.020
pH	6
Prot	Neg
Gluc	Neg
Ketones	Neg
Bili	Neg
Blood	Neg
LE	Neg
Nitrite	Neg
Color	Yellow

Arterial blood gas:

pH	7.3
PO_2	80 mmHg
PCO_2	65 mmHg
HCO_3	24 mmol/L

a. Urine toxicology results not available

b. Alcohol, acetaminophen, salicylates negative

c. CPK, carboxyhemoglobin levels normal (if ordered)

d. CXR (Figure 45.2)

Figure 45.2

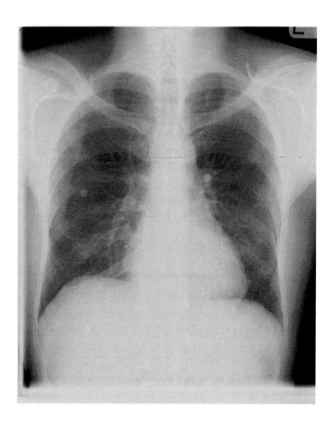

L. Action

a. Meds

    i. Naloxone IV until status improves

    ii. If naloxone not given, suffers respiratory depression, requires intubation and ICU admission – or codes in the ER

b. Observation for 12 hours if repeated doses of naloxone given, consider admission

    i. With repeated escalating doses of naloxone if mental status declines, or administer naloxone IV drip

c. Consult Poison Center and discharge with referral for substance abuse counseling

M. Diagnosis

a. Opioid overdose

N. Critical actions

- Finger stick glucose
- Naloxone administration
- EKG
- CXR
- Reassessment after interventions

O. Examiner instructions

a. This is a case of opioid (narcotic) intoxication from access to client's medications, which included fentanyl patches and oxycodone tablets. The patient presents with the "classic triad" of opioid overdose – coma, miosis (small pupils), and decreased respiratory rate. Important early actions include administering naloxone incrementally, as a large initial dose can precipitate withdrawal, vomiting, and possibly aspiration. Prolonged delay, (as if waiting for urine toxicology screen results) will result in respiratory depression and necessitate intubation to prevent death. Failure to monitor and observe after naloxone administration will result in recurrence of obtundation and respiratory depression. If this patient is sent outside of the ED (for CXR, CT scan) without intubation, inform candidate that the "patient has stopped breathing." The patient will be found apneic, hypoxic, and bradycardic, requiring ACLS.

P. Pearls

a. While opioid withdrawal alone is not life threatening, suddenly precipitating withdrawal with high-dose naloxone can pose significant risk. Withdrawal symptoms can be managed with clonidine, antiemetics, antidiarrheals, and methadone.

b. A titrated dose of naloxone is warranted in patients who maintain appropriate airway patency and ventilation. A naloxone dose of up to 2.0 mg IV may be necessary in patients with significant respiratory depression, and may be repeated every 3 minutes until 10 mg have been administered or respiratory depression is reversed. If no improvement, bag-valve-mask ventilation and/or endotracheal intubation is indicated.

c. The duration of action of naloxone IV is 20 to 60 minutes, shorter than most opioids. Thus, it may be necessary to re-dose, especially in the setting of sustained-release opioid ingestions.

d. Gastric decontamination should be considered in toxic ingestions, particularly when less than one hour after ingestion (especially beta-blockers, calcium channel blockers and cyclic antidepressants). However, the risks of aspiration in a comatose patient must be balanced with potential gains. Gastric decontamination rarely affects clinical outcomes in the undifferentiated poisoned patient and should not be used routinely

e. Urine toxicology screens are time-consuming, highly prone to false readings, and will not change emergent management of adult patients.

f. A finger stick blood sugar test is key to eliminating a common cause of altered mental status, and should be performed immediately on every altered patient.

g. Some states mandate reporting of impaired healthcare workers and reporting intoxication cases to Poison Control Centers, which can aid in management and outpatient follow-up.

Q. References
a. Tintinalli's: Chapter 180. Opioids
b. Rosen: Chapter 162. Opioids

CASE 46: Diarrhea (Nicholas Genes, MD, PhD)

A. Chief complaint
a. 34-year-old man with abdominal pain and diarrhea

B. Vital signs
a. BP: 122/77 HR: 92 RR: 18 T: 37.5°C Sat: 99% on RA

C. What does the patient look like?
a. Patient appears stated age, comfortably lying on his stretcher.

D. Primary survey
a. Airway: speaking in full sentences
b. Breathing: no respiratory distress, no cyanosis
c. Circulation: warm and dry skin, normal capillary refill

E. History
a. HPI: a 34-year-old man with no significant past medical history presents with persistent diarrhea over the past few weeks. He denies fever. He defecates more than six times a day, producing a watery brown stool with a foul odor and no signs of blood or flecks of mucus. His abdomen feels bloated and occasionally diffusely painful. Symptoms were initially worse, then seemed to resolve, but have returned and persisted. He thinks he has lost 10 lbs.
b. PMHx: as a teen, had asthma, but has "outgrown it"
c. PSHx: none
d. Allergies: none
e. Meds: none
f. Social: lives alone, consumes alcohol socially, no smoking, no IV drug use
g. FHx: father with diabetes; brother with Crohn's disease
h. PMD: none

F. Secondary survey

a. General: alert and oriented, no apparent distress
b. HEENT: mucous membranes dry
c. Neck: normal
d. Chest: lungs clear to auscultation, no wheezes
e. Heart: borderline tachycardic, no murmurs or rubs
f. Abdomen: soft, nontender, mild distension, active bowel sounds, no hepatosplenomegaly
g. Rectal: hemoccult negative brown stool
h. Urogenital: normal
i. Back: normal
j. Extremities: normal
k. Neuro: normal
l. Skin: warm, dry, no edema, no clubbing
m. Lymph: normal

G. Action

a. Further history: The patient denies recent illness and has never had unprotected sex, anal sex, or sex with high-risk partners. He has not been exposed to blood-borne pathogens. Denies antibiotic use in recent months. The patient admits to traveling outside the country about 6 weeks ago; he visited several eastern European countries.
b. Obtain stool sample for ova and parasites, fecal leukocytes, stool culture, *Clostridium difficile* toxin, Giardia antigen
c. Send electrolyte panel

H. Nurse

a. BP: 125/73 HR: 92 RR: 18 T: 37.5°C Sat: 99% on RA

I. Results

Complete blood count:

WBC	10.9×10^3/uL
Hct	43%
Plt	220×10^3/uL

Basic metabolic panel:

Na	133 mEq/L
K	3.2 mEq/L
Cl	105 mEq/L
CO_2	16 mEq/L
BUN	28 mEq/dL
Cr	1.1 mg/dL
Gluc	99 mg/dL

Coagulation panel:

PT	12.7 sec
PTT	28.3 sec
INR	1.0

Liver function panel:

AST	44 U/L
ALT	38 U/L
Alk Phos	110 U/L
T bili	0.9 mg/dL
D bili	0.1 mg/dL
Amylase	55 U/L
Lipase	28 U/L
Albumin	3.9 g/dL

Urinalysis:

SG	1.030
pH	7
Prot	Neg
Gluc	Neg
Ketones	Neg
Bili	Neg
Blood	Neg
LE	Neg
Nitrite	Neg
Color	Yellow

a. Ova and parasites analysis reveals cysts and motile, pear-shaped trophozoites
b. Fecal leukocytes not seen
c. Other tests pending

J. Action

a. Oral rehydration using a glucose-containing beverage, or IV fluids such as NS with supplementary potassium
b. Prescribe antibiotics – Ciprofloxacin PO for 3 days, Trimethoprim/sulfamethoxazole, or non-gastrointestinally absorbed agent such as rifaximin for presumed infectious diarrhea
c. Administer loperamide as needed for loose stools
d. Arrange for outpatient follow-up
e. Report case to the Centers for Disease Control

K. Diagnosis

a. Traveler's diarrhea – strongly suggestive of giardiasis, but may not be definitively diagnosed in a single encounter

L. Critical actions

▓ Elicit social history – travel, risk factors for immune compromise, recent antibiotic use
▓ Send stool sample with ova and parasites, fecal leukocytes, Giardia antigen, *C. difficile* toxin
▓ Rehydrate and replete electrolyte deficiencies
▓ Prescribe antibiotics
▓ Arrange for follow-up

M. Examiner instructions

a. This is a case of traveler's diarrhea, resulting from *Giardia lamblia* infection. The patient's symptoms are vague, mild, and his clinical course in the ED is stable and unchanging. Important early actions are to elicit a travel history, risk factors for immunocompromised state, and other important causes of diarrhea and abdominal symptomatology. Critical actions include sending a stool sample for laboratory analysis, rehydrating the patient, prescribing antibiotics, and arranging for follow-up. Imaging is of no benefit in this case, and requests to consult gastroenterologists or infectious disease specialists will yield no additional information.

N. Pearls

a. Approximately 40% of Americans traveling to developing countries are affected by diarrhea or gastroenteritis in the first two weeks of travel.
b. *G. lamblia* is the most commonly identified cause of *chronic* traveler's diarrhea, as in this case (*Escherichia coli* being the most common acute cause). Giardia is a protozoan infection of the proximal gut, typically transmitted by contaminated water, commonly in Eastern Europe (though food or fecal–oral transmission is possible and accounts for occasional daycare epidemics in the USA). Infected patients are usually asymptomatic or self-limited after an acute phase, but in some patients, symptoms can persist for years. A course of metronidazole is more than 90% effective in achieving cure.

c. *Entamoeba histolytica* amebiasis is a culprit for long-term travelers to Africa, Asia, and Latin America. Like Giardia, amebiasis is a protozoan infection identified by antigen or ova and parasite testing. Unlike Giardia, *E. histolytica* can invade the colon wall and liver, causing fevers, pain, and potentially fatal abscesses.

d. Acute diarrheal illness (less than 2 weeks) is usually caused by bacteria or their toxins, with common organisms including *E. coli*, *Campylobacter jejuni*, *Salmonella*, *Shigella*, *Vibrio*, and *C. difficile*.

e. *Vibrio cholera* is rarely imported into the USA, causing only 80 cases per year. It presents as a profuse, painless watery diarrhea ("rice-water stools") in tropical travelers that can result in profound dehydration and requires aggressive fluid resuscitation.

f. Though loperamide use has been traditionally discouraged, large randomized trials have demonstrated its efficacy in shortening symptom duration for infectious diarrhea, when given in conjunction with antibiotics.

O. References
a. Tintinalli's: Chapter 156. World Travelers
b. Rosen: Chapter 94. Gastroenteritis

CASE 47: Seizure (Shefali Trivedi, MD)

A. Chief complaint
a. 45-year-old male with seizure prior to arrival

B. Vital signs
a. BP: 122/80 HR: 102 RR: 18 T: 38.6°C Sat: 99% on RA

C. What does the patient look like?
a. Patient appears stated age, sleeping comfortably on stretcher and in no acute distress.

D. Primary survey
a. Airway: patent, speaks in full sentences
b. Breathing: no apparent respiratory distress, no cyanosis
c. Circulation: warm, dry skin, normal capillary refill

E. Action
a. Oxygen via NC or non rebreather mask
b. Two large-bore peripheral IV lines
c. Labs
   i. CBC, BMP, LFTs, Calcium, Magnesium, +/- Prolactin, toxicology panel
d. 1 L NS
e. Blood cultures
f. EKG and monitored bed

F. History
a. HPI: a 45-year-old male with a past medical history of hypertension presents after a seizure witnessed by his wife about 1 hour before arrival. According to his wife, the

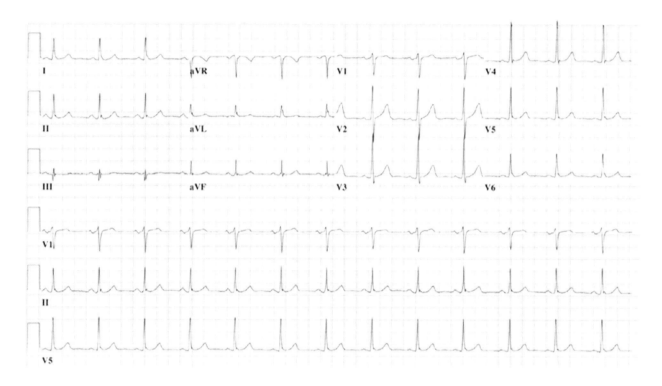

Figure 47.1

seizure was generalized tonic-clonic and lasted about 30 seconds with no postictal state. There was no head trauma associated with the event. This was his first seizure. The patient does not recall the seizure, but does note that he has had subjective fever associated with generalized mild abdominal pain for the past 3 days. He denies chest pain, shortness of breath, headache, chills, upper respiratory infection symptoms, nausea, vomiting, diarrhea, urinary symptoms, trauma, sick contacts, or travel history.

b. PMHx: hypertension

c. PSHx: none

d. Allergies: none

e. Meds: hydrochlorathiazide

f. Social: lives with wife and two children at home; denies smoking, alcohol, drug use; sexually active with his wife only

g. FHx: noncontributory

h. PMD: Dr. Parker, who he sees at least annually

G. Nurse

a. BP: 129/87 HR: 88 RR: 16 Sat: 100% on O_2, remains febrile

b. EKG (Figure 47.1)

H. Secondary survey

a. General: alert and oriented, no acute distress

b. HEENT: pale conjunctivae, otherwise normal

c. Neck: normal

d. Chest: normal

e. Heart: normal

    f. Abdomen: normal

    g. Rectal: hemoccult negative brown stool, normal rectal tone

    h. Urogenital: normal

    i. Extremities: normal

    j. Back: normal

    k. Neuro: normal

    l. Skin: petechiae and bruising noted on upper and lower extremities bilaterally

  m. Lymph: normal

I. Action

    a. CT head without contrast

    b. Acetaminophen PO

J. Nurse

    a. BP: 117/75 HR: 82 RR: 16 Sat: 100% on RA

K. Results

Complete blood count:

WBC	9.9×10^3/uL
Hct	19.4%
Plt	20×10^3/uL

Basic metabolic panel:

Na	137 mEq/L
K	3.9 mEq/L
Cl	102 mEq/L
CO_2	25 mEq/L
BUN	13 mEq/dL
Cr	1.9 mg/dL
Gluc	110 mg/dL

Coagulation panel:

PT	13.8 sec
PTT	30 sec
INR	1.0

Liver function panel:

AST	33 U/L
ALT	13 U/L
Alk Phos	75 U/L
T bili	1.2 mg/dL
D bili	0.4 mg/dL
Amylase	47 U/L
Lipase	25 U/L
Albumin	4.0 g/dL

Urinalysis:

SG	1.020
pH	6
Prot	+
Gluc	Neg
Ketones	Neg
Bili	Neg
Blood	Neg
LE	Neg
Nitrite	Neg
Color	Yellow

    a. CT head (Figure 47.2)

L. Action

    a. Ask for a peripheral smear

    b. Consult hematology

    c. Prednisone

    d. Plasma exchange

M. Diagnosis

    a. Thrombotic thrombocytopenic purpura

Figure 47.2

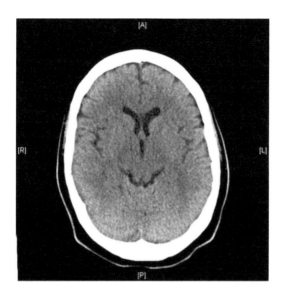

N. Critical actions

■ Note petechiae on physical examination
■ Obtain CBC
■ Steroids
■ Plasmapheresis
■ Hematology consultation (noting possible diagnosis of TTP)
■ Admission

O. Examiner instructions

a. This is a case of thrombotic thrombocytopenic purpura (TTP), where platelets aggregate in small blood vessels abnormally. This may lead to bleeding complications and multiorgan system complications. A thorough search into the cause of seizure is important in this case, especially laboratory evaluation and head CT to investigate intracranial complication such as bleeding.

b. Curveball: The patient could present actively seizing, or seize during the secondary survey, requiring the candidate to alter focus on the primary survey and seizure control. Benzodiazepines (such as lorazepam, midazolam) should be the first-line agents used to treat the seizures. After two doses, the seizures should stop.

P. Pearls

a. The classic pentad of TTP includes: fever, microangiopathic hemolytic anemia, thrombocytopenia, renal impairment, and CNS impairment. However, it is uncommon to have all components of the pentad (only 40% of patients present with all five components) and the presence of all five indicates that severe end organ ischemia or damage has taken place.

b. TTP is a clinical diagnosis, but characteristic laboratory findings include severe anemia, thrombocytopenia (<20,000 platelets/μL), schistocytes, helmet cells, fragmented RBCs on the peripheral smear. Decreased haptoglobin, elevated reticulocyte count, elevated indirect bilirubin are also common findings.

c. Neurologic findings can include headache, seizure activity, coma, CVA, or paresthesias.

d. Dialysis, anticonvulsants, or benzodiazepines may need to be ordered if the patient is suffering from severe renal impairment or seizure activity, respectively, and there is an anticipated delay before the effect of plasma exchange will take place.

e. Avoid platelet transfusions in TTP unless there is a risk of intracranial bleeding or hemorrhage, as added platelets can augment the platelet aggregation and cause worsening thrombosis and eventual ischemia.If plasmapheresis and steroid therapy are unsuccessful interventions, splenectomy may be required.

Q. References
a. Tintinalli's: Chapter 232. Acquired Hemolytic Anemia
b. Rosen: Chapter 122. Disorders of Hemostasis

CASE 48: Toothache (Shefali Trivedi, MD)

A. Chief complaint
a. 36-year-old male with infected tooth

B. Vital signs
a. BP: 141/79 HR: 107 RR: 18 T: 38.0°C Sat: 99% on RA

C. What does the patient look like?
a. Patient appears stated age, sitting up in stretcher, holding left side of face, uncomfortable in mild distress.

D. Primary survey
a. Airway: patent, speaking in full sentences
b. Breathing: no apparent distress, no cyanosis
c. Circulation: warm, dry skin, normal capillary refill

E. History
a. HPI: a 36-year-old male with no past medical history presents with left jaw pain and left lower molar pain for 7 days and swelling associated with difficulty opening his mouth for 2 days. The patient states he was going to try to make an appointment with his dentist, but the pain was so severe that he needed to come to the emergency department first. The patient states that the swelling appears to be worsening over the past 2 days and he has noted a foul smell from his mouth. He also notes subjective fever and chills for 2 days. He denies nausea, vomiting, diarrhea, constipation, trauma, or previous similar symptoms.
b. PMHx: none
c. PSHx: none
d. Allergies: no known drug allergies
e. Social: lives with his wife at home; denies smoking, drug use; drinks alcohol socially; sexually active with his wife only
f. FHx: noncontributory
g. PMD: Dr. Taylor, who he does not see regularly for routine visits

F. Secondary survey

a. General: alert and oriented, sitting up on stretcher, holding left side of face, uncomfortable in mild painful distress

b. HEENT: normocephalic, atraumatic, ocular examination normal, ears normal to inspection, tympanic membranes clear; nose examination normal; + left external jaw swelling, + trismus (unable to open mouth greater than 2 cm), + left submandibular area tense/indurated, erythematous, tender to palpation, + whitish discoloration of gum below left lower molars

c. Neck: normal

d. Chest: normal

e. Heart: normal

f. Abdomen: normal

g. Extremities: normal

h. Back: normal

i. Neuro: normal

j. Skin: normal

k. Lymph: normal

G. Action

a. Oxygen via NC or nonrebreather mask

b. Two large-bore peripheral IV lines

c. Prepare intubation equipment (may be needed if condition worsens)

d. Labs

   i. CBC, BMP, PT/PTT, blood type and hold

e. 1 L NS bolus

f. Monitor: BP: 138/82 HR: 98 RR: 16 Sat: 100% on 2 L NC

g. Acetaminophen PO

H. Action

a. Meds

   i. Clindamycin IV

   ii. Morphine IV

b. Consult ear, nose, and throat (ENT) specialist

I. Nurse

a. BP: 135/79 HR: 89 RR: 16 Sat: 99% on 2 L NC

b. Patient: symptoms improving, but pain is still present

J. Results

Complete blood count:

WBC	24.3×10^3/uL	BUN	18 mEq/dL
Hct	43.50%	Cr	1.1 mg/dL
Plt	225×10^3/uL	Gluc	126 mg/dL

Basic metabolic panel:

		Coagulation panel:	
Na	138 mEq/L	PT	13.3 sec
K	3.8 mEq/L	PTT	32 sec
Cl	104 mEq/L	INR	1.1
CO_2	24 mEq/L		

K. Action
a. ENT consult

b. Admission for administration of IV antibiotics and monitoring of airway patency

L. Diagnosis
a. Ludwig's angina

M. Critical actions
▨ Airway management, assessment for difficult airway characteristics and anticipate advanced airway management techniques

▨ Antibiotics

▨ ENT consult – Consult should not be delayed for diagnostic imaging

▨ Admission

N. Examiner instructions
a. This is a case of Ludwig's angina, which is a deep soft tissue infection in the neck, usually caused by a dental infection. Early antibiotics, airway monitoring, and surgical consultation are paramount.

b. Ludwig's angina is a clinical diagnosis. Although, diagnostic imaging such as soft tissue plain films of the neck, US, CT, or MRI may aid in the diagnosis of Ludwig's angina and its complications. Unless the candidate describes a specific concern for Ludwig's angina (based on induration of the submandibular space and concerning patient presentation), the ENT consultant will simply advise that the patient should follow-up with a dentist the next day. If antibiotics are not administered in a timely manner, patient may develop increasing airway swelling, difficulty breathing, increased heart rate and respiratory distress, and require emergency intubation.

c. Curveball: This case could be used to review advanced airway management strategies. The examiner should have the patient present in more acute distress with significant airway swelling, or progress rapidly during the secondary survey. Thus, the primary survey will reveal a patient in significant respiratory distress, unable to swallow his oral secretions. The candidate will have to manage the airway using advanced techniques (fiberoptic intubation, "awake" intubation, surgical airway, or others). This should be addressed before any other intervention (in parallel with establishing IV access). If the candidate chooses rapid sequence intubation with paralysis in the setting of this significant airway edema, they will NOT be successful in viewing the vocal cords and the intubation attempt will fail.

O. Pearls
a. A recently extracted or infected lower molar tooth is often present in the history of patients with Ludwig's angina.

b. The most common physical examination findings include bilateral submandibular swelling and elevation or protrusion of the tongue.

c. Ludwig's angina is a clinical diagnosis and includes the following five criteria: cellulitis with little or no pus in the submandibular space; bilateral cellulitis; gangrene with serosanguinous putrid fluid; involvement of connective tissue, fascia, and muscles, but sparing of glandular tissue; and cellulitis spread by continuity and not by lymphatics.

d. Airway compromise can occur suddenly and especially if action is not taken immediately. Posterior displacement of the tongue often leads to obstruction of the airway and patients may require endotracheal intubation. However, this often is difficult given the altered anatomy from the infection. Fiberoptic oral intubation or nasotracheal intubation may be necessary.

e. Preferred antibiotic choices include high-dose penicillin with metronidazole; clindamycin; cefoxitin; ampicillin-sulbactam; ticaricillin-clavulanate; or piperacillin-tazobactam.

f. Incision and drainage may be indicated if the patient does not respond to antibiotics.

P. References
a. Tintinalli's: Chapter 241. Infections and Disorders of the Neck and Upper Airway
b. Rosen: Chapter 70. Oral Medicine

CASE 49: Penetrating chest trauma (Abiola Fasina, MD)

A. Chief complaint
a. 24-year-old male stabbed in the chest

B. Vital signs
a. BP: 115/62 HR: 120 RR: 30 T: 97°C Sat: 97% on RA

C. What does the patient look like?
a. Young male with pale clammy skin, supine on a stretcher. Patient is somnolent with slow speech. Large gauze is present over the left mid-chest soaked in blood with emergency medical technician applying pressure.

D. Primary survey
a. Airway: speaking, no stridor
b. Breathing: tachypneic, using accessory muscles in obvious distress, equal breath sounds
c. Circulation: pale, clammy skin with thready radial pulses bilaterally, which disappear while examining patient

E. Action
a. Oxygen via non rebreather mask
b. Preparations for intubation, for airway protection and impending respiratory collapse
c. Two large-bore peripheral IV lines
d. Labs
   i. CBC, BMP, PT/PTT, blood type and cross-match, and lactate sent
e. NS boluses started wide open
f. Monitor: BP: 90/50 HR: 135 RR: 32 Sat: 95% on non rebreather mask
g. Intubate with appropriate RSI, e.g. etomidate and succinylcholine or rocuronium; placement confirmed with capnography
h. Order portable CXR
i. Call blood bank for 2 units uncross-matched O negative blood
j. Page surgical/trauma team

F. History
a. HPI: a 24-year-old male picked up by EMS outside bar after being stabbed in the chest with a knife during a bar brawl. Patient was found sitting on the curb clutching his chest and complaining of pain. Patient denied any medical problems but admitted to having several drinks during the course of the evening.
b. PMHx: none
c. PSHx: none
d. Allergies: none
e. Meds: none
f. Social: social alcohol use
g. FHx: noncontributory
h. PMD: none

G. Nurse
a. NS/LR wide open
b. Repeat vital signs: BP: 90/52 HR: 145 RR: 24 Sat: 100% on ventilator
c. CXR (Figure 49.1)

H. Secondary survey
a. General: unconscious and intubated
b. HEENT: normal; no facial lacerations or bruises are noted. Pupils equal, round, reactive and 3 mm bilaterally
c. Neck: distended neck veins
d. Chest: 2 cm wide laceration over the left anterior chest wall at approximately fifth intercostal space actively bleeding; equal breath sounds heard
e. Heart: muffled heart sounds – tachycardic
f. Abdomen: soft, nontender, no cuts, or hematomas noted
g. Rectal: good tone with hemoccult negative stool
h. GU: normal
i. Back: normal
j. Extremities: good tone; weak radial pulses, no palpable dorsalis pedis pulses; cool clammy hands and feet
k. Neuro: withdraws to pain; unable to assess further

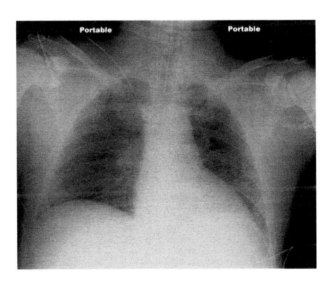

Figure 49.1

l. Skin: pale, no rashes or lesions

m. Lymph: normal

I. Action

a. Establish adequate IV access – two large-bore peripheral IV, intraosseus vascular access, or central venous access. Transfusion of uncross-matched blood initiated.

b. Focused assessment with sonography in trauma (FAST) examination (Figure 49.2). Examiner may allow transient improvement if pericardiocentesis is attempted, then progress to loss of vitals.

c. CXR: heart silhouette unremarkable; endotracheal tube in correct position above the carina

J. Nurse

a. Patient has lost vital signs, unable to palpate a pulse

K. Action

a. ED thoracotomy is performed (describe procedure) with presumptive diagnosis of acute pericardial tamponade due to penetrating chest wall injury. Once patient has lost pulses, there should be no delay for US or any imaging modality by the candidate prior to initiating this procedure.

b. Tetanus shot administered, cefazolin IV

c. Surgery/trauma team arrives and prepares to take patient to OR

d. Foley catheter

Figure 49.2 A, B, C and D

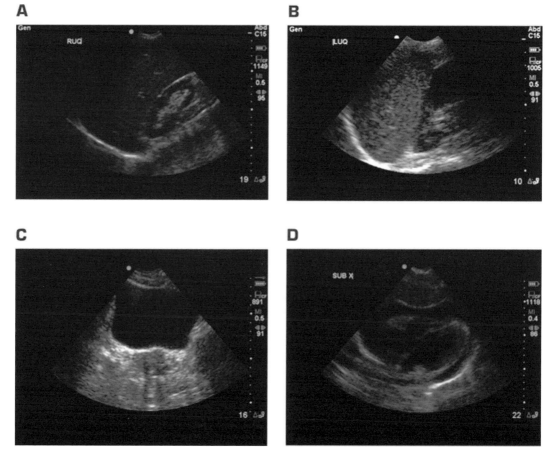

L. Results

Complete blood count:

WBC	12.0×10^3/uL
Hct	24.0%
Plt	250×10^3/uL

Basic metabolic panel:

Na	141 mEq/L
K	5.0 mEq/L
Cl	111 mEq/L
CO_2	24 mEq/L
BUN	29 mEq/dL
Cr	0.9 mg/dL
Gluc	100 mg/dL

Coagulation panel:

PT	14.6 sec
PTT	30 sec
INR	1.1

Urinalysis:

SG	1.010
pH	5
Prot	Neg
Gluc	Neg
Ketones	Neg
Bili	Neg
Blood	Neg
LE	Neg
Nitrite	Neg
Color	Yellow

Arterial blood gas:

pH	7.4
PO_2	85 mmHg
PCO_2	40 mmHg
HCO_3	24 mmol/L

M. Action

a. Thoracotomy reveals large amount of blood and clot in pericardium, 1 cm hole in right ventricle with active bleeding

b. Tamponade ventricular bleeding with finger, Foley catheter, or by oversewing

c. Patient taken emergently to OR by surgical team

N. Diagnosis

a. Acute pericardial tamponade due to penetrating chest wall trauma

O. Critical actions

▨ Intubating patient for airway protection

▨ Starting fluid resuscitation immediately

▨ Diagnosing pericardial tamponade (recognizing Beck's triad of distended neck veins, muffled heart sounds, and hypotension on performing US)

▨ Starting blood transfusion

▨ Surgical consultation for emergent OR repair

P. Examiner instructions

a. This is a case of acute pericardial tamponade due to ongoing bleeding within the pericardium (fibrous sac around the heart). This constricts the heart and prevents normal pumping of blood, causing a rapid heart rate and low blood pressure. This patient's condition will rapidly deteriorate (heart rate will rise, blood pressure and oxygen saturation fall) until the pressure is relieved. Loss of vital signs is an indication for emergency thoracotomy in the ED. If pericardiocentesis is attempted, blood will be obtained but the patient's condition will only slightly improve. Because of the volume and rate of bleeding, the fact that some of the blood is clotting, a needle is insufficient to drain enough blood to alleviate the condition. In this case, an open approach (thoracotomy) is warranted. Pericardiocentesis is not helpful in this setting because of a high incidence of false negatives, risk of further injury to the heart, and delay in definitive management.

b. Once thoracotomy is performed, the patient should be taken to the OR by trauma/ surgery for surgical repair.

Q. Pearls

a. ABCs: Airway, breathing, and circulation always come first in the management of trauma patients. Securing the airway is the first step in appropriate management of this patient.

b. Beck's triad of hypotension, distended neck veins, and muffled heart sounds raise concern for pericardial effusion, though they are all present in only about one-third of cases. Beck's triad can also be seen in tension pneumothorax or systemic air embolism.

c. CXR is frequently unremarkable in pericardial effusion; do not depend on imaging to make the diagnosis. The CXR in this case served to confirm ETT tube position.

d. Tamponade can also cause Kussmaul's breathing (distension of neck veins during inspiration) and pulsus paradoxus (drop in systolic blood pressure of more than 10 to 15 mmHg during inspiration).

R. References

a. Tintinalli's: Chapter 259. Cardiac Trauma
b. Rosen: Chapter 45. Thoracic Trauma

CASE 50: Animal bite (Shefali Trivedi, MD)

A. Chief complaint

a. 35-year-old male presents with cat bite to right hand 4 hours ago

B. Vital signs

a. BP: 128/82 HR: 78 RR: 16 T: 98.0°F Sat: 98% on RA

C. What does the patient look like?

a. Patient appears stated age, comfortable, sitting on stretcher, and in no acute distress.

D. Primary survey

a. Airway: speaking in full sentences
b. Breathing: no apparent respiratory distress, no cyanosis
c. Circulation: warm, dry skin, normal capillary refill

E. History

a. HPI: a 35-year-old male with a past medical history of hypertension, presents with a cat bite to the right hand 4 hours ago while playing with his neighbor's cat. The patient reports minimal bleeding and mild pain with making a fist. He denies fever, chills, nausea, vomiting, diarrhea, or constipation. He is right hand dominant. He states that his neighbor informed him that the cat is a house cat, has received all appropriate vaccinations, and has been healthy and acting normally. He denies other injuries and his last tetanus is unknown.
b. PMHx: hypertension
c. PSHx: none

d. Allergies: none

e. Meds: amlodipine

f. Social: lives with his wife and daughter at home; denies alcohol use, smoking, or illicit drug use; sexually active with his wife only

g. FHx: no relevant history

h. PMD: Dr Fox

F. Secondary survey

a. General: alert, oriented × 3, comfortable

b. Head: normocephalic, atraumatic

c. Eyes: extraocular movement intact, pupils equal, reactive to light

d. Ears: normal tympanic membranes

e. Nose: no discharge

f. Neck: full range of motion, no jugular vein distension, no stridor

g. Pharynx: normal dentition, no lesions, no swelling

h. Chest: nontender

i. Lungs: clear bilaterally

j. Heart: rate and rhythm regular, no murmurs, rubs, or gallops

k. Abdomen: normal bowel sounds, soft, nontender, or distended

l. Extremities: puncture wound on right index finger over the MCP joint not actively bleeding; full range of motion at all joints, mild pain with flexion at MCP joint, neurovascularly intact; no erythema, swelling, foreign body, streaking; normal capillary refill; left hand and bilateral lower extremities within normal limits

m. Back: nontender

n. Neuro: cranial nerves II to XII intact; normal sensation, strength; normal reflexes and gait, right index finger with normal flexion and extension at DIP, PIP, MCP joint with normal sensation

o. Skin: warm and dry (normal other than noted earlier)

p. Lymph: no lymphadenopathy

G. Action

a. Wound care

   i. Irrigation

b. Meds

   i. Amoxicillin/clavulanate or cefuroxime, initiated in ED

   ii. Tetanus toxoid

c. Follow-up

   i. Wound check in 48 hours in ED or PMD

d. Discussion regarding rabies – low risk, have friend monitor for unusual behavior

e. Imaging

   i. X-ray of finger to rule out foreign body

H. Diagnosis

a. Cat bite

I. Critical actions

▪ Appropriate antibiotics

▪ Tetanus immunization

▪ Follow-up for wound check

J. Examiner instructions

a. This is a case of cat bite from a known healthy cat, with verifiable immunization records, without evidence of neurovascular injury by exam. The candidate should ask about the cat to identify risk for rabies and perform a thorough examination to assess for tendon injury and infection. An x-ray of the finger may be helpful to evaluate for foreign body since it is a puncture wound and difficult to directly visualize. The candidate should also request for follow-up for the patient because 60% to 80% of wounds caused by cat bites tend to become infected.

K. Pearls

a. Prophylactic antibiotics are indicated for all cat bites, as these wounds tend to be deep and difficult to adequately irrigate. Cefuroxime or amoxicillin-clavulanate is recommended for prophylactic treatment, and therapy should be initiated in the ED for high-risk bites, such as cat bites to the hand. A dose of IV antibiotic therapy may be preferable for high-risk bites, but even a PO dose is acceptable since a prescription may not be filled for 24 hours.

b. Infection tends to be polymicrobial. The most common organisms isolated from cat bites include *Staphylococcus* species, *Streptococcus* species, and most often, *Pasteurella multocida*.

c. Prophylaxis is also recommended in bites in immunocompromised hosts, deep dog bite wounds, hand wounds, and any lacerations being sutured.

d. Consider rabies vaccination, active and passive, in all high-risk animal bites according to CDC guidelines.

L. References

a. Tintinalli's: Chapter 50. Puncture Wounds and Bites

b. Rosen: Chapter 61. Mammalian Bites

CASE 51: Abdominal pain: female (Shefali Trivedi, MD)

A. Chief complaint

a. 24-year-old female brought in by mother with complaint of lower abdominal pain for the past 4 days

B. Vital signs

a. BP: 110/75 HR: 110 RR: 14 T: 102.4°F Sat: 99% on RA

C. What does the patient look like?

a. Patient appears stated age, lying supine in stretcher, in moderate discomfort due to pain.

D. Primary survey

a. Airway: speaking in full sentences

b. Breathing: no apparent respiratory distress, no cyanosis

c. Circulation: warm, dry skin, normal capillary refill

E. Action

a. Oxygen via NC or non rebreather mask

b. Two large-bore peripheral IV lines

c. Labs

   i. CBC, BMP, LFT, coagulation studies, blood type and cross-match

   ii. Lactate, blood cultures, UA, urine culture, urine pregnancy test

d. 1 L NS bolus

e. Monitor: BP: 115/76 HR: 98 RR: 16 Sat: 99% on O_2 or RA

F. History

a. Ask mother to step out of room during the examination. Candidate may begin the interview with mother present, but should ask to conduct at least part of interview with mother out of the room.

b. HPI: a 24-year-old female with no past medical history presents with lower abdominal pain for 4 days. Patient states that the pain is a constant, nonradiating, sharp pain in the left lower quadrant that has worsened over the past 4 days. She also notes that she has had a thick malodorous yellowish/greenish vaginal discharge for the past 1 week for which she has not sought medical attention. She also notes fever to 102°F at home yesterday associated with chills. She is sexually active with two partners and admits that she is inconsistent with using protection. She denies urinary symptoms, nausea, vomiting, diarrhea, constipation, sick contacts, travel history, unusual food intake, trauma, or previous similar symptoms.

c. PMHx: none

d. PSHx: none

e. Allergies: none

f. Meds: oral contraceptive

g. Social: lives with her mother, father, and younger sister at home; social smoker and drinks alcohol socially; denies drug use; sexually active with two partners

h. FHx: no relevant history

i. PMD: none

G. Secondary survey

a. General: alert, oriented × 3, mild distress secondary to pain

b. Head: normocephalic, atraumatic

c. Eyes: extraocular movement intact, pupils equal, reactive to light

d. Ears: normal tympanic membranes

e. Nose: no discharge

f. Neck: full range of motion, no jugular vein distension, no stridor

g. Pharynx: normal dentition, no lesions, no swelling

h. Chest: nontender

i. Lungs: clear bilaterally

j. Heart: rate and rhythm regular, no murmurs, rubs, or gallops

k. Abdomen: soft, positive tenderness left suprapubic area with voluntary guarding, no rebound, nontender McBurney's point, no hepatosplenomegaly, no masses, no hernias, no peritoneal signs, positive bowel sounds

l. Rectal: normal tone, brown stool, occult blood negative

m. Urogenital: normal external genitalia, positive moderate amount of dark yellowish/greenish malodorous discharge in the vaginal vault, no blood in vaginal vault; positive friable cervix, os closed, positive cervical motion tenderness, positive left adnexal tenderness, normal right adnexal examination

n. Extremities: full range of motion, no deformity, normal pulses
o. Back: nontender, no CVA tenderness
p. Neuro: cranial nerves II to XII intact; normal sensation, strength; normal reflexes and gait
q. Skin: warm and dry
r. Lymph: no lymphadenopathy

H. Nurse
a. Labs
　　i. Urine pregnancy test negative

I. Action
a. Meds
　　i. Cefoxitin
　　ii. Doxycycline
　　iii. Acetaminophen
　　iv. Morphine
b. Reassess
　　i. Morphine: pain improved
　　ii. No morphine: pain persists
c. Consult
　　i. Gynecology
d. Imaging
　　i. Pelvic US
e. Labs
　　i. Gonorrhea and chlamydia culture (send specimen during pelvic examination for culture)

J. Nurse
a. BP: 112/76 HR: 84 RR: 14 T: 100.2°F Sat: 100% on RA
b. Patient: still with mild discomfort
c. Pelvic US (Figure 51.1)

Figure 51.1

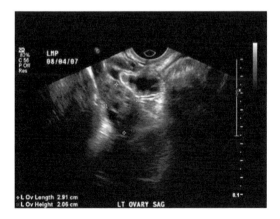

K. Results

Complete blood count:

WBC	13.2×10^3/uL
Hct	43.8%
Plt	289×10^3/uL

Basic metabolic panel:

Na	142 mEq/L
K	4.2 mEq/L
Cl	105 mEq/L
CO_2	24 mEq/L
BUN	15 mEq/dL
Cr	0.9 mg/dL
Gluc	110 mg/dL

Coagulation panel:

PT	12.2 sec
PTT	27.2 sec
INR	0.89

Liver function panel:

AST	25 U/L
ALT	23 U/L
Alk Phos	56 U/L
T bili	0.6 mg/dL
D bili	0.4 mg/dL
Amylase	64 U/L
Lipase	28 U/L
Albumin	4.2 g/dL

Urinalysis:

SG	1.010–1.030
pH	5–8
Prot	Neg mg/dL
Gluc	Neg mg/dL
Ketones	Neg mg/dL
Bili	Neg
Blood	Neg
LE	Neg
Nitrite	Neg
Color	Yellow

L. Action

a. Gynecology consult

   i. Discuss need for admission for IV antibiotics for tubo-ovarian abscess

b. Discussion with patient and PMD regarding need for admission for IV antibiotics

M. Diagnosis

a. Tubo-ovarian abscess

N. Critical actions

▓ Urine pregnancy test

▓ Pelvic US

▓ Antibiotics

▓ Gynecology consult

▓ Pain medications

▓ Urogenital examination

O. Examiner instructions

a. This is a case of tubo-ovarian abscess (TOA), a serious infection of the female upper genital tract affecting the ovaries. TOA is a type of sexually transmitted disease caused typically by *Chlamydia trachomatis* or *Neisseria gonorrhoeae* that starts from an infection of the cervix and spreads to the upper genital tract. The patient's symptoms of lower abdominal pain and fever should prompt the candidate to order urine pregnancy test early in the encounter. Important actions include urogenital examination, early antibiotics, pain control, and pelvic US. Ultimately the patient will complain of increased pain and fever if antibiotics and pain medication are not ordered. The patient should be admitted for IV antibiotics and pain control.

P. Pearls

a. TOA is part of the admission criteria for patients with pelvic inflammatory disease.

b. Sixty to eighty percent of patients with TOAs improve with IV antibiotics alone, but those that do not improve may need to have drainage of the abscess laparoscopically, percutaneously, or surgically, or other pathologies need to be considered.

c. Patients may present with a bleeding pelvic mass that may be secondary to a bleeding vessel due to erosion or rupture of the abscess.

d. When considering pathologies other than TOA, the patient may require a CT abdomen/pelvis with PO and IV contrast to rule out other causes of the patient's symptoms (such as appendicitis).

Q. References

a. Tintinalli's: Chapter 107. Pelvic Inflammatory Disease

b. Rosen: Chapter 98. Sexually Transmitted Diseases

CASE 52: Headache (Bing Shen, MD)

A. Chief complaint

a. 55-year-old male brought in by wife with worsening headache, fever, and eye pain

B. Vital signs

a. BP: 138/88 HR: 110 RR: 16 T: 101.2°F Sat: 99% on RA FS: 109

C. What does the patient look like?

a. Patient appears stated age, moderately uncomfortable secondary to pain, lying supine on stretcher.

D. Primary survey

a. Airway: speaking in full sentences

b. Breathing: no respiratory distress, no cyanosis

c. Circulation: warm skin, normal capillary refill

E. Action

a. Oxygen via NC

b. Two large-bore peripheral IV lines

c. Labs

   i. CBC, BMP, LFT, coagulation studies, blood type and cross-match

   ii. Lactate

d. 1 L NS bolus

e. Monitor: BP: 128/76 HR: 115 RR: 16 Sat: 100% on 2 L NC

f. EKG

F. History

a. HPI: a 55-year-old male states that he has had a "bad cold" over the past week with worsening headache and fever over the past 2 days and now pain in the left eye. He reports having cold-like symptoms over the past week with yellowish-green nasal discharge, and mild facial fullness and pain. Today, the headache is severe, frontal, and nonradiating. His left eye is now irritated and painful. He feels chills and has

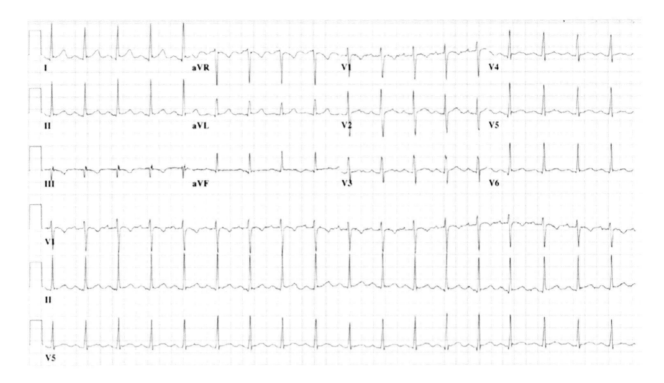

Figure 52.1

had subjective fevers. He has also been experiencing some sensitivity to light today
and weakness from being ill.

b. PMHx: hypercholesterolemia
c. PSHx: none
d. Allergies: none
e. Meds: simvastatin
f. Social: lives with wife and children; denies alcohol use, smoking, or illicit drug use;
   sexually active with wife only
g. PMD: none

G. Nurse
a. Repeat vitals if given 1 L NS
   i. BP: 125/88 HR: 105 RR: 16 Sat: 100% on 2 L
b. Repeat vitals without fluids
   i. BP: 115/70 HR: 120 RR: 16 Sat: 100% on 2 L
c. EKG (Figure 52.1)

H. Secondary survey
a. General: alert, oriented, uncomfortable, ill-appearing
b. Head: normocephalic, atraumatic, no erythema on face; mild tenderness over the
   left maxilla
c. Eyes:
   i. Left eye: conjunctiva + injection and chemosis, slight ptosis on left, pupil 5 mm
       reactive, + papilledema
   ii. Right eye: normal examination, pupil 3 mm reactive
d. Ears: normal tympanic membranes
e. Nose: no discharge

  f. Neck: full range of motion, no jugular vein distension, no stridor, Brudzinski's and Kernig's negative.

  g. Pharynx: normal

  h. Chest: nontender

  i. Lungs: clear bilaterally

  j. Heart: rate and rhythm regular, no murmurs, rubs, or gallops

  k. Abdomen: normal bowel sounds, soft, nontender or distended

  l. Rectal: normal

  m. Urogenital: normal external genitalia
    i. Male: no discharge, normal testicular examination.

  n. Extremities: full range of motion, no deformity, normal pulses

  o. Back: nontender

  p. Neuro: normal mental status; CN: visual acuity 20/40 bilaterally; decreased abduction of left eye; slightly less sensation to touch periorbitally on left; + papilledema on left; + photophobia; otherwise nonfocal neurological examination with normal cerebellar, gait, strength, reflexes, and tone

  q. Skin: warm and dry

  r. Lymph: no lymphadenopathy

I. Action

  a. Lumbar puncture, consider d-dimer

  b. Meds
    i. Ceftriaxone
    ii. Vancomycin
    iii. Dexamethasone
    iv. Acetaminophen
    v. Morphine

  c. Consult
    i. Neurology
    ii. Ophthalmology

  d. Imaging
    i. Head CT without contrast
    ii. MRI/MRV of head

J. Nurse

  a. BP: 115/75 HR: 110 RR: 16 T: 101°F O_2, Sat: 100% on 2 L

  b. Patient: continues to have severe headache, nausea, fever

K. Results

Complete blood count:

WBC	16.7×10^3/uL	BUN	30 mEq/dL
Hct	44.4%	Cr	1.2 mg/dL
Plt	244×10^3/uL	Gluc	130 mg/dL

Basic metabolic panel:

Na	140 mEq/L	PT	13.5 sec
K	4.0 mEq/L	PTT	27.0 sec
Cl	104 mEq/L	INR	1.1
CO_2	24 mEq/L		

Coagulation panel:

Liver function panel:		Urinalysis:	
AST	20 U/L	SG	1.010–1.030
ALT	15 U/L	pH	5–8
Alk Phos	110 U/L	Prot	Neg mg/dL
T bili	0.7 mg/dL	Gluc	Neg mg/dL
D bili	0.2 mg/dL	Ketones	Neg mg/dL
Amylase	110 U/L	Bili	Neg
Lipase	72 U/L	Blood	Neg
Albumin	4.3 g/dL	LE	Neg
Lactate	2.0 mmol/L	Nitrite	Neg
		Color	Yellow
		D-Dimer:	0.93 mcg/mL

a. CSF-WBC: 40, RBC: 100, protein: 35, glucose: 50, clear, Gram stain negative
b. Head CT – (Figure 52.2) sinusitis bilaterally in the maxillary sinuses; no other acute intracerebral abnormality
c. MRI – signal hyperintensities within the left cavernous sinus suggestive of cavernous sinus thrombosis

L. Action

a. Consult
   i. Neurology
   ii. Ophthalmology
   iii. MICU
b. Meds
   i. IV antibiotics (if not previously given)
      1. 3rd or 4th generation cephalosporin
      2. Vancomycin or nafcillin
      3. Metronidazole
   ii. Heparin infusion, with consultation
   iii. Dexamethasone (if not given earlier)

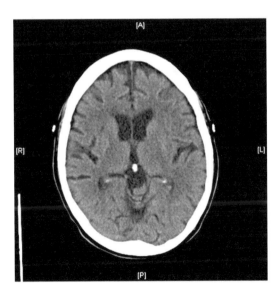

Figure 52.2

M. Diagnosis

a. Cavernous venous sinus thrombosis (CVST)

N. Critical actions

▨ Early antibiotics and steroids

▨ Lumbar puncture

▨ MRI for diagnosis

▨ ICU

O. Examiner instructions

a. This is a case of CVST that likely developed from a sinus infection. This is a serious infection of the veins within the brain that can be life-threatening if untreated. The important early actions are to start antibiotics and steroids to treat presumed meningitis, obtain neuroimaging, and perform an LP. A head CT should be obtained before performing the LP due to the focal neurological deficits. The patient's severe pain should continue despite treatment and this should guide the examinee to more definitive testing such as MRI or MRV. Elevated d-dimer is present in approximately 90% of cases of CVST, and can be used, along with clinical findings, to guide the need for further diagnostic testing. If the MRI is not ordered, the patient should develop continued pain in the left eye, worsening vision, and ophthalmoplegia (difficulty moving the eye). If the MRI is not ordered, or examiner feels that the candidate will not order it, the case will proceed to the neurologist/ophthalmologist's recommendation of an MRI or MRV.

P. Pearls

a. Headache is the most common chief complaint. Fever, eye pain, photophobia, orbital congestion, proptosis, ptosis, nausea, vomiting, somnolence, ophthalmoplegia (cranial nerves III, IV, and VI) are common. Sensory deficits in the 1st and 2nd branches (ophthalmic and maxillary branches) of the trigeminal nerve may be present. Papilledema, retinal hemorrhage, and decreased visual acuity may occur from venous congestion within the retina. Symptoms are initially unilateral but may become bilateral as infection and thrombosis spreads.

b. Causes: acute infections are usually Gram positive (*Staphylococcus aureus* most common), arising from frontal, sphenoid, or ethmoid sinus infections, and dental infections; less commonly from infections of tonsils, soft palate, middle ear, or orbit. Gram negative and anaerobes can occur as well.

c. LP reveals inflammatory cells in 75% of cases.

d. Steroids should be administered to treat thrombus and prevent possible long-term neurological deficits.

e. Anticoagulation should be considered with neurology consultation, though evidence is limited.

Q. References

a. Tintinalli's: Chapter 159. Headache and Facial Pain

b. Rosen: Chapter 103. Headache Disorders

CASE 53: Pediatric fever (Bing Shen, MD)

A. Chief complaint

a. 20-month-old male brought in by mother with the complaint of fever for the past 5 days

B. Vital signs

a. BP: 85/63 HR: 120 RR: 24 T: 40.2°C Sat: 100% on RA Wt: 10 kg

C. What does the patient look like?

a. Patient appears stated age, uncomfortable, fussy, in mother's arms.

D. Primary survey

a. Airway: able to speak words

b. Breathing: no apparent respiratory distress, no cyanosis

c. Circulation: warm skin, normal capillary refill.

E. Action

a. Oxygen supplementation (blow-by O_2)

b. One peripheral IV line

c. Labs

  i. CBC, BMP, LFT, coagulation studies, blood type and cross-match

  ii. Blood cultures, UA, urine culture

d. Monitor: BP: 85/63 HR: 120 RR: 24

F. History

a. HPI: a 20-month-old male, normal birth history and up-to-date with vaccines, is brought in by his mother for a persistent fever for the past 5 days and a new rash that the mother noticed earlier during the day. The child is feeding well, but is less active generally because of this illness. The fever has been as high as 103°F at home orally. The child has a slight dry cough, no diarrhea, and no vomiting.

b. PMHx: normal full-term birth at 39 weeks; up-to-date vaccinations

c. PSHx: none

d. Allergies: none

e. Meds: none

f. Social: lives at home with mother and father; no siblings

g. FHx: no relevant history.

h. PMD: Dr. Alvarez, who he sees regularly for routine visits

G. Secondary survey

a. General: alert, in no distress, irritable but consoled in mother's arms

b. Head: normocephalic, atraumatic, full fontanelle

c. Eyes: bilateral injection, extraocular movement grossly intact, pupils equal, reactive to light

d. Ears: normal tympanic membranes

e. Nose: no discharge

f. Neck: + cervical lymphadenopathy, full range of motion, no jugular vein distension, no stridor

g. Pharynx: slight edema, reddened tongue, dry red lips

    h. Chest: nontender

    i. Lungs: clear bilaterally

    j. Heart: rate and rhythm regular, no murmurs, rubs, or gallops

    k. Abdomen: normal bowel sounds, soft, nontender or distended

    l. Rectal: normal tone, brown stool, occult blood negative

   m. Urogenital: normal external genitalia

      i. Male: no discharge, normal testicular examination

    n. Extremities: full range of motion, no deformity, normal pulses

    o. Back: nontender

    p. Neuro: moving all extremities symmetrically

    q. Skin: scarlatiniform rash on perineum, erythema of palms and feet

    r. Lymph: no lymphadenopathy

H. Action

    a. Meds

      i. Initiate IV fluids:20 ml/kg bolus or maintenance fluids or saline lock

    b. Imaging

      i. CXR

    c. Reassess

      i. Patient still irritable

    d. Testing

      i. Rapid Strep test, throat culture

      ii. CRP, ESR

I. Nurse

    a. BP: 85/63 HR: 125 RR: 25 T: 39.6°C Sat: 100% on 2 L

    b. Patient: still irritable

Complete blood count:

WBC	$14.1 \times 10^3/uL$
Hct	36.5%
Plt	$410 \times 10^3/uL$

Basic metabolic panel:

Na	139 mEq/L
K	4.2 mEq/L
Cl	101 mEq/L
CO_2	22 mEq/L
BUN	21 mEq/dL
Cr	1.0 mg/dL
Gluc	100 mg/dL

Coagulation panel:

PT	13.1 sec
PTT	26.0 sec
INR	1.0

Liver function panel:

AST	21 U/L
ALT	19 U/L
Alk Phos	106 U/L

T bili	0.5 mg/dL
D bili	0.1 mg/dL
Amylase	32 U/L
Lipase	53 U/L
Albumin	3.6 g/dL

Urinalysis:

SG	1.010–1.030
pH	5–8
Prot	Neg mg/dL
Gluc	Neg mg/dL
Ketones	Neg mg/dL
Bili	Neg
Blood	Neg
LE	Neg
Nitrite	Neg
Color	Yellow

Arterial blood gas:

pH	7.35–7.45
PO_2	80–100 mmHg
PCO_2	35–45 mmHg
HCO_3	22–26 mmol/L

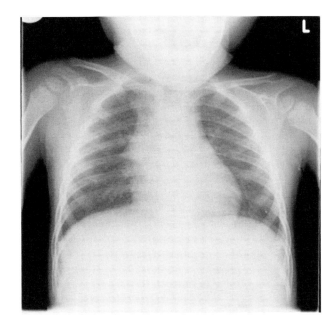

Figure 53.1

J. Results

a. ESR: 40, CRP: 3

b. Rapid Strep test: negative

c. CXR (Figure 53.1)

K. Action

a. Consult

   i. Pediatric rheumatology

   ii. Infectious disease

b. Discuss with family regarding diagnosis and management

c. Meds

   i. IVIG: 2 g/kg IV over 8 to 12 hours

   ii. Aspirin 100 mg/kg/day divided q 6 hours

L. Diagnosis

a. Kawasaki disease

M. Critical actions

▨ Treatment of Kawasaki: ASA and IVIG

▨ Discussion with family regarding diagnosis and management

▨ Consultation with infectious disease or rheumatology

N. Examiner instructions

a. This is a case of Kawasaki disease, an acute febrile vasculitis of childhood. The cause is unknown but affects the small and medium-sized blood vessels of the body and can lead to complications if undiagnosed and untreated. This patient presents early on in the course of the disease. His clinical presentation warrants an infectious work-up. A lumbar puncture would be appropriate if suspicious for meningitis. IV fluids and symptomatic relief may be given, however the definitive course of therapy should be IVIG and aspirin. Antibiotics can be started if the diagnosis is not certain; however, the patient cannot be discharged as Kawasaki disease has significant morbidity if not treated appropriately. The candidate should keep the patient's mother up-to-date with his condition throughout the course of the encounter.

O. Pearls

a. Kawasaki disease is the leading cause of acquired heart disease in North American children. There are no pathognomonic laboratory findings – the diagnosis must be established clinically, as detailed below:

b. Diagnostic criteria

  i. Fever of at least 5 days' duration

  ii. Four out of five of the following

    1. Conjunctival injection

    2. Lips and oral mucosal findings (dry, red, fissured lips, strawberry tongue, oropharyngeal erythema)

    3. Extremity findings (erythema of palms and soles, edema of hands and feet, periungual desquamation)

    4. Polymorphous rash

    5. Cervical lymphadenopathy

c. Lab abnormalities: ESR and CRP may be elevated; CBC may show elevated WBC and left shift; UA often shows a sterile pyuria; thrombocytosis (Plt count >650,000/microliter) is associated with an increased risk of coronary artery thrombosis.

d. Twenty percent of untreated patients develop coronary aneurysms between 2 to 6 weeks after disease onset. With treatment this is reduced to 4% to 5%.

e. Dysrhythmias and myocardial infarction can cause sudden death in 1% to 2% of patients, usually in the 3rd or 4th week.

f. Some patients will present with "incomplete KD," which occurs when not all diagnostic criteria are met. These children are still at risk for complications and should be monitored closely.

P. References

a. Tintinalli's: Chapter 122B. Pediatric Heart Disease: Acquired Heart Disease

b. Rosen: Chapter 167 – Pediatric Fever

CASE 54: Back pain (Bing Shen, MD)

A. Chief complaint

a. 42-year-old male with back pain and right leg pain

B. Vital signs

a. BP: 139/83 HR: 92 RR: 14 T: 36.2°C Sat: 100% on RA

C. What does the patient look like?

a. Patient appears stated age, in moderate to severe pain, sitting on stretcher.

D. Primary survey

a. Airway: speaking full sentences

b. Breathing: no apparent respiratory distress, no cyanosis

c. Circulation: warm and dry skin, normal capillary refill

E. Action

a. Oxygen via NC or nonrebreather mask

b. Two large-bore peripheral IV lines

c. Labs

    i. CBC, BMP, coagulation studies, blood type and cross-match

    ii. UA

d. Monitor: BP: 135/85 HR: 90 RR: 12 Sat: 100% on RA or on 2 L NC

F. History

a. HPI: a 42-year-old male presents with severe lumbar back pain that began as moderate back pain 1 month ago after falling off his bike. The back pain at that time was managed successfully with ibuprofen. However, 7 days ago the pain returned much more severely and was associated with right posterior leg pain, numbness and tingling to the thigh, leg, and feet, and slight weakness of the right leg. Yesterday he had difficulty voiding and has, on occasion, wet himself. He denies bowel changes or fever.

b. PMHx: hypertension

c. PSHx: none

d. Allergies: none

e. Meds: ibuprofen, does not remember blood pressure medication

f. Social Hx: ten pack per year smoker, social EtOH, no illicit drug use.

g. FHx: no relevant history.

h. PMD: none

G. Secondary survey

a. General: alert, oriented × 3, comfortable

b. Head: normocephalic, atraumatic

c. Eyes: extraocular movement intact, pupils equal, reactive to light

d. Ears: normal tympanic membranes

e. Nose: no discharge

f. Neck: full range of motion, no jugular vein distension, no stridor

g. Pharynx: normal dentition, no lesions, no swelling

h. Chest: nontender

i. Lungs: clear bilaterally

j. Heart: rate and rhythm regular, no murmurs, rubs, or gallops

k. Abdomen: normal bowel sounds, soft, mild suprapubic tenderness and fullness, no rebound, guarding, or rigidity

l. Rectal: slightly diminished tone, brown stool, occult blood negative

m. Urogenital: normal external genitalia

    i. Male: no discharge, normal testicular examination

n. Extremities: full range of motion, no deformity, normal pulses

o. Back: tenderness low right paralumbar and lumbar area

p. Neuro: normal mental status, normal cranial nerves; reflexes +2 patellar bilateral; +1 ankle jerk on right; +2 on left; right lateral leg/foot sensory deficit; mildly decreased perianal and perineal sensation; strength 4/5 right big toe, ankle plantar flexion; 4/5 quadriceps; 4/5 left-sided lower extremities; + straight leg raise on right; unable to rise from bed because of back pain

q. Skin: warm and dry

r. Lymph: no lymphadenopathy

H. Action

a. Foley catheter placement with post-void residual assessment

b. Meds

    i. Pain control

        1. Ketorolac

        2. Morphine or alternative

c. Consult

    i. Neurosurgery

d. Reassess

    i. Pain improved after analgesia.

e. Imaging

    i. MRI

    ii. CT lumbar spine (does not obviate MRI)

    iii. X-ray of lumbar sacral spine (unnecessary)

I. Nurse

a. Vitals: BP: 135/85 HR: 90 RR: 12 Sat: 100% on RA

b. Patient: with mild pain

J. Results

Complete blood count:	
WBC	12.1×10^3/uL
Hct	41.5%
Plt	253×10^3/uL

Coagulation panel:	
PT	13.1 sec
PTT	26 sec
INR	1.0

Basic metabolic panel:	
Na	139 mEq/L
K	4.0 mEq/L
Cl	101 mEq/L
CO_2	18.9 mEq/L
BUN	52 mEq/dL
Cr	1.6 mg/dL
Gluc	202 mg/dL

Urinalysis:	
SG	1.010–1.030
pH	5–8
Prot	Neg mg/dL
Gluc	Neg mg/dL
Ketones	Neg mg/dL
Bili	Neg
Blood	Neg
LE	Neg

a. Post-void residual: 600 ml

b. X-ray (Figure 54.1)

c. CT: (if ordered): herniation of the L5-S1 intervertebral disk with posterolateral protrusion impinging upon the thecal sac

d. MRI: large L5-S1 disk herniation, causing bilateral recess obliteration and moderate thecal sac stenosis; likely compression of bilateral S1 nerve roots

K. Action

a. Admission and preparation for operating room decompression of nerve

b. Meds

    i. Consider dexamethasone IV, in consultation with neurosurgeon

L. Diagnosis

a. Cauda equina syndrome

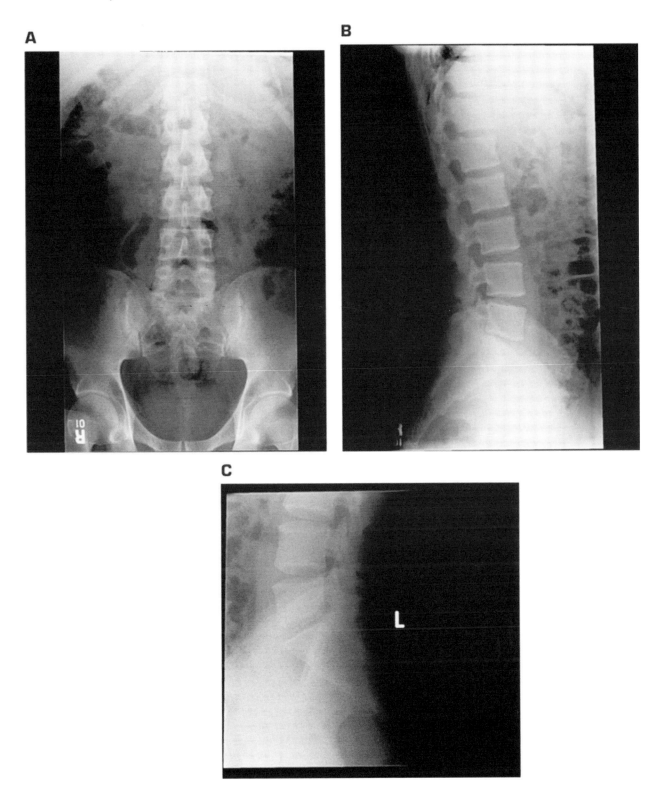

Figure 54.1 A, B, and C

M. Critical actions

▨ Pain control
▨ Complete neurological examination
▨ MRI

▧ Neurosurgical consult for decompression surgery
▧ Consider dexamethasone, in consultation with neurosurgeon

N. Examiner instructions

a. This is a case of cauda equina syndrome, caused by lumbar disk herniation. Cauda equina is a condition when a mass, most often the lumbar disk, protrudes to compress the spinal nerve roots. Serious complications include paralysis. Thorough physical examination is key in this case. When asked for the neurological examination, examiner should inquire what part of the examination specifically the candidate is interested in (mental status, sensory, reflexes, motor, cranial nerve, cerebellar) as well as which part of the body he/she is interested in. Preoperative labs should be sent because the patient may need to go to the OR. Adequate pain control should be administered as needed for patient comfort. If CT myelogram is ordered, report not possible at this time due to resources. After obtaining the MRI, immediate admission to neurosurgery and operating room preparations should be made.

O. Pearls

a. Cauda equina arises from massive midline disk herniation; it is a surgical emergency.
b. Most commonly L4-L5, then L5-S1 and L3–4 disks are affected.
c. Most common findings: combined motor weakness and sensory deficits. Positive straight leg raise, decreased deep tendon reflexes, saddle anesthesia and bowel/bladder retention/overflow incontinence also very common.
d. Assess sphincter tone (60%-80% of cases have decreased tone), diminished perineal sensation (75% sensitivity for cauda equina), and post-void residual. If residual is greater than 100–200 mL then urinary retention is present. Within the clinical picture of cauda equina, urinary retention is 90% sensitive and 95% specific for the diagnosis.
e. MRI of the entire spinal column is the gold standard for diagnosis. CT myelogram is an alternative if MRI is not available or contraindicated. CT of the spine will delineate bony structures, and may give some indication of cord compressive when other modalities are unavailable.
f. Dexamethasone dosing is controversial, but should be considered to relieve edema caused by acute radiculopathy.

P. References

a. Tintinalli's: Chapter 255. Spine and Spinal Cord Trauma
b. Rosen: Chapter 106. Spinal Cord Disorders

CASE 55: Cardiac arrest (Bing Shen, MD)

A. Chief complaint

a. 7-month-old male is brought in by mother and EMS after noticing that the child was unresponsive, not breathing, and blue in color. EMS is bagging patient with 100% nonrebreather mask and chest compressions.

B. Vital signs

a. BP: not obtainable HR: 0 RR: 0 T: 34.2°C (rectal) O$_2$ Sat not obtainable wt ~ 8 kg FS: 60

C. What does the patient look like?

a. Patient appears cyanotic, not responsive, and limp.

D. Primary survey

a. Airway: unresponsive, patent airway
b. Breathing: no spontaneous breaths
c. Circulation: no carotid, femoral, or brachial pulses; no capillary refill

E. Action

a. PALS resuscitation
  i. Intubation with straight laryngoscope blade, 3.5 uncuffed tube; verify placement
  ii. Oxygen – continuous bag 8 to 10 breaths/min
  iii. Chest compressions (thumb-encircling hands) 100/min
b. IV – two 22- to 24-gauge IV or intraosseous lines
c. IVF – 20 ml/kg (160 cc) warm NS bolus
d. Rewarming (heater, warm saline, etc)
e. Monitor: No pulse, asystole
f. Asystole PALS algorithm; 0.01 mg/kg (1:10,000) epinephrine; repeat every 3 to 5 minutes; continue CPR with rhythm checks every 5 cycles of CPR
g. Consider reversible causes: The H's & T's (Hypovolemia, Hypoxia, Hydrogen ion [acidosis], Hypoglycemia, Hyperglycemia, Hypokalemia, Hyperkalemia, Hypothermia, Tension pneumothorax, Tamponade, Toxins, Thrombosis [coronary, pulmonary embolus])

F. History

a. HPI: a 7-month-old male with normal full-term birth and no past medical history was found in the crib by his mother in the middle of the evening to be unresponsive and blue in color. The patient appeared well before being put to sleep. EMS was called immediately (~ 25 minutes ago) and child was brought immediately to the ED. CPR was initiated by EMS and no medications were given.
b. PMHx: none
c. PSHx: none
d. Allergies: none
e. Meds: none
f. Social: lives at home with mother and three siblings, ages 2, 5, 10 years old
g. PMD: Dr Young

G. Nurse

a. Monitor: no pulse, continued asystole: T: 35.2°C
b. Obtain health-care worker (such as a social worker), to talk to mother, locate other children

H. Secondary survey

a. General: unresponsive
b. HEENT: dilated and fixed pupils; intubated
c. Neck: normal
d. Chest: no spontaneous respirations; breath sounds equal post-intubation
e. Heart: no beat auscultated
f. Abdomen: normal

g. Back: normal

h. Extremities: normal

i. Neuro: no reflexes

j. Skin: cool, no signs of trauma

I. Action

a. Reassess:

    i. T: 37.2°C, no other vital signs

b. Pronouncement of death after significant resuscitation time

J. Action

a. Informing family of child's death

b. Involve clergy, social support, pediatrician

c. Blood and urine collection for postmortem testing

K. Diagnosis

a. Sudden infant death syndrome

L. Critical actions

▪ Initiate appropriate PALS life support

▪ Assess for signs of abuse

▪ Resuscitation and ensure that the temperature is within normal limits before pronouncement of death

▪ Provide psychosocial support to the family

M. Examiner instructions

a. This is a case of sudden infant death syndrome (SIDS); however, that is impossible to ascertain on presentation. SIDS is a syndrome that leads to sudden death of an infant under 1 year of age without known cause. Pediatric acute life support should be initiated until futility – significant time of resuscitation, loss of brainstem reflexes, normothermia. Reflexes should be assessed. Warm NS and an infant heater can help rewarm the patient. The family should be offered all forms of psychosocial support. For all cases of unexpected death in a child, abuse should be considered and excluded. In this case, no evidence of abuse is found.

N. Pearls

a. Sudden infant death syndrome is the sudden death of an infant under 1 year of age, which remains unexplained after a thorough case investigation, performance of a complete autopsy, examination of the death scene, and review of the clinical history.

b. The "Back to Sleep" campaign (which instructs parents to put their infants to sleep on their backs) has reduced the rate of SIDS by greater than 40%.

c. As the cause of death is unknown, blood and urine should be sent to facilitate postmortem examination and autopsy.

d. Social and psychological support should be offered immediately to help the family come to terms with the loss and to initiate the process of grieving.

O. References

a. Rosen's: Chapter 8

b. Tintinalli's: Chapters 15, 112

c. 2010 AHA PALS Guidelines

CASE 56: Knee pain (Bing Shen, MD)

A. Chief complaint
a. 54-year-old female with right knee pain and swelling for the past 2 days

B. Vital signs
a. BP: 149/83 HR: 88 RR: 12 T: 38.4°C Sat: 100% on RA FS: 120

C. What does the patient look like?
a. Patient appears stated age, in moderate pain, and sitting on stretcher.

D. Primary survey
a. Airway: speaking full sentences
b. Breathing: no apparent respiratory distress, no cyanosis
c. Circulation: warm and dry skin, normal capillary refill

E. Action
a. One large-bore peripheral IV line
b. Labs
   i. CBC, BMP, coagulation studies, blood type and cross-match
   ii. ESR, CRP, blood cultures
c. Monitor: BP: 145/85 HR: 90 RR: 12 Sat: 100%

F. History
a. HPI: a 54-year-old female with a history of hypercholesterolemia, gout, and obesity, states that she has had worsening right knee pain over the past 2 days. She has never had pain in the knee before and states that she has had gout pain in her left big toe in the past. The pain is localized to the right knee and has steadily increased in intensity over the past few days. She denies any fevers, but states she does feel chills. She is mostly concerned about the pain, which prevents her from doing her daily activities. She took ibuprofen 800 mg × 2 Q6 without relief, last dose 1 hour prior. She has no other complaints; denies trauma to the knee.
b. PMHx: hypercholesterolemia, gout, and obesity
c. PSHx: none
d. Allergies: none
e. Meds: ibuprofen and acetaminophen, simvastatin, colchicine
f. Social: some alcohol use – "socially"; nonsmoker; denies drugs; sexually active; lives with husband; works in computer programming

G. Secondary survey
a. General: alert, oriented × 3, moderate pain
b. Head: normocephalic, atraumatic
c. Eyes: extraocular movement intact, pupils equal, reactive to light
d. Ears: normal tympanic membranes
e. Nose: no discharge
f. Neck: full range of motion, no jugular vein distension, no stridor
g. Pharynx: normal dentition, no lesions, no swelling
h. Chest: nontender
i. Lungs: clear bilaterally

j. Heart: rate and rhythm regular, no murmurs, rubs, or gallops

k. Abdomen: normal bowel sounds, soft, nontender or distended

l. Extremities: right knee swollen with palpable effusion; very tender to palpation and ranging; nonerythematous; patient unable to walk without extreme pain; hip and ankle both normal; distal pulses normal, equal bilaterally

m. Back: nontender

n. Neuro: cranial nerves II to XII intact; normal sensation, strength; normal reflexes and gait

o. Skin: warm and dry

p. Lymph: no lymphadenopathy

H. Action

a. Procedure

   i. Right knee arthrocentesis

      1. Informed consent with explanation of risks, benefits, and alternatives

      2. Time out to identify side, done under aseptic conditions

      3. Cloudy fluid obtained – send for culture, Gram stain, cell count

      4. Crystals/wet prep, glucose, lactate

b. Meds

   i. Morphine (opiate)

c. Reassess

   i. Patient's pain is much improved after pain medication and arthrocentesis, but is still present

d. Imaging: x-ray right knee

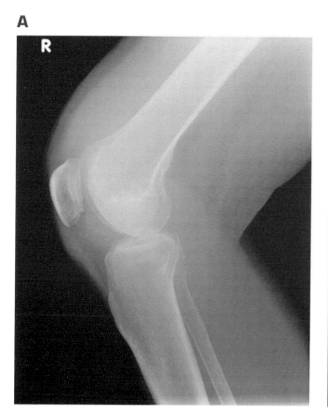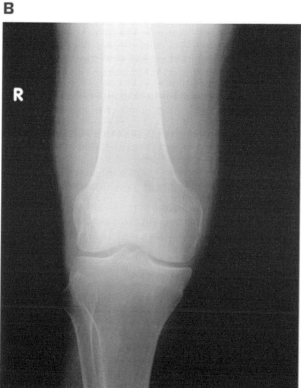

Figure 56.1 A and B

I. Nurse

a. Vitals: BP: 130/78 HR: 88 RR: 12 O_2 Sat: 100% on O_2.

b. Patient: with mild pain

c. X-ray right knee (Figure 56.1)

J. Results

a. PT/PTT: 13.1/26, INR: 1.0

b. ESR: if ordered – 20 mm/h; CRP: if ordered – 18 mg/L

c. Synovial fluid results

    i. Color: cloudy, WBC: 100,000, RBC: 300, Poly: 93%

    ii. Gram stain: Gram positive cocci

    iii. Crystals: no crystals seen

    iv. If ordered (glucose depressed, protein elevated)

Complete blood count:

WBC	11.9×10^3/uL	CO_2	24.2 mEq/L
Diff	83.6/9.1/5.0	BUN	23 mEq/dL
Hct	41.5%	Cr	1.2 mg/dL%
Plt	553×10^3/uL	Gluc	135 mg/dL

Basic metabolic panel: **Coagulation panel:**

Na	139 mEq/L	PT	12.3–15.5 sec
K	4.0 mEq/L	PTT	25.4–35.0 sec
Cl	101 mEq/L	INR	0.9–1.3

K. Action

a. Consult

    i. Orthopedics – for possible joint irrigation in OR

b. Admission for IV antibiotics

c. Antibiotics: nafcillin or vancomycin if clinical suspicion for MRSA

L. Diagnosis

a. Septic arthritis

M. Critical actions

▨ Pain management

▨ Joint aspiration for Gram stain, cultures, crystals, WBC

▨ Antibiotics after Gram stain, fluid results

▨ X-ray to assess for osteomylitis

N. Examiner instructions

a. This is a case of septic arthritis involving the right knee; a bacterial infection that can cause severe damage to the joint if left undiagnosed and untreated. The patient is otherwise healthy and clinically appears well, so an appropriate work-up for the right knee pain and fever can be done without the concern for starting early sepsis management. IV fluids and antipyretics can be initiated as needed, however, the patient should receive pain medication. Her pain will persist until an appropriate dose of opioid, such as morphine, is given. A diagnostic arthrocentesis (joint aspiration) should be performed before all other studies (x-ray is allowable if done quickly, but should not hold up the arthrocentesis). A Gram stain should be obtained before initiating antibiotics.

O. Pearls
a. Most patients with a monoarticular arthritis, even with a history of gout, require an arthrocentesis.
b. Synovial Gram stain, cultures, and WBC are the most important studies. The serum WBC, ESR, and CRP have poor sensitivities and specificities. A joint aspirate with a WBC of > 50,000 with PMNs greater than 80% is highly suggestive of infection.
c. An x-ray should be obtained to rule out osteomyelitis.
d. Antibiotics should be tailored to Gram stain results. Ceftriaxone should be given for gonorrheal infection, nafcillin or vancomycin for *Staphylococcus* infection. For gram-negative bacilli infection, treat with 3rd or 4th generation cephalosporin with antipseudomonal coverage.
e. Lyme titers, rheumatoid factor, ANA, lupus-anticoagulant may be helpful in follow-up management of joint pain.

P. References
a. Tintinalli's: Chapter 281
b. Rosen's: Chapters 114, 134
c. Ferri F. *Ferri's Clinical Advisor 2008*. 10th ed. Elsevier: Mosby, Philadelphia, PA; 2007.

CASE 57: Rash (Braden Hexom, MD)

A. Chief complaint
a. 14-year-old male brought in by parents with the complaint of rash, fever, mild headache, abdominal pain with vomiting, and diarrhea for 2 days; 1 day history of rash

B. Vital signs
a. BP: 105/82 HR: 105 RR: 16 T: 38.6°C Sat: 100% on RA FS: 87 wt: 55 kg

C. What does the patient look like?
a. Patient appears stated age, awake and alert responding to questions but is pale, listless, and uncomfortable.

D. Primary survey
a. Airway: speaking in full sentences
b. Breathing: no respiratory distress
c. Circulation: pale, clammy skin

E. Action
a. Two large-bore peripheral IV lines
b. Labs
    i. CBC, BMP, LFT, coagulation studies, blood type and cross-match

   c. 1 L NS bolus

   d. Monitor: BP: 100/80 HR: 105 RR: 16 Sat: 100% on RA

F. History

  a. HPI: a 14-year-old male with no past medical history developed fever 2 days ago associated with abdominal pain, vomiting, and diarrhea requiring him to stay home from school. Today, his mother noticed a rash on his hands and wrists that has been steadily spreading to the chest and back. Vomiting and diarrhea (nonbloody, nonbilious) have been intermittent 3 to 4 times each day. He is able to keep down thin liquids; fever to 102°F at home orally. Mother has tried acetaminophen 500 mg with some improvement. Initially the parents thought it was "just the flu" until they noticed the rash. The season is fall.

  b. PMHx: none, immunizations up-to-date

  c. PSHx: lives with married parents, does well in school, active in Boy Scouts, no drugs/alcohol/smoking, not sexually active

  d. FHx: not relevant

  e. Allergies: none

  f. Meds: none

  g. PMD: Dr Kim

  h. Travel history (if asked): last weekend went on camping trip with Boy Scouts, does not remember insect bite

G. Nurse

  a. Fluids

    i. BP: 112/88 HR: 87 RR: 16 Sat: 99%

  b. No fluids

    i. BP: 101/72 HR: 105 RR: 16 Sat: 99%

    ii. Patient will develop continued vomiting until given fluids.

  c. Meds

    i. Antiemetic may be given but will not affect the case

H. Secondary survey

  a. General: alert, oriented × 3, listless, in no acute distress

  b. Head: normocephalic, atraumatic

  c. Eyes: pale conjunctivae, extraocular movement intact, pupils equal, reactive to light

  d. Ears: normal tympanic membranes

  e. Nose: no discharge

  f. Neck: full range of motion, no jugular vein distension, no stridor

  g. Pharynx: normal dentition, no lesions, no swelling

  h. Chest: nontender

  i. Lungs: clear bilaterally

  j. Heart: rate and rhythm regular, no murmurs, rubs, or gallops

  k. Abdomen: mild hepatosplenomegaly, nondistended, nontender, soft, no rebound/guarding, no masses/hernias, no rigidity

  l. Rectal: normal tone, brown stool, occult blood negative

  m. Urogenital: normal external genitalia

    i. Male: no discharge, normal testicular examination

n. Extremities: full range of motion, no deformity, normal pulses, maculopapular rash over palms, soles, and extremities to the trunk

o. Back: nontender

p. Neuro: cranial nerves II to XII intact; normal sensation, strength; normal reflexes and gait

q. Skin: warm and dry, maculopapular rash over complete extremities and front of chest, including palms and soles

r. Lymph: no lymphadenopathy

I. Action

a. Meds (any of the following)
   i. Doxycycline
   ii. Tetracycline
   iii. Chloramphenicol (especially in pregnancy, risk of myelosuppression should be considered)

b. Reassess
   i. GI symptoms improving, appears more alert (if given fluids)
   ii. No fluids: still vomiting, uncomfortable

c. Consultation
   i. Dermatology for skin biopsy

d. Imaging
   i. CXR
   ii. X-ray abdomen obstructive series

e. Labs
   i. Antibody titer for Rocky Mountain spotted fever and Lyme disease

J. Nurse

a. CXR (Figure 57.1)

b. Obstructive series (Figure 57.2)

K. Results

a. Titer – will not return for several days

b. Skin biopsy – will not return for several days

Complete blood count:		Coagulation panel:	
WBC	13.9×10^3/uL	PT	13 sec
Diff	89.5/6.7/1.2	PTT	25 sec
Hct	43%	INR	1.0
Plt	75×10^3/uL		
		Liver function panel:	
Basic metabolic panel:		AST	168 U/L
Na	128 mEq/L	ALT	182 U/L
K	4.2 mEq/L	Alk Phos	210 U/L
Cl	101 mEq/L	T bili	0.6 mg/dL
CO_2	18.9 mEq/L	D bili	0.1 mg/dL
BUN	23 mEq/dL	Amylase	79 U/L
Cr	0.7 mg/dL%	Lipase	46 U/L
Gluc	94 mg/dL	Albumin	4.1 g/dL

Urinalysis:

SG	1.010–1.030	Bili	Neg
pH	5–8	Blood	Neg
Prot	Neg mg/dL	LE	Neg
Gluc	Neg mg/dL	Nitrite	Neg
Ketones	Neg mg/dL	Color	Yellow

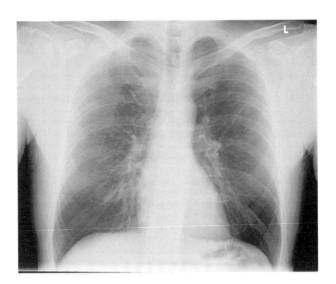

Figure 57.1

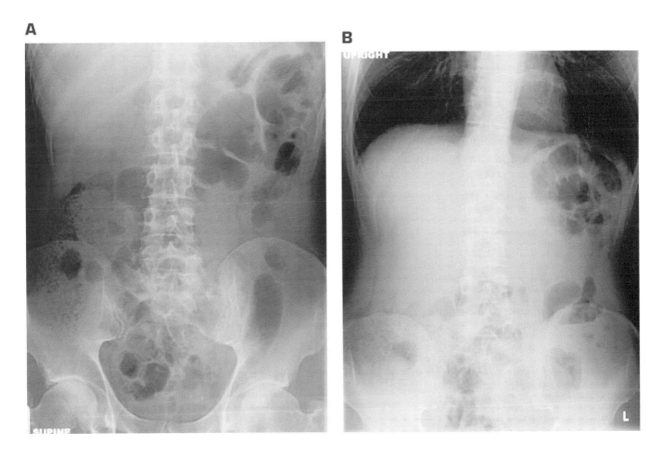

Figure 57.2 A and B

L. Diagnosis

a. Rocky Mountain spotted fever

M. Critical actions

▦ Obtaining travel history – camping

▦ Examination of rash

▦ CBC, BMP, LFT

▦ Complete physical examination including chest, lungs, abdomen, and neurological examination

▦ Antibiotics

N. Examiner instructions

a. This is a case of Rocky Mountain spotted fever (RMSF), a tick-borne illness usually involving a triad of fever, headache, rash in a patient with a recent history of tick bite. Only about 50% of cases involve a history of tick bite, so it is often treated on the basis of a clinical suspicion and exposure history, in this case the recent history of camping. Symptoms can involve multiple organs and can be serious, so a thorough examination is necessary, including neurological, chest, lungs, and abdomen. Early actions in this case include fluid resuscitation and administration of antibiotics. If fluids are not given, the patient will continue to have an elevated heart rate until fluids are given. Laboratory tests required for the case include CBC, chemistry, and LFTs, although the results are not sufficiently serious to warrant admission. Antibody titers and/or a skin biopsy are acceptable, but the results will not be available and do not affect the case. A chest and/or abdomen x-ray is also acceptable but again will not affect the case.

O. Pearls

a. Rash beginning on the palms and soles and spreading to the trunk is pathognomonic for Rocky Mountain spotted fever.

b. A history that raises suspicion for a tick bite, whether actually observed or not, is suspicious for RMSF.

c. RMSF can cause serious vasculitis, resulting in meningitis, pulmonary edema, liver or renal failure, or myocarditis, so a thorough physical examination is necessary to rule out end-organ damage.

d. A high WBC count, hyponatremia, and elevated LFTs support the diagnosis.

e. When any single tick-borne illness is encountered, consider the possibility of co-infection with the others (including Lyme disease, ehrlichiosis, and babesiosis)

P. References

a. Tintinalli's: Chapters 155, 245

b. Rosen's: Chapter 132

CASE 58: Sickle-cell disease (Braden Hexom, MD)

A. Chief complaint

a. 18-year-old male, with a history of sickle-cell disease, brought in by mother with the complaint of 3 days of left shoulder and left-sided chest pain

B. Vital signs

a. BP: 96/53 HR: 110 RR: 24 T: 37.6°C Sat: 92% on RA FS: 93 wt: 60 kg

C. What does the patient look like?

a. Patient appears stated age, awake, and alert responding to questions but appears in severe pain and mildly tachypneic.

D. Primary survey

a. Airway: speaking full sentences

b. Breathing: mild respiratory distress

c. Circulation: dry and cool skin, normal capillary refill

E. Action

a. Oxygen via NC or nonrebreather mask

b. Two large-bore peripheral IV lines

c. Labs

    i. CBC, BMP, LFT, coagulation studies, blood type and cross-match

    ii. Lactate, blood cultures, UA, urine culture, reticulocyte count

d. 1 L NS bolus

e. CXR

f. Meds

    i. IV morphine

F. History

a. HPI: an 18-year-old male with history of sickle cell (SS type) developed pain in the left shoulder 3 days ago; pain has now become worse and is extending to the scapula and left chest. He took hydrocodone at home without improvement. He is well known to the ED and is noted to have multiple visits in the past few months for pain crises and is admitted about two to three times per year. Today he notes mild shortness of breath; denies diarrhea, vomiting, headache, or neck pain. Chest pain is sharp, nonradiating, worse with inspiration.

b. PMHx: History of sickle cell with multiple ED visits and admissions. If asked about previous episodes, the patient will explain that most painful crises are in the hips and legs and this is the first visit for chest pain. The mother states, "he has never had pain like this before." Normally pain responds to 2 mg dilaudid or 16 mg morphine.

c. PSHx: none

d. Allergy: none

e. Meds: hydrocodone

f. Social: lives with single mother, no drugs/alcohol/smoking

g. FHx: mother and father with SS trait

h. PMD: pediatric hematologist – Dr Weber

G. Nurse

a. EKG (Figure 58.1)

b. Oxygen

    i. BP: 102/62 HR: 100 RR: 20 T: 37°C Sat: 95% on RA

c. No oxygen

    i. BP: 101/72 HR: 105 RR: 28 Sat: 89%

    ii. Patient will develop worsening shortness of breath until oxygen is applied

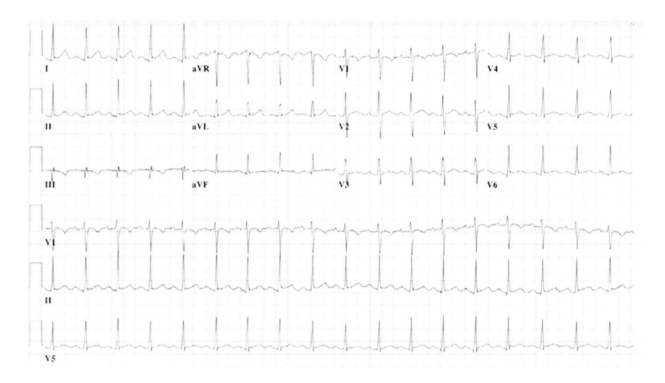

Figure 58.1

H. Secondary survey

a. General: alert, oriented × 3, in distress because of pain and mild shortness of breath

b. Head: normocephalic, atraumatic

c. Eyes: extraocular movement intact, pupils equal, reactive to light

d. Ears: normal tympanic membranes

e. Nose: no discharge

f. Neck: full range of motion, no jugular vein distension, no stridor

g. Pharynx: normal dentition, no lesions, no swelling

h. Chest: nontender

i. Lungs: diminished breath sounds at left base, + crackles, dull to percussion, normal breath sounds right lung

j. Heart: rate and rhythm regular, no murmurs, rubs, or gallops

k. Abdomen: normal bowel sounds, soft, nontender or distended

l. Rectal: normal tone, brown stool, occult blood negative

m. Extremities: no deformity, normal pulses, + pain to range of motion of left shoulder, right upper and bilateral lower extremities with full range of motion

n. Back: nontender

o. Neuro: cranial nerves II to XII intact; normal sensation, strength; normal reflexes and gait

p. Skin: warm and dry

q. Lymph: no lymphadenopathy

I. Action

a. Meds

   i. Morphine or dilaudid

   ii. Ceftriaxone and azithromycin or levofloxacin

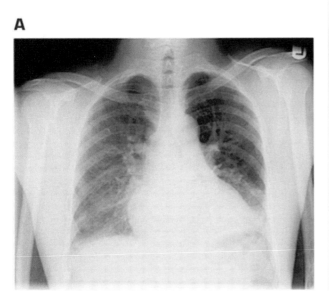

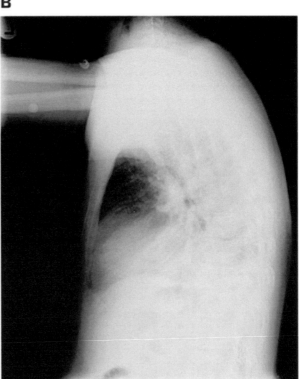

Figure 58.2 A and B

b. Reassess
  i. If less than a total of 10 mg morphine or 2 mg dilaudid, pain continues
  ii. If total 10 mg morphine or 2 mg dilaudid, pain improves
c. Consultation
  i. Hematology – recommends consideration for exchange transfusion, suggest discussing ICU for admission
d. Imaging
  i. CXR
e. Fluids

J. Nurse
a. CXR (Figure 58.2)

K. Results
a. Reticulocyte count 10.6
b. Smear – occasional sickled cells, Howell-Jowell bodies, occasional target cells

Complete blood count:	
WBC	18.9×10^3/uL
Diff	93/6/1
Hct	23.2%
Plt	75×10^3/uL

Basic metabolic panel:	
Na	134 mEq/L
K	4.9 mEq/L
Cl	108 mEq/L
CO_2	18.9 mEq/L
BUN	23 mEq/dL
Cr	0.7 mg/dL%
Gluc	94 mg/dL

Coagulation panel:

PT	13 sec
PTT	25 sec
INR	1.0

Liver function panel:

AST	43 U/L
ALT	40 U/L
Alk Phos	75 U/L
T bili	2.6 mg/dL
D bili	0.1 mg/dL
Amylase	35 U/L
Lipase	23 U/L
Albumin	4.5 g/dL
LDH	356

Urinalysis:

SG	1.010–1.030
pH	5–8
Prot	Neg mg/dL
Gluc	Neg mg/dL
Ketones	Neg mg/dL
Bili	Neg
Blood	Neg
LE	Neg
Nitrite	Neg
Color	Yellow

Arterial blood gas:

pH	7.35
PO_2	65 mmHg
PCO_2	32 mmHg
HCO_3	19 mmol/L

L. Diagnosis

a. Acute chest syndrome

M. Critical actions

▒ Oxygen
▒ IVF to prevent hypovolemia
▒ Pain control with IV opiate
▒ CXR and identification of pulmonary infiltrate
▒ Antibiotics
▒ Exchange transfusion or hematology consult
▒ Admission to medical ICU

N. Examiner instructions

a. This is a case of acute chest syndrome in a sickle-cell patient, a condition of unclear etiology thought to be caused by infection or lack of oxygen supply to the lung tissue that can lead to respiratory failure and death. This is a more serious diagnosis than the more common pain crises, and can lead to rapid deterioration of respiratory status. Symptoms that identify acute chest syndrome are chest pain, respiratory complaints, fever, or cough. Oxygen, administration of IV pain control, and antibiotics are critical actions for this case. If oxygen is not given, the patient will have progressively worse breathing. If adequate IV pain medicine (less than 10 mg of morphine or equivalent total) is not given, the patient will continue to have severe pain. Antibiotics should be given after identification of an infiltrate on CXR. A CBC and reticulocyte count should be obtained to evaluate the level of anemia and type and hold.

b. Curveball: the nurse approaches the candidate and states, "This guy is here all the time, and complains about pain here or there until he gets his fix of narcotics." The nurse will be reluctant to give any narcotics until the MD reassures that the patient is experiencing pain common in sickle-cell crisis, and that his chronic use of narcotics (as part of his prescribed treatment) will raise his tolerance to this class of medicines significantly.

O. Pearls

a. Rapid identification of painful crises that are not typical of the patient's usual symptoms should elicit a search for more serious complications of sickle cell including acute chest, aplastic crisis, splenic sequestration, hemolytic crisis, serious infection, stroke, or other end-organ infarct.

b. IV pain medication, oxygen, aggressive fluid rehydration, and/or blood transfusion are mainstays of treatment.

c. In severe cases of acute chest, exchange transfusion is warranted.

d. Since acute chest syndrome with pneumonia cannot reliably be distinguished from acute chest syndrome with**out** pneumonia on clinical grounds, empiric antibiotics for community-acquired pneumonia are usually warranted.

P. References

a. Tintinalli's: Chapters 135, 231

b. Rosen's: Chapter 119

CASE 59: Headache (Braden Hexom, MD)

A. Chief complaint

a. 22-year-old male brought in by friends with the complaint of fever and headache

B. Vital signs

a. BP: 118/84 HR: 105 RR: 16 T: 38.9°C Sat: 100% on RA FS: 87

C. What does the patient look like?

a. Patient appears stated age, somewhat lethargic, appears ill, responding slowly to questions.

D. Primary survey

a. Airway: speaking in full sentences

b. Breathing: no respiratory distress, no cyanosis

c. Circulation: pale, clammy skin

E. Action

a. Oxygen via NC or nonrebreather mask

b. Two large-bore peripheral IV lines

  i. CBC, BMP, LFT, coagulation studies, blood type and cross-match

  ii. Lactate, blood cultures, UA, urine culture, alcohol level, acetaminophen level, salicylate level, urine toxicology screen

c. 1 L NS bolus

d. Monitor: BP: 118/84 HR: 105 RR: 16 T: 38.9°C Sat: 100% on O_2

F. History

a. HPI: a 22-year-old male college student with no past medical history developed fever and headache this morning after attending an all-night drinking party. He denies any drug use but admits to drinking "a few drinks the night before." He woke up with a headache last night that he attributed to alcohol. He did not want to come to the hospital, but his roommate insisted when he developed a fever and was "not very awake." He describes a headache that does not go away and is bilaterally radiating down to the neck and shoulders. He has tried acetaminophen for the headache without improvement. Not the worst headache of life but significant pain, not sudden onset or thunderclap, no nausea, vomiting, blurry vision; + photophobia, + neck pain.

b. PMHx: none, immunizations up-to-date
c. PSHx: lives with roommate in college dormitory, does well in school, social drinking and smoking, no drugs
d. Allergy: none
e. Meds: none
f. FHx: no relevant history
g. PMD: school health services
h. Travel history (if asked): none

G. Nurse
a. With fluids
   i. BP: 112/88 HR: 87 RR: 16 Sat: 99%
b. no fluids
   i. BP: 90/70 HR: 110 RR: 16 Sat: 99%
c. Meds
   i. Ibuprofen or acetaminophen
      1. Does not improve headache or fever
   ii. Antiemetic
      1. Does not improve headache
d. Place patient into an isolation room, droplet precautions

H. Secondary survey
a. General: mildly lethargic but arousable, oriented × 3
b. Head: normocephalic, atraumatic
c. Eyes: extraocular movement intact, pale conjunctivae, + photophobia, equal and reactive pupils, unable to visualize fundus
d. Ears: normal tympanic membranes
e. Nose: no discharge
f. Neck: pain and stiffness with flexion, no jugular vein distension, no stridor
g. Pharynx: normal dentition, no lesions, no swelling
h. Chest: nontender
i. Lungs: clear bilaterally
j. Heart: rate and rhythm regular, no murmurs, rubs, or gallops
k. Abdomen: normal bowel sounds, soft, nontender or distended
l. Rectal: normal tone, brown stool, occult blood negative
m. Urogenital: normal external genitalia
   i. Male: no discharge, normal testicular examination
n. Extremities: full range of motion, no deformity, normal pulses
o. Back: nontender
p. Neuro: cranial nerves II to XII intact; normal sensation, strength; normal reflexes and gait
q. Skin: warm and dry, diffuse petechial rash over complete trunk
r. Lymph: no lymphadenopathy

Figure 59.1

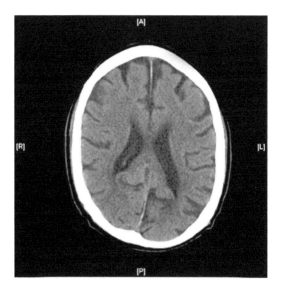

I. Action
a. Meds
    i. Dexamethasone
    ii. Ceftriaxone IV
    iii. Vancomycin IV
b. Imaging
    i. CT head (will take 20 minutes to obtain if candidate does not order antibiotics)
    ii. CXR

J. Nurse
a. CT head (Figure 59.1)

K. Action
a. Lumbar puncture
    i. Sent for Gram stain, culture, cell count, glucose, protein

L. Nurse
a. CXR (Figure 59.2)

M. Results
a. Serum and urine toxicology negative
b. Cerebral spinal fluid
    i. WBC: 1600
    ii. PMNs: 95%
    iii. RBC: 20
    iv. Glucose: 34
    v. Protein: 198
    vi. Gram stain: Gram-negative diplococci

Complete blood count:

WBC	17.3×10^3/uL
Diff	89.5/6.7/1.2
Hct	43%
Plt	75×10^3/uL

Basic metabolic panel:

Na	121 mEq/L
K	4.2 mEq/L
Cl	101mEq/L
CO_2	18.9 mEq/L
BUN	23 mEq/dL
Cr	0.7 mg/dL%
Gluc	94 mg/dL

Coagulation panel:

PT	13 sec
PTT	25 sec
INR	1.0

Liver function panel:

AST	25 U/L
ALT	26 U/L
Alk Phos	220 U/L
T bili	0.6 mg/dL
D bili	0.1 mg/dL
Amylase	79 U/L
Lipase	46 U/L
Albumin	3.9 g/dL

Urinalysis:

SG	1.010–1.030
pH	5–8
Prot	Neg mg/dL
Gluc	Neg mg/dL
Ketones	Neg mg/dL
Bili	Neg
Blood	Neg
LE	Neg
Nitrite	Neg
Color	Yellow

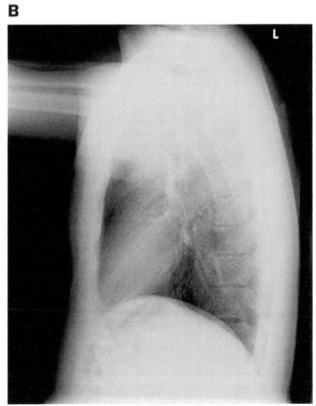

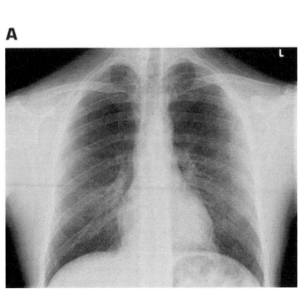

Figure 59.2 A and B

N. Action
a. Admission to ICU setting, isolation bed
b. Public heath
    i. Discussion with friends regarding prophylaxis
    ii. Call to dean of college regarding possible health concern
    iii. Prophylaxis to all exposed health providers
    iv. Report case to Department of Public Health

O. Diagnosis
a. Bacterial meningitis

P. Critical actions
▢ Appropriate antibiotic therapy before imaging or lumbar puncture
▢ Lumbar puncture
▢ Admission to isolation bed and ICU
▢ Assessment of public health concerns

Q. Examiner instructions
a. This is a case of bacterial meningitis, a serious infection of the tissues surrounding the brain and usually fatal if not treated promptly. Classic symptoms are headache, fever, neck stiffness, and a petechial or purpuric rash. Seizure and altered mental status are common. Treatment must begin immediately with IV antibiotics as soon as the diagnosis is suspected. Antibiotics should be administered before CT and lumbar puncture if there will be an expected delay as these are diagnostic tests. If steroids are given, they should be administered before or with the antibiotic. The candidate should isolate the patient early in the course of the case and get in contact with college health services regarding prophylaxis of students and staff for meningitis.

R. Pearls
a. Petechial/purpuric rash in the setting of headache and fever is sufficient to begin treatment.
b. CT does not necessarily need to be performed if the patient is without focal neurological deficits, papilledema, immunocompromise, or recent seizure.
c. Kernig's (contraction of hamstrings in response to knee extension) or Brudzinski's (flexion of hips/knees in response to neck flexion) signs are often insensitive but may aid in the diagnosis.
d. In patients with high suspicion of bacterial meningitis, IV steroids are recommended before or with antibiotics, which should include vancomycin 1 g and ceftriaxone 2 g.
e. Immunocompromised patients require additional CSF testing and broader-spectrum antibiotics, as they are susceptible to a wider range of organisms including tuberculosis, cryptococcus, staphylococcus, and listeria. Antibiotic therapy should include vancomycin, ampicillin, and ceftazidime.

S. References
a. Tintinalli's: Chapter 168
b. Rosen's: Chapters 107, 173

CASE 60: Chest pain (Braden Hexom, MD)

A. Chief complaint

a. 34-year-old male with chest pain

B. Vital signs

a. BP: 146/98 HR: 78 RR: 14 T: 37.9°C Sat: 98% on RA FS: 74

C. What does the patient look like?

a. Patient appears stated age, alert, oriented × 3, sitting up on stretcher, in no acute distress.

D. Primary survey

a. Airway: speaking full sentences

b. Breathing: no apparent respiratory distress, no cyanosis

c. Circulation: dry and cool skin, normal capillary refill

E. Action

a. Oxygen via NC or nonrebreather mask

b. Two large-bore peripheral IV lines

c. Labs

    i. CBC, BMP, LFT, coagulation studies, blood type and cross-match

d. 1 L NS bolus

e. EKG

F. History

a. HPI: A 34-year-old male with no past medical history presenting with chest pain for the past 4 hours. He describes the pain as slow in onset, gradually worsening throughout the day. The pain is localized to the mid chest, and is sharp, nonradiating, worse with inspiration. There is associated mild shortness of breath. There is no fever, chills, diaphoresis, nausea, or vomiting. If asked, he reports it is made worse with lying down, and made better by sitting forward. If asked about recent illnesses, he states that he had "a cold" about a week ago that resolved on its own; no recent travel; no swelling or pain in leg.

b. PMHx: none

c. PSHx: lives with wife and young child, social drinking, no smoking or drugs

d. Allergies: none

e. Meds: none

f. FHx: no family history of heart disease, MI, or stroke

g. PMD: none

G. Nurse

a. EKG (Figure 60.1)

b. Medication

    i. Ibuprofen or indomethacin – pain improves

    ii. Codeine – no improvement

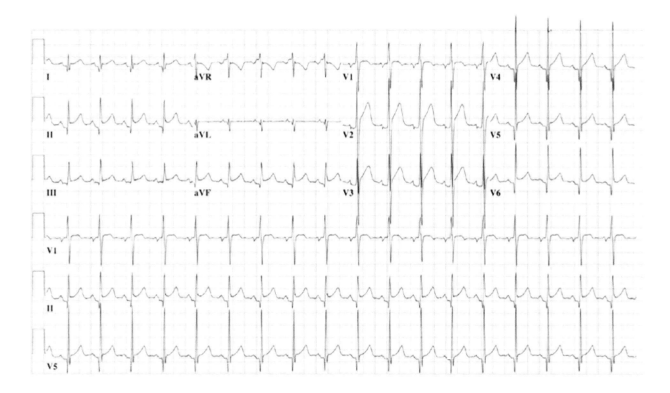

Figure 60.1

H. Secondary survey
  a. General: alert, oriented × 3, sitting forward on stretcher, in no acute distress
  b. Head: normocephalic, atraumatic
  c. Eyes: extraocular movement intact, pupils equal, reactive to light
  d. Ears: normal tympanic membranes
  e. Nose: no discharge
  f. Neck: full range of motion, no jugular vein distension, no stridor
  g. Pharynx: normal dentition, no lesions, no swelling
  h. Chest: nontender
  i. Lungs: clear bilaterally
  j. Heart: friction rub is heard over the left apex (must ask), normal rate and rhythm
  k. Abdomen: normal bowel sounds, soft, nontender or distended
  l. Rectal: normal tone, brown stool, occult blood negative
  m. Extremities: full range of motion, no deformity, normal pulses
  n. Back: nontender
  o. Neuro: cranial nerves II to XII intact; normal sensation, strength; normal reflexes and gait
  p. Skin: warm and dry
  q. Lymph: no lymphadenopathy

I. Action
  a. Imaging
      i. Echocardiogram official (bedside ED US machine unavailable)
      ii. CXR

b. Labs
  i. Add on cardiac enzymes and D-dimer
c. Disposition
  i. Admit for serial echocardiography

J. Results

Complete blood count:

WBC	10.3×10^3/uL
Hct	43%
Plt	75×10^3/uL

Basic metabolic panel:

Na	133 mEq/L
K	4.6 mEq/L
Cl	105 mEq/L
CO_2	19 mEq/L
BUN	24 mEq/dL
Cr	0.9 mg/dL%
Gluc	77 mg/dL

Coagulation panel:

PT	12.5 sec
PTT	26.1 sec
INR	1.0

Liver function panel:

AST	45 U/L
ALT	44 U/L
Alk Phos	54 U/L
T bili	0.5 mg/dL
D bili	0.2 mg/dL
Amylase	65 U/L
Lipase	23 U/L
Albumin	4.5 g/dL

Urinalysis:

SG	1.010–1.030
pH	5–8
Prot	Neg mg/dL
Gluc	Neg mg/dL
Ketones	Neg mg/dL
Bili	Neg
Blood	Neg
LE	Neg
Nitrite	Neg
Color	Yellow

a. Cardiac enzymes
  i. Troponin 0.3
  ii. CK: 63
  iii. MB: 4.8
b. D-dimer – negative
c. Echocardiogram – moderate amount of pericardial effusion, normal EF, no wall motion abnormality, no evidence of cardiac tamponade
d. CXR (Figure 60.2)

K. Diagnosis
a. Pericarditis

L. Critical actions
▪ EKG
▪ Cardiac examination
▪ Echocardiogram
▪ NSAID
▪ Admission

M. Examiner instructions
a. This is a case of pericarditis, an acute inflammation of the lining of the heart. Often caused by viral illnesses or idiopathic, it is not an acute coronary syndrome, and

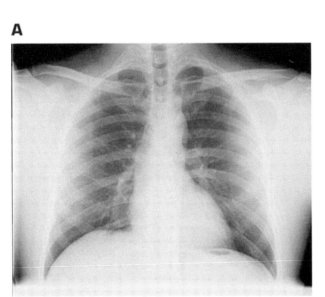

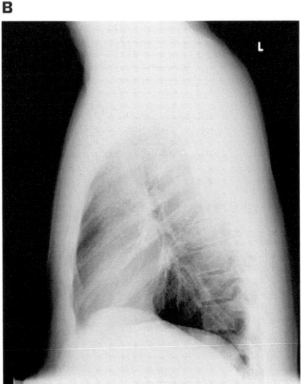

Figure 60.2 A and B

rarely requires admission. Early actions include obtaining an EKG, NSAID, and echocardiogram. Once the candidate diagnoses pericardial effusion, the patient should be admitted for observation and management to watch for cardiac tamponade. The candidate should still consider other differentials such as pulmonary embolism or myocardial infarction by reviewing risk factors such as family history of cardiac disease and recent travel history. Ultimately the patient has no risk factors for either pulmonary embolism or myocardial infarction and improves with NSAID.

N. Pearls

a. Pericarditis may be caused by viral or bacterial illnesses, malignancy, radiation, or a variety of other causes.

b. Patients often present with chest pain, made worse with lying down and improved with sitting forward. Additional symptoms can include dysphagia, dyspnea, and intermittent low-grade fevers. A friction rub heard over the left side of the chest is the most frequently encountered physical finding.

c. Physical examination and EKG analysis are usually sufficient to confirm the diagnosis.

d. ST-elevation and T-wave inversion are the most common EKG findings for pericarditis and are typically diffuse and rarely correspond to typical MI zones of infarction. PR-depression is the most pathognomonic EKG finding, but is not necessary to make the diagnosis of pericarditis.

e. Test such as laboratory tests, chest radiographs, and echocardiogram can aid in ruling out other causes of chest pain.

f. Cardiac tamponade must be considered and ruled out before discharge.

g. Once a thorough search for other causes of chest pain, including acute MI, pulmonary embolism, myocarditis, or pneumothorax is completed, patients with pericarditis can usually be managed as outpatients with 1 to 3 weeks of NSAID therapy unless there is evidence of myocarditis or pericardial fluid.

O. References
a. Tintinalli's: Chapter 59
b. Rosen's: Chapter 82

CASE 61: Altered mental status (Braden Hexom, MD)

A. Chief complaint
a. 73-year-old female brought in by basic life support ambulance with complaint of confusion and facial droop, rule out stroke

B. Vital signs
a. BP: 153/104 HR: 105 RR: 16 T: 36.8°C Sat: 100% on RA FS: pending (if requested by candidate)

C. What does the patient look like?
a. Patient appears stated age, confused, garbled response to questions, with obvious facial droop on right side.

D. Primary survey
a. Airway: awake, garbled vocalizations
b. Breathing: no respiratory distress
c. Circulation: diaphoretic, pale, clammy skin

E. Action
a. Oxygen via NC or nonrebreather mask
b. Two large-bore peripheral IV lines
c. Labs
   i. CBC, BMP, LFT, coagulation studies, blood type and cross-match
   ii. Finger stick glucose: 22 (if requested by candidate)
d. 1 L NS bolus
e. EKG
f. Meds
   i. D50 1–2 AMPS
   ii. Naloxone and thiamine

F. History
a. HPI: a 73-year-old female is brought in by her husband who found her on the sofa around 10 AM with confusion and slurred speech. She was brought immediately to the ED by ambulance (now 10:30 AM). Husband states he last saw his wife around 7 AM when she was at her baseline. She has a history of hypertension, high cholesterol, diabetes, and hypothyroid disease. The husband reports no recent illnesses or complaints. She suffers from mild dementia and forgetfulness, but is

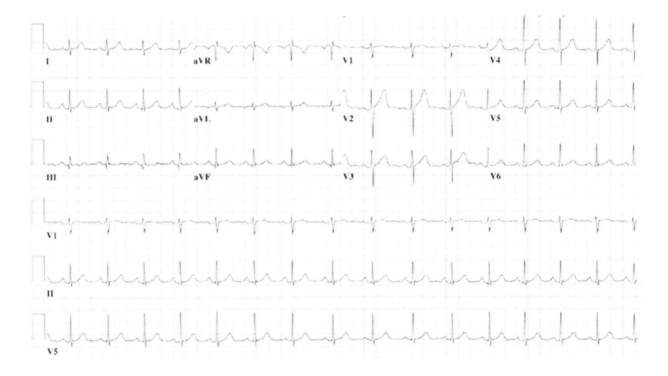

Figure 61.1

otherwise active, walks frequently, and is usually alert and conversational. Patient is confused and unable to answer questions.

b. EMS: no relevant history, only gave O_2 by mask

c. PMHx: hypertension, high cholesterol, diabetes (noninsulin dependent), hypothyroid

d. PSHx: none

e. Allergies: none

f. Meds: lovastatin, metoprolol, aspirin, glyburide, metformin, levothyroxine

g. Social: lives with husband, no smoking/alcohol/drugs

h. FHx: no relevant history

G. Nurse

a. D50 push IV

  i. Patient's symptoms resolve completely. Patient is now awake, alert, and becomes oriented with supportive care. Upon questioning she states she took her regular medications but did not eat breakfast because she had a doctor's appointment at 1 PM.

b. If D50 is not given, patient will continue to be confused with focal neurological findings

c. EKG (Figure 61.1)

H. Secondary survey

a. General

  i. Dextrose – A & O × 3, in no acute distress

  ii. No dextrose – patient remains confused

b. Head: normocephalic, atraumatic

   c. Eyes: pale conjunctivae, extraocular movement intact, pupils equal, reactive to light
   d. Ears: normal tympanic membranes
   e. Nose: no discharge
   f. Neck: full range of motion, no jugular vein distension, no stridor
   g. Pharynx: normal dentition, no lesions, no swelling
   h. Chest: nontender
   i. Lungs: clear bilaterally
   j. Heart: rate and rhythm regular, no murmurs, rubs, or gallops
   k. Abdomen: normal bowel sounds, soft, nontender or distended
   l. Rectal: normal tone, brown stool, occult blood negative
   m. Urogenital: normal external genitalia
   n. Extremities: full range of motion, no deformity, normal pulses
   o. Back: nontender
   p. Neuro:
      i. Dextrose – cranial nerves II to XII intact; normal sensation, strength; normal reflexes and gait
      ii. No dextrose – facial droop with garbled speech, does not cooperate with examination, reflexes normal, Babinski reflex normal, withdraws to pain
   q. Skin: clammy
   r. Lymph: no lymphadenopathy

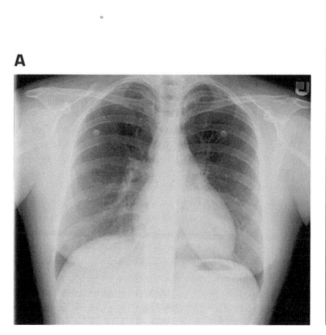
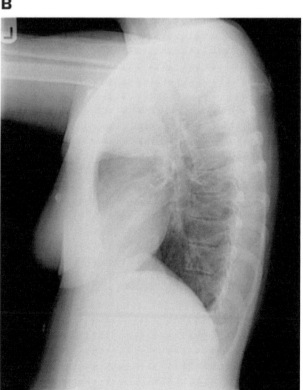

Figure 61.2 A and B

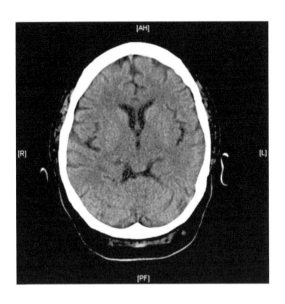

Figure 61.3

I. Action

a. Further action required (candidate may opt for any combination, must do one)

   i. Option 1: feed the patient

   ii. Option 2: D5 or D10 fluid administration at maintenance rate

   iii. Option 3: octreotide 50 to 125 mcg subcutaneously

b. Imaging

   i. CXR (Figure 61.2)

c. Admission

J. Nurse

a. CT head (Figure 61.3) if ordered – not necessary

K. Results

Complete blood count:

WBC	11.0×10^3/uL
Hct	32%
Plt	155×10^3/uL

Basic metabolic panel:

Na	138 mEq/L
K	4.3 mEq/L
Cl	111 mEq/L
CO_2	21 mEq/L
BUN	23 mEq/dL
Cr	0.9 mg/dL%
Gluc	234 mg/dL

Coagulation panel:

PT	13 sec
PTT	25 sec
INR	1.0

Liver function panel:

AST	45 U/L
ALT	44 U/L
Alk Phos	54 U/L
T bili	0.5 mg/dL
D bili	0.2 mg/dL
Amylase	65 U/L
Lipase	23 U/L
Albumin	4.5 g/dL

Urinalysis:

SG	1.010–1.030
pH	5–8
Prot	Neg mg/dL
Gluc	Neg mg/dL
Ketones	Neg mg/dL
Bili	Neg
Blood	Neg
LE	Neg
Nitrite	Neg
Color	Yellow

L. Disposition

a. Admission for observation

M. Diagnosis

a. Hypoglycemia secondary to sulfonylurea

N. Critical actions

▧ IV access

▧ Finger stick glucose

▧ IV dextrose

▧ Further antihypoglycemic intervention (dextrose fluids, oral feeding, or octreotide)

▧ Admission

O. Examiner instructions

a. This is a case of altered mental status with neurological deficits as a result of hypoglycemia. Hypoglycemia (low blood glucose) can mimic stroke syndromes presenting with weakness and confusion, and can typically be reversed with the administration of dextrose. The hypoglycemia in this scenario is due to not eating breakfast after taking a diabetes medicine (glipizide, a sulfonylurea). Upon this patient's initial presentation, she exhibited signs of an acute stroke, which may lead the candidate to misdiagnose this patient and initiate a stroke protocol including head CT, neurology consultation, intubation, or even thrombolysis. Obtaining an immediate blood glucose level is crucial to the diagnosis. With the ingestion in this case, further action is required beyond a rapid correction of blood glucose with dextrose in the case. Blood sugar levels must be maintained because sulfonylurea drugs can cause delayed or rebound hypoglycemia for many hours. Feeding, fluids with dextrose, or octreotide are all adequate options for this, with two or all three sometimes required. Admission is mandatory.

P. Pearls

a. Symptoms of hypoglycemia are due to both the effects on the brain and a reflex sympathetic surge. Neurological effects include confusion, altered mental status, agitation, seizures, unresponsiveness, and symptoms that may mimic acute stroke such as focal neurological deficits. Peripheral effects due to a sympathetic output of catacholamines cause anxiety, irritability, vomiting, palpitations, tremor, and sweating. One amp of D50 is about 100 calories, which is insufficient to maintain adequate blood glucose beyond a few minutes.

b. Rapid blood glucose determination is essential in all patients with altered mental status.

c. Additional intervention is required to maintain blood glucose levels. Often food is sufficient, but additional infusions of dextrose may be required

d. Long-acting oral hypoglycemics require admission and observation.

e. The elderly and severely malnourished (i.e., alcoholics) can present with hypoglycemia in the absence of sympathetic signs or even awareness of hypoglycemia, often mimicking intoxication, unresponsiveness, or stroke.

f. Octreotide inhibits release of insulin and has been shown to be effective in the treatment of sulfonylurea ingestions, given at a dose of 50 to 125 mcg SQ with continuous infusions of 125 mcg/hr. It is only recommended after initial glucose therapy has been initiated, as it primarily reduces the risk of recurrent hypoglycemia.

g. Glucagon 1 mg IM/IV may be used when IV access is unattainable, but response is generally slower and is often not useful for patient with depleted glycogen stores such as alcoholics.

Q. References
a. Tintinalli's: Chapters 218, 219
b. Rosen's: Chapter 126

CASE 62: Headache (Ravi Kapoor, MD, MPH)

A. Chief complaint
a. 42-year-old male presents with weakness, headache, and nausea for 1 day

B. Vital signs
a. BP: 150/90 HR: 105 RR 20 T 37.2°C Sat: 99% on RA

C. What does the patient look like?
a. Patient appears stated age, uncomfortable, and well-nourished.

D. Primary survey
a. Airway: speaking in full sentences
b. Breathing: no respiratory distress, no cyanosis
c. Circulation: dry and cool skin, normal capillary refill

E. Action
a. Oxygen via 100% nonrebreather mask
b. Two large-bore peripheral IV lines
c. Labs
   i. CBC, BMP, LFT, coagulation studies, blood type and cross-match
d. Monitor: BP: 150/90 HR: 100 RR: 22 Sat: 100%

F. History
a. HPI: a 42-year-old male with no past medical history presents to your community ED (located high in the mountains) with a 1-day history of "flu-like" illness with headache, weakness, and nausea. His friend brought him into the ED after he woke up this morning with a feeling of unsteadiness. They had arrived 2 days before to go skiing for the week and the symptoms started yesterday morning after waking up. This morning, they were planning to go skiing but the patient complained of worsening headache and unsteadiness; no chest pain, shortness of breath, palpitations, vomiting, diarrhea, fever, or blurry vision. Nobody else in the ski party has similar symptoms. The friend states that they arrived yesterday by helicopter, ascending 10,000 feet.
b. PMHx: none
c. PSHx: none
d. Allergies: none
e. Meds: none
f. Social: lives with wife at home, smokes one pack of cigarettes a day for 20 years, denies alcohol, drugs, not sexually active; works as an investment banker
g. FHx: no relevant history
h. PMD: Dr Miller

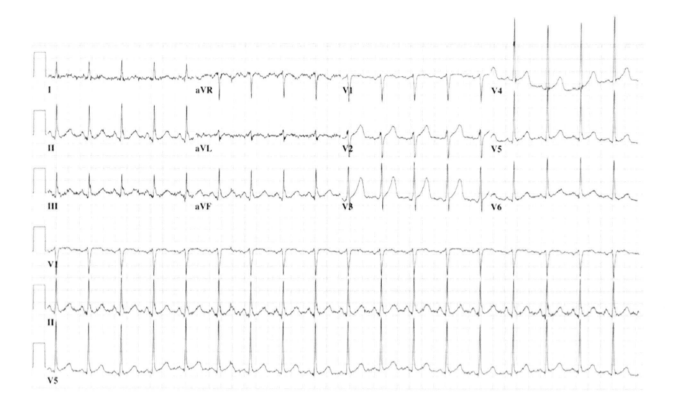

Figure 62.1

i. Travel history: arrived yesterday to the mountains by helicopter, ascended 10,000 feet

G. Nurse
a. EKG (Figure 62.1)

H. Secondary survey
a. General: appears sleepy but arousable, oriented × 3, uncomfortable
b. Head: normocephalic, atraumatic
c. Eyes: extraocular movement intact, pupils equal, reactive to light, no papilledema on fundoscopic examination
d. Ears: normal tympanic membranes
e. Nose: no discharge
f. Neck: full range of motion, no jugular vein distension, no stridor
g. Pharynx: normal dentition, no lesions, no swelling
h. Chest: nontender
i. Lungs: clear bilaterally
j. Heart: rate and rhythm regular, no murmurs, rubs, or gallops
k. Abdomen: normal bowel sounds, soft, nontender or distended
l. Rectal: normal tone, brown stool, occult blood negative
m. Extremities: full range of motion, no deformity, normal pulses
n. Back: nontender
o. Neuro: intact reflexes throughout, ataxic on tandem gait, poor finger to nose, positive Romberg's test, no focal weakness, no sensory deficit
p. Skin: warm and dry
q. Lymph: no lymphadenopathy

I. Action

a. Meds

    i. Acetazolamide

    ii. Dexamethasone

    iii. Ondansetron

b. Reassess

    i. Patient still uncomfortable, now with worsening headache (HA) and nausea.

c. Imaging

    i. CT head without contrast

    ii. CXR

J. Nurse

a. BP: 130/90 HR: 90 RR: 16 O_2 Sat: on NRB 100%

b. Patient: mildly confused, with continued HA

c. Imaging

    i. CT head (Figure 62.2)

    ii. CXR (Figure 62.3)

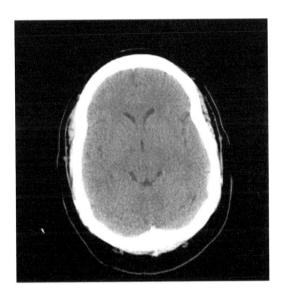

Figure 62.2

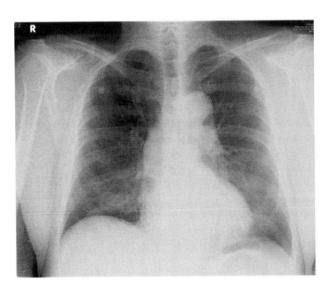

Figure 62.3

K. Results

Complete blood count:

WBC	9×10^3/uL
Hct	42%
Plt	300×10^3/uL

Basic metabolic panel:

Na	138 mEq/L
K	4.9 mEq/L
Cl	106 mEq/L
CO_2	22 mEq/L
BUN	18 mEq/dL
Cr	1.0 mg/dL%
Gluc	90 mg/dL

Coagulation panel:

PT	13 sec
PTT	39 sec
INR	1.2

Liver function panel:

AST	45 U/L
ALT	44 U/L
Alk Phos	54 U/L
T bili	0.5 mg/dL
D bili	0.2 mg/dL
Amylase	65 U/L
Lipase	23 U/L
Albumin	4.5 g/dL

Urinalysis:

SG	1.010–1.030
pH	5–8
Prot	Neg mg/dL
Gluc	Neg mg/dL
Ketones	Neg mg/dL
Bili	Neg
Blood	Neg
LE	Neg
Nitrite	Neg
Color	Yellow

L. Action

a. Hyperbaric chamber

b. Arrange for transfer/decent to lower altitude

M. Diagnosis

a. High altitude cerebral edema

N. Critical actions

▨ Treatment with dexamethasone

▨ Rapid descent

▨ Oxygen

O. Examiner instructions

a. This is a case of acute mountain sickness that progresses to high altitude cerebral edema (HACE) without high altitude pulmonary edema (HAPE). HACE and HAPE are the most severe forms of high-altitude illnesses and are life-threatening. They can occur after a rapid ascent in altitude, progressing from acute mountain sickness. Our patient presents with flu-like symptoms 1 day after rapid ascent to the mountains by helicopter, which precipitates his illness. The history of being on a ski vacation can be given early in the case, but the candidate must ask specifically how he got to the resort to elicit the history of rapid ascent. Important early actions include recognition, oxygen, acetazolamide, steroids, and rapid descent. If the candidate does not recognize that the patient has HACE and initiate treatment, the patient will rapidly become more lethargic and confused, ultimately requiring intubation. With appropriate management, the patient will do well and will be stable for transfer to a low-altitude medical center.

P. Pearls

a. High-altitude illness typically occurs within the first 48 hours after rapid ascent above altitudes of 2000 m.

b. Acute mountain sickness (AMS) presents with flu-like or hangover-like symptoms including nausea, vomiting, anorexia, headache, weakness, and decreased urination.

c. As symptoms of AMS worsen, it may progress to high altitude cerebral edema with vomiting, altered mental status, and ataxia. Neurologic findings distinguish acute mountain sickness (absent) from HACE (present).

d. Treatment of HACE is rapid decent and steroids. Hyperbarics may be used as a temporizing measure, but may delay definitive descent (unless a portable hyperbaric bag is employed).

Q. References

a. Tintinalli's: Chapter 216

b. Rosen's: Chapters 101, 142

c. UpToDate: "Acute Mountain Sickness and High Altitude Cerebral Edema"

CASE 63: Altered mental status (Ravi Kapoor, MD, MPH)

A. Chief complaint

a. 79-year-old male brought in by EMS for altered mental status, nausea, and weakness

B. Vital signs

a. BP: 100/50 HR: 48 RR: 16 T: 37.4°C O$_2$ Sat: RA 99% FS: 120 (must ask)

C. What does the patient look like?

a. Patient appears stated age, speaking in full sentences, nauseous, and inattentive.

D. Primary survey

a. Airway: speaking in full sentences

b. Breathing: no respiratory distress, no cyanosis

c. Circulation: warm dry skin, normal capillary refill

E. Action

a. Oxygen via NC or nonrebreather mask

b. Two large-bore peripheral IV lines

c. Labs

   i. CBC, BMP, LFT, coagulation studies, blood type and cross-match

   ii. Lactate, blood cultures, UA, urine culture, troponin

d. Monitor: BP: 100/50 HR: 48 RR: 16 T: 37.4°C (rectal) FS: 120 Sat: 99% on 100% FM nonrebreather mask

e. EKG

F. History

a. HPI: a 79-year-old male with known history of congestive heart failure (CHF), hypertension (HTN), and hypercholesterolemia presents with confusion at home per his wife. The patient's wife states that her husband has had increasing confusion over the past few days, and has complained of nausea, weakness, and dizziness. He has also stated that things look funny (if asked, he states that "things have yellowish hue"). He denies chest pain, shortness of breath, fever, cough, urinary symptoms, headache, or pain. His baseline mental status is good and he is able to go to the store on his own. His wife notes that he was placed on erythromycin several days ago for bronchitis that has now resolved.

b. PMHx: HTN, hypercholesterolemia, CHF
c. PSHx: none
d. Allergies: none
e. Meds: digoxin, furosemide, simvastatin, aspirin, erythromycin
f. Social: lives with wife at home, leaving apartment less these days, denies alcohol, smoking, drugs, not sexually active
g. FHx: no relevant history
h. PMD: Dr Johnson

G. Nurse
a. BP: 90/45 HR: 40 RR: 16 Sat 99% on O_2
  i. Lab
    1. Add digoxin level
b. Patient states he feels dizzy and nauseous (diaphoretic)
c. EKG (Figure 63.1)

H. Secondary survey
a. General: alert, oriented × 2 (person, place, patient thinks it is 1978), comfortable
b. Head: normocephalic, atraumatic

Figure 63.1

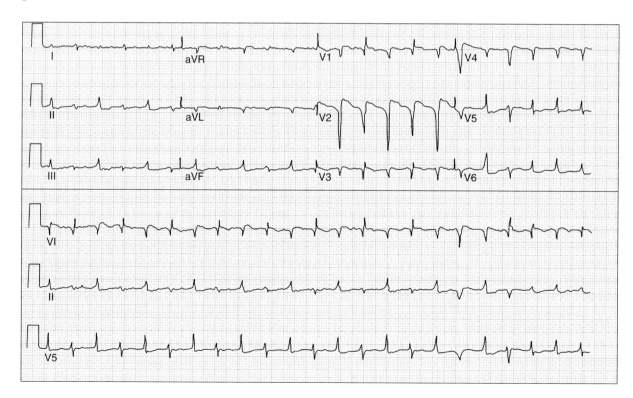

  c. Eyes: extraocular movement intact, pupils equal, reactive to light
  d. Ears: normal tympanic membranes
  e. Nose: no discharge
  f. Neck: full range of motion, no jugular vein distension, no stridor
  g. Pharynx: normal dentition, no lesions, no swelling
  h. Chest: nontender
  i. Lungs: clear bilaterally
  j. Heart: bradycardic, regular, no murmurs, rubs, or gallops
  k. Abdomen: normal bowel sounds, soft, nontender or distended
  l. Rectal: normal tone, brown stool, occult blood negative
  m. Extremities: full range of motion, no deformity, normal pulses, 1+ pitting edema
  n. Back: nontender
  o. Neuro: cranial nerves II to XII intact; normal sensation, strength; normal reflexes and gait
  p. Skin: warm and dry
  q. Lymph: no lymphadenopathy

I. Action
  a. Meds
     i. Atropine IV
     ii. Digibind 6 vials over 30 minutes (if digibind not given, patient will continue to be bradycardic and more confused)
  b. Imaging
     i. CXR
     ii. Repeat EKG
  c. IV fluids
     i. NS 1 L bolus
  d. Poison control
  e. Transcutaneous pacer pads placed on patient

J. Nurse
  a. If digibind given, BP: 100/59 HR: 60 RR: 18 Sat: 98% on O_2
  b. Patient: dizziness and nausea improved (less diaphoretic)

K. Results

Complete blood count:	
WBC	9×10^3/uL
Hct	33.5%
Plt	321×10^3/uL

Basic metabolic panel:	
Na	139 mEq/L
K	6.0 mEq/L
Cl	108 mEq/L
CO_2	22 mEq/L
BUN	25 mEq/dL
Cr	1.9 mg/dL%
Gluc	122 mg/dL

Coagulation panel:	
PT	13.1 sec
PTT	26 sec
INR	1.0

Liver function panel:	
AST	45 U/L
ALT	44 U/L
Alk Phos	54 U/L
T bili	0.5 mg/dL
D bili	0.2 mg/dL
Amylase	65 U/L
Lipase	23 U/L
Albumin	4.5 g/dL

Urinalysis:

SG	1.010–1.030	Bili	Neg
pH	5–8	Blood	Neg
Prot	Neg mg/dL	LE	Neg
Gluc	Neg mg/dL	Nitrite	Neg
Ketones	Neg mg/dL	Color	Yellow

    a. Lactate 1.1 mmol/L

    b. Troponin 0

    c. Digoxin level 2.4

    d. CXR (Figure 63.2)

    e. EKG (Figure 63.3)

L. Action

a. Meds

    i. Calcium gluconate 1000 mg (1 AMP)**

    ii. Dextrose 25 g (1 AMP)

    iii. Insulin 10U IV push

    iv. Bicarbonate 50 meq (1 AMP)

    v. Sodium polystyrene sulfonate 30 g PO

b. CCU consult

c. EKG

d. Speak to wife to explain patient's condition

M. Nurse

a. Accepted to CCU

Figure 63.2

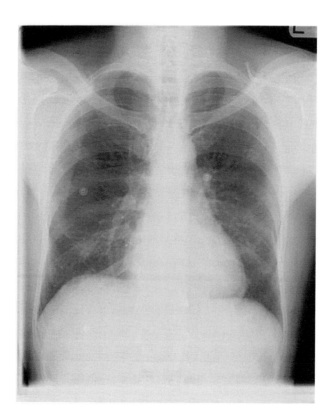

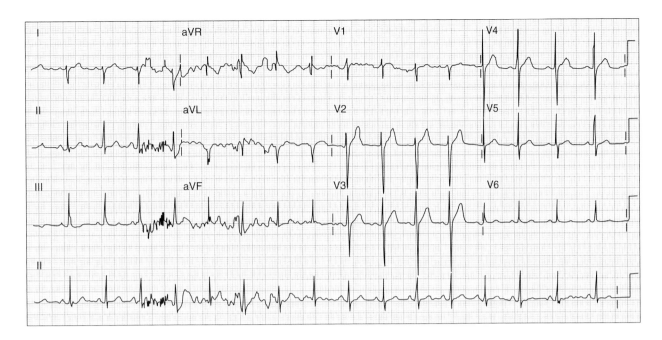

Figure 63.3

N. Diagnosis
a. Digoxin toxicity

O. Critical actions
- EKG
- Atropine or pacer pads requested (+/− pacing)
- Digoxin-specific Fab
- Treatment for hyperkalemia
- CCU

P. Examiner instructions
a. This is a case of digoxin (digitalis) toxicity caused by an increase in serum levels secondary to being placed on erythromycin and new renal insufficiency. Cardioactive steroids have been used to control irregular cardiac rhythms since William Withering described their effects in 1785. In excess, digoxin can lead to life-threatening abnormalities in heart conduction. The patient presents with nonspecific complaints of nausea, confusion, and dizziness but also has classic disturbances in color vision that can occur with digoxin toxicity. The candidate should initially cast a broad differential to exclude causes of altered mental status such as hypoglycemia, hypoxia, stroke, myocardial infarction, and infection. A thorough history should elicit his current medications, including digoxin, and a level should be ordered. As the case progresses, the patient will become increasingly diaphoretic, bradycardic, and hypotensive, and complain of dizziness. At this time, the patient should be empirically treated with the antidote, digoxin-specific Fab.

Q. Pearls
a. The mortality of digoxin toxic patients correlates with serum potassium levels, and patients with levels over 5.5 meq/L have a mortality of 50%, if untreated.

b. The digoxin level itself, does not correlate with toxicity, especially in chronic toxicity.

c. Digoxin-specific Fab causes a sharp decrease in free serum digoxin concentration, an (clinically unimportant) increase in total serum digoxin, and a decrease in serum potassium.

d. Caution should be used if hyperkalemia is treated before being given the digoxin-specific Fab, as profound HYPOkalemia may occur.

e. β-blockers and calcium channel blockers are contraindicated as they may worsen AV block.

f. Symptoms of digoxin toxicity are nonspecific and include weakness, dizziness, shortness of breath, confusion, disturbances in color vision (yellow-green tendency), nausea, vomiting, and headache.

g. The three methods for calculating the required number of vials of digoxin-specific Fab:

1. Dose unknown: Adult – 10 vials

   Child – 5 vials

   (may repeat q30° or earlier if severe symptoms)

2. Dose known: $\dfrac{\text{Dose(mg)} \times 0.8(\text{bioavailability})}{0.5}$

3. Digoxin level known: $\dfrac{\text{Level(ng/ml)} \times \text{Weight(kg)}}{100}$

** There is increasing evidence calcium does not adversely affect the heart in digoxin toxicity (Fenton F, *et al.*, Hyperkalemia and digoxin toxicity in a patient with kidney failure. *Ann Emerg Med* 1996; Hack JB, *et al.*, The effect of calcium chloride in treating hyperkalemia due to acute digoxin toxicity in a porcine model. *J Toxicol Clin Toxicol* 2004) as opposed to the three case reports that describe the adverse effects of calcium in this setting. Rosen's explicitly states calcium can be given for the treatment of hyperkalemia in this setting. Tintinalli states calcium administration "is controversial."

R. References

a. Tintinalli's: Chapters 23, 187

b. Rosen's: Chapter 152

c. Nelson *et al.*, (2010). *Goldfrank's Toxicologic Emergencies* (9th ed.). McGraw-Hill. Chapter 64.

d. UpToDate: "Digitalis (Cardiac Glycoside) Poisoning"

CASE 64: Shortness of breath (Ravi Kapoor, MD, MPH)

A. Chief complaint

a. 82-year-old female brought in by EMS for sudden onset of shortness of breath for 30 minutes

B. Vital signs

a. BP: 230/90 HR: 120 RR: 28 T: 37.2°C Sat: 92% on nonrebreather mask

C. What does the patient look like?

a. Patient appears stated age, uncomfortable, sitting upright to breathe, cannot speak in full sentences, and diaphoretic.

D. Primary survey
a. Airway: unable to speak in full sentences but able to say name
b. Breathing: severe respiratory distress with cyanosis
c. Circulation: pale, cool, diaphoretic skin

E. Action
a. Oxygen via NC or nonrebreather mask
b. Two large-bore peripheral IV lines
c. Labs
   i. CBC, BMP, coagulation studies, blood type and cross-match
   ii. Troponin, brain natriuretic peptide (BNP), lactate
d. Monitor: BP: 220/90 HR: 120 RR: 35 Sat: 94% on nonrebreather mask
e. EKG
f. CXR

F. History
a. HPI: an 82-year-old female presents, but is unable to give history secondary to her labored breathing. Her husband states she has a history of hypertension, diabetes, and hypercholesterolemia and says that she has been feeling short of breath for the past 2 days. She has had difficulty sleeping at night because she gets short of breath if she lies flat. She has not left the apartment recently, as they live on the third floor of a walk-up. She was fearful that she would not be able to make it back up the stairs if she went out. The patient is able to deny nausea, vomiting, leg swelling, cough, fever, or chest pain. This morning she woke up with acute worsening shortness of breath.
   i. EMS: bilateral crackles on chest examination. The patient was given 1 sublingual nitroglycerine, oxygen, and 40 mg of furosemide.
b. PMHx: hypertension, diabetes, and hypercholesterolemia, no prior cardiac work-up
c. PSHx: none
d. Allergies: none
e. Meds: does not know except a water pill
f. Social: lives with husband at home, leaving apartment less these days, denies alcohol, smoking, drugs, not sexually active
g. FHx: not relevant
h. PMD: Dr Johnson

G. Nurse
a. BP: 220/90 HR: 120 RR: 35 Sat: 94% on 100% nonrebreather mask
b. EKG (Figure 64.1)
c. CXR (Figure 64.2)

H. Action
a. Nitroglycerin 1 tablet sublingual
b. Furosemide IV

I. Secondary survey
a. General: severe respiratory distress, awake, unable to speak
b. Head: normocephalic, atraumatic

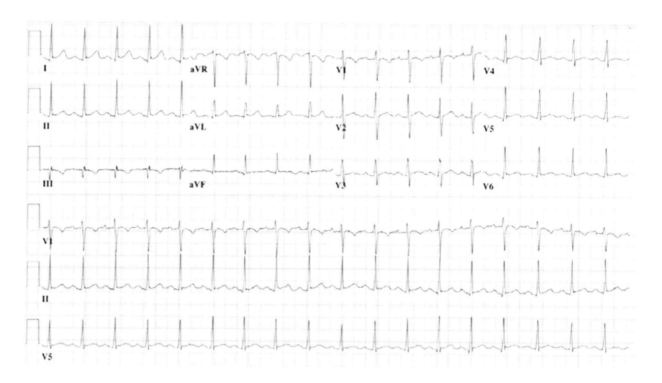

Figure 64.1

Figure 64.2

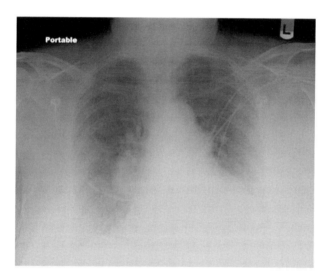

c. Eyes: extraocular movement intact, pupils equal, reactive to light
d. Ears: normal tympanic membranes
e. Nose: no discharge
f. Neck: full range of motion, + jugular vein distension, no stridor
g. Pharynx: normal dentition, no lesions, no swelling
h. Chest: nontender
i. Lungs: diffuse crackles, minimal air movement
j. Heart: tachycardia, regular rhythm, no murmurs, rubs, or gallops
k. Abdomen: normal bowel sounds, soft, nontender or distended
l. Rectal: normal tone, brown stool, occult blood negative

m. Urogenital: deferred
n. Extremities: full range of motion, no deformity, normal pulses, 2 + pitting edema
o. Back: nontender
p. Neuro: cranial nerves II to XII intact; normal sensation, strength; normal reflexes and gait
q. Skin: warm and dry
r. Lymph: no lymphadenopathy

J. Action
a. Noninvasive ventilation
  i. CPAP/BiPAP – improvement of symptoms, vital signs
    1. BP: 170/70 HR: 110 RR: 20 Sat: 97% on 100%
b. Meds
  i. Nitroglycerin high dose – shortness of breath mild improvement
    1. Greater than 10 mcg/min of IV nitroglycerine and titrate to relief of SOB
    2. Greater than 2 tablets nitroglycerine 0.4 mg SL (sequentially)
       BP: 170/70 HR: 110 RR: 26 Sat: 97% on 100%
  ii. Nitroglycerin inappropriately low dose – worsening shortness of breath requiring intubation
    1. Less than 10 mcg/min of IV nitroglycerine
    2. Less than 2 tablets nitroglycerine 0.4 mg SL (sequentially)
       BP: 220/90 HR: 130 RR: 46 Sat: 90% on 100%
  iii. Furosemide 1 mg/kg IV
  iv. Aspirin 325 mg PO
c. Foley catheter placement
d. CCU consult

K. Nurse
a. BP: 150/90 HR: 90 RR: 20 O_2 Sat: 100% with noninvasive ventilation and after high dose nitro
b. Patient: is significantly less short of breath

L. Results

Complete blood count:

WBC	18×10^3/uL
Hct	27%
Plt	300×10^3/uL

Basic metabolic panel:

Na	139 mEq/L
K	4.9 mEq/L
Cl	119 mEq/L
CO_2	12 mEq/L
BUN	30 mEq/dL
Cr	1.8 mg/dL%
Gluc	90 mg/dL

Coagulation panel:

PT	13 sec
PTT	39 sec
INR	1

Liver function panel:

AST	1–50 U/L
ALT	1–53 U/L
Alk Phos	30–110 U/L
T bili	0.1–1.2 mg/dL
D bili	0.0–0.8 mg/dL
Amylase	30–300 U/L
Lipase	23–300 U/L
Albumin	3.5–4.9 g/dL

Urinalysis:

SG	1.010–1.030
pH	5–8
Prot	Neg mg/dL
Gluc	Neg mg/dL
Ketones	Neg mg/dL
Bili	Neg

Urinalysis *(continued)*:		Arterial blood gas:	
Blood	Neg	pH	7.35–7.45
LE	Neg	PO$_2$	80–100 mmHg
Nitrite	Neg	PCO$_2$	35–45 mmHg
Color	Yellow	HCO$_3$	22–26 mmol/L

a. Lactate 1.6 mmol/L

b. Troponin 2.0, BNP 4000

M. Action

a. If intubated, continue management, with adequate sedation

b. Admit to CCU

N. Diagnosis

a. Congestive heart failure, exacerbation

O. Critical actions

▓ Oxygen

▓ High-dose nitroglycerin drip / sequential SL 0.4 mg NTG tablets initiated immediately

▓ Furosemide

▓ Aspirin

▓ CCU consult

P. Examiner instructions

a. This is a case of acute pulmonary edema (APE) in the setting of a patient with congestive heart failure (CHF). This results primarily from increased LV and pulmonary capillary hydrostatic pressures forcing a plasma ultrafiltrate across the pulmonary capillary membrane. This fluid then enters the pulmonary interstitium and alveoli causing difficulty breathing. This patient presents with severe respiratory distress from APE that must be managed aggressively to avoid intubation. If nitrates are started (either high-dose IV or sequential sublingual doses) the patient will do well. If no nitrates or inappropriately small doses are administered, the patient will continue to worsen and require intubation. Noninvasive ventilation strategies such as continuous positive airway pressure (CPAP) may be used with patient improvement as long as adequate doses of nitrates are used. Once the patient is improving, a search of the cause of CHF (such as myocardial infarction, medication non-compliance, dietary indiscretion, or infection), must begin.

Q. Pearls

a. Patients will often present with difficulty breathing on exertion.

b. The physical exam often outperforms diagnostic tests in this condition. Physical findings include pitting edema, crackles, wheezing ("not all that wheezes is asthma"), hypoxia, jugular venous distension, S3 or S4 on cardiac examination.

c. Five-year survival for patients with the diagnosis of CHF is 60% in men and 45% in women.

d. It is important to search for the root cause of exacerbation (such as MI, PNA, PE).

e. BNP is highly sensitive for CHF and can be sent in equivocal cases.

   f. Treatment includes preload reduction with nitroglycerin, positive pressure ventilation, and diuresis.

   g. CPAP may be beneficial in severe exacerbations to prevent intubation.

R. References
a. Tintinalli's: Chapter 57
b. Rosen's: Chapter 169
c. UpToDate: "Treatment of acute decompensated heart failure: Components of therapy"

CASE 65: Shortness of breath (Christopher Strother, MD)

A. Chief complaint
a. 10-day-old male with shortness of breath, "pulling," poor feeding

B. Vital signs
a. BP: 110/80, RUE HR: 175 RR: 90 T: 36.2°C Sat: 95% on RA FS: 70 wt: 3 kg

C. What does the patient look like?
a. Patient appears stated age, lethargic, tachypneic, mild intercostal and subcostal retractions.

D. Primary survey
a. Airway: patent, weak cry
b. Breathing: respiratory distress, diffuse mild crackles bilaterally
c. Circulation: capillary refill 2 seconds, diminished femoral pulses

E. Action
a. Oxygen supplementation (nonrebreather mask)
b. IV placement
c. Labs
   i. CBC, BMP, blood gas, blood culture, LFT, PT/PTT, blood type, UA, urine culture
d. 20 ml/kg NS (60 ml) bolus
e. Monitor: BP: 110/80, RUE HR: 175 RR: 85 Sat: 97% on O_2
   i. Unable to obtain LE blood pressure
f. EKG, CXR

F. History
a. HPI: a 10-day-old male, born full term via normal spontaneous vaginal delivery born at home. He is breastfed with some difficulty often "tiring out" while feeding. He "sleeps a lot," and mother reports he "always breathes that fast." He was doing well until his tenth day of life (today) when he developed worsening shortness of breath, tachypnea, retractions, and refusing to breastfeed. He has exhibited worsening lethargy over the past few hours; denies fever, no vomiting or diarrhea, no cough, no rash, no sick contacts, and no medications given at home now or at birth.
b. PMHx: none
c. PSHx: none

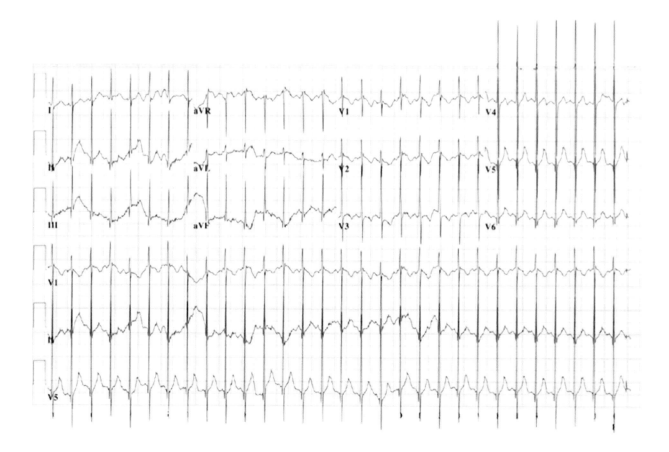

Figure 65.1

d. Allergies: none
e. Social: lives with parents at home, no pets or siblings
f. FHx: not relevant
g. PMD: Dr Chris

G. Nurse
a. EKG (Figure 65.1)
b. Lower extremity blood pressures
   i. BP: 50/palp

H. Secondary survey
a. General: lethargic, mild respiratory distress, severe tachypnea
b. HEENT: normal
c. Neck: normal
d. Chest: mild diffuse rales, mild retractions, tachypnea
e. Heart: S1S2, + systolic murmur at left sternal border and scapula
f. Abdomen: liver palpable at 3 cm below costal margin, soft, nontender
g. Rectal: normal
h. Urogenital: normal
i. Extremities: normal
j. Back: normal

  k. Neuro: lethargic, nonfocal
  l. Skin: mottled, cyanotic
 m. Lymph: normal

I. Action
 a. Procedures
   i. Endotracheal intubation via rapid sequence intubation
   ii. Ventilator settings: volume 10 ml/kg (30 ml) or with chest rise, O_2 100%, rate of 40
   iii. Consider central line placement
 b. Meds
   i. Prostaglandin E1
 c. Reassess
   i. Patient still with significant distress if not intubated, will begin to improve only after prostaglandin administration
 d. Consult
   i. Cardiology
 e. Imaging
   i. CXR
 f. Labs
   i. UA, Ucx

J. Nurse
 a. Repeat vital signs
   i. If intubated: BP: 100/70 HR: 160
   ii. If not intubated: BP: 80/50 HR: 170 RR: 80 Sat: 92% on O_2
 b. Patient: still in distress if not intubated

K. Results

Complete blood count:

WBC	9.5×10^3/uL	T bili	1.0 mg/dL
Hct	52.5%	D bili	0.3 mg/dL
Plt	150×10^3/uL	Amylase	44 U/L
		Lipase	18 U/L
Basic metabolic panel:		Albumin	3.4 g/dL
Na	139 mEq/L		
K	4.2 mEq/L	**Urinalysis:**	
Cl	110 mEq/L	SG	1.010
CO_2	20 mEq/L	pH	6
BUN	9 mEq/dL	Prot	Neg
Cr	0.6 mg/dL%	Gluc	Neg
Gluc	90 mg/dL	Ketones	Neg
		Bili	Neg
Coagulation panel:		Blood	Neg
PT	11.1 sec	LE	Neg
PTT	28 sec	Nitrite	Neg
INR	1.0	Color	Yellow
Liver function panel:		**Arterial blood gas:**	
AST	25 U/L	pH	7.45
ALT	12 U/L	PO_2	140 mmHg
Alk Phos	115 U/L	PCO_2	46 mmHg
		HCO_3	28 mmol/L

Figure 65.2

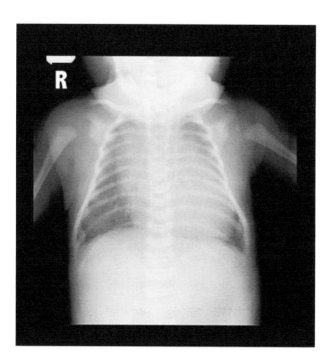

a. Lactate 1.2 mmol/L
b. Portable CXR (Figure 65.2)

L. Action
a. Meds
    i. Antibiotics to cover sepsis (ampicillin and cefotaxime or gentamycin)
    ii. Prostaglandin drip
b. Cardiology consult
    i. For cardiac echo and admission: echo demonstrates critical aortic coarctation
    ii. Emergent operative repair needed
c. Discussion with family and PMD need for ICU admission and urgent repair of lesion

M. Diagnosis
a. Critical aortic coarctation

N. Critical actions
▨ Recognition of respiratory distress
▨ Oxygen administration, intubation
▨ IV access
▨ EKG, CXR
▨ Recognition of cardiomegaly and cardiac cause of respiratory distress
▨ Cardiology consult
▨ Prostaglandin administration

O. Examiner instructions
a. This is a case of critical congenital heart disease that is dependent upon a patent ductus arteriosis to maintain blood flow to the body. A structural abnormality in the heart prevents blood from being oxygenated properly by the lungs. A fetal bypass pathway (the ductus arteriosis) allows some oxygenation to occur; when this closes, patients rapidly deteriorate. It is often clinically unrecognizable at birth, but

patients develop obstructive heart failure which acutely worsens when the duct closes (normally at about one week). The newborn will have distress, and will have difficulty feeding due to the increased energy required to breathe. Infants often are described as "tired," "wears out" or "gets sweaty" when feeding. Important initial actions are oxygenation, IV access, CXR, and cardiology consultation. A congenital heart lesion must be considered in any newborn with shock or severe distress and prostaglandin should be given in case the lesion is duct-dependent. This patient will slowly improve with prostaglandin administration, but needs definitive intervention for true resolution of symptoms. Without prostaglandin the patient will develop steadily worsening heart failure and shock (blood pressure and oxygen level will fall, heart rate and respiratory rate will rise).

P. Pearls
a. Congenital heart disease should be considered in any newborn in shock or severe distress.
b. Early recognition of possible heart disease and initiation of prostaglandin and cardiology involvement is important.
c. Infants in extremis should also be treated for possible infection/sepsis. Sepsis work-up should be done with lumbar puncture performed only if the infant is stable enough to tolerate it.
d. Differential blood pressure and oxygen saturation from upper to lower extremities is a clue to congenital heart disease with a patent ductus arteriosis.

Q. References
a. Tintinalli's: Chapters 34, 122
b. Rosen's: Chapter 169

CASE 66: Flank pain (Ravi Kapoor, MD, MPH)

A. Chief complaint
a. 30-year-old male presents with flank pain for 2 days, worse today

B. Vital signs
a. BP: 140/90 HR: 125 RR: 16 T: 37.4°C O_2 sat RA 99% FS: 100

C. What does the patient look like?
a. Patient appears stated age, speaking in full sentences, vomiting, uncomfortable, and writhing in bed.

D. Primary survey
a. Airway: speaking in full sentences
b. Breathing: no respiratory distress, no cyanosis
c. Circulation: normal skin, warm

E. Action
a. Oxygen via NC or nonrebreather mask
b. Two large-bore peripheral IV lines

   c. Labs

       i. CBC, BMP, coagulation studies, blood type and cross-match

       ii. UA

   d. 1 L NS bolus

   e. Monitor: BP: 140/90 HR: 125 RR: 16 T: 37.4°C O_2 sat RA 99%

   f. Meds

       i. Ketorolac IV or ibuprofen PO

       ii. Morphine IV

       iii. Metoclopramide or equivalent antiemetic

F. History

a. HPI: a 30-year-old male with no past medical history presents with left flank pain for 1 day. The pain is characterized as 10/10 in the left flank radiating to the groin. Patient states the pain began last night suddenly on the left side and was intermittent and associated with nausea. He took ibuprofen with mild relief but states that the pain returned this morning much worse than before with three episodes of vomiting in the past 4 hours precipitating his visit. Patient states that he has never had this sensation before. Patient denies fever, chills, chest pain, shortness of breath, or headache; no hematemsis, no chest pain.

b. PMHx: none

c. PSHx: none

d. Allergies: none

e. Meds: daily vitamin A and vitamin C

f. Social: lives with wife at home; denies alcohol use, smoking, or illicit drug use, sexually active with one partner

g. FHx: not relevant

h. PMD: none

G. Nurse

a. If analgesia is given

       i. BP: 130/80 HR: 105 RR: 16 T: 37.4°C Sat: 99% on O_2

       ii. Patient: feels significantly improved—mild dull pain to left flank

b. Without analgesia

       i. BP: 160/100 HR: 120 RR: 16 T: 37.4°C Sat: 99% on O_2

       ii. Patient: still writhing in bed in significant pain

c. UA large blood, negative leukocyte esterase, negative nitrites

H. Secondary survey

a. General: alert, oriented

       i. Analgesia – appears more comfortable

       ii. No analgesia – writhing in bed in pain

b. Head: normocephalic, atraumatic

c. Eyes: extraocular movement intact, pupils equal, reactive to light

d. Ears: normal tympanic membranes

e. Nose: no discharge

f. Neck: full range of motion, no jugular vein distension, no stridor

g. Pharynx: normal dentition, no lesions, no swelling

  h. Chest: nontender

  i. Lungs: clear bilaterally

  j. Heart: rate and rhythm regular, no murmurs, rubs, or gallops

  k. Abdomen: normal bowel sounds, soft, not tender or distended

  l. Rectal: normal tone, brown stool, occult blood negative

  m. Urogenital: normal external genitalia, no hernia

    i. Male: no discharge, normal testicular examination

  n. Extremities: full range of motion, no deformity, normal pulses

  o. Back: + costovertebral angle tenderness on the left

  p. Neuro: cranial nerves II to XII intact; normal sensation, strength; normal reflexes and gait

  q. Skin: warm and dry

  r. Lymph: no lymphadenopathy

I. Action

  a. Meds

    i. Analgesia as above if not given before

  b. Imaging

    i. CT without contrast

J. Nurse

  a. BP: 110/70 HR: 72 RR: 16 Sat 98% on O_2 after pain medicine

  b. Patient: no longer in pain, tachycardia resolved

  c. Imaging

    i. CT (Figure 66.1) – 3 mm stone in the left ureterovesicular junction (UVJ) with moderate hydronephrosis

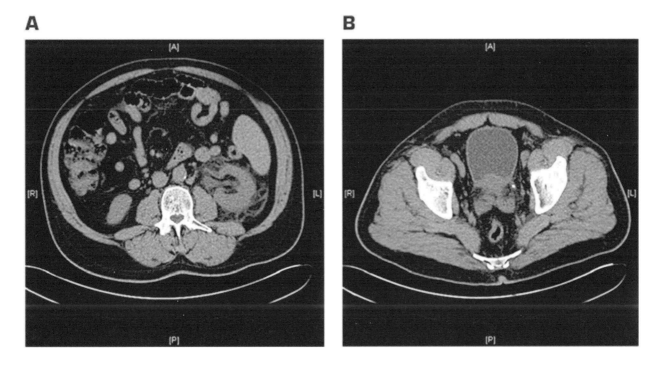

Figure 66.1 A and B

K. Results

Complete blood count:

WBC	8×10^3/uL
Hct	41.5%
Plt	253×10^3/uL

Basic metabolic panel:

Na	139 mEq/L
K	4.2 mEq/L
Cl	101 mEq/L
CO_2	18.9 mEq/L
BUN	20 mEq/dL
Cr	1.0 mg/dL%
Gluc	99 mg/dL

Coagulation panel:

PT	12.3–15.5 sec
PTT	25.4–35.0 sec
INR	0.9–1.3

Urinalysis:

SG	1.010–1.030
pH	5–8
Prot	Neg mg/dL
Gluc	Neg mg/dL
Ketones	Neg mg/dL
Bili	Neg
Blood	large
LE	Neg
Nitrite	Neg
Color	Yellow

L. Action

a. Consult
  i. Urology or PMD for follow-up
b. Discuss with patient regarding the diagnosis of kidney stone, need for straining urine, and hydration with pain medications as needed
c. Disposition
  i. Home
  ii. Pain medications

M. Diagnosis

a. Renal colic

N. Critical actions

▨ Large-bore IV access and hydration with greater than 1 L NS
▨ Early pain control
▨ Confirmation of diagnosis of renal colic with CT without contrast given first episode of colic
▨ UA
▨ Temperature

O. Examiner instructions

a. This is a case of flank pain secondary to renal colic. This is an extremely painful condition caused by the passage of small stones from the kidney to the bladder. The patient has significant pain initially and appears extremely uncomfortable from the start. The candidate should address the patient's pain early in the encounter. No history is obtainable from the patient, except allergies, unless the pain is addressed. The key to diagnosing the patient's pain is in the history of symptoms and UA. The history in this case is classic for renal colic. In addition, he has a reason to have stones (vitamin A, C intake) and has physical findings suggesting the diagnosis with costovertebral angle tenderness in the absence of abdominal pain or tenderness.

P. Pearls

a. The ureterovesicular junction is the most common place to find stones on CT.

b. Likelihood of the stone passing spontaneously is loosely related to the size of the stone. At 4 mm pass 90%, 4 to 6 mm 50% pass, and > 6 mm 10% pass.

c. Flank pain in absence of abdominal tenderness should suggest renal colic. However, aortic and iliac aneurysms or dissection may mimic the symptoms of renal colic. In addition, surgical emergencies such as appendicitis and cholecystitis which should be considered in the differential.

d. Pain control should be initiated early.

e. Indications for admission for kidney stones include high-grade obstruction, intractable pain or vomiting, associated urinary tract infection, solitary or transplanted kidney.

f. Obtain urology consult for any stone over 6 mm, as they will likely need lithotripsy to pass.

g. Consider US as diagnostic tool instead of CT scan if indicated (pregnancy).

Q. References

a. Tintinalli's: Chapter 97

b. Rosen's: Chapter 97

CASE 67: Seizure (Satjiv Kohli, MD, MBA)

A. Chief complaint

a. 45-year-old male brought in by EMS seizing despite lorazepam IM

B. Vital signs

a. BP: 175/110 HR: 130 RR: 18 T: 36.6°C Sat: 98% on RA FS: 85 (must ask)

C. What does the patient look like?

a. Patient in ED with tonic-clonic movements; bleeding from mouth.

D. Primary survey

a. Airway: bleeding from mouth

b. Breathing: no apparent respiratory distress, no cyanosis

c. Circulation: normal capillary refill

E. Action

a. Oxygen via NC or nonrebreather mask

b. Two large-bore peripheral IV lines

c. Labs

   i. CBC, BMP, LFT, coagulation studies, blood type and cross-match

   ii. Lactate, alcohol level, acetaminophen level, salicylate level, urine toxicology screen.

d. 1 L NS bolus

e. Monitor: BP: 170/90 HR: 110 RR: 18 Sat: 98% on 2 L NC

f. EKG

g. Suction mouth

    h. Meds

       i. Lorazepam 4 mg IVP (less than 8 mg)

          1. No improvement, continues to seize

       ii. Lorazepam 4 mg + 4 mg IVP (greater than 8 mg)

          1. Stops seizing

F. History

a. HPI: according to EMS, patient's family called in EMS because he started to seize ~15 minutes ago. He is a heavy alcohol user but has not been drinking for the last 3 days, due to not feeling well from a cold. He denies any prior seizures; denies fevers, chills, vomiting, or abdominal pain; no sick contacts or recent travel.

b. PMHx: HTN, DM, Tuberculosis (treated)

c. PSHx: none

d. Allergies: NKDA

e. Social: alcohol abuse; otherwise unknown; unemployed and lives at home with wife, two children, and aunt

f. FHx: none

g. PMD: none

G. Secondary survey

a. General: somnolent, minimally responsive

b. Lungs: clear, fair air movement

c. Heart: tachycardic but regular

d. Abdomen: soft, nontender, nondistended; normoactive bowel sounds

e. Rectal: occult blood positive with brown stool

f. Urogenital: normal

g. Extremities: normal

h. Back: normal

i. Neuro: + gag reflex; GCS 9

j. Skin: pale, no rashes, no edema, no cellulitis

k. Lymph: normal

H. Nurse

a. EKG (Figure 67.1)

I. Action

a. Imaging

    i. CT head

    ii. CXR

J. Results

Complete blood count:

WBC	15.1 × 103/uL	BUN	35 mEq/dL
Hct	41.5%	Cr	1.6 mg/dL%
Plt	253 × 103/uL	Gluc	202 mg/dL

Basic metabolic panel:

Na	128 mEq/L	**Coagulation panel:**	
K	4.2 mEq/L	PT	13.1 sec
Cl	101 mEq/L	PTT	26 sec
CO$_2$	18.9 mEq/L	INR	1.0

Liver function panel:

AST	22 U/L	Gluc	Neg mg/dL
ALT	20 U/L	Ketones	Neg mg/dL
Alk Phos	100 U/L	Bili	Neg
T bili	0.5 mg/dL	Blood	Neg
D bili	0.2 mg/dL	LE	Neg
Amylase	84 U/L	Nitrite	Neg
Lipase	50 U/L	Color	Yellow
Albumin	4.5 g/dL		

Arterial blood gas:

Urinalysis:

		pH	7.35–7.45
SG	1.010–1.030	PO_2	80–100 mmHg
pH	5–8	PCO_2	35–45 mmHg
Prot	Neg mg/dL	HCO_3	22–26 mmol/L

a. Lactate 10 mmol/L

b. CT head (Figure 67.2)

c. CXR – normal

d. EtOH level < 10, ASA 0, acetaminophen 0

e. Patient starting to seize again, generalized tonic-clonic

K. Action

a. Consult

   i. Neurology for EEG

   ii. ICU

b. Discussion with family regarding status

Figure 67.1

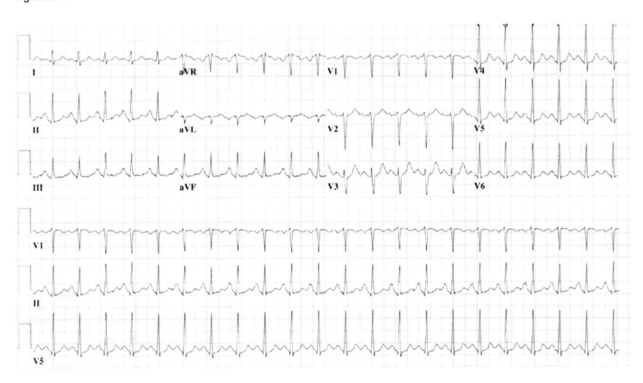

Figure 67.2

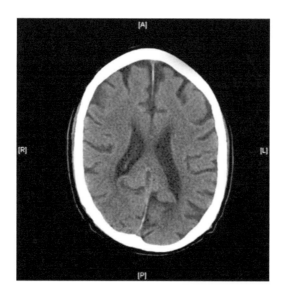

    c. Meds
        i. Lorazepam 4 mg IVP – seizure stops
        ii. Phenytoin or fosphenytoin 10 mg/kg load over 10 minutes

L. Diagnosis

a. Status epilepticus

M. Critical actions

▨ Finger stick blood glucose
▨ IV access
▨ IV benzodiazepine
▨ Head CT to evaluate for intracranial pathology
▨ Labs to exclude metabolic pathology
▨ Serum toxicology
▨ Neurology consult for new onset seizure/status epilepticus

N. Examiner instruction

a. Status epilepticus represents a true medical emergency, defined by intractable seizures. The longer the seizure continues, the worse the damage to the brain and ultimate prognosis. The patient's seizure is likely due to alcohol withdrawal secondary to not feeling well over the past few days. As such, his seizures are difficult to control and will not break until at least 8 mg of lorazepam is given in total. The patient will be able to maintain his airway unless doses of lorazepam exceed 20 mg or its equivalent. If less than 8 mg of lorazepam is given, the patient will continue to seize. If other sedating agents are given such as propofol or phenobarbital without maximizing the dose of benzodiazepines, the patient will require intubation. Once the seizure stops, the candidate should search for seizure etiology by discussing with EMS and family members. The patient should be positioned to maximize ventilation and to prevent physical injury. Oxygen should be administered via NC or face mask, and a large suction catheter should be available to suction the patient's secretions. If the airway cannot otherwise be maintained, there is respiratory failure, or there is clinical evidence of increased ICP, the patient should be intubated using RSI. In our patient, monitoring should include cardiovascular (heart rate, blood pressure) and pulmonary (respiratory rate, pulse oximetry) function.

O. Clinical pearls
a. A rapid blood glucose level should be determined in all patients with seizure.
b. The main principle of treatment of status epilepticus is to stop the seizure as rapidly as possible and prevent recurrence.
c. In the younger patient, the tongue may obstruct the airway. In this case, placement of a nasopharyngeal airway may improve the patient's respiratory status.
d. The three most commonly used agents to treat convulsive status epilepticus are benzodiazepines, phenytoin, and barbiturates.
e. Consider INH overdose or tricyclic antidepressant overdose in patient unresponsive to treatment.
f. If trauma is suspected, always use C-spine precautions.
g. Hyperthermia should be treated with antipyretics and cooling blankets if necessary.
h. If the cause of the seizure is unknown, blood should be obtained for determination of serum electrolytes, glucose, sodium, calcium, magnesium, renal function, toxicology, antiepileptic levels (if indicated), and CBC.
i. If necessary, an intraosseous line can be used to administer all medications, including anticonvulsants.

P. References
a. Rosen's: Chapter 100
b. Tintinalli's: Chapter 165

CASE 68: Fever (Satjiv Kohli, MD, MBA)

A. Chief complaint
a. 70-year-old male sent from nursing home with fever

B. Vital signs
a. BP: 105/70 HR: 110 RR: 20 T: 38.4°C Sat: 98% on RA

C. What does the patient look like?
a. Patient appears diaphoretic; warm to touch.

D. Primary survey
a. Airway: patent
b. Breathing: no apparent respiratory distress; no cyanosis
c. Circulation: wet and warm skin, normal capillary refill

E. Action
a. Oxygen via NC or nonrebreather mask
b. Two large-bore peripheral IV lines
c. Labs
   i. CBC, BMP, LFT, coagulation studies, blood type and cross-match
   ii. Lactate, blood cultures, UA, urine culture

   d. 1 L NS bolus

   e. Monitor: BP: 100/70 HR: 110 RR: 20 T: 38.4°C Sat: 98% on RA

   f. EKG

   g. Medicine

      i. Acetaminophen

F. History

   a. HPI: a 70-year-old male with a history of peripheral vascular disease, coronary artery disease, diabetes, and Alzheimer's dementia is sent to the ED from local nursing home with fever. Patient is nonverbal at baseline and is unable to provide history. According to the nursing home chart, he has been having a fever for 3 days, and is at baseline mental status (nonverbal).

   b. PMHx: described as above

   c. PSHx: CABG s/p 5 years ago, R orchiectomy s/p 10 years ago, femoral-popliteal bypass s/p 2 years ago

   d. Allergies: none

   e. Meds: aspirin, insulin, colace, haloperidol,

   f. Social: lives at nursing home

   g. FHx: unavailable

   h. PMD: Dr Gold

G. Nurse

   a. EKG (Figure 68.1)

   b. Fluids

      i. BP: 110/80 HR: 90 RR: 20 T: 38.1°C Sat: 99% on O_2

   c. No fluids

      i. BP: 88/60 HR: 125 RR: 22 T: 38.1°C Sat: 99% on O_2

Figure 68.1

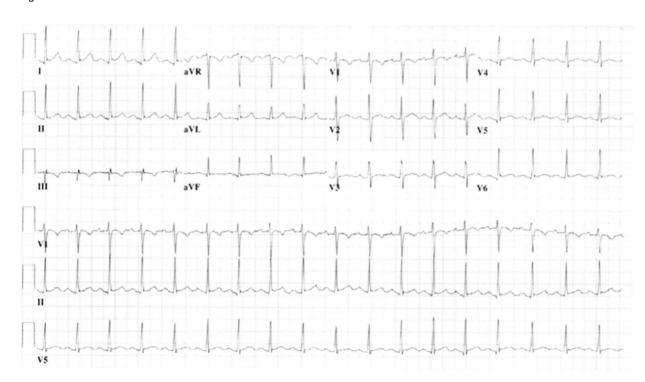

H. Secondary survey

a. General: lethargic, disoriented

b. Head: normocephalic, atraumatic

c. Eyes: extraocular movement intact, pupils equal, reactive to light

d. Ears: normal tympanic membranes

e. Nose: no discharge

f. Neck: full range of motion, no jugular vein distension, no stridor

g. Pharynx: normal dentition, no lesions, no swelling

h. Chest: nontender

i. Lungs: clear bilaterally

j. Heart: tachycardic rate, rhythm regular, no murmurs, rubs, or gallops

k. Abdomen: normal bowel sounds, soft, not tender or distended

l. Rectal: normal tone, brown stool, occult blood negative

m. Urogenital (must ask)

   i. Male: left scrotum erythematous and swollen; fluctuance extending to the perineum posteriorly; crepitance noted on examination

n. Extremities: full range of motion, no deformity, normal pulses

o. Back: nontender

p. Neuro: cranial nerves II to XII intact; normal sensation, strength; normal reflexes and gait

q. Skin: warm and dry

r. Lymph: no lymphadenopathy

I. Action

a. Preoperative CXR

b. Medication

   i. Ampicillin

   ii. Gentamycin

   iii. Metronidazole

c. General surgery and/or urology consult

   i. OR for debridement

d. Discussion with family regarding emergency surgical debridement

J. Nurse

a. CXR (Figure 68.2)

b. Labs pending

c. Surgery ready to take patient to the operating room

K. Diagnosis

a. Fournier gangrene

L. Critical actions

▨ Full physical examination looking for source of fever

▨ Adequate fluid resuscitation

▨ Emergency surgical consult

▨ Broad-spectrum antibiotics

Figure 68.2

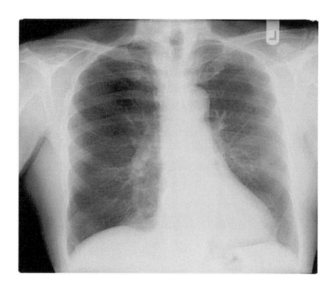

M. Examiner instructions

a. This is a case of Fournier gangrene, a serious bacterial infection of the perineum, the area between the genital area and rectum. It is rapidly spreading and fatal if untreated. Important early actions included recognizing the fever and tachycardia and starting fluids, getting cultures, and administering an antipyretic. Additionally, a complete physical examination is imperative in this febrile, nonverbal patient, to look for source of fever. If a complete physical examination does not include a skin or GU examination looking for cellulitis or Fournier, the patient will continue to decompensate by becoming more lethargic, hypotensive, and tachycardic, ultimately requiring vasopressors and intubation. After making the diagnosis, it is essential to give broad-spectrum antibiotics and obtain immediate surgical consult for definitive treatment in the OR.

N. Pearls

a. Fournier syndrome is a subcutaneous infection of the perineum that occurs primarily in men, usually between 20 and 50 years of age, and usually involves the penis or scrotum.

b. The inflammation may involve the entire abdomen, back, and thighs.

c. There is frequently crepitance on palpation, indicating subcutaneous gas.

d. Systemic symptoms include nausea and vomiting, changes in sensorium, and lethargy.

e. Cultures demonstrate bacteria of the distal colon, with a complex picture of aerobic and anaerobic bacteria. *Bacteroides fragilis* tends to be the predominant anaerobe and *Escherichia coli* the predominant aerobe.

f. Bacterial invasion of the subcutaneous tissues of the perineum causes obliteration of the small branches of the pudendal arteries that supply the perineal or scrotal skin, resulting in acute dermal gangrene.

g. The combination of erythema, edema, inflammation, and infection in a closed space stimulates anaerobic growth. Identification of the offending organism can be done with Gram stain and wound cultures.

h. The most common causal factors are infection or trauma to the perianal area, including anal intercourse, scratches, chemical or thermal injury, and diabetes.

i. Local trauma and perianal disease precede approximately one-third of all cases.

j. Emergency management includes antibiotic therapy against anaerobes and Gram-negative enterics and wide incision and drainage of the area to remove all the necrotic tissue.

k. The mortality rate is ~3% to 38%.

O. References

a. Rosen's: Chapter 135

b. Tintinalli's: Chapter 96

CASE 69: Vomiting (Satjiv Kohli, MD, MBA)

A. Chief complaint

a. 7-month-old boy brought in by mother for abdominal pain and vomiting

B. Vital signs

a. BP: 80/50 HR: 150 RR: 28 T: 38°C, Sat: 97% on RA wt: 8.5 kg FS: 80

C. What does the patient look like?

a. Patient sleeping in mother's arms; listless.

D. Primary survey

a. Airway: patent

b. Breathing: rapid breaths but expanding chest symmetrically

c. Circulation: 2+ distal pulses bilaterally; capillary refill intact

E. Action

a. Establish IV access

b. 20 ml/kg NS bolus (160–200 ml)

c. Labs

   i. CBC, BMP, UA

F. History

a. HPI: patient's mother reports that the patient has not been "feeling well" for 5 days. He has not been feeding and has been having episodic fits associated with non-bloody, nonbilious vomiting for 1 day. During these fits, the patient is inconsolable. They last ~10 to 15 minutes. Also having decreased urine output; no fever, chills, cough, diarrhea, melena, hematemesis, or rashes. Mother denies sick contacts or inhalation/ingestion of foreign bodies.

b. PMHx: born at term; immunizations up-to-date.

c. PSHx: none

d. Social: lives at home with parents and older sister

e. FHx: not relevant

f. PMD: Dr Long

G. Nurse

a. If no fluids are given

   i. BP: 80/50 HR: 170 RR: 30, 98% on RA

b. After fluid bolus

   i. BP: 90/50 HR: 140 RR: 30, 98% on RA

H. Secondary survey

a. General: lethargic, sleeping in mother's arms; arousable to verbal stimuli

b. HEENT: anterior fontanelle sunken; mucous membranes dry; throat without exudates or erythema; TMs intact bilaterally

c. Neck: supple without lymphadenopathy

d. Lungs: clear to auscultation bilaterally

e. Heart: tachycardic but regular; no murmurs, rubs, or gallops

f. Abdomen: soft, moderately tender diffusely; nondistended; no rebound or guarding; normoactive bowel sounds

g. Rectal: guiac +; no gross blood

h. Extremities: normal

i. Back: normal

j. Neuro: normal

k. Skin: no rashes, no edema, no cellulites

l. Lymph: normal

I. Action

a. Abdominal x-ray

b. Abdominal US

c. Reevaluate

 i. Monitor: BP: 95/60 HR: 140

J. Results

Complete blood count:

WBC	$12.1 \times 10^3/uL$
Hct	41.5%
Plt	$253 \times 10^3/uL$

Basic metabolic panel:

Na	139 mEq/L
K	4.2 mEq/L
Cl	101 mEq/L
CO_2	18.9 mEq/L
BUN	10 mEq/dL
Cr	0.3 mg/dL%
Gluc	80 mg/dL

Coagulation panel:

PT	12.3–15.5 sec
PTT	25.4–35.0 sec
INR	0.9–1.3

Liver function panel:

AST	10 U/L
ALT	11 U/L
Alk Phos	20 U/L
T bili	0.5 mg/dL
D bili	0.1 mg/dL
Amylase	22 U/L
Lipase	20 U/L
Albumin	4.1 g/dL

Urinalysis:

SG	1.010–1.030
pH	5–8
Prot	Neg mg/dL
Gluc	Neg mg/dL
Ketones	Neg mg/dL
Bili	Neg
Blood	Neg
LE	Neg
Nitrite	Neg
Color	Yellow

a. Abdominal x-ray (Figure 69.1)

b. Abdominal US (Figure 69.2)

K. Action

a. Surgery consult

b. Admit to PICU

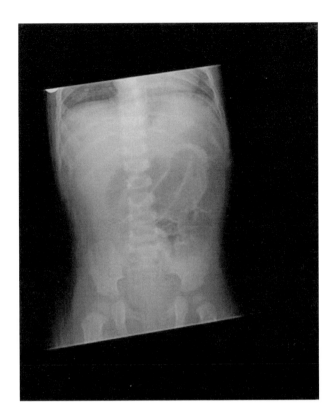

Figure 69.1

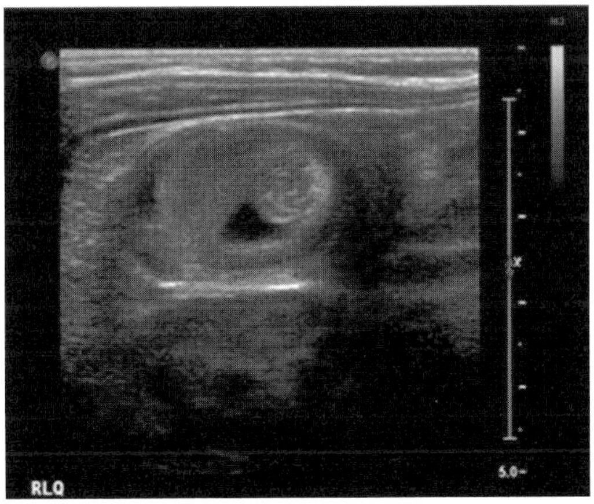

Figure 69.2

c. Discussion with family and PMD regarding possibility for emergent OR if no improvement with barium enema

d. Therapeutic study
   i. Barium enema

L. Nurse

a. Barium enema – (Figure 69.3) with resolution of intussusception

M. Diagnosis

a. Intussusception

N. Critical actions

▓ NS bolus (20 ml/kg)

▓ Complete physical examination

Figure 69.3

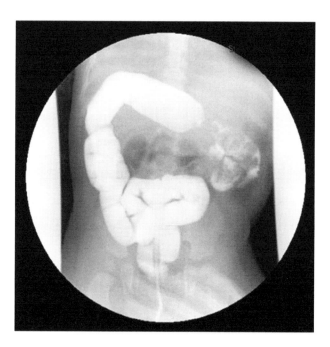

■ Barium enema
■ Pediatric surgical consult

O. Examiner instructions

a. This is a case of intussusception, a serious condition resulting from the patient's intestine involuting into itself. If untreated, the patient can become obstructed or develop a perforation of the intestine. Early actions include IV access, prompt surgical consultation, and either an initial US or barium enema. In this patient, the mother was concerned because the patient has been having intermittent episodes of inconsolable crying and vomiting which is consistent with intussusception in this age group. The infant should intermittently appear well but then have sudden episodes where he is inconsolable. Unless the diagnosis is established by US or enema, the patient's physical examination will progress to peritonitis requiring emergent surgical intervention. If the diagnosis is made with rapid reduction by enema, the patient will do well with observation.

P. Pearls

a. Intussusception is the most common cause of intestinal obstruction in children younger than 2 years old and occurs most commonly in infants 5 to 12 months old.
b. The exact etiology is unclear, but the most prevalent theory relates to a lead point that causes telescoping of one segment of intestine into another. As the process continues and intensifies, edema develops and obstructs venous return, resulting in ischemia of the bowel wall. As ischemia of the bowel wall continues, peritoneal irritation ensues, and perforation may occur.
c. The classic triad of symptoms in intussusception is abdominal pain, vomiting, and bloody stools. All three symptoms occur in less than one-third of patients; however, three-quarters of patients with intussusception have two findings, and 13% have either none or only one.
d. In a typical case, the child presents with cyclical episodes of severe abdominal pain. The pain typically lasts 10 to 15 minutes and has a periodicity of 15 to

30 minutes. During the painful episodes, the child is inconsolable, often described as drawing the legs up to the abdomen and screaming in pain.

e. Diarrhea containing mucus and blood constitutes the classic "currant jelly" stool.

f. Dance's sign: palpation of the abdomen may reveal a sausage-like mass in the right upper quadrant representing the actual intussusception and an empty space in the right lower quadrant representing the movement of the cecum out of its normal position. This finding is pathagnomonic for intussusception.

g. Ill-appearing or febrile children require broad-spectrum, triple-antibiotic coverage with ampicillin, gentamycin, and either clindamycin or metronidazole.

Q. References
a. Rosen's: Chapters 93, 170
b. Tintinalli's: Chapter 123

CASE 70: Fever (Satjiv Kohli, MD, MBA)

A. Chief complaint
a. 45-year-old male arrives to the ED complaining of fever

B. Vital signs
a. BP: 105/50 HR: 110 RR: 24 T: 39.4°C Sat 88% on RA

C. What does the patient look like?
a. Patient is warm to touch and diaphoretic.

D. Primary survey
a. Airway: speaking in full sentences
b. Breathing: no apparent respiratory distress, no cyanosis
c. Circulation: warm and wet skin, normal capillary refill

E. Action
a. Oxygen via nonrebreather mask
b. Two large-bore peripheral IV lines
c. Labs
  i. CBC, BMP, LFT, coagulation studies, blood type and cross-match
  ii. Lactate, blood cultures, UA, urine culture, LDH, stool culture, stool ova and parasites
d. Meds
  i. Acetaminophen
e. 1 L NS bolus
f. Monitor: BP: 95/60 HR: 115 RR: 24 O_2 Sat: 95% on O_2
g. EKG
h. Imaging
  i. CXR

F. History
a. HPI: a 45-year-old male with HIV-AIDS with last known CD 4 count of 150 and medically noncompliant who states that he has been coughing with green sputum

for the last 3 days. He is also complaining of fever, shortness of breath, pleuritic chest pain, and nonbloody diarrhea. He denies headache, hemoptysis, night chills, vomiting, abdominal pain, or melena; no recent travel, camping or sick contacts.

b. PMHx: AIDS

c. PSHx: none

d. Allergies: bactrim

e. Meds: noncomplaint, does not know

f. Social: lives in apartment alone; daily smoker and occasional EtOH use but denies illicit drug use; not sexually active

g. FHx: not relevant

h. PMD: clinic

G. Nurse

a. EKG normal sinus tachycardia

b. CXR (Figure 70.1)

H. Secondary survey

a. General: alert, oriented × 3, mild respiratory distress

b. Head: cachectic, atraumatic

c. Eyes: extraocular movement intact, pupils equal, reactive to light

d. Ears: normal tympanic membranes

e. Nose: no discharge

f. Neck: full range of motion, no jugular vein distension, no stridor

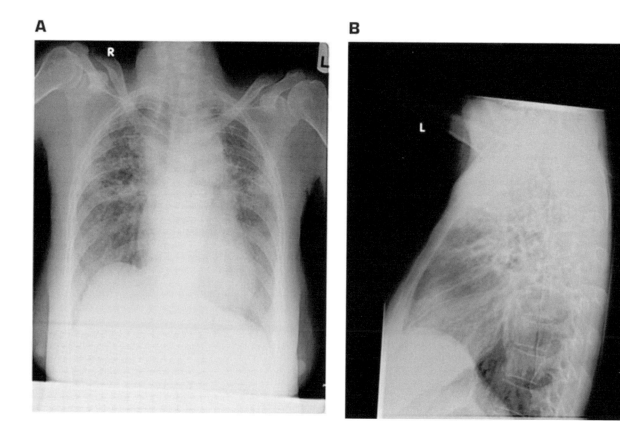

Figure 70.1

g. Pharynx: poor dentition, throat without exudates, + thrush
h. Chest: nontender
i. Lungs: decreased breath sounds bilaterally with crackles
j. Heart: rate and rhythm regular, no murmurs, rubs, or gallops
k. Abdomen: normal bowel sounds, soft, nontender, or distended
l. Rectal: normal tone, brown stool, occult blood negative
m. Urogenital: normal external genitalia
   i. Male: no discharge, normal testicular examination
n. Extremities: full range of motion, no deformity, normal pulses
o. Back: nontender
p. Neuro: cranial nerves II to XII intact; normal sensation, strength; normal reflexes and gait
q. Skin: warm and dry
r. Lymph: no lymphadenopathy

I. Action

a. Move patient to negative pressure isolation room (droplet precautions)
b. Meds
   i. Prednisone
   ii. Ceftriaxone
   iii. Azithromycin
   iv. Atorvaquone-consult pharmacy about alternatives when patient is allergic to bactrim
c. Reassess
   i. Patient with continued shortness of breath mildly improved.

J. Nurse

a. 1 L NS
   i. BP: 105/60 HR: 105 RR: 24 Sat: 95% on O_2

K. Results

Complete blood count:

WBC	1.1×10^3/uL
Diff	88.6/8.4/1.8
Hct	41.5%
Plt	253×10^3/uL

Basic metabolic panel:

Na	139 mEq/L
K	4.2 mEq/L
Cl	101 mEq/L
CO_2	18.9 mEq/L
BUN	52 mEq/dL
Cr	1.6 mg/dL%
Gluc	202 mg/dL

Coagulation panel:

PT	12.3–15.5 sec
PTT	25.4–35.0 sec
INR	0.9–1.3

Liver function panel:

AST	1–50 U/L
ALT	1–53 U/L
Alk Phos	30–110 U/L
T bili	0.1–1.2 mg/dL
D bili	0.0–0.8 mg/dL
Amylase	30–300 U/L
Lipase	23–300 U/L
Albumin	3.5–4.9 g/dL
LDH	420

Urinalysis:

SG	1.010–1.030
pH	5–8
Prot	Neg mg/dL
Gluc	Neg mg/dL
Ketones	Pos
Bili	Neg
Blood	Neg

Urinalysis *(continued)*:		Arterial blood gas:	
LE	Neg	pH	7.3
Nitrite	Neg	PO_2	56 mmHg
Color	Yellow	PCO_2	35 mmHg
		HCO_3	19 mmol/L

a. Lactate 3.6 mmol/L

L. Actions
a. Admit to isolation with a monitored bed
b. Discuss with patient issues regarding advanced directives

M. Diagnosis
a. HIV pneumonia, likely PCP

N. Critical actions
▓ Oxygen supplementation
▓ IV fluids
▓ CXR
▓ UA
▓ Antibiotics
▓ Respiratory isolation

O. Examiner instructions
a. This is a case of fever in an AIDS patient, likely caused by pneumonia. Important early actions included recognizing the fever, tachycardia, and hypoxia and providing IV fluids, O_2 supplementation, and acetaminophen. The patient has significant shortness of breath secondary to his diffuse interstitial pneumonia and hypoxia. Supplemental oxygen improves his symptoms. With early antibiotics and steroids, the patient's symptoms and oxygen saturation will improve. If pneumonia is not recognized and the patient does not receive antibiotics early, the patient will continue to complain of worsening shortness of breath and cough and ultimately become septic, with increased heart rate and hypotension. Given the patient's risk for tuberculosis, he should be placed in a room with respiratory precautions to prevent spread to health-care workers.

P. Pearls
a. Fever is a common presenting complaint for patients with AIDS brought to the ED. Evidence of an infectious cause or other reason for fever should be sought by careful history and physical examination.
b. Tests ordered should include complete blood count, electrolytes, liver function tests, urinalysis and culture, blood cultures (aerobic, anaerobic, and fungal), and CXR. If the patient has diarrhea, stool culture and stool examination for ova and parasites should be sent. If PCP is suspected, LDH and ABG can be sent.
c. If there are neurologic signs or symptoms or if no other source of fever is identified, lumbar puncture (LP) should be performed after a noncontrast head CT.
d. Development of pulmonary disorders is often related to CD4 counts. In patients with pulmonary involvement and CD4 counts > 500, encapsulated bacteria, tuberculosis (TB), and malignancies are common. With lower CD4 counts, PCP, atypical

mycobacteria, fungal infections, CMV, lymphoma, lymphoproliferative disorders, and Kaposi's Sarcoma may also be seen.

e. A focal infiltrate on plain chest radiography often suggests bacterial pneumonia.

f. A diffuse interstitial or perihilar, granular pattern on chest radiography is associated with PCP.

Q. References
a. Rosen's: Chapter 130
b. Tintinalli's: Chapter 149

CASE 71: Palpitations (Shawn Zhong, MD)

A. Chief complaint
a. 39-year-old female with history of hypertension brought in by EMS with the complaint of palpitations

B. Vital signs
a. BP: 161/112 HR: 160 RR: 18 T: 35.1°C Sat: 99% on RA

C. What does the patient look like?
a. Patient appears stated age, slightly apprehensive, and sitting up on stretcher.

D. Primary survey
a. Airway: speaking in full sentences
b. Breathing: mildly increased respiratory rate, no respiratory distress, no cyanosis
c. Circulation: extremities warm and well perfused

E. Action
a. Oxygen via NC or nonrebreather mask
b. Two large-bore peripheral IV lines
    i. CBC, BMP
    ii. Urine pregnancy test
c. 1 L NS bolus
d. Monitor: BP: 152/65 HR: 162 RR: 18 Sat: 100% on O_2
e. EKG

F. History
a. HPI: a 39-year-old female with history of hypertension states that she has had palpitations for the last hour; denies any chest pain; slightly short of breath and dizzy; denies any nausea, vomiting, fevers, chills, headache, neck pain, or pain in other parts of body; no recent illnesses
b. PMHx: hypertension
c. PSHx: none
d. Allergies: none
e. Meds: hydrochlorothiazide
f. Social: lives with husband and children at home; drinks alcohol socially; denies any smoking; denies any cocaine or other illicit drugs; is sexually active with husband only

g. FHx: mother had heart attack at age 68; father has diabetes

h. PMD: Dr Fischer

G. Nurse

a. BP: 150/112 HR: 160 RR: 23 Sat: 99% on 2 L

b. Patient: complaints of mild shortness of breath and dizziness

c. EKG (Figure 71.1)

H. Secondary survey

a. General: alert, oriented × 3, mildly increased respiratory rate

b. Head: normocephalic, atraumatic

c. Eyes: extraocular movement intact, pupils equal, reactive to light

d. Ears: normal tympanic membranes

e. Nose: no discharge

f. Neck: full range of motion, no jugular vein distension, no stridor, no carotid bruit

g. Pharynx: normal dentition, no lesions, no swelling

h. Chest: nontender

i. Lungs: clear bilaterally

j. Heart: tachycardiac, rhythm regular, no murmurs, rubs, or gallops

k. Abdomen: normal bowel sounds, soft, nontender, or distended

l. Rectal: normal tone, brown stool, occult blood negative

m. Extremities: full range of motion, no deformity, normal pulses

n. Back: nontender

o. Neuro: cranial nerves II to XII intact; normal sensation, strength; normal reflexes, normal gait

Figure 71.1

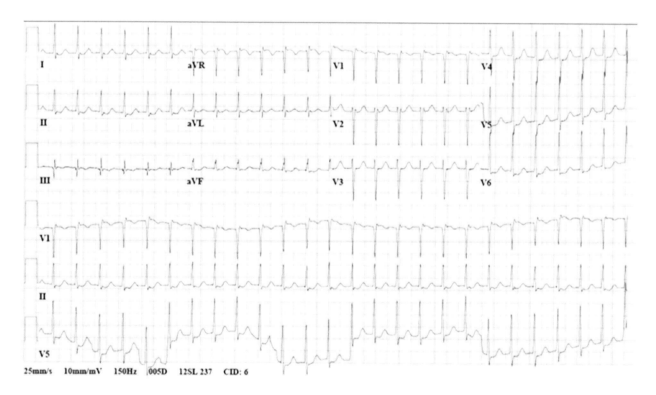

25mm/s   10mm/mV   150Hz   005D   12SL 237   CID: 6

p. Skin: warm and dry

q. Lymph: no lymphadenopathy

I. Action

a. Maneuvers

    i. Vagal maneuvers (no response)

        1. Carotid massage

        2. Ice packs on face

        3. Valsalva maneuver

b. Meds

    i. Adenosine 6 mg rapid IVP (three way stop-cock or other method to ensure a rapid delivery)

    ii. Rhythm strip running; defibrillator at bedside

    iii. Warn patient of side effects

J. Nurse

a. BP: 152/98 HR: 150 RR: 20 Sat: 97% on 2 L

b. Patient felt nauseous during injection of adenosine, but now again feels mildly dizzy and with palpitations

K. Action

a. Medication

    i. Adenosine 12 mg rapid IVP

    ii. Rhythm strip running; defibrillator at bedside

    iii. Warn patient of side effects

L. Nurse

a. BP: 152/98 HR: 95 RR: 16 Sat: 98% on 2 L

M. Results

a. Urine pregnancy test negative

Complete blood count:

WBC	5.3×10^3/uL
Hct	41.5%
Plt	350×10^3/uL

Basic metabolic panel:

Na	138 mEq/L
K	4.3 mEq/L
Cl	105 mEq/L
CO_2	30 mEq/L
BUN	12 mEq/dL
Cr	1.1 mg/dL%
Gluc	100 mg/dL

Coagulation panel:

PT	12.6 sec
PTT	26.0 sec
INR	1.0

Liver function panel:

AST	23 U/L
ALT	26 U/L
Alk Phos	42 U/L
T bili	1.0 mg/dL
D bili	0.3 mg/dL
Amylase	50 U/L
Lipase	25 U/L
Albumin	4.7 g/dL

Urinalysis:

SG	1.010–1.030
pH	5–8
Prot	Neg mg/dL
Gluc	Neg mg/dL
Ketones	Neg mg/dL
Bili	Neg
Blood	Neg

Urinalysis _(continued)_:

LE	Neg
Nitrite	Neg
Color	Yellow

Arterial blood gas:

pH	7.4
PO_2	95 mmHg
PCO_2	41 mmHg
HCO_3	24 mmol/L

b. Patient with significant improvement and resolution of symptoms
c. EKG (Figure 71.2)

N. Action
a. Discussion with patient regarding diagnosis and instruction on vagal maneuvers
b. Follow-up with cardiology and PMD for further work-up

O. Diagnosis
a. Supraventricular tachycardia (SVT)

P. Critical actions
▨ Large-bore IV access
▨ EKG
▨ Discussion with patient regarding side effects of adenosine
▨ Adenosine with rhythm strip – must specify a rapid push of adenosine
▨ Repeat EKG and vitals after breaking rhythm

Q. Examiner instructions
a. This is a case of hemodynamically stable supraventricular tachycardia that responds to adenosine. This is a type of irregular rapid heart rate that is typically

Figure 71.2

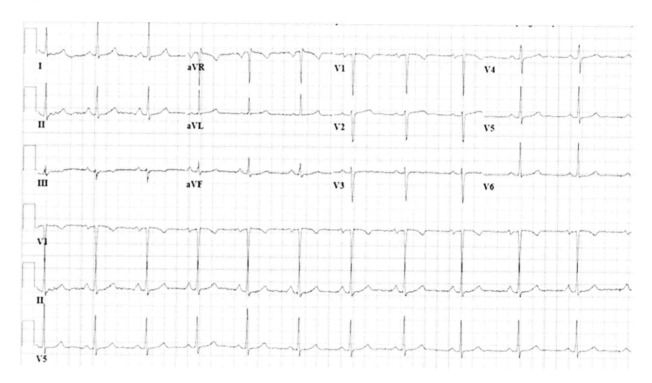

not dangerous and responds to treatment. The patient's main symptoms are palpitations and dizziness with stable vitals. Important early actions include large-bore IV access and EKG. After obtaining an EKG, decision must be made to determine the rhythm. Upon conversion of the rhythm to a slow rate, the candidate must repeat the EKG and vital signs to ensure stability. The patient can be safely discharged once the rate is normal and referred to a cardiologist for further assessment for the cause of the arrhythmia.

R. Pearls
a. Vagal maneuvers can be used before adenosine.
b. Adenosine must be given IV push rapidly in a large-gauge IV, as close to the heart as possible.
c. Should warn patient of adenosine side effects – flushing, sense of impending doom, dizziness.
d. Calcium channel blockers are another class of drugs that can be used.
   i. Diltiazem can be pushed.
   ii. Verapamil should be given at slower rate (no IVP) and has more potential for blood pressure effects.
e. β-blockers is another class of drugs that can be used.
   i. Esmolol drip or propanolol.
f. Cardioversion is required for unstable SVT (refer to appendix).
g. If there is concern for myocardial ischemia as a cause for SVT, consider cardiac enzymes and admission or cardiology consult.

S. References
a. Tintinalli's: Chapter 22
b. Rosen's: Chapter 77

CASE 72: Cough (Shawn Zhong, MD)

A. Chief complaint
a. 45-year-old female brought in by friend, with shortness of breath, cough, and fever

B. Vital signs
a. BP: 78/32 HR: 125 RR: 30 T: 40.2°C Sat: 90% on RA

C. What does the patient look like?
a. Patient appears stated age, tachypneic, moderate respiratory distress, somnolent, but awakens easily.

D. Primary survey
a. Airway: speaking in full sentences
b. Breathing: increased respiratory rate, moderate distress, no cyanosis
c. Circulation: warm, increased capillary refill

E. Action
a. Oxygen via NC or nonrebreather mask
b. Two large-bore peripheral IV lines

    c. Labs
        i. CBC, BMP, LFT, coagulation studies, blood type and cross-match
        ii. Lactate, blood cultures, UA, urine culture
    d. 2 L NS bolus
    e. Monitor: BP: 77/40 HR: 112 RR: 26 Sat: 100% on nonrebreather mask (NRM)
    f. EKG
    g. CXR

F. History

    a. HPI: a 45-year-old female with no past medical history here with fever and shortness of breath for 3 days. Patient states symptoms started with a cough for 2 days but since yesterday with fevers of 40.2°C and chills; at times feels like her entire body is shaking; also today with increased shortness of breath, had difficulty sleeping last night secondary to cough and shortness of breath; denies any headache, nausea, vomiting, abdominal pain, or diarrhea; recent visit to Mexico City 1 month ago.
    b. PMHx: none
    c. PSHx: none
    d. Allergies: none
    e. Meds: none
    f. Social: denies alcohol use or illicit drug use; smokes one pack per day for 30 years; lives with boyfriend in apartment; sexually active without protection; tested negative for HIV 6 months ago
    g. FHx: not relevant
    h. PMD: none

G. Secondary survey

    a. General: somnolent but arousable, oriented × 3, tachypneic, mild respiratory distress on oxygen
    b. Head: normocephalic, atraumatic
    c. Eyes: extraocular movement intact, pupils equal, reactive to light
    d. Ears: normal tympanic membranes
    e. Nose: no discharge
    f. Neck: full range of motion, no jugular vein distension, no stridor
    g. Pharynx: normal dentition, no lesions, no swelling
    h. Chest: nontender
    i. Lungs: crackles bilaterally, no wheezes/rhonchi
    j. Heart: tachycardic, rhythm regular, no murmurs, rubs, or gallops
    k. Abdomen: normal bowel sounds, soft, nontender or distended
    l. Rectal: normal tone, brown stool, occult blood negative
    m. Urogenital: normal external genitalia
        i. Female: no blood or discharge, cervical os closed, no cervical motion tenderness, no adnexal tenderness
    n. Extremities: full range of motion, no deformity, normal pulses
    o. Back: nontender
    p. Neuro: cranial nerves II to XII intact; normal sensation, strength; normal reflexes and gait
    q. Skin: warm and clammy
    r. Lymph: no lymphadenopathy

H. Nurse
a. 2 L fluids
   i. BP: 110/78 HR: 110 RR: 20 Sat: 97% on NRM
b. 1 L fluids
   i. BP: 80/68 HR: 120 RR: 24 Sat: 97% on NRM
c. No fluids
   i. BP: 62/48 HR: 130 RR: 28 Sat: 97% on NRM

I. Results

Complete blood count:

WBC	17.2×10^3/uL
Diff	92% N/6 bands
Hct	39.5%
Plt	350×10^3/uL

Basic metabolic panel:

Na	138 mEq/L
K	4.3 mEq/L
Cl	105 mEq/L
CO_2	30 mEq/L
BUN	32 mEq/dL
Cr	1.1 mg/dL%
Gluc	100 mg/dL

Coagulation panel:

PT	12.6 sec
PTT	26.0 sec
INR	1.0

Liver function panel:

AST	23 U/L
ALT	26 U/L
Alk Phos	42 U/L

T bili	1.0 mg/dL
D bili	0.3 mg/dL
Amylase	50 U/L
Lipase	25 U/L
Albumin	4.7 g/dL

Urinalysis:

SG	1.010–1.030
pH	5–8
Prot	Neg mg/dL
Gluc	Neg mg/dL
Ketones	Neg mg/dL
Bili	Neg
Blood	Neg
LE	Neg
Nitrite	Neg
Color	Yellow

Arterial blood gas:

pH	7.35
PO_2	65 mmHg
PCO_2	35 mmHg
HCO_3	20 mmol/L

a. Lactate 2 mmol/L
b. CXR (Figure 72.1)
c. EKG normal sinus tachycardia

J. Action
a. Meds
   i. Levofloxacin OR
   ii. Ceftriaxone and azithromycin
b. Admit patient for IV antibiotics (patient's pneumonia severity index is 115 placing them in class IV. This is associated with a 9.5% mortality risk.)

K. Diagnosis
a. Community-acquired pneumonia

L. Critical actions
▨ IV access
▨ NS fluid bolus > 2 L

A

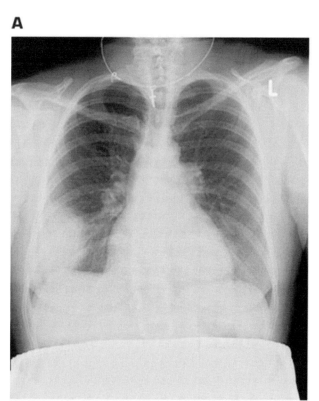

B

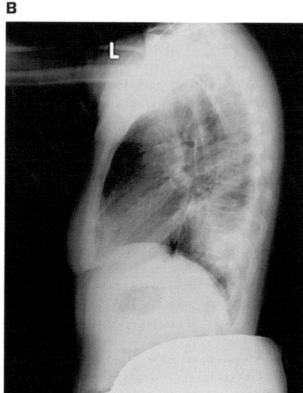

Figure 72.1 A and B

▪ CXR
▪ Antibiotics
▪ Admission

M. Examiner instructions

a. This is a case of community-acquired pneumonia in a healthy patient without medical problems. Pneumonia is most commonly a bacterial infection of the lungs that needs treatment with antibiotics. The seriousness of the infection relates to both the type of bacteria and the patient's ability to fight infection (medical history and age). Early actions with our patient include the recognition and treatment of abnormal vital signs, low blood pressure, high pulse, and low oxygen saturation despite supplemental oxygen and generous IV fluids. CXR should be taken, antibiotics should be given early, and the patient will need to be admitted for antibiotics given the severity of pneumonia represented by vital signs.

N. Pearls

a. Antibiotics should be given early.

b. If blood cultures are sent, antibiotics should be started ideally after the cultures are drawn.

c. Obtain CXR early.

d. In a patient who appears septic, use lactate to help guide treatment.

e. Risk classification guides such as the pneumonia severity index can be used to help identify patients at risk for mortality, but ultimately clinical judgment should be used.

O. References
a. Tintinalli's: Chapter 68
b. Rosen's: Chapter 74

CASE 73: Drowning (Shawn Zhong, MD)

A. Chief complaint
a. 27-year-old male brought in by EMS after diving into the shallow end of a pool and losing consciousness, was immediately rescued by lifeguards, no CPR needed, unable to move arms and legs immediately after, complains of neck pain, immobilized with C collar and backboard

B. Vital signs
a. BP: 90/40 HR: 93 RR: 15 T: 36.2°C Sat: 98% on RA

C. What does the patient look like?
a. Patient appears stated age, lying on stretcher, wet from the pool, and not moving.

D. Primary survey
a. Airway: speaking in full sentences
b. Breathing: no apparent respiratory distress, no cyanosis
c. Circulation: warm and well perfused
d. Disability
    i. Opens eyes to commands, able to abduct arms and flex biceps but minimal extension of arms; no other movement in 4 extremities; CN2–10 grossly intact
    ii. Sensations intact in all extremities
e. Exposure
    i. No other obvious injuries/deformities noted

E. Action
a. Oxygen via NC or nonrebreather mask
b. Two large-bore peripheral IV lines
c. Labs
    i. CBC, BMP, LFT, coagulation studies, blood type and cross-match
d. 2 L LR
e. Monitor: BP: 93/50 HR: 80 RR: 26 Sat: 100% on 2 L
f. FAST (Figure 73.1)
g. Imaging
    i. CT scan of head and C-spine
    ii. CT scan of neck, chest, abdomen, and pelvis with IV contrast
    iii. CXR
    iv. Pelvis x-ray

F. History
a. HPI: a 27-year-old male with no past medical history. Patient was at local pool and dove into the shallow end. He lost consciousness, was rescued by lifeguard, and awoke unable to move. Bystanders called EMS; currently states that he cannot

Figure 73.1
A, B, C and D

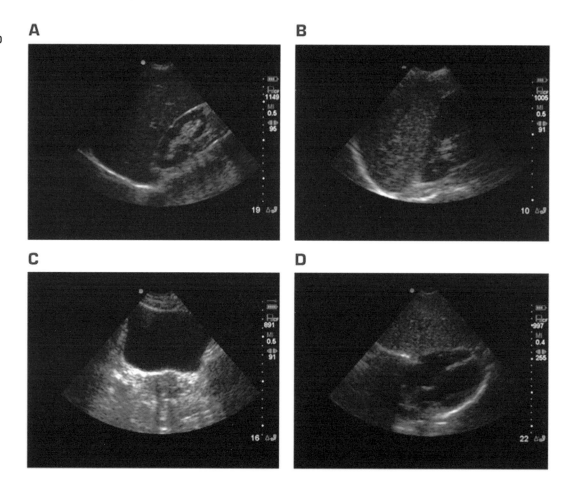

move his extremities below his shoulders; denies headache, nausea, vomiting, blurry vision, chest pain, or shortness of breath.

b. PMHx: none

c. PSHx: none

d. Allergies: NKDA

e. Social: lives with wife, no children; denies smoking; drinks socially; denies illicit drug use

f. FHx: DM

G. Secondary survey

a. General: alert, oriented × 3, very anxious

b. Head: 4 cm contusion to forehead, no stepoff

c. Eyes: extraocular movement intact, pupils equal, reactive to light

d. Ears: normal tympanic membranes

e. Nose: no discharge

f. Neck: no stridor, C collar in place

g. Pharynx: normal dentition, no lesions, no swelling

h. Chest: no evidence of trauma

i. Lungs: clear bilaterally

j. Heart: rate and rhythm regular, no murmurs, rubs, or gallops

k. Abdomen: normal bowel sounds, soft, nontender, distended suprapubically

l. Rectal: no tone, brown stool, occult blood negative, incontinent of stool

m. Urogenital: normal external genitalia
    i. Male: no discharge, normal testicular examination
n. Extremities: no deformity, normal pulses
o. Back: no evidence of trauma; unable to feel
p. Neuro: cranial nerves II to XII intact; opens eyes to commands, able to abduct arms and flex biceps but minimal extension of arms bilaterally; 0/5 motor strength of lower extremities, no sensation of lower extremities, decreased sensation below C5 dermatome, upgoing toes bilaterally
q. Skin: warm and dry (cover patient with blanket)
r. Lymph: no lymphadenopathy

H. Nurse
a. Vitals
    i. BP: 92/50 HR: 75 RR: 28 Sat: 98% on O_2; increase use of intercostals

I. Results

Complete blood count:		Coagulation panel:	
WBC	5.3×10^3/uL	PT	12.6 sec
Hct	41.5%	PTT	26.0 sec
Plt	350×10^3/uL	INR	1.0
Basic metabolic panel:		Liver function panel:	
Na	138 mEq/L	AST	23 U/L
K	4.3 mEq/L	ALT	26 U/L
Cl	105 mEq/L	Alk Phos	42 U/L
CO_2	30 mEq/L	T bili	1.0 mg/dL
BUN	12 mEq/dL	D bili	0.3 mg/dL
Cr	1.1 mg/dL%	Amylase	50 U/L
Gluc	100 mg/dL	Lipase	25 U/L
		Albumin	4.7 g/dL
Urinalysis:		Bili	Neg
SG	1.010–1.030	Blood	Neg
pH	5–8	LE	Neg
Prot	Neg mg/dL	Nitrite	Neg
Gluc	Neg mg/dL	Color	Yellow
Ketones	Neg mg/dL		

a. CXR (Figure 73.2)
b. Pelvic x-ray (Figure 73.3)
c. CT C-spine (Figure 73.4)
    i. C4 burst fracture into canal
d. CT head, chest, abdomen, pelvis – negative
e. Repeat vitals
    i. BP: 90/48 HR: 70 RR: 32 Sat: 98% on O_2; shallow breaths; intercostal muscles use very visible

J. Action
a. Discussion with patient regarding results of CT and need for intubation give concern for inability of the diaphragm to sustain breathing

Figure 73.2

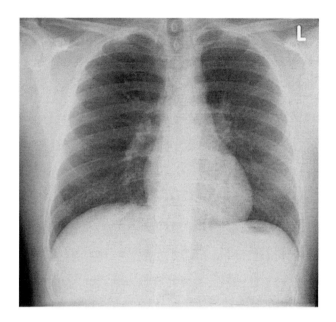

Figure 73.3

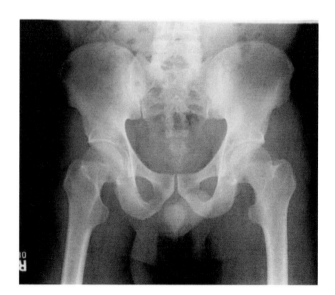

b. Consult
    i. Neurosurgery
c. Intubate
    i. C-spine immobilization

K. Nurse
a. BP: 88/46 HR: 48 Sat: 100% on mechanical ventilation

L. Action
a. ICU consult
b. Central line
    i. CVP = 9
c. Start pressors

A   **B**   Figure 73.4
A and B

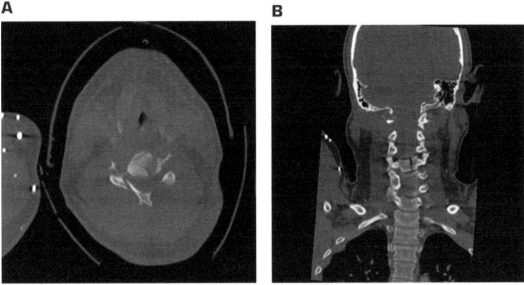

M. Diagnosis
a. C-spine fracture
b. Spinal cord injury
c. Neurogenic shock

N. Critical actions
- Large-bore IV access and fluid bolus
- C-spine precautions
- CT C-spine
- Neurosurgery consult
- Intubation
- Pressors for neurogenic shock

O. Examiner instructions
a. This is a case of spinal cord injury and neurogenic shock after a cervical spine fracture. This is a devastating injury to the neck that leads to quadriplegia. In this patient, the injury to the spinal cord has led to damage of associated nerves that maintain blood pressure and breathing. Initial actions should be aimed at the trauma assessment of this injured patient including FAST, surgery consult, CT of the head, neck, chest, abdomen, and pelvis. All work-up will be negative except for the cervical spine injury that should necessitate an emergent neurosurgery consultation. The use of steroids is controversial and should only be given if asked by the neurosurgery consult, who will not recommend it. The patient will become hypotensive secondary to neurogenic shock and will need fluids and ultimately vasopressors. If the patient is not started on vasopressors, he should become more hypotensive. The patient will also need intubation given increased work of breathing from lack of function of the diaphragm from his spinal cord injury. If

the patient is not intubated, he will become more short of breath and hypoxic. The patient will need to be admitted to the ICU.

P. Pearls
a. In blunt trauma, spinal injuries should be presumed and should be treated as unstable until proven otherwise.
b. Nexus and Canadian C-spine rules are helpful in determining if imaging is needed.
c. Neurogenic shock can occur in injuries above T6 – hypotension and bradycardia.
d. Diaphragm involvement (caused by phrenic nerve injury from lesions above L5) can occur and respiratory failure must be anticipated.
e. Steroids remain controversial but if used, must be initated early.

Q. References
a. Tintinalli's: Chapter 25
b. Rosen's: Chapter 40

CASE 74: Abdominal pain (Sheler Sadati, MD)

A. Chief complaint
a. 54-year-old man brought in by EMS for severe epigastric pain for 6 hours as well as nausea and vomiting

B. Vital signs
a. BP: 85/59 HR: 112 RR: 20 T: 38.3°C O$_2$ Sat: 97% on RA

C. What does the patient look like?
a. Patient appears in moderate distress due to pain; does not want to lie down on the stretcher.

D. Primary survey
a. Airway: speaks full sentences
b. Breathing: no apparent respiratory distress; no cyanosis
c. Circulation: slightly diaphoretic; normal capillary refill

E. Action
a. Oxygen via NC or nonrebreather mask
b. Two large-bore peripheral IV lines
c. Labs
   i. CBC, BMP, LFT, coagulation studies, blood type and cross-match
   ii. Lactate, blood cultures, UA, urine culture, EtOH level
d. 1 L NS bolus
e. Monitor: BP: 85/59 HR: 112 RR: 20 T: 38.3°C O$_2$ Sat: 97% on HRA
f. EKG
g. Image
   i. Upright CXR

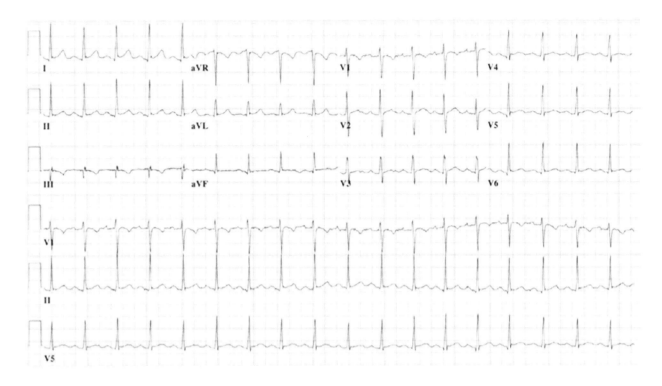

Figure 74.1

F. History

a. HPI: a 54-year-old man with past medical history of hypertension and heavy alcohol consumption (weekend drinker, for years) and hypertriglyceridemia presents with severe epigastric pain for the past 6 hours. The pain started in the middle of the night and woke the patient from sleep. Patient reports that he was at some friend's house for a poker game and they were drinking and having fun and he felt ok when he went to sleep. Patient describes the pain as sharp and stabbing, radiating to his back associated with nausea. He reports four episodes of nonbilious, nonbloody vomiting since the pain started; no diarrhea; no blood per rectum; denies fever or chills; denies any urinary symptoms or flank pain; denies similar episodes of pain in the past. Denies scorpion bite.
b. PMHx: hypertension, hypertriglyceridemia
c. PSHx: inguinal hernia repair in 2002
d. Allergies: none
e. Meds: noncompliant
f. Social: recently divorced; smoker (30 packs/year), drinks alcohol when he parties with friends on weekends; denies any drug abuse
g. FHx: mother with hypertension
h. PMD: Dr Gonzalez

G. Nurse

a. Fluids
   a. BP: 96/67 HR: 110 RR: 20 Sat: 97% on O_2
b. No fluids
   a. BP: 76/67 HR: 120 RR: 20 Sat: 97% on O_2
c. EKG (Figure 74.1)
d. CXR (Figure 74.2) negative for free air under diaphragm

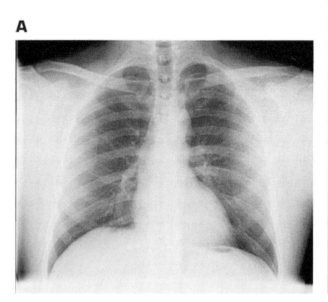

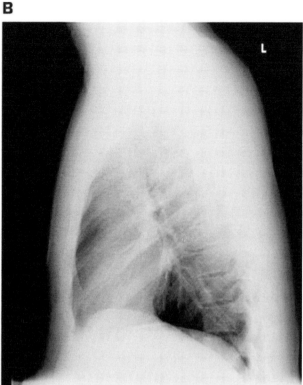

Figure 74.2 A and B

H. Secondary survey

a. General: alert, oriented × 3, appears in severe distress due to pain
b. Head: normocephalic, atraumatic
c. Eyes: extraocular movement intact, pupils equal, reactive to light
d. Ears: normal tympanic membranes
e. Nose: no discharge
f. Neck: full range of motion, no jugular vein distension, no stridor
g. Pharynx: normal dentition, no lesions, no swelling
h. Chest: nontender
i. Lungs: clear bilaterally
j. Heart: tachycardic rate, rhythm regular, no murmurs, rubs, or gallops
k. Abdomen: bowel sounds hypoactive, mildly distended, obese, tenderness in epigastric area with guarding; no rebound; no rigidity
l. Rectal: normal tone, brown stool, occult blood negative
m. Urogenital: normal external genitalia
   i. Male: no discharge, normal testicular examination
n. Extremities: full range of motion, no deformity, normal pulses
o. Back: nontender
p. Neuro: cranial nerves II to XII intact; normal sensation, strength; normal reflexes and gait
q. Skin: warm and dry
r. Lymph: no lymphadenopathy

I. Results

Complete blood count:

WBC	17.4×10^3/uL	Alk Phos	42 U/L
Hct	38%	T bili	1.0 mg/dL
Plt	350×10^3/uL	D bili	0.3 mg/dL
		Amylase	1103 U/L
Basic metabolic panel:		Lipase	2120 U/L
Na	138 mEq/L	Albumin	4.7 g/dL
K	4.3 mEq/L		
Cl	105 mEq/L	**Urinalysis:**	
CO_2	30 mEq/L	SG	1.010–1.030
BUN	34 mEq/dL	pH	5–8
Cr	1.1 mg/dL%	Prot	Neg mg/dL
Gluc	256 mg/dL	Gluc	Neg mg/dL
		Ketones	Neg mg/dL
Coagulation panel:		Bili	Neg
PT	12.6 sec	Blood	Neg
PTT	26.0 sec	LE	Neg
INR	1.0	Nitrite	Neg
		Color	Yellow
Liver function panel:			
AST	23 U/L		
ALT	26 U/L		

a. Calcium 7.8

J. Action
a. Meds
   i. Morphine
   ii. Acetaminophen
b. Imaging
   i. CT abdomen and pelvis with contrast (optional)
   ii. US – bedside (optional)
c. NPO
d. 2 L NS

K. Nurse
a. BP: 100/67 HR: 90 RR: 20 Sat: 97% on O_2
b. Patient: improvement of pain
c. CT abdomen/pelvis – normal
d. US – normal

L. Action
a. Admission
b. Discussion with patient regarding alcohol cessation and diagnosis

M. Diagnosis
a. Pancreatitis

N. Critical actions

- ▨ 2 L IV NS
- ▨ Type and hold
- ▨ Pain medications: opiates
- ▨ Discussion regarding alcohol cessation

O. Examiner instructions

a. This is a case of pancreatitis in a patient with a history of heavy alcohol consumption for years and recent binge drinking. Pancreatitis is an inflammation of the pancreas typically caused by heavy alcohol consumption or gallstones in the USA. As in our patient, the pain is typically sharp and constant in nature and radiating to back associated with nausea and vomiting. If the patient does not get pain medications, he should start getting more upset and agitated. If the patient does not get at least 2 L of fluids, the blood pressure will decline and the patient will become more agitated. The patient should ultimately get admitted to the hospital and kept NPO, no food or drinks by mouth to allow the pancreas to rest.

P. Pearls

a. The degree of elevation in amylase and lipase does not correlate with severity of the disease.
b. Ranson's criteria is just a tool for prognosis and does not change the emergency management of these patients.
c. These patients require aggressive fluid resuscitation due to sequestration of large volumes of fluid in the retroperitoneum.
d. Bluish discoloration in the left flank (Turner's sign) and around the umbilicus (Cullen's sign) are rarely seen, but indicate hemorrhagic pancreatitis.
e. CT scan is not a sensitive test to diagnose pancreatitis. It is most useful to rule out complications such as pancreatic phlegmon or abscess.
f. Patients with chronic pancreatitis do not usually have elevation of pancreatic enzymes due to chronic damage to the organ.
g. Most common cause of acute pancreatitis are ethanol and gallstones.
h. Most common electrolyte abnormality is hypocalcemia.
i. Causes of mortality include ARDS, hemorrhagic shock, sepsis, and DIC.

Q. References

a. Rosen's: Chapters 89, 170
b. Tintinalli's: Chapter 82

CASE 75: Abdominal pain (Sheler Sadati, MD)

A. Chief complaint

a. 84-year-old female presents with intermittent crampy abdominal pain and diarrhea since last night

B. Vital signs

a. BP: 168/84 HR: 94 RR: 16 T: 37.8°C O$_2$ Sat: 97% on RA FS: 112

C. What does the patient look like?

a. Patient agitated and ill-appearing; in no acute respiratory distress; appears very uncomfortable due to pain, changing her position constantly in stretcher to find a comfortable position.

D. Primary survey

a. Airway: speaking in full sentences

b. Breathing: no apparent respiratory distress, no cyanosis

c. Circulation: does not appear pale; normal capillary refill

E. Action

a. Oxygen via NC or nonrebreather mask

b. Two large-bore peripheral IV lines

c. Labs

    i. CBC, BMP, LFT, coagulation studies, blood type and cross-match

    ii. Lactate

d. 1 L NS bolus

e. Monitor: BP: 165/96 HR: 95 RR: 18 Sat: 100% on O_2

    i. Irregular rhythm on monitor, narrow complex

f. EKG

F. History

a. HPI: a 84-year-old female with history of hypertension, paroxysmal atrial fibrillation on amiodarone, presents with crampy abdominal pain starting in the middle of night about 6 hours before arrival to ED. Patient describes a severe 10/10 pain which is intermittent, diffuse but mostly in lower abdomen associated with nausea and diarrhea. Patient reports 6–8 episodes of watery diarrhea. She noticed bloody diarrhea twice (red blood mixed with stool). Patient denies any vomiting. She is unsure of fever; denies any urinary symptoms or other complaints.

b. PMHx: hypertension, atrial fibrillation which caused syncope a few months ago and was admitted to the hospital, but converted to sinus rhythm upon discharge, and was discharged on amiodarone, no coumadin; TIA 6 months ago

c. PSHx: cholecystectomy, hysterectomy

d. Allergies: none

e. Meds: amiodarone, aspirin

f. Social: denies alcohol use, smoking, or illicit drug use

g. FHx: father with hypertension

G. Nurse

a. EKG (Figure 75.1)

b. Patient still with pain

H. Secondary survey

a. General: alert, oriented × 3, appears agitated and in severe distress due to abdominal pain

b. Head: normocephalic, atraumatic

c. Eyes: extraocular movement intact, pupils equal, reactive to light

d. Ears: normal tympanic membranes

e. Nose: no discharge

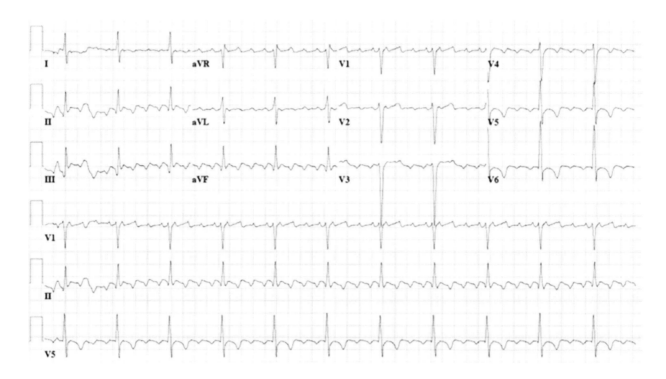

Figure 75.1

   f. Neck: full range of motion, no jugular vein distension, no stridor

   g. Pharynx: normal dentition, no lesions, no swelling

   h. Chest: nontender

   i. Lungs: clear bilaterally

   j. Heart: irregular rhythm, no murmurs, rubs, or gallops

   k. Abdomen: obese; soft. Bowel sounds hypoactive, mild distention, mild tenderness diffusely, more prominently in lower abdomen without rebound or guarding

   l. Rectal: normal tone, brown stool, occult blood positive

   m. Urogenital: normal external genitalia

      i. Female: no blood or discharge, cervical os closed, no cervical motion tenderness, no adnexal tenderness

   n. Extremities: full range of motion, no deformity, normal pulses

   o. Back: nontender

   p. Neuro: cranial nerves II to XII intact; normal sensation, strength; normal reflexes and gait

   q. Skin: warm and dry

   r. Lymph: no lymphadenopathy

I. Action:

   a. Medication

      i. Morphine

      ii. Ciprofloxacin

      iii. Metronidazole

   b. Imaging

      i. Upright CXR with obstructive series

      ii. CT of abdomen and pelvis with IV and oral contrast (angiography unavailable)

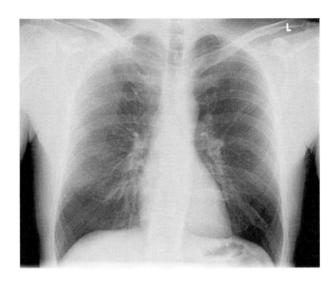

Figure 75.2

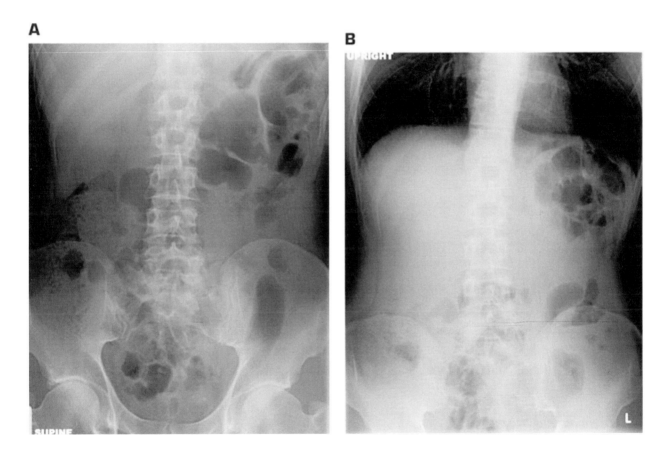

Figure 75.3 A and B

J. Nurse

a. CXR (Figure 75.2)

b. Obstructive series (Figure 75.3)

c. CT – superior mesenteric arterial thrombus, pneumatosis intestinalis and bowel wall thickening along ascending and transverse colon

K. Results
a. Lactate 4.8 mmol/L

Complete blood count:

WBC	14.9×10^3/uL	D bili	0.3 mg/dL
Hct	38%	Amylase	120 U/L
Plt	350×10^3/uL	Lipase	65 U/L
		Albumin	4.7 g/dL

Basic metabolic panel:

Na	138 mEq/L	**Urinalysis:**	
K	3.3 mEq/L	SG	1.010–1.030
Cl	105 mEq/L	pH	5–8
CO_2	18 mEq/L	Prot	Neg mg/dL
BUN	32 mEq/dL	Gluc	Neg mg/dL
Cr	1.2 mg/dL%	Ketones	Neg mg/dL
Gluc	120 mg/dL	Bili	Neg
		Blood	Neg
Coagulation panel:		LE	Neg
PT	12.6 sec	Nitrite	Neg
PTT	26.0 sec	Color	Yellow
INR	1.0		
		Arterial blood gas:	
Liver function panel:		pH	7.4
AST	23 U/L	PO_2	95 mmHg
ALT	26 U/L	PCO_2	41 mmHg
Alk Phos	42 U/L	HCO_3	24 mmol/L
T bili	1.0 mg/dL		

L. Action
a. Consult
  i. Surgery or vascular surgery for possible embolectomy
  ii. Interventional radiology for possible procedure
b. Discussion with patient regarding diagnosis
c. Meds
  i. Morphine

M. Diagnosis
a. Ischemic bowel, embolism to superior mesenteric artery

N. Critical actions
▪ NS 2 L
▪ CT of abdomen and pelvis with contrast
▪ Antibiotics
▪ Surgery consult or interventional radiology consult
▪ Pain medication

O. Examiner instructions
a. This is a case of bowel ischemia secondary to an embolic clot from atrial fibrillation. The patient's symptoms are due to a lack of blood supply to the intestines secondary to a blood clot which has occluded one of the major blood vessels to the

intestines. Atrial flutter, an irregular heart rhythm, has predisposed her to developing blood clots. This patient presented to ED with sudden onset of abdominal pain out of proportion to examination which is typical of this condition. Early actions include pain control, recognition of diagnosis with initiation of work-up including CT scan, IV antibiotics, and surgery and/or interventional radiology consult once the diagnosis is known. Both services initially do not want to take the patient for definitive treatment and the candidate will need to be persistent. If the patient is allowed to be admitted to the ICU without treatment (embolectomy or papaverine infusion or lysis) the patient will become hypotensive and complaint of severe pain with new peritoneal signs on abdominal examination – rebound, guarding, and rigidity.

P. Pearls

a. Mesenteric ischemia/infarction is typically seen in the elderly population with cardiovascular disease such as atrial fibrillation, congestive heart failure, and coronary artery disease.

b. The most common cause of ischemic bowel is mesenteric artery occlusion as a result of embolus from the heart in atrial fibrillation (65%-75% of cases).

c. CT scan findings may demonstrate bowel wall thickening, pneumatosis intestinalis, or air within portal venous system.

d. Angiography is the gold standard.

e. Patients often have severe abdominal pain out of proportion to examination.

f. Lactate may be elevated but is a late finding.

Q. References

a. Rosen's: Chapter 90

b. Tintinalli's: Chapter 79

CASE 76: Shortness of breath (Sheler Sadati, MD)

A. Chief complaint

a. 59-year-old male with history of COPD brought in by EMS for severe respiratory distress

B. Vital signs

a. BP: 168/84 HR: 94 RR: 30 T: 37.8°C Sat: 92% on O_2

C. What does the patient look like?

a. Patient alert and awake with anxious affect; moderate respiratory distress; using accessory muscle to breathe.

D. Primary survey

a. Airway: able to speak in one-word sentences only, secondary to shortness of breath

b. Breathing: moderate respiratory distress, cyanotic around lips and fingertips; diffuse wheezing

c. Circulation: does not appear pale; normal capillary refill

E. Action

a. Oxygen via NC or nonrebreather mask

b. Two large-bore peripheral IV lines

c. Labs

    i. CBC, BMP, LFT, coagulation studies, blood type and cross-match

d. 1 L NS bolus

e. Monitor: BP: 168/84 HR: 94 RR: 30 Sat: 92% on O_2

f. EKG

g. Meds

    i. Albuterol via nebulizer, continuous treatment

    ii. Ipatropium bromide via nebulizer, continuous treatment

    iii. Methylprednisolone or equivalent steroids, IV

    iv. Magnesium IV

h. Imaging

i. CXR

F. History

a. HPI: a 59-year-old male, morbidly obese with history of hypertension and COPD with dry cough and runny nose over the past 3 days. Patient has been taking his albuterol treatment via nebulizer at home, but today despite multiple treatments developed severe SOB and called FMS. The patient denies fever, chills, headache, nausea, vomiting, diarrhea, chest pain.

b. PMHx: COPD, hypertension

c. PSHx: none

d. Allergies: none

e. Meds: hydrochlorothiazide, albuterol, aspirin

f. Social: heavy smoker (30 packs per year) recently decreased the number of cigarettes to 6 to 7 per day; denies alcohol or drug abuse; lives at home alone

g. FHx: unsure; patient is adopted

G. Nurse

a. Patient: mild improvement of symptoms but still in moderate distress

b. BP: 168/84 HR: 94 RR: 25 Sat 93% on O_2

c. EKG (Figure 76.1)

d. CXR (Figure 76.2)

H. Secondary survey

a. General: moderate respiratory distress, diaphoretic and anxious

b. Head: normocephalic, atraumatic

c. Eyes: extraocular movement intact, pupils equal, reactive to light

d. Ears: normal tympanic membranes

e. Nose: no discharge

f. Neck: full range of motion, no jugular vein distension, no stridor

g. Pharynx: normal dentition, no lesions, no swelling

h. Chest: nontender

i. Lungs: tachypneic, using accessory muscles to breathe, diffuse wheezing bilaterally, scattered rhonchi

j. Heart: tachycardic rate, rhythm regular, no murmurs, rubs, or gallops

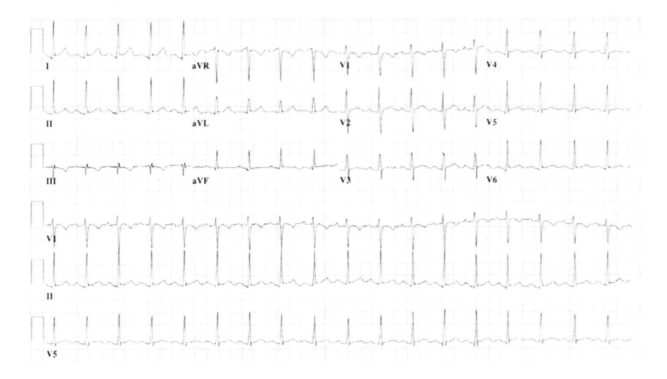

Figure 76.1

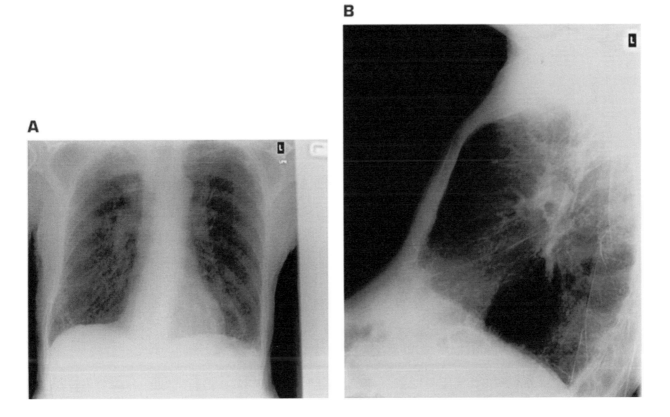

Figure 76.2 A and B

   k. Abdomen: normal bowel sounds, soft, nontender or distended

   l. Rectal: normal tone, brown stool, occult blood negative

m. Extremities: full range of motion, no deformity, normal pulses

   n. Back: nontender

   o. Neuro: cranial nerves II to XII intact; normal sensation, strength; normal reflexes

   p. Skin: warm and dry

   q. Lymph: no lymphadenopathy

I. Action

   a. BiPAP or CPAP

   b. Prepare for possible intubation

   c. Meds

      i. Continuous albuterol and ipatropium bromide nebulizer treatment

      ii. Levofloxacin OR

      iii. Ceftriaxone and azithromycin

J. Results

Complete blood count:

WBC	11.8×10^3/uL	D bili	0.3 mg/dL
Hct	41.5%	Amylase	50 U/L
Plt	350×10^3/uL	Lipase	25 U/L
		Albumin	4.7 g/dL

Basic metabolic panel:

Na	138 mEq/L	**Urinalysis:**	
K	4.3 mEq/L	SG	1.010–1.030
Cl	105 mEq/L	pH	5–8
CO_2	38 mEq/L	Prot	Neg mg/dL
BUN	12 mEq/dL	Gluc	Neg mg/dL
Cr	1.1 mg/dL%	Ketones	Neg mg/dL
Gluc	100 mg/dL	Bili	Neg
		Blood	Neg
Coagulation panel:		LE	Neg
PT	12.6 sec	Nitrite	Neg
PTT	26.0 sec	Color	Yellow
INR	1.0		
		Arterial blood gas:	
Liver function panel:		pH	7.2
AST	23 U/L	PO_2	65 mmHg
ALT	26 U/L	PCO_2	65 mmHg
Alk Phos	42 U/L	HCO_3	30 mmol/L
T bili	1.0 mg/dL		

K. Nurse

   a. Patient's breathing improved significantly on BiPAP O_2 Sat 98%; mental status improved. Patient appears more comfortable

L. Action

   a. Continue BiPAP or CPAP

   b. Continuous albuterol treatment

   c. Medical ICU consult

M. Diagnosis
a. Chronic obstructive pulmonary disease (COPD) exacerbation

N. Critical actions
▨ O_2 supplementation
▨ β-agonist and anticholinergic treatment via nebulizer
▨ Steroids
▨ CXR
▨ BiPAP or CPAP or intubation

O. Examiner instructions
a. This is a case of COPD, likely secondary to viral infection versus pneumonia. COPD is a disease affecting the lungs, causing difficulty with air exchange. In severe exacerbations, patients can stop breathing. This patient's COPD was worsened because of a recent lung infection and comes into the ED in significant respiratory distress. Unless aggressive management is instituted with albuterol, Atrovent, steroids, and magnesium, the patient's shortness of breath will worsen. If noninvasive ventilatory support such as BiPAP or CPAP is given, the patient will not need to be intubated. If BiPAP or CPAP is not attempted, the patient will become more confused and lethargic, retaining CO_2, and becoming unresponsive with low oxygenation. The patient will require intubation and admission to the medical ICU.

P. Pearls
a. Antibiotics should be administered to all COPD patients with possible associated respiratory infection even if it is thought to be acute bronchitis versus pneumonia.
b. Anticholinergic agents such as ipratropium bromide work on larger central airways as opposed to β-agonists agents, such as albuterol, that work on the small peripheral airways. Ipratropium bromide has a synergistic effect when used with albuterol, although has slower onset of action.
c. Magnesium sulfate at a dose of 2 g has been shown to be effective in some cases of COPD exacerbation, although the mechanism of action is not well known and its use is still controversial.
d. Steroid use is less compelling compared to asthma exacerbation, but still should be given in all acute exacerbation.
e. If the patient requires intubation, the ventilator setting should be adjusted such as lower tidal, higher RR, low or no PEEP, minimizing complications such as pneumothorax.
f. The risk of oxygen-induced apnea if the patient is tachypneic is less compared to when the patient is bradypneic. Regardless if the patient is in respiratory distress, oxygen should be given in high concentrations.

Q. References
a. Rosen's: Chapter 72
b. Tintinalli's: Chapter 73

CASE 77: Altered mental status (Sheler Sadati, MD)

A. Chief complaint

a. 48-year-old male with unknown history brought in by EMS with altered mental status. The patient was found on the sidewalk unresponsive and was given 1 amp of D50, 0.4 mg of naloxone, and 100 mg of thiamine with minimal improvement.

B. Vital signs

a. BP: 183/105 HR: 136 RR: 20 T: 38.0°C O_2 Sat: 97% on RA FS: 254 (must ask)

C. What does the patient look like?

a. Patient appears unkempt and is covered in urine; appears confused, but awake; uncooperative with staff; agitated.

D. Primary survey

a. Airway: speaking and maintaining his airway
b. Breathing: no apparent respiratory distress, no cyanosis
c. Circulation: diaphoretic, skin warm with normal capillary refill

E. Action

a. Oxygen via NC or nonrebreather mask
b. Two large-bore peripheral IV lines
   i. While trying to place an IV line, patient becomes verbally and physically abusive to nursing staff (The candidate will be unable to move on from this step until the patient is restrained and/or medication is given for sedation.)
   ii. Any attempt to talk to the patient does not work
c. EKG
d. Meds
   i. Lorazepam or haloperidol
e. Restraints
f. Imaging
g. CT head

F. Nurse

a. Patient more cooperative with sedation
b. Labs
   i. CBC, BMP, LFT, coagulation studies, blood type and cross-match
   ii. Alcohol level, acetaminophen level, salicylate level, urine toxicology screen
c. Monitor: BP: 183/105 HR: 136 RR: 20 Sat: 97% on RA (refusing O_2)

G. History

a. HPI: The patient was found sleeping on the sidewalk. Police tried to question him and EMS was called because the patient was minimally arousable.
   i. EMS: (must ask) As per EMS, this patient is well-known to them and typically is brought to various hospitals for intoxication. Today he looks much different because he is confused. There were no signs of trauma or drug ingestion; there was an empty vodka bottle at the scene.
b. PMHx: unknown
c. PSHx: unknown

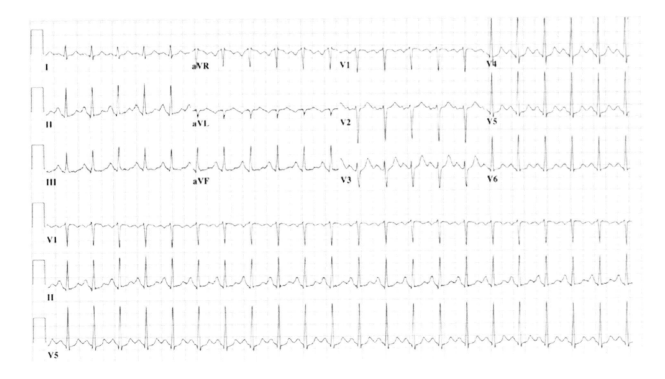

Figure 77.1

d. Allergies: unknown
e. Meds: unknown
f. Social: unknown
g. FHx: unknown

H. Nurse
a. EKG (Figure 77.1)

I. Secondary survey
a. General: agitated, confused, abusive to staff; uncooperative with the history and examination
b. Head: normocephalic, atraumatic
c. Eyes: extraocular movements intact, pupils equal, reactive to light
d. Ears: normal tympanic membranes
e. Nose: no discharge, no septal hematoma
f. Neck: nontender
g. Pharynx: normal dentition, no lesions, no swelling, small laceration on tongue with minimal bleeding
h. Chest: nontender
i. Lungs: clear bilaterally
j. Heart: rate and rhythm regular, no murmurs, rubs, or gallops
k. Abdomen: normal bowel sounds, soft, nontender and nondistended
l. Rectal: deferred
m. Urogenital: deferred
n. Extremities: full range of motion, no deformity, normal pulses
o. Back: nontender

   p. Neuro: uncooperative with examination; patient is confused and awake; appears to be oriented to person; unsure of date or location; affect agitated; no focal deficits noted

   q. Skin: diaphoretic and warm

   r. Lymph: no lymphadenopathy

J. Nurse

   a. Patient: develops a grand mal seizure

K. Action

   a. Oxygen via NC or nonrebreather mask

   b. Meds

      i. Lorazepam (will need a total of 8 mg for patient to stop seizing)

L. Nurse

   a. BP: 173/90 HR: 105 RR: 14 Sat: 97% on O_2

M. Results

Complete blood count:

WBC	14.3×10^3/uL	Alk Phos	42 U/L
Hct	34%	T bili	1.0 mg/dL
Plt	126×10^3/uL	D bili	0.3 mg/dL
		Amylase	50 U/L
Basic metabolic panel:		Lipase	25 U/L
Na	138 mEq/L	Albumin	4.7 g/dL
K	3.4 mEq/L		
Cl	105 mEq/L	**Urinalysis:**	
CO_2	22 mEq/L	SG	1.010–1.030
BUN	21 mEq/dL	pH	5–8
Cr	1.1 mg/dL%	Prot	Neg mg/dL
Gluc	241 mg/dL	Gluc	Neg mg/dL
		Ketones	Neg mg/dL
Coagulation panel:		Bili	Neg
PT	12.6 sec	Blood	Neg
PTT	26.0 sec	LE	Neg
INR	1.0	Nitrite	Neg
		Color	Yellow
Liver function panel:			
AST	23 U/L		
ALT	26 U/L		

   a. Lactate: 1.7 mmol/L

   b. Urine tox: negative, alcohol 56, acetaminophen 0, aspirin 0

   c. CXR (Figure 77.2)

   d. CT of head (Figure 77.3) negative for hemorrhage or mass; mild atrophy reported

N. Actions

   a. Admit to ICU for alcohol withdrawal seizures

   b. Meds

      i. MVI

      ii. Folic acid

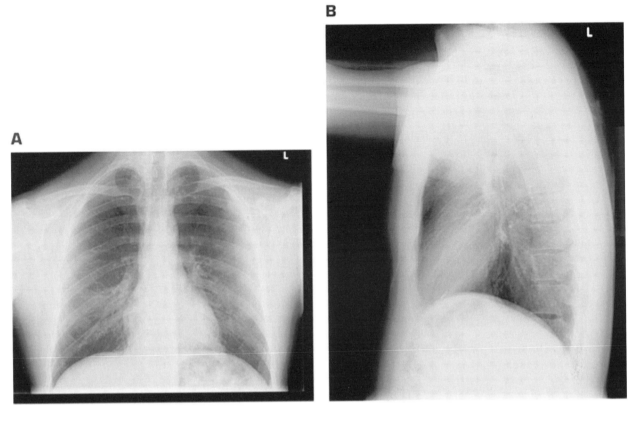

Figure 77.2 A and B

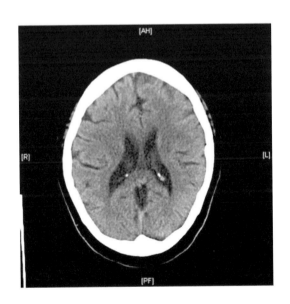

Figure 77.3

O. Diagnosis
a. Alcohol withdrawal with seizure

P. Critical actions
- Benzodiazepine until seizure stops
- FS glucose

▪ Head CT

▪ Management of agitated patient (sedation or restraints)

Q. Examiner instructions

a. This is a case of an alcohol withdrawal seizure. Seizure secondary to the cessation of alcohol in a chronic user can be a life-threatening condition if left untreated. The patient was found by EMS in the postictal period with minimal response to the coma cocktail. The candidate must get the history from EMS of alcohol use by the patient. The patient is confused and agitated because of a recent unwitnessed seizure in the field and will continue to become more agitated and abusive to staff until proper medication or restraints are applied. If haloperidol is given, the patient will initially calm down, but will seize a few minutes later. Early actions include finger stick glucose, IV access, CT head, and blood tests including toxicology screens. The patient will proceed to have a generalized tonic-clonic seizure that will only respond to lorazepam, 8 mg, or equivalent. The patient should be admitted to a monitored bed and continued on benzodiazepines for withdrawal.

R. Pearls

a. Benzodiazepines are the medication of choice for alcohol withdrawal syndrome.

b. Any patient with seizure activity should be assessed for possible alcohol-related seizures.

c. Alcoholic patients are prone to hypoglycemia due to decreased reservoir of glycogen secondary to chronic liver damage; blood glucose should be assessed for all alcoholics with mental status changes.

d. Administration of glucose should not be given before thiamine in suspected alcoholics since it can precipitate Wernicke's encephalopathy or Korsakoff's syndrome with potentially irreversible brain damage.

e. Always assess alcoholics fully for trauma, infection, and metabolic abnormalities.

f. Alcohol withdrawal syndrome usually develops 6 to 24 hours after the reduction of alcohol intake and can last up to 7 days. Monitoring these patients closely in inpatient units is recommended until the signs and symptoms of withdrawal resolve completely.

S. References

a. Rosen's: Chapter 185

b. Tintinalli's: Chapter 165

CASE 78: Weakness (Matthew Constantine, MD)

A. Chief complaint

a. 66-year-old male brought in by EMS with sudden-onset right-sided paralysis and slurred speech

B. Vital signs

a. BP: 192/109 HR: 85 RR: 18 T: 36.9°C Sat: 98% on RA FS: 89 (must ask)

C. What does the patient look like?

a. Patient appears stated age, comfortable and in no apparent distress, with a right facial droop.

D. Primary survey

a. Airway: speaking in full sentences, however, speech is slurred

b. Breathing: no apparent respiratory distress, no cyanosis

c. Circulation: warm and dry skin, normal capillary refill

E. Action

a. Oxygen via NC or nonrebreather mask

b. Two large-bore peripheral IV lines

c. Labs

    i. CBC, BMP, LFT, coagulation studies, blood type and cross-match

    ii. Troponin

d. Monitor: BP: 187/115 HR: 75 RR: 18 Sat: 100% on O_2 2 L NC

e. EKG

F. History

a. HPI: This is a 66-year-old male with no significant PMHx who states that he awoke from sleep normally this morning; however, he was unable to get out of bed. He states that he felt paralyzed on his entire right side. His wife called EMS. EMS notes that they found the patient in bed and unable to move his right side. The patient also notes a right-sided facial droop. He feels as if his right arm and leg are numb, as he could not feel EMS move them. He states that the last time that he felt normal was when he went to sleep at 11:00 PM. He awoke in his normal routine at 6:00 AM. He presently denies any other symptoms including headache, nausea, vomiting, vertigo, vision or hearing changes, left-sided symptoms, fevers, chills, chest pain or shortness of breath. He reports that he had one episode of similar symptoms 1 week ago. He states that he was watching TV when he felt weakness on the right arm greater than leg; however, the symptoms only lasted for 2 to 4 minutes. He was about to call EMS when the symptoms resolved.

b. PMHx: no significant past medical history

c. PSHx: none

d. Allergies: none

e. Meds: none

f. Social: lives with wife at home, 28 pack-year smoking history, social EtOH use

g. FHx: father with CAD, mother with CVA at age 66

h. PMD: none, patient has not seen MD in 5+ years

G. Nurse

a. EKG (Figure 78.1)

b. No fluids

    i. BP: 205/120 HR: 64 RR: 20 Sat: 99% on O_2

H. Secondary survey

a. General: A & O × 3, NAD, right-sided facial droop and slurred speech obvious when talking to patient

b. Head: right facial droop, normocephalic, atraumatic

c. Eyes: extraocular movement intact, pupils equal, reactive to light

d. Ears: normal tympanic membranes

e. Nose: no discharge

f. Neck: full range of motion, no jugular vein distention, no stridor

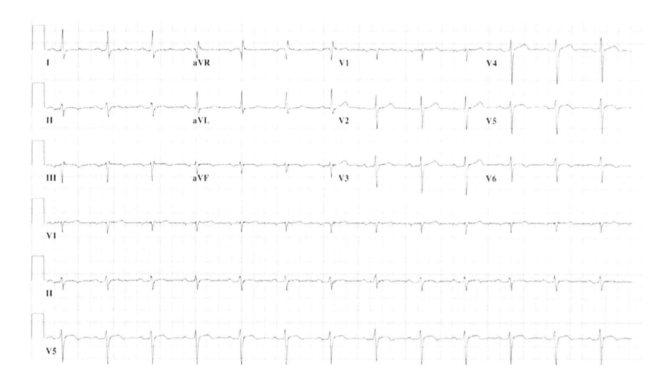

Figure 78.1

g. Pharynx: normal dentition, no lesions, no swelling
h. Chest: nontender
i. Lungs: clear bilaterally
j. Heart: rate and rhythm regular, no murmurs, rubs, or gallops
k. Abdomen: normal bowel sounds, soft, nontender or distended
l. Rectal: normal tone, brown stool, occult blood negative
m. Urogenital: normal external genitalia
   i. Male: no discharge, normal testicular examination
n. Extremities: no deformity, normal pulses
o. Back: nontender
p. Neuro: Cranial nerves: right-sided facial droop with forehead sparing, otherwise CNs intact. 0/5 motor strength in right upper and lower extremities. Loss of fine touch and pain on right upper and lower extremities. Unable to cooperate with right-sided cerebellar examination, or gait/Romberg testing. Does not acknowledge MD's presence when on the patient's right side and does not voluntarily turn or look to right. When filling in clock face, he only writes numbers on the left side. Memory is intact; however, he notes lack of ability to concentrate or maintain attention for longer than several minutes.
q. Skin: warm and dry
r. Lymph: no lymphadenopathy

I. Action
a. Imaging
   i. Head CT without contrast

b. Meds
    i. Aspirin should not be given until after CT
    ii. BP control is optional at this point and may await reassessment after CT scan
c. Consult
    i. Neurology/stroke service if available
d. Imaging (additional but only after patient return from CT scanner)
    i. CXR

J. Nurse
a. BP: 235/139 HR: 69 RR: 18 Sat: 98% on O_2
b. Patient: without change in appearance or paralysis

K. Results

Complete blood count:

WBC	5.3×10^3/uL	D bili	0.3 mg/dL
Hct	41.5%	Amylase	50 U/L
Plt	350×10^3/uL	Lipase	25 U/L
		Albumin	4.7 g/dL

Basic metabolic panel:

Na	138 mEq/L	**Urinalysis:**	
K	4.3 mEq/L	SG	1.010–1.030
Cl	105 mEq/L	pH	5–8
CO_2	30 mEq/L	Prot	Neg mg/dL
BUN	12 mEq/dL	Gluc	Neg mg/dL
Cr	1.1 mg/dL%	Ketones	Neg mg/dL
Gluc	100 mg/dL	Bili	Neg
		Blood	Neg
Coagulation panel:		LE	Neg
PT	12.6 sec	Nitrite	Neg
PTT	26.0 sec	Color	Yellow
INR	1.0		

Arterial blood gas:

Liver function panel:		pH	7.4
AST	23 U/L	PO_2	95 mmHg
ALT	26 U/L	PCO_2	41 mmHg
Alk Phos	42 U/L	HCO_3	24 mmol/L
T bili	1.0 mg/dL		

a. Troponin
b. Head CT (Figure 78.2) negative for acute hemorrhage, mass, or edema; ischemic changes in the left MCA distribution with hyperdense MCA sign (see image)
c. CXR (Figure 78.3)

L. Action
a. Neurology consult
    i. Admission for further assessment/observation and further imaging
b. Discussion with family

Figure 78.2 A,
B and C

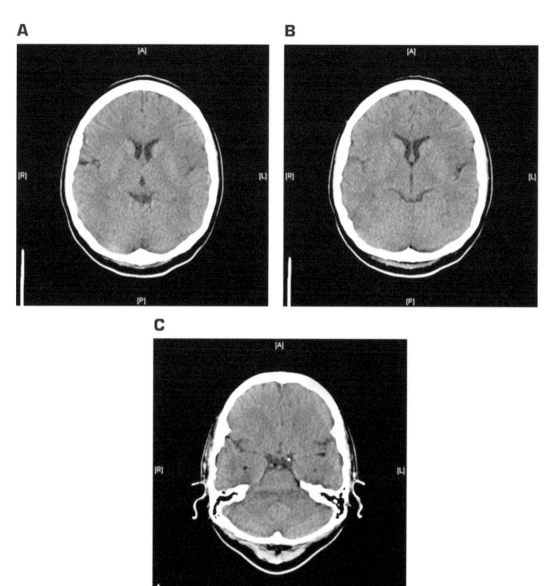

c. Meds
  i. Aspirin
  ii. Antihypertensives at this point may be given considering that SBP is > 230 and/or DBP is >130; options include but are not limited to
    1. β-blockers such as labetolol or esmolol
    2. Calcium channel blockers such as nicardipine
    3. Nitro agents such as nitroprusside/nitroglycerin
  iii. tPA is not indicated at this time because time of onset cannot be established at less than 3–4.5 hours as the patient was last seen before sleep

M. Diagnosis
a. Stroke: left MCA

N. Critical actions
▇ Finger stick glucose
▇ Head CT

Figure 78.3

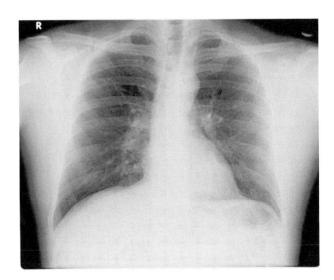

- Neurology/stroke team notification
- Neurological examination
- BP control with IV agents

O. Examiner instructions
a. This is a case of a left middle cerebral artery stroke, a condition caused by a cessation of flow to one of the arteries supplying the brain, resulting in death of the tissue. The patient's symptoms include neurological deficits that are consistent with the left motor and sensory centers in the brain (nondominant hemisphere) which are fed by this artery. Early critical actions include establishing the time of onset (or time last known to be without deficit), IV access, monitoring, immediate head CT and neurology consult. Because the CT is negative for signs of intracranial hemorrhaging, the symptoms are assumed to be the result of a thromboembolic process. Subsequently, antiplatelet, anticoagulation, and thrombolytic therapies are considered. Blood pressure monitoring and management is important throughout the case.

P. Pearls
a. Approximately 80% of strokes are ischemic as opposed to hemorrhagic.
b. Time of symptom onset is key to treatment consideration as tPA protocols call for administration within 3 hours (with extended window parameters) of symptoms onset.
c. Patient must have an immediate CT of the head to rule out intracranial hemorrhage.
d. Thromboembolic strokes may be preceded by TIAs.
e. Blood pressure control is a constant consideration not only for the pathologic processes involved but also for administration of tPA. Generally BP of >210/130 should be treated; however, exact goals and pharmacologic agents are variable. Additionally, patients that are to be receiving tPA should have a BP <185/110.

Q. References
a. Tintinalli's: Chapter 161
b. Rosen's: Chapter 101

CASE 79: Pedestrian struck (Matthew Constantine, MD)

A. Chief complaint

a. 57-year-old female brought in by EMS after being struck by an automobile. Patient complains of right leg pain and lower back pain. She is immobilized with a backboard and collar.

B. Vital signs

a. BP: 145/77 HR: 105 RR: 25 T: 36.2°C Sat: 98% on RA FS: 131

C. What does the patient look like?

a. Patient appears stated age, uncomfortable-appearing and in moderate distress, lying supine on the backboard and in a cervical collar.

D. Primary survey

a. Airway: speaking in full sentences
b. Breathing: mildly tachypneic, no cyanosis
c. Circulation: warm and dry, normal capillary refill
d. Disability/deformity
   i. Open right ankle fracture noted; multiple ecchymoses on right leg, thigh, and hip

E. Action

a. Oxygen via NC or nonrebreather mask
b. Two large-bore peripheral IV lines
c. Labs
   i. CBC, BMP, LFTs, coagulation studies, blood type and cross-match two units
   ii. Point of care hematocrit
d. 2 L NS bolus
e. Monitor: BP: 139/91 HR: 120 RR: 20 Sat: 100% on O_2
f. EKG
g. FAST (Figure 79.1)
h. Imaging
   i. CXR
   ii. Pelvic x-ray
   iii. C-spine x-ray
i. Consults
   i. Surgery/trauma
   ii. Orthopedics

F. History

a. HPI: This is a 57-year-old female who was struck by a car at low speed (~10 mph) while crossing an intersection. The patient was struck on the right side, knocked onto the hood and then landed ~4 feet in front of the vehicle. She presently complains of pain in her right lower extremity at the ankle as well as at the right hip and lower back. She denies LOC, vision or hearing changes, vertigo, neck pain, chest pain, shortness of breath, nausea, vomiting, or abdominal pain. She denies recent alcohol or drug use. Her last tetanus is unknown.

A

B

Figure 79.1 A, B, C and D

C

D

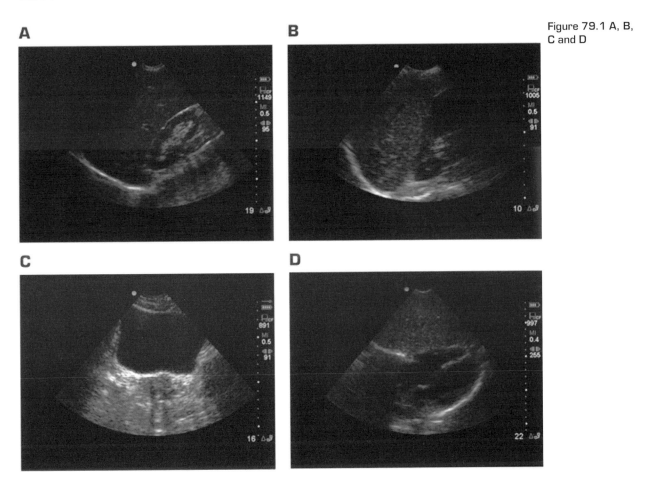

b. PMHx: hypertension

c. PSHx: none

d. Allergies: none

e. Meds: amlodipine

f. Social: lives alone, social EtOH, denies smoking or drug use.

g. FHx: not relevant

h. PMD: Dr Pine

G. Nurse

a. EKG (Figure 79.2.)

b. Hematocrit 32%

c. 2 L NS

    i. BP: 100/66 HR: 120 RR: 22 Sat: 98% on O_2

d. If no fluids given then

    i. BP: 80/45 HR: 125 RR: 22 Sat: 98% on O_2

H. Secondary survey

a. General: alert, oriented × 3, moderate distress secondary to pain

b. Head: contusion to left forehead, no scalp lacerations or bony deformities noted

c. Eyes: extraocular movement intact, pupils equal, reactive to light

d. Ears: normal tympanic membranes

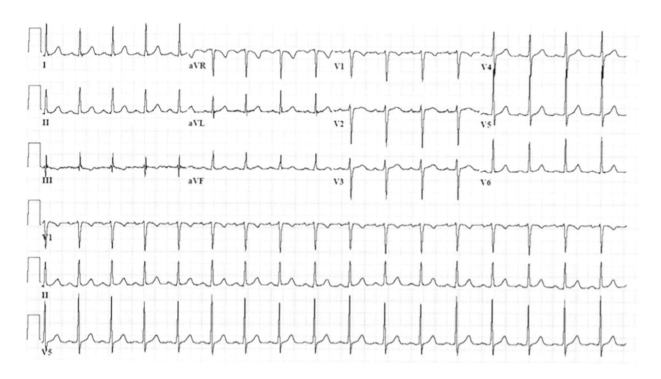

Figure 79.2

    e. Nose: no discharge

    f. Neck: full range of motion, no stridor, C collar in place

    g. Pharynx: normal dentition, no lesions, no swelling

    h. Chest: nontender, no contusions/abrasions

    i. Lungs: clear bilaterally

    j. Heart: tachycardic rate, rhythm regular, no murmurs, rubs, or gallops

    k. Abdomen: normal bowel sounds, soft, nontender, nondistended, no ecchymosis

    l. Pelvis: 4 cm movement when inward pressure is applied to both femoral heads with both hands

    m. Rectal: normal tone, brown stool, occult blood negative

    n. Urogenital: normal external genitalia

       i. Female: no urethral blood

    o. Extremities: open nonangulated fracture of the medial right ankle with swelling and ecchymosis with minimal bleeding. Right knee and femur are nontender to palpation. Palpation of right hip reproduces same right-sided pelvic and back pain that was elicited on pelvic examination. ROM at ankle, knee, and hip are limited due to patient discomfort

    p. Back: no midline tenderness, no ecchymosis noted; patient complains of right paraspinal tenderness

    q. Neuro: GCS – eyes open spontaneously, moves upper and left lower extremities on commands and without discomfort, responds appropriately to questions, GCS = 15; no sensory deficits noted; CNs 2–12 intact; cerebellar testing is normal.

    r. Skin: pale and cool now (different from primary survey), other lesions as noted elsewhere on examination

    s. Lymph: no lymphadenopathy

Figure 79.3

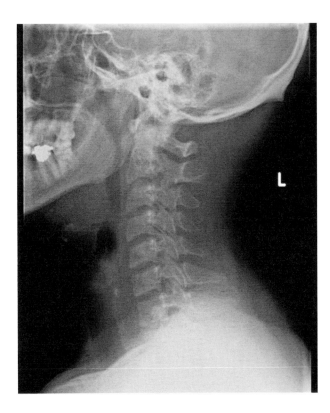

I. Nurse

a. BP: 72/25 HR: 140 RR: 25 Sat 98% on O_2

b. C-spine x-ray (Figure 79.3)

c. CXR (Figure 79.4)

d. AP pelvis (Figure 79.5)

J. Action

a. Central access through two 16-gauge IVs is acceptable – best choice is 8Fr; introducer in the subclavian vein

   i. Avoid femoral access as patient with obvious RLE injury and suspected pelvic fracture

   ii. IJ difficult to access secondary to C collar

b. Orthopedics reductions

   i. The pelvis requires stabilization either with external fixator applied by orthopedics or a sheet wrapped/tied around pelvis. With pelvic laxity and dropping BP in the setting of a negative FAST and CXR, pelvic hemorrhage is high on the differential

c. Meds

   i. Tetanus

   ii. Cephalexin

   iii. Morphine (Opioid medication)

d. Consult

   i. Interventional radiology for emergent pelvic angiography

e. Imaging

   i. Patient will require head CT and CT of chest, abdomen, and pelvis (currently unavailable given hemodynamic instability of patient)

Figure 79.4

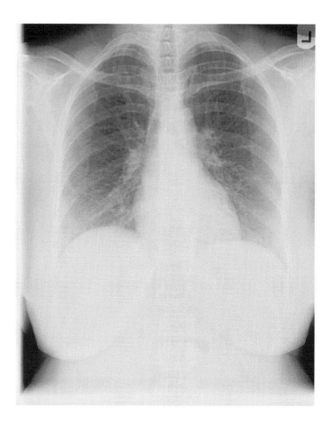

Figure 79.5

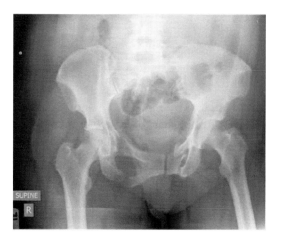

　　　ii. Right lower extremity films (these are not critical at this point and can wait until the patient is stable)
　f. IV fluids
　　i. 2 L NS
　g. Blood products
　　i. Two units packed red blood cells (no type specific available, must ask for O + or − blood)

K. Nurse
a. Reassess
　i. Patient: still with pain
　ii. Vitals

1. 2 U blood
   a. Vitals: BP: 100/61 HR: 110 RR: 25 Sat: 98% on 100% NRB O_2
2. No blood
   a. Vitals: BP: 70/25 HR: 150 RR: 30 Sat: 98% on O_2

L. Results

Complete blood count:

WBC	10×10^3/uL	Alk Phos	42 U/L
Hct	30.5%	T bili	1.0 mg/dL
Plt	251×10^3/uL	D bili	0.3 mg/dL
		Amylase	50 U/L
Basic metabolic panel:		Lipase	25 U/L
Na	138 mEq/L	Albumin	4.7 g/dL
K	4.3 mEq/L		
Cl	105 mEq/L	**Urinalysis:**	
CO_2	30 mEq/L	SG	1.010–1.030
BUN	12 mEq/dL	pH	5–8
Cr	1.1 mg/dL%	Prot	Neg mg/dL
Gluc	100 mg/dL	Gluc	Neg mg/dL
		Ketones	Neg mg/dL
Coagulation panel:		Bili	Neg
PT	12.6 sec	Blood	Neg
PTT	26.0 sec	LE	Neg
INR	1.0	Nitrite	Neg
		Color	Yellow
Liver function panel:			
AST	23 U/L		
ALT	26 U/L		

a. Lactate 2.7 mmol/L

M. Action

a. Discussion with family and PMD about the need for emergent embolization for presumed pelvic fracture with bleeding
b. Meds
   i. Morphine or other pain medication
c. Interventional radiology for emergent embolization
d. Surgery to continue management with further imaging and admission to SICU

N. Diagnosis

a. Pelvic fracture with hemorrhage
b. Open right ankle fracture

O. Critical actions

▨ IV access with at least 2 large-bore catheters
▨ Blood transfusion
▨ Immediate activation of surgery/trauma service
▨ FAST examination
▨ X-ray: chest and pelvis

■ Reduction and fixation of pelvis
■ Consulting IR for angiographic intervention

P. Examiner instructions

a. This is a case of a pelvic fracture secondary to trauma, a serious condition due to the proximity of many large blood vessels that can be injured as a result of the fracture. Initially our patient had outward signs of significant lower extremity trauma and a mechanism severe enough to cause such an injury. The patient although injured appears stable initially, in terms of mental status, GCS, and vital signs. However, over the course of the case the patient becomes more hypotensive and tachycardic. Immediate actions after ensuring adequate airway, breathing and circulation are to establish adequate IV access with large-bore catheters, fluid boluses, and to activate any trauma service available or consult surgery. The secondary survey shows that the patient has no evidence of significant injuries other than the right lower extremity and the pelvis. The candidate will need to address the likely source of bleeding in the pelvis with definitive treatment: embolization by interventional radiology. If the candidate attempts to wait for CT of the head, chest, abdomen, and pelvis, the patient should become more hypotensive and the surgery consult should indicate that the patient appears too unstable to go to the scanner.

Q. Pearls

a. Mechanism of injury is a key historical factor in predicting clinical course.
b. Pelvic injury carries a significant mortality and evaluation is a key part of the trauma work-up.
c. Pelvic fractures associated with instability require immediate intervention.
d. Early consultation of trauma services, orthopedics, and possibly interventional radiology should be obtained as pelvic fractures may decompensate quickly.

R. References

a. Tintinalli's: Chapter 269
b. Rosen's: Chapter 55

CASE 80: Back pain (Matthew Constantine, MD)

A. Chief complaint

a. 29-year-old female presents to the emergency room with complaint of back pain.

B. Vital signs

a. BP: 115/68 HR: 112 RR: 16 T: 37.8°C (oral) Sat: 98% on RA FS: 105

C. What does the patient look like?

a. Patient appears stated age, is ill-appearing, and in mild distress. She is lying on her left side.

D. Primary survey

a. Airway: speaking in full sentences
b. Breathing: no apparent respiratory distress, no cyanosis
c. Circulation: warm and dry skin, normal capillary refill

E. Action

a. Two large-bore peripheral IV lines

b. Labs

   i. CBC, BMP

   ii. UA, urine culture, urine pregnancy test

c. 1 L NS bolus

d. Rectal temperature: 38.5°C

e. Meds

   i. Acetaminophen

f. Vitals

   i. BP: 115/70 HR: 115 RR: 18 Sat: 99%

F. History

a. HPI: This is a 29-year-old female with a past medical history significant for mild intermittent asthma who complains of right-sided back pain. The pain is located in the right midback, radiates to the right flank and has been getting progressively worse for the past 2 days. She states that she has been febrile for the past 3 days, with 3 episodes of nausea and vomiting over the past 2 days. She is not presently nauseous and is tolerating PO intake. One week ago she had noted some slight burning with urination and increased urinary frequency. These symptoms have abated after increasing hydration with cranberry juice but have not completely resolved. She had similar urinary symptoms 1 month ago that improved with hydration only. She denies other symptoms except for a mild intermittent cough that is relieved by her bronchodilator inhaler. She states that this is her baseline "asthma" cough that has not changed over the past several months. Additionally, she has been sexually active with three different male partners over the past 6 months. She states that she does not always use condoms; however, she does use birth control. The patient denies any vaginal discharge or itching. Her LMP was 3 weeks ago.

b. PMHx: asthma

c. PSHx: none

d. Allergies: none

e. Meds: albuterol MDI

f. Social: lives alone at home, social EtOH, denies smoking and drug use

g. FHx: not relevant

h. PMD: Dr Diaz

G. Nurse

a. Vitals

   i. After 1 L NS

      1. BP: 110/75 HR: 95 RR: 18 Sat: 99%

   ii. If no fluids

      1. BP: 110/75 HR: 120 RR: 18 Sat: 99%

b. Patient

   i. Still with pain, shaking chills

c. Urine pregnancy test negative

H. Secondary survey

 a. General: alert, oriented × 3, moderate distress secondary to pain
 b. Head: normocephalic, atraumatic
 c. Eyes: extraocular movements intact, pupils equal, reactive to light
 d. Ears: normal tympanic membranes
 e. Nose: no discharge
 f. Neck: full range of motion, no jugular vein distention, no stridor
 g. Pharynx: normal dentition, no lesions, no swelling
 h. Chest: nontender
 i. Lungs: clear bilaterally
 j. Heart: rate and rhythm regular, no murmurs, rubs, or gallops
 k. Abdomen: normal bowel sounds, soft, nontender, nondistended
 l. Rectal: normal tone, brown stool, occult blood negative
 m. Urogenital: normal external genitalia
   i. Female: no blood or discharge, cervical os closed, no cervical motion tenderness, no adnexal tenderness or masses
 n. Extremities: full range of motion, no deformity, normal pulses
 o. Back: right-sided CVA tenderness
 p. Neuro: cranial nerves II to XII intact; normal sensation, strength; normal reflexes and gait
 q. Skin: warm and dry
 r. Lymph: no lymphadenopathy

I. Action

 a. Meds
   i. Morphine or other pain medications
   ii. 1 L NS bolus
 b. Reassess
   i. Patient slightly improved after IVF, antipyretic, and pain medicine
 c. Imaging
   i. CXR

J. Nurse

 a. BP: 120/65 HR: 75 RR: 18 Sat: 98% on RA

K. Results

Complete blood count:

WBC	15.1×10^3/uL
Diff	92.4/7.4/1.8
Hct	39.0%
Plt	301×10^3/uL

Basic metabolic panel:

Na	138 mEq/L
K	4.3 mEq/L
Cl	105 mEq/L
CO_2	30 mEq/L
BUN	31 mEq/dL
Cr	1.2 mg/dL%
Gluc	98 mg/dL

Coagulation panel:

PT	12.6 sec
PTT	26.0 sec
INR	1.0

Liver function panel:

AST	23 U/L
ALT	26 U/L
Alk Phos	42 U/L
T bili	1.0 mg/dL
D bili	0.3 mg/dL
Amylase	50 U/L
Lipase	25 U/L
Albumin	4.7 g/dL

Urinalysis:

SG	1.010–1.030	Bili	Neg
pH	5–8	Blood	large
Prot	Neg mg/dL	LE	pos
Gluc	Neg mg/dL	Nitrite	pos
Ketones	pos	Color	Yellow

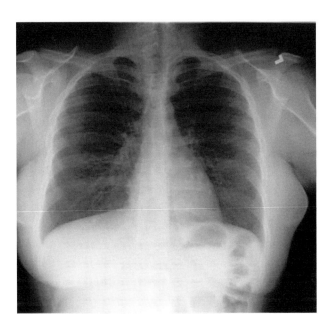

Figure 80.1

a. Urine culture pending

b. CXR (Figure 80.1)

L. Action

a. Meds

   i. Ciprofloxacin IV or other appropriate antibiotic

b. Optional – CT without and with contrast – r/o nephrolithiasis and abscess

   i. CT (Figure 80.2)

c. Disposition

   i. Discharge to home, however, must ensure proper follow-up of patient within 2 to 3 days

   ii. Discharge plan

      1. Ciprofloxacin PO × 10 to 14 days

      2. Pain control

      3. Instructions for proper hydration as she is tolerating PO

      4. Instructions to return if symptoms worsen or if she is unable to tolerate PO, and to call back for culture results

M. Diagnosis

a. Pyelonephritis

Figure 80.2

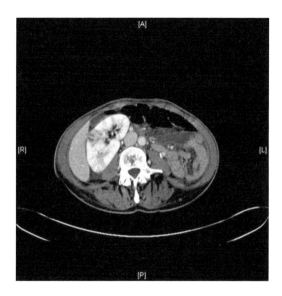

N. Critical actions

▨ Pain control

▨ Urine pregnancy test

▨ IV fluids

▨ Antibiotics

▨ Ensuring proper outpatient treatment, instructions, and follow-up

O. Examiner instructions

a. This is a case of acute pyelonephritis, a bacterial infection of the urinary system affecting the kidneys. The patient has had preceding symptoms consistent with a UTI. Her symptoms of flank pain, fever, and urinary symptoms are classic. Early actions for this patient include hydration, pain management, and antibiotics. A pregnancy test is also necessary since medications such as ciprofloxacin are harmful to the fetus. The candidate should perform a thorough examination and history to exclude other causes of fever and vomiting such as appendicitis and pelvic disease. Once the patient receives pain medications, fluids, and antipyretics, she can be safely discharged home with antibiotics, follow-up, and thorough discharge instructions.

P. Pearls

a. The diagnosis of acute pyelonephritis can be made based on clinical presentation with a supportive UA. It is important to remember that in the setting of overwhelming historical and physical examination findings, a negative UA does not rule out the diagnosis.

b. ED treatment is aimed at starting antibiotics and providing supportive care.

c. Additional work-up (CT scan or ultrasound) as well as disposition are based on comorbidities, patient age and severity of symptoms, immune status, previous treatment failures, and patient's ability to comply with outpatient treatment and follow-up.

Q. References

a. Tintinalli's: Chapter 94

b. Rosen's: Chapter 99

CASE 81: Altered mental status (Matthew Constantine, MD)

A. Chief complaint
a. 39-year-old female brought in by EMS with altered mental status

B. Vital signs
a. BP: 152/50 HR: 140 RR: 24 T: 39°C oral Sat: 98% on RA FSG: 120 (must ask)

C. What does the patient look like?
a. Patient, appears stated age, moderately agitated with muttering speech lying on stretcher.

D. Primary survey
a. Airway: speaking in full sentences; however, statements are inappropriate to context
b. Breathing: mildly tachypneic, no cyanosis
c. Circulation: warm and moist skin, normal capillary refill

E. Action
a. Oxygen via NC or nonrebreather mask
b. Two large-bore peripheral IV lines
c. Labs
  i. CBC, BMP, Mg, Phos, LFTs, coagulation studies, blood type and cross-match
  ii. Lactate, blood cultures, UA, urine culture, urine pregnancy test, alcohol level, acetaminophen level, salicylate level, urine toxicology screen, TSH, free T4
d. 1 L NS bolus
e. Monitor: BP: 160/60 HR: 144 RR: 24 T: 39.9°C rectal (must ask) Sat: 100% on 2 L NC
f. EKG
g. CXR

F. History
a. HPI: This is a 39-year-old female with no significant PMHx who presents with altered mental status per EMS. Her husband, who called EMS, accompanied her to the ED. He states that over the past 1 day, the patient has evolved from mild memory loss and confusion to frank psychosis and now has inappropriate speech. The last time that the patient was seen with a normal mental status by the husband was 2 days ago before going to sleep. The husband is unsure of other symptoms that may have been present over the past 2 days except a cough. The patient had previously complained of a productive cough with mild right-sided chest pain that started about a week ago. The patient had previously told her husband that she felt as if she had a "cold." Today, the patient started to have diarrhea and vomiting, holding her stomach at times. The husband denies any drug use, alcohol use or other chemical exposures by the patient. When asked about past medical history the husband states that she has recently found out from an employee health screen that she had high blood pressure however she has not followed up with a doctor. In addition, over the past several months the patient has considered seeing a psychiatrist. She had previously complained about increasing anxiety with associated insomnia, occasional palpitations, and decreased appetite with weight loss. The patient had attributed these symptoms to the stress of her job and was planning to see a psychiatrist referred by her employer.

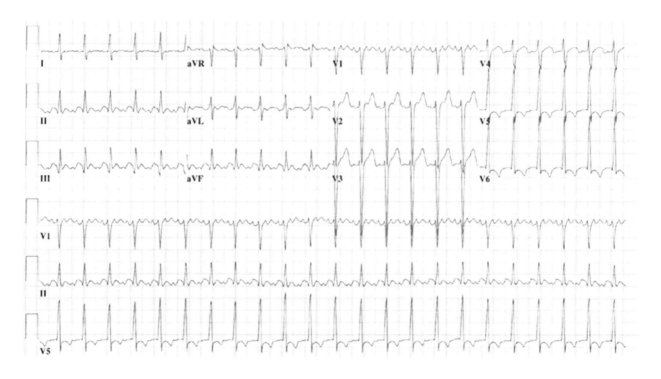

Figure 81.1

    i. EMS: concurs that they did not find any pill bottles, open chemical containers, drug paraphernalia, or other environmental factors that would account for the patient's condition

b. PMHx: none

c. PSHx: none

d. Allergies: none

e. Meds: none

f. Social: lives with husband and 11-year-old child at home; no alcohol, smoking, or drugs per husband; employed as a police officer

g. FHx: no significant family history

h. PMD: Dr Chan

G. Nurse

a. EKG (Figure 81.1)

b. CXR (Figure 81.2)

c. 1 L NS bolus

    i. BP: 157/100 HR: 139 RR: 22 Sat: 100% on O_2

d. No fluids

    i. BP: 95/30 HR: 160 RR: 26 Sat: 100% on O_2

H. Secondary survey

a. General: patient continues to mutter inappropriate statements; patient can, however, be prompted to answer basic yes/no questions such as presence of pain

b. Head: normocephalic, atraumatic

c. Eyes: extraocular movements intact, pupils equal, reactive to light, conjunctivae can be seen above and below iris bilaterally (eyes appear to be protruding)

d. Ears: normal tympanic membranes

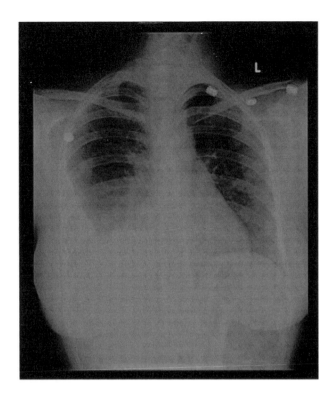

Figure 81.2

e. Nose: no discharge
f. Neck: supple with negative meningeal signs, + midline enlarged mass, non-tender, no stridor (must ask)
g. Pharynx: normal dentition, no lesions, no swelling
h. Chest: nontender
i. Lungs: mild tachypnea, clear bilaterally
j. Heart: tachycardic rate, rhythm regular, no murmurs, rubs, or gallops
k. Abdomen: normal bowel sounds, soft, nontender, nondistended, bowel sounds slightly hyperactive
l. Rectal: normal tone, brown stool, occult blood negative
m. Urogenital: normal external genitalia
  i. Female: no blood or discharge, cervical os closed, no cervical motion tenderness, no adnexal tenderness
n. Extremities: full range of motion, no deformity, normal pulses
o. Back: nontender
p. Neuro: A + O × 1, patient not able to comply with examination; however, is moving all four extremities without gross deficit; no facial droop or slurred speech; gait not tested; no clonus or rigidity; DTRs brisk, symmetric
q. Skin: warm to touch and diaphoretic, no rash, erythema, or petechiae noted
r. Lymph: no lymphadenopathy

I. Action
a. Lumbar puncture after CT head
b. Meds
  i. Ceftriaxone IV
  ii. Azithromycin IV
  iii. 1 L NS bolus

   c. Reassess

      i. Patient condition including vitals unchanged

   d. Imaging

      i. CXR

      ii. CT head noncontrast

J. Nurse

   a. BP: 98/59 HR: 90 RR: 18 Sat 98% on O_2 (after 1 L)

   b. Patient: still agitated

   c. Nurse notes that patient has had 1 episode of watery diarrhea

K. Results

Complete blood count:

WBC	18.0×10^3/uL
Hct	41.5%
Plt	421×10^3/uL

Basic metabolic panel:

Na	138 mEq/L
K	3.5 mEq/L
Cl	105 mEq/L
CO_2	30 mEq/L
BUN	21 mEq/dL
Cr	1.1 mg/dL%
Gluc	105 mg/dL

Coagulation panel:

PT	12.6 sec
PTT	26.0 sec
INR	1.0

Liver function panel:

AST	23 U/L
ALT	26 U/L
Alk Phos	42 U/L
T bili	1.0 mg/dL
D bili	0.3 mg/dL
Amylase	50 U/L
Lipase	25 U/L
Albumin	4.7 g/dL

Urinalysis:

SG	1.010–1.030
pH	5–8
Prot	Neg mg/dL
Gluc	Neg mg/dL
Ketones	Neg mg/dL
Bili	Neg
Blood	Neg
LE	Neg
Nitrite	Neg
Color	Yellow

   a. Lactate 1.5 mmol/L

   b. Urine toxicology negative

   c. Urine pregnancy test negative

   d. CT (Figure 81.3)

   e. LP (once CT noted to be negative)

      i. Cell count: tube 1: RBC: 40, WBC: 1; tube 4: RBC: 12, WBC: 0

      ii. Glucose 59

      iii. Protein 41

      iv. Gram stain negative

      v. Culture pending

   f. Phos 3.0

   g. Mag 2.0

   h. Alcohol negative

   i. Acetaminophen negative

   j. Aspirin negative

   k. TSH pending

   l. T3 and T4 pending

A 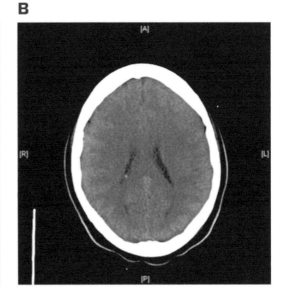 **B**

Figure 81.3
A and B

L. Action
a. Consult
   i. ICU
b. Discussion with family
c. Meds
   i. Propanolol
   ii. PTU
   iii. Iodine

M. Diagnosis
a. Thyrotoxicosis
b. Pneumonia

N. Critical actions
▨ NS fluid bolus, 1 L
▨ Finger stick glucose
▨ CXR
▨ Antibiotics – for possible meningitis
▨ CT and LP for r/o CNS pathology
▨ Serum toxicology assays
▨ Propanolol, PTU, and iodine treatments
▨ ICU consult

O. Examiner instructions
a. This is a case of thyrotoxicosis or thyroid storm. This is a condition caused by an overactive thyroid that leads to a serious state of overstimulation of the body including fast heart rate and breathing, fever, as well as symptoms such as vomiting, diarrhea, and confusion. This event, however, is usually secondary to a stressor or pathological process, the most common being a respiratory infection. In this case, the patient had an undiagnosed hyperthyroid condition that had been manifesting

symptoms such as anxiety, insomnia, palpitations, and weight loss. She had attributed these symptoms to emotional stress. Additionally the patient had exophthalmos on examination. The respiratory infection had been developing over the last week and contributed to the onset of the thyroid storm. The presenting signs and symptoms in this case were altered mental status, diarrhea, hypertension, tachycardia, hyperthermia, and diaphoresis. The differential for this set of symptoms, however, is quite extensive and includes other serious conditions including sepsis, CNS infection, sympathomimetic overdose, EtOH withdrawal, and neuroleptic malignant syndrome. The early critical actions were aimed at several of these possible diagnoses. For this reason the patient received antibiotics with coverage for pneumonia and meningitis. The patient also required a head CT, LP, and toxicology assays for aspirin and acetaminophen to exclude other causes of altered mental status. Based on her presentation, physical examination findings including vital signs as well as history, she required immediate treatment for thyrotoxicosis. The latter critical actions of propanolol, propylthiouracil, iodine, and ICU consult were aimed at treating this diagnosis. The diagnosis of thyrotoxicosis is generally a clinical diagnosis with treatment started empirically as thyroid function testing is often not typically available before the need to begin treatment. As thyrotoxicosis carries a high mortality rate even with treatment, the patient will require admission to a monitored setting, preferably an ICU.

P. Pearls

a. Patients will usually have a history of thyroid disease or prior symptoms that would suggest an undiagnosed condition.
b. A metabolic stressor such as an infection, diabetic ketoacidosis, myocardial infarction, stroke, trauma, or even emotional stress typically induces thyrotoxicosis.
c. Early evaluation includes ruling out other entities that may present with similar signs and symptoms.
d. Thyrotoxicosis is a clinical diagnosis that needs to be treated before confirmatory testing, which can often take hours.

Q. References

a. Tintinalli's: Chapter 224
b. Rosen's: Chapter 128

CASE 82: Abdominal pain (Christopher Strother, MD)

A. Chief complaint

a. 3-year-old male brought in by his mother with the complaint of abdominal pain and vomiting after falling off a stool at home

B. Vital signs

a. BP: 115/73 HR: 155 RR: 32 (crying) T: 36.8°C Sat: 100% on RA

C. What does the patient look like?

a. Patient appears stated age, uncomfortable-appearing and holding his abdomen.

D. Primary survey
a. Airway: patent, speaking normally, crying
b. Breathing: no apparent respiratory distress, no cyanosis
c. Circulation: pink, warm skin, normal capillary refill

E. Action
a. No immediate actions indicated

F. History
a. HPI: This is a 3-year-old male who presents with moderate to severe diffuse abdominal pain. His mother states that the child fell off a stool in the kitchen onto a marble floor, or possibly onto another chair, cried initially, calmed down, then fell asleep for a couple of hours. The incident was not witnessed by his mother as she was not home at the time. He awoke crying and has been crying about stomach pain for the past 30 minutes. He is refusing to eat or drink. There has been no vomiting or diarrhea. He denies pain anywhere else.
b. PMHx: none
c. PSHx: none
d. Allergies: none
e. Social: lives with mother and mother's boyfriend; no smoking or pets in the house
f. FHx: not relevant
g. PMD: Dr Kaufmann

G. Secondary survey
a. General: alert but very fussy, moderate distress secondary to pain
b. HEENT: normal
c. Neck: normal, supple
d. Chest: normal
e. Heart: normal
f. Abdomen: diffuse tenderness and guarding, nondistended, no masses, no hernias, bowel sounds present, limited examination due to patient uncooperativeness due to pain
g. Rectal: hemoccult negative brown stool
h. Urogenital: normal
i. Extremities: normal, scattered bruises on forearms, upper arms, and thighs
j. Back: normal, no tenderness
k. Neuro: normal
l. Skin: normal except minor bruising as above
m. Lymph: normal

H. Action
a. Meds
   i. Pain control
   ii. NS 20 ml/kg
b. Consult
   i. Surgery
   ii. Social work
c. Imaging
   i. CT abdomen

  ii. Focused assessment with sonography in trauma (FAST): negative for free fluid

 d. Monitor

 e. One large-bore peripheral IV line

 f. Labs

  i. CBC, BMP, blood type, PT/PTT

I. Nurse

 a. BP: 98/75 HR: 125 RR: 26 Sat: 100% on RA

 b. Patient: still with significant pain unless opioid given

J. Results

Complete blood count:

WBC	20.1×10^3/uL
Hct	34.5%
Plt	553×10^3/uL

Basic metabolic panel:

Na	142 mEq/L
K	4.0 mEq/L
Cl	110 mEq/L
CO_2	21 mEq/L
BUN	8 mEq/dL
Cr	0.6 mg/dL%
Gluc	120 mg/dL

Coagulation panel:

PT	13.1 sec
PTT	26 sec
INR	1.0

Liver function panel:

AST	14 U/L
ALT	28 U/L
Alk Phos	220 U/L
T bili	0.4 mg/dL
D bili	0.2 mg/dL
Amylase	68 U/L
Lipase	35 U/L
Albumin	3.5 g/dL

Urinalysis:

SG	1.025
pH	7
Prot	Neg
Gluc	Neg
Ketones	Neg
Bili	Neg
Blood	Neg
LE	Neg
Nitrite	Neg
Color	Yellow

 a. CT abdomen (Figure 82.1) demonstrates splenic laceration

K. Action

 a. Surgery consult

  i. Admit for serial examinations, observation

 b. Social work consult

  i. The patient has an injury due to abuse. The police and child protective services need to be contacted, they will likely temporarily remove the child from his home. The mother seems appropriate currently and is also a victim of abuse by her boyfriend.

 c. Ophthalmology consult

  i. No retinal hemorrhages

 d. Discussion with family regarding need for admission, social work, child services due to severity of injury with inconsistent story (discussed sensitively with mother)

 e. Meds

  i. Morphine

 f. Radiology

  i. Skeletal survey for occult fractures

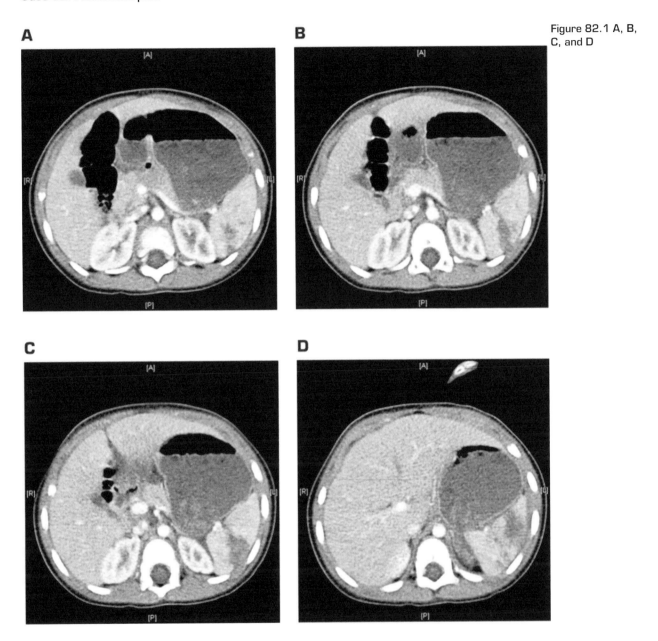

Figure 82.1 A, B, C, and D

L. Diagnosis
a. Nonaccidental abdominal trauma
b. Splenic laceration

M. Critical actions
▪ Recognition of potentially serious abdominal injury
▪ CT abdomen
▪ Recognition of inconsistent story, possible abuse
▪ Surgery consult
▪ Social work/child services consult

N. Examiner instructions
a. This is a case of nonaccidental trauma, or abuse. The key to the case is the story of
falling off a chair is inconsistent with a serious abdominal injury. Also, the physical

examination reveals bruising that is inconsistent with a typical 3-year-old's rough-housing. Knee and elbow scrapes and similar findings are expected at this age, but soft tissue bruising of arms and thighs is concerning. A 3-year-old is easily influenced and will likely agree with whatever story the mother gives initially. The real history is that the mother's abusive boyfriend kicked him when he dropped and broke a dish in the kitchen. The mother will only admit this if a social worker is called to speak with her, or if directly asked about the possibility of the boyfriend causing the injury.

b. The severe tenderness of the abdomen should prompt CT evaluation. Social work or child services should be notified in any case of suspected abuse. If highly suspicious or confirmed nonaccidental trauma, ophthalmology should be consulted to evaluate for retinal hemorrhage as a sign of shaken baby syndrome. Particularly in younger children and infants, a full skeletal survey should be done to rule out occult injury and identify old injury patterns.

O. Pearls

a. Physicians are mandated reporters – if abuse is suspected, authorities must be notified.

b. The story should corroborate the injury.

c. Mothers who are abused often have children at risk and vice versa.

d. CT scan is the gold standard for diagnosis of blunt abdominal injury in children.

e. Splenic lacerations in stable children often do well with minimal intervention; immediate laparotomy is NOT indicated. However, surgery should always be consulted.

P. References

a. Tintinalli's: Chapter 290

b. Rosen's: Chapter 66

CASE 83: Abdominal pain (Lisa Jacobson, MD)

A. Chief complaint

a. 5-year-old boy presents with mild abdominal pain, cola-colored urine, and diarrhea

B. Vital signs

a. BP: 115/70 HR: 90 RR: 18 T: 38.0°C

C. What does the patient look like?

a. A well-developed, interactive child with a pale complexion, in mild distress.

D. Primary survey

a. Airway: speaking in full sentences

b. Breathing: regular rate

c. Circulation: distal pulses bounding

E. Action

a. Labs

i. CBC, BMP, LFTs, coagulation studies, blood type and cross-match

b. IV access

c. Acknowledge hypertension by repeating blood pressure

F. History

a. HPI: This is a 5-year-old boy with 10 days of watery diarrhea and occasional nonbilious, nonbloody vomiting. His mother has noticed that he feels warm on occasion and has given him acetaminophen. He has consistently complained of lower abdominal pain that she thought was related to the diarrhea and she thought he just had the "stomach flu." When he started complaining that his urine looked funny she brought him to the ER. The child endorses red material in his diarrhea at times over the past few days.

b. PMHx: none

c. PSHx: none

d. Allergies: penicillin

e. Social: lives with mom and dad, has one younger sister; attends kindergarten

f. FHx: maternal grandmother has diabetes; father has high blood pressure

g. PMD: Dr Kline

G. Nurse

a. Repeat BP: 117/75

H. Secondary survey

a. General: pale, normally developed boy in mild distress

b. HEENT: pupils equal and reactive, mucous membranes moist, TMs clear

c. Neck: normal

d. Chest: CTA bilaterally, no wheeze/rhonchi/rales

e. Heart: RRR no murmurs

f. Abdomen: soft, nondistended, mild tenderness in lower abdomen

g. Rectal: occult blood positive

h. Urogenital: circumcised, no lesions, bilateral descended testes, no hernias

i. Extremities: full range, no edema

j. Back: normal

k. Neuro: normal

l. Skin: occasional petechiae and ecchymoses on shins

m. Lymph: normal

I. Action

a. Labs: stool culture

b. IV hydration

J. Nurse

a. Vitals remain the same

b. Patent: still with abdominal discomfort; has had diarrhea during the visit

K. Results

a. Helmet and burr cells seen on CBC

Complete blood count:			
WBC	13.1×10^3/uL	K	4.8 mEq/L
Hct	21.5%	Cl	101 mEq/L
Plt	35×10^3/uL	CO$_2$	18.9 mEq/L
		BUN	18 mEq/dL
Basic metabolic panel:		Cr	1.1 mg/dL%
Na	139 mEq/L	Gluc	89 mg/dL

Coagulation panel:

PT	12.6 sec
PTT	26.0 sec
INR	1.0

Liver function panel:

AST	23 U/L
ALT	26 U/L
Alk Phos	42 U/L
T bili	1.6 mg/dL
D bili	0.3 mg/dL
Amylase	50 U/L
Lipase	25 U/L
Albumin	4.7 g/dL

Urinalysis:

SG	1.010–1.030
pH	5–8
Prot	Positive
Gluc	Neg mg/dL
Ketones	Neg mg/dL
Bili	Positive
Blood	Positive
LE	Neg
Nitrite	Neg
Color	Yellow

L. Action

a. Consult

   i. Hematology, possible plasmapheresis if symptoms worsen

   ii. Nephrology

b. Admit

c. Discuss diagnosis with family

d. Meds

   i. IV hydration

e. EKG (Figure 83.1)

f. NPO

g. May type and cross for platelets although this is unnecessary

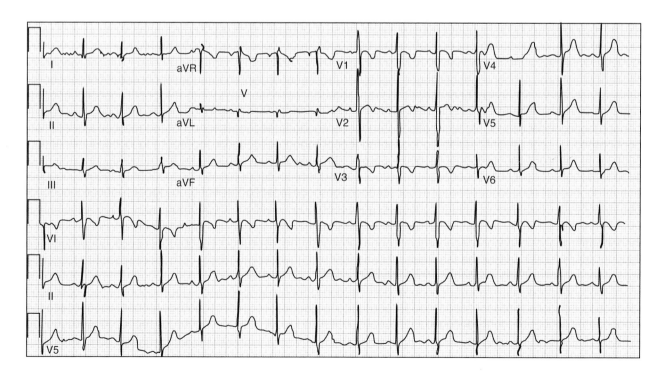

Figure 83.1

M. Diagnosis
a. Hemolytic uremic syndrome (HUS)

N. Critical actions
▨ Large-bore IV access and fluid bolus
▨ Discussion with family
▨ Admission
▨ Pediatric hematology consult

O. Examiner instructions
a. This is a case of HUS in a child following an episode of *Escherichia coli* O157:H7-mediated diarrheal illness. This condition is typically caused by ingesting bacteria from sources such as uncooked meats and causes severe low red blood cell and platelet count and kidney problems. Early actions include IV access, CBC, and fluids. The use of antimotility agents is contraindicated in patients with *E. coli* infectious diarrhea. In children, advanced measures such as plasma exchange or infusion are rarely used as mortality is so low. Antibiotics are not indicated. The patient should be admitted for observation and hydration.

P. Pearls
a. Treatment with antimotility agents may lead to toxic megacolon.
b. Treatment with antibiotics may enhance toxin release.
c. Treat hyperkalemia.
d. Consider plasmapheresis if symptoms are severe.
e. Ninety percent recover with supportive treatment alone.
f. Up to 40% of patients may develop seizures from CNS involvement.
g. Consider thrombocytopenic purpura and disseminated intravascular coagulation in your differential.

Q. References
a. Tintinalli's: Chapter 232
b. Rosen's: Chapter 174

CASE 84: Respiratory distress (Lisa Jacobson, MD)

A. Chief complaint
a. 2-year-old female with respiratory distress

B. Vital signs
a. BP: 90/60 HR: 125 RR: 40 T: 37.1°C Sat: 90% on RA

C. What does the patient look like?
a. A well-developed, interactive child with pale complexion in mild respiratory distress.

D. Primary survey
a. Airway: crying
b. Breathing: labored, fast
c. Circulation: distal pulses bounding

E. Action

   a. Oxygen supplementation (blow-by O_2)

   b. Airway management preparation

      i. Bag valve mask and intubation tray

   c. Peripheral IV lines

   d. Monitor: BP: 90/60 HR: 125 RR: 40 Sat: 93% on blow-by O_2

F. History

   a. HPI: This is a 2-year-old girl brought in by her anxious mother who states that her daughter suddenly started to cry while she was playing in her room unattended for 5 minutes. The girl has appeared agitated and short of breath since. The mother states she only went to the other room to answer the phone. She thinks her daughter's lips look a little blue. The episode occurred 30 minutes ago and the daughter has been inconsolable since, which is not like her.

   b. PMHx: none, normal delivery full term, immunizations up-to-date

   c. PSHx: none

   d. Allergies: none

   e. Meds: none

   f. Social: lives with her parents, has one older sister; attends daycare

   g. FHx: maternal grandmother has diabetes; father has high blood pressure

   h. PMD: Dr Stern

G. Nurse

   a. BP: 90/69 Sat: 92% on blow-by O_2

H. Examination

   a. General: alert, interactive, mild respiratory distress

   b. Head: normocephalic, atraumatic

   c. Eyes: extraocular movements intact, pupils equal, reactive to light

   d. Ears: normal tympanic membranes

   e. Nose: no discharge

   f. Pharynx: no obvious foreign body in posterior pharynx (must ask), no exudates or injection of tonsils, cyanotic lips

   g. Neck: full range of motion, no jugular vein distention, no stridor

   h. Chest: nontender

   i. Lungs: breath sounds clear and equal bilaterally, severe increased work of breathing, significant respiratory effort grunting, air exchange fair

   j. Heart: tachycardic, pulses 2 + equal bilaterally, no murmurs

   k. Abdomen: soft, nontender, bowel sounds normal

   l. Genital examination: Tanner I girl

   m. Extremities: full range of motion, no deformity, normal pulses

   n. Back: normal inspection

   o. Neuro: awake, alert appropriate for age

   p. Skin: warm and dry; no rash

   q. Lymph: no lymphadenopathy

I. Action

   a. Portable CXR

Figure 84.1

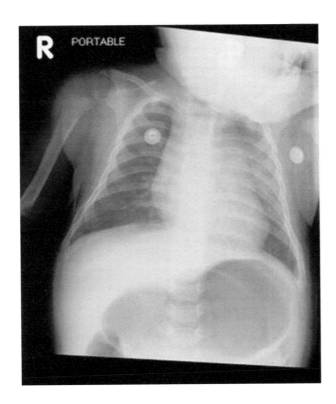

b. ENT consult (ENT initially says they will be down in 1 hour – candidate must be persistent.)

c. Conversation with mother to explain concern for foreign body

J. Nurse

a. CXR (Figure 84.1)

K. Action

a. ENT is able to remove the foreign body (Examinee must have visualized the foreign body on x-ray – ENT should ask what they saw on x-ray.)

b. Repeat vital signs: BP: 90/60 HR: 115 RR: 22 Sat: 100%

c. Admit for observation or observe in ED and discharge with precautions

L. Diagnosis

a. Foreign body aspiration

M. Critical actions

▨ Airway management preparation

▨ Oxygen supplementation

▨ CXR

▨ ENT consult

N. Examiner instructions

a. This is a case of aspiration of a foreign body found in the posterior larynx. The child was left alone by her mother and swallowed something that has partially obstructed the airway. The candidate should prepare to manage the airway but should not intubate. A foreign body is visualized on x-ray and ENT consult can come immediately to remove the object but initially the ENT consult will be resistant. In this case there is only one x-ray, but the candidate should ask for inspiratory and expiratory films. Foreign body management may also consist of abdominal thrusts in the upright or supine position, as the child is older than 1 year.

O. Pearls

a. Radiographs are completely normal in one of three cases of foreign body aspiration.
b. Most commonly aspirated objects by children are food and toys.
c. Aspirated foreign bodies should be in the differential in respiratory distress and pneumonia for all small children.
d. Blind airway sweeps should never be performed.

P. References

a. Tintinalli's: Chapter 119
b. Rosen's: Chapter 168

CASE 85: Overdose (Lisa Jacobson, MD)

A. Chief complaint

a. 45-year-old female with foot pain and depression

B. Vital signs

a. BP: 115/70 HR: 90 RR: 16 T: 37.0°C C Sat: 100% on RA wt: 50 kg

C. What does the patient look like?

a. Patient is a thin, Caucasian woman with a flat affect.

D. Primary survey

a. Airway: speaking in full sentences
b. Breathing: no apparent respiratory distress, no cyanosis
c. Circulation: dry and cool skin, normal capillary refill

E. History

a. HPI: This is a 45-year-old female who sustained an ankle fracture 7 days ago and has been feeling frustrated by her current immobility. Eight hours ago, she was at home drinking wine and feeling sad and frustrated when she decided to take the remaining 29 of her 50 oxycodone/APAP tablets with the intention to commit suicide. She then went to bed. When she awoke this morning, she felt guilty and scared. Not wanting to die, she told her husband what had happened and was brought to the ER. She denies headache, nausea, vomiting, abdominal pain, chest pain, shortness of breath, numbness, tingling, or weakness. She has had no recent illness and denies co-ingestions or previous suicide attempts. She was in the ED 1 week ago for placement of a cast for her left ankle fracture.
b. PMHx: none
c. PSHx: none
d. Allergies: none
e. Meds: received Rx for 50 oxycodone/acetaminophen (5/325 mg) 7 days ago
f. Social: denies tobacco, drinks wine daily, denies illicit drug use
g. FHx: none

F. Action
  a. Oxygen via NC or nonrebreather mask
  b. Two large-bore peripheral IV lines
  c. Labs
    i. CBC, BMP, LFTs, coagulation studies, blood type and cross-match
    ii. Urine pregnancy test, alcohol level, acetaminophen level, salicylate level, urine toxicology screen
  d. Monitor: BP: 115/70 HR: 90 RR: 16 Sat: 100% on O_2
  e. EKG
  f. CXR
  g. Meds
    i. Charcoal can be given though unlikely to provide benefit 8 hours post-ingestion
  h. Psychiatric hold

G. Secondary survey
  a. General: alert, oriented x 3, comfortable, gaze evading
  b. Head: normocephalic, atraumatic
  c. Eyes: extraocular movements intact, pupils pinpoint bilaterally
  d. Ears: normal tympanic membranes
  e. Nose: no discharge
  f. Neck: full range of motion, no jugular vein distention, no stridor
  g. Pharynx: normal dentition, no lesions, no swelling
  h. Chest: nontender
  i. Lungs: clear bilaterally
  j. Heart: rate and rhythm regular, no murmurs, rubs, or gallops
  k. Abdomen: normal bowel sounds, soft, nontender, nondistended
  l. Rectal: normal tone, brown stool, occult blood negative
  m. Extremities: normal pulses, full range, no edema, left lower extremity casted to mid calf
  n. Back: nontender
  o. Neuro: cranial nerves II to XII intact; normal sensation, strength; normal reflexes and gait
  p. Skin: warm and dry
  q. Lymph: no lymphadenopathy

H. Action
  a. Call Poison Control Center
  b. Start *N*-acetylcysteine (NAC)
  c. Psychiatry consult
  d. Admit

I. Nurse
  a. EKG (Figure 85.1)

J. Results
  a. Urine pregnancy test negative
  b. UTox negative
  c. Alcohol level 252
  d. Salicylate level <5
  e. Acetaminophen 167

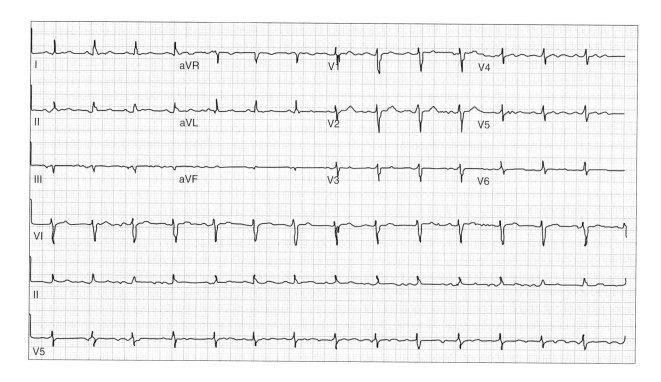

Figure 85.1

Complete blood count:

WBC	5.3×10^3/uL	D bili	0.3 mg/dL
Hct	41.5%	Amylase	50 U/L
Plt	350×10^3/uL	Lipase	25 U/L
		Albumin	4.7 g/dL

Basic metabolic panel:

Na	138 mEq/L	**Urinalysis:**	
K	4.3 mEq/L	SG	1.010–1.030
Cl	105 mEq/L	pH	5–8
CO_2	30 mEq/L	Prot	Neg mg/dL
BUN	12 mEq/dL	Gluc	Neg mg/dL
Cr	1.1 mg/dL%	Ketones	Neg mg/dL
Gluc	100 mg/dL	Bili	Neg
		Blood	Neg
Coagulation panel:		LE	Neg
PT	12.6 sec	Nitrite	Neg
PTT	26.0 sec	Color	Yellow
INR	1.0		

Liver function panel:

		Arterial blood gas:	
		pH	7.4
AST	23 U/L	PO_2	95 mmHg
ALT	26 U/L	PCO_2	41 mmHg
Alk Phos	42 U/L	HCO_3	24 mmol/L
T bili	1.0 mg/dL		

f. CXR (Figure 85.2)

Figure 85.2

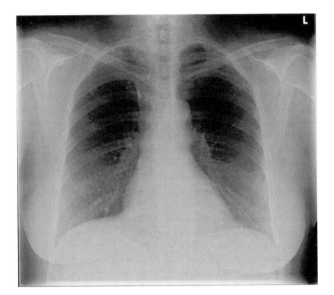

K. Diagnosis
a. Acetaminophen overdose

L. Critical actions
▓ Determine timing of ingestion
▓ Check acetaminophen level and potentially co-ingested substance levels
▓ Start NAC immediately based on calculated dose greater than 140 mg/kg
▓ Check EKG
▓ Place patient on suicide watch

M. Examiner instructions
a. This is a case of acetaminophen overdose that presents at approximately 8 hours post-ingestion. This is a serious overdose given the amount of medication ingested and has a high risk for liver failure and death. Thus the candidate needs to assess either for quantity of ingestion or check an immediate level and begin NAC, the antidote. As in any overdose or ingestion case, the candidate must also evaluate for co-ingestants and toxidromes. GI decontamination is not necessary so many hours post-ingestion.

N. Pearls
a. Toxic exposure to acetaminophen is likely with greater than 140 mg/kg ingestion in a single dose or when greater than 7.5 g is ingested within a 24-hour period.
b. Acetaminophen is typically metabolized mainly via glucuronidation and sulfation, but following overdose these mechanisms are easily saturated. A larger proportion of acetaminophen instead cycles through cytochrome P450 to NAPQI which depletes glutathione stores. If stores are sufficiently depleted, NAPQI binds to other hepatic macromolecules causing necrosis.
c. There are four stages of toxicity:
    i. First 24 hours – minimal signs and symptoms
    ii. 24 to 48 hours – RUQ pain, abnormal LFTs
    iii. 72 to 96 hours – fulminant hepatic failure for some patients causing metabolic acidosis, renal failure, encephalopathy

iv. End of first week – recovery in survivors to full hepatic function

d. Children have increased hepatic sulfation and may be at decreased risk of hepato-toxicity compared to adults.

O. References

a. Rosen's: Chapter 148

b. Tintinalli's: Chapter 184

CASE 86: Chest pain (Lisa Jacobson, MD)

A. Chief complaint

a. 59-year-old male with chest pain

B. Vital signs

a. BP: 115/70 HR: 90 RR: 16 T 98.5°F

C. What does the patient look like?

a. Patient is an obese man, diaphoretic and clutching his chest.

D. Primary survey

a. Airway: speaking in full sentences

b. Breathing: no apparent respiratory distress, no cyanosis

c. Circulation: dry and cool skin, normal capillary refill

E. Action

a. Oxygen via NC or nonrebreather mask

b. Two large-bore peripheral IV lines

c. Labs

   i. CBC, BMP, LFTs, coagulation studies, blood type and cross-match

   ii. Troponin

d. Monitor: BP: 115/70 HR: 90 RR: 16 T: 98.5°F

e. EKG

F. History

a. HPI: This is a 59-year-old who presents with sudden onset chest pressure (8/10) radiating down his left arm for the past 2 hours. He has associated nausea and diaphoresis. He denies shortness of breath, vomiting, back pain, fever, chills, or cough. He has no history of cardiac disease. He reports decreased exercise tolerance for the past 2 weeks.

b. PMHx: hypercholesterolemia

c. PSHx: none

d. Allergies: none

e. Meds: atorvastatin

f. Social: denies drug or alcohol use, smokes one pack per day for 30 years, no cocaine

g. FHx: father with MI at 53

h. PMD: Dr Silverstein

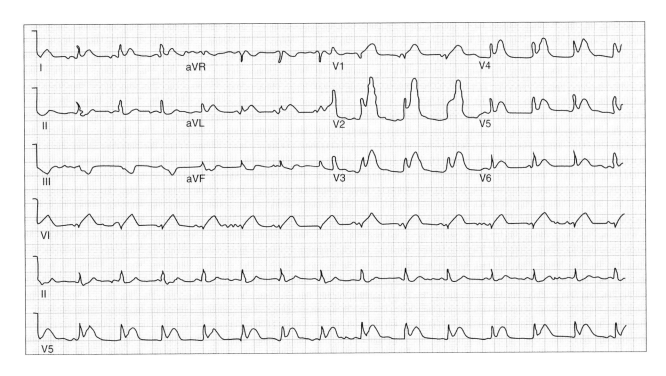

Figure 86.1

G. Nurse
a. EKG (Figure 86.1)

H. Secondary survey
a. General: alert, oriented × 3, uncomfortable, diaphoretic
b. Head: normocephalic, atraumatic
c. Eyes: extraocular movements intact, pupils equal, reactive to light
d. Ears: normal tympanic membranes
e. Nose: no discharge
f. Neck: full range of motion, no jugular vein distention, no stridor
g. Pharynx: normal dentition, no lesions, no swelling
h. Chest: nontender
i. Lungs: clear bilaterally
j. Heart: rate and rhythm regular, no murmurs, rubs, or gallops
k. Abdomen: normal bowel sounds, soft, nontender, nondistended
l. Rectal: normal tone, brown stool, occult blood negative
m. Extremities: full range of motion, no deformity, normal pulses
n. Back: nontender
o. Neuro: cranial nerves II to XII intact; normal sensation, strength; normal reflexes and gait
p. Skin: warm and diaphoretic
q. Lymph: no lymphadenopathy

I. Action
a. Consult
   i. Cardiology for catherization
b. Discussion with patient regarding EKG results

    c. Meds

       i. Aspirin chewable

      ii. Sublingual nitroglycerin and/or morphine 4 to 6 mg IV for pain control

      iii. β-blocker such as metoprolol IV

      iv. Heparin drip

    d. CXR

J. Nurse

    a. Nitroglycerin or morphine

       i. Vitals unchanged, pain improved 4/10

    b. No nitroglycerin

       i. Vitals unchanged, pain worsens to 10/10

K. Results

Complete blood count:

WBC	7.3×10^3/uL
Hct	41.5%
Plt	330×10^3/uL

Basic metabolic panel:

Na	146 mEq/L
K	4.0 mEq/L
Cl	105 mEq/L
CO_2	27 mEq/L
BUN	12 mEq/dL
Cr	1.1 mg/dL%
Gluc	89 mg/dL

Coagulation panel:

PT	12.6 sec
PTT	26.0 sec
INR	1.0

Liver function panel:

AST	23 U/L
ALT	26 U/L
Alk Phos	42 U/L
T bili	1.0 mg/dL
D bili	0.3 mg/dL
Amylase	50 U/L
Lipase	25 U/L
Albumin	4.7 g/dL

Urinalysis:

SG	1.010–1.030
pH	5–8
Prot	Neg mg/dL
Gluc	Neg mg/dL
Ketones	Neg mg/dL
Bili	Neg
Blood	Neg
LE	Neg
Nitrite	Neg
Color	Yellow

    a. Troponin normal

    b. Cardiac catheterization lab is ready for patient

L. Diagnosis

    a. Anterolateral myocardial infarction

M. Critical actions

▨ Cardiac monitoring

▨ EKG within 10 minutes of arrival

▨ Cardiology catheterization

▨ Aspirin

▨ Pain control with morphine or nitroglycerin

N. Examiner instructions

    a. This is a case of anterolateral wall myocardial infarction (heart attack), in which there is a clot in the coronary artery preventing oxygen delivery to the heart muscle causing cell death. The candidate should recognize this immediately upon seeing the EKG and should activate the cardiac catheterization lab to open the clot and deliver treatment and medications including aspirin, nitroglycerin, and oxygen. There is no need to wait for laboratory results, and the candidate may successfully complete the examination without asking for these results.

O. Pearls
a. Patients with myocardial infarction may present anywhere on the spectrum from well to extremely distressed and toxic.
b. Cardiac catherization is currently the management of choice but in hospitals without access to coronary angioplasty and without the option to transfer the patient to a catherization-capable center, thrombolytic treatment is indicated in the absence of contraindications.
c. The anatomy of the heart is such that the circumflex artery is most likely responsible for lateral wall ischemia as it wraps around the sulcus toward the right coronary artery territory. The left anterior descending artery is most often the source of anterior and septal oxygen supply.

P. References
a. Tintinalli's: Chapter 53
b. Rosen's: Chapter 78
c. PT O'Gara,. 2013 ACCF/AHA Guideline for the Management of ST-Elevation Myocardial Infarction. *Circulation* 2013; 127 : e362-e425.

CASE 87: Fever (Edward R. Melnick, MD, MHS)

A. Chief complaint
a. 89-year-old female brought in by EMS from a nursing home for evaluation of fever and altered mental status

B. Vital signs
a. BP: 134/87 HR: 94 RR: 24 T: 38.7°C Sat: 93% on RA FS: 209 (must ask)

C. What does the patient look like?
a. Patient appears stated age, pale, drowsy, and incoherent

D. Primary survey
a. Airway: speaking several words at a time
b. Breathing: increased respiratory rate and work of breathing, but no apparent respiratory distress and no cyanosis
c. Circulation: pale and very warm skin, normal capillary refill

E. Action
a. Oxygen via NC or nonrebreather mask
b. Two large-bore peripheral IV lines
c. Labs
  i. CBC, BMP, LFTs, coagulation studies, blood type and cross-match
  ii. Lactate, troponin, blood cultures, UA, urine culture

d. 1 L NS IV bolus

e. Monitor: BP: 128/91 HR: 96 RR: 24 Sat: 100% on 4 L NC

f. EKG

g. Imaging

   i. CXR

F. History

a. HPI: This is an 89-year-old female brought in by EMS from a nursing home for evaluation of fever and altered mental status. The patient cannot give a history due to her dementia and mental status changes. The nursing home transfer summary states that the patient has a history of diabetes, hypertension, and dementia. Yesterday, she was at her baseline of being alert and conversant but was noted today to be less coherent, drowsy, and febrile to 103°F.

b. PMHx: diabetes, hypertension, and dementia

c. PSHx: none

d. Allergies: none

e. Meds: insulin, diltiazem, aspirin

f. Social: lives in nursing home, no family contact information listed in nursing home transfer summary

g. FHx: not relevant

h. PMD: nursing home staff physician

G. Nurse

a. EKG (Figure 87.1)

b. With or without fluids

   i. BP: 111/73 HR: 100 RR: 24 Sat; 100% on 4 L NC

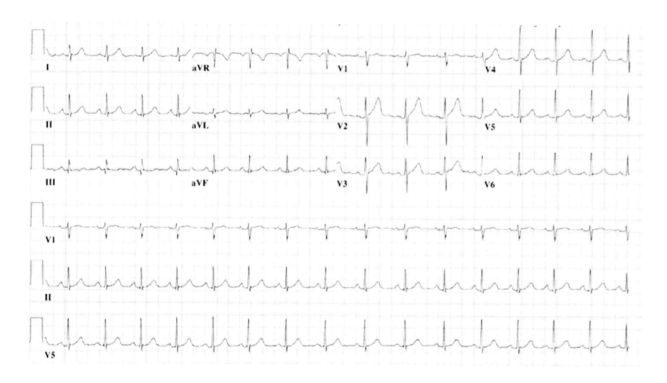

Figure 87.1

H. Secondary survey

a. General: pale, warm skin, drowsy, incoherent, not oriented to person, place, or time, increased work of breathing

b. Head: normocephalic, atraumatic

c. Eyes: extraocular movements intact, pupils equal, reactive to light

d. Ears: normal tympanic membranes

e. Nose: no discharge

f. Neck: full range of motion, no jugular vein distention, no stridor

g. Pharynx: normal dentition, no lesions, no swelling

h. Chest: nontender

i. Lungs: increased respiratory rate and work of breathing, no respiratory distress, focal rhonchi at the right base otherwise clear lungs

j. Heart: tachycardic rate, rhythm regular, no murmurs, rubs, or gallops

k. Abdomen: normal bowel sounds, soft, nontender, nondistended

l. Rectal: normal tone, brown stool, occult blood negative

m. Urogenital: normal external genitalia

   i. Female: no blood or discharge, cervical os closed, no cervical motion tenderness, no adnexal tenderness

n. Extremities: full range of motion, no deformity, normal pulses

o. Back: nontender

p. Neuro: cranial nerves II to XII intact; normal sensation, strength; normal reflexes and gait

q. Skin: warm and dry

r. Lymph: no lymphadenopathy

I. Nurse

a. BP: 101/67 HR: 104 RR: 24 Sat: 98% on 4 L NC

b. Labs sent but radiology is delayed because of technical problems – both portable and PA/lateral chest x-rays are unavailable

J. Action

a. Meds

   i. Broad-spectrum antibiotics to cover nosocomial infection of unknown source; for example, cefepime and vancomycin

   ii. Additional IV fluid bolus of 1L NS

b. Reassess

   i. Patient appears unchanged from prior examination

K. Nurse

a. With antibiotics

   i. BP: 112/75 HR: 90 RR: 18 Sat: 100% on 4 L NC

b. Without antibiotics

   i. BP: 89/57 HR: 117 RR: 26 Sat: 98% on 4 L NC

c. CXR (Figure 87.2)

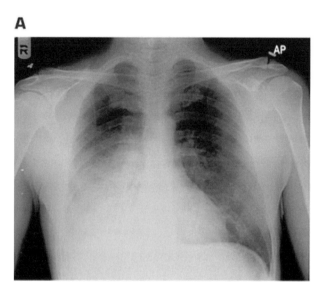

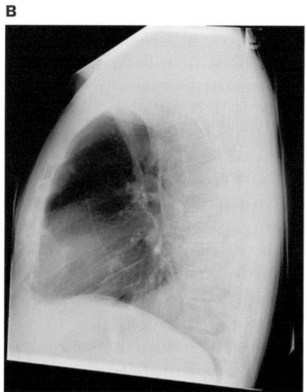

Figure 87.2 A and B

L. Results

Complete blood count:

WBC	16.7×10^3/uL
Hct	41.5%
Plt	250×10^3/uL

Basic metabolic panel:

Na	148 mEq/L
K	4.3 mEq/L
Cl	115 mEq/L
CO_2	21 mEq/L
BUN	49 mEq/dL
Cr	2.1 mg/dL%
Gluc	100 mg/dL

Coagulation panel:

PT	12.6 sec
PTT	26.0 sec
INR	1.0

Liver function panel:

AST	23 U/L
ALT	26 U/L
Alk Phos	42 U/L
T bili	1.0 mg/dL
D bili	0.3 mg/dL
Amylase	50 U/L
Lipase	25 U/L
Albumin	4.7 g/dL

Urinalysis:

SG	1.0.20
pH	7
Prot	Neg mg/dL
Gluc	Neg mg/dL
Ketones	Neg mg/dL
Bili	Neg
Blood	Neg
LE	Neg
Nitrite	Neg
Color	Yellow

a. Lactate 1.2 mmol/L with antibiotics (5.1 if no antibiotics given empirically)

M. Action

a. MICU contact for admission

b. If no antibiotics given empirically, initiate early goal-directed therapy (EGDT) with central venous access and central venous pressure monitoring

N. Nurse

a. Radiology machine fixed, CXR obtained (Figure 87.2A and 87.2B)

O. Diagnosis

a. Systemic inflammatory response syndrome (SIRS) due to pneumonia

P. Critical actions

▨ Large-bore IV access and fluid bolus

▨ Lactate

▨ CBC

▨ Blood and urine culture

▨ CXR

▨ Evaluate for sources of fever including cellulitis, decubitus ulcers, UA

▨ Early antibiotics – alternatively, aggressively resuscitate if not given early and patient decompensates

Q. Examiner instructions

a. This is a case of systemic inflammatory response syndrome (SIRS), a severe inflammatory state of the body caused by an infection, due to nosocomial pneumonia. The patient's temperature, heart rate, respiratory rate, and WBC count all fulfill SIRS. Important early actions include obtaining appropriate IV access and IV fluid resuscitation, giving broad-spectrum antibiotics, and checking lactate, urinalysis, CBC, cultures, and CXR. Since the CXR is not immediately available, the candidate must decide whether to give antibiotics early on the basis of the clinical diagnosis of pneumonia. If antibiotics are not given, the patient begins to manifest signs of septic shock. At this point, in addition to giving broad-spectrum antibiotics, the candidate must also initiate early goal-directed therapy by obtaining central access and central venous pressure monitoring.

R. Pearls

a. Systemic inflammatory response syndrome is a systemic inflammatory response to a variety of severe clinical insults. It is not a diagnosis, but rather a stratification tool for patients with systemic inflammation and can used in cases of trauma, burns, and pancreatitis in addition to infection.

b. SIRS is manifested by two or more of the following conditions: (1) temperature $>38°C$ or $<36°C$; (2) heart rate >90 beats/min; (3) respiratory rate >20 breaths/min or $PaCO_2$ <32 mmHg; and (4) white blood cell count $>12,000/$ L, $<4000/L$, or $>10\%$ immature (band) forms.

c. Meeting more of these criteria has been associated with an increase in mortality rates in prospective analysis of both medical and surgical patients.

d. Sepsis defines the state in which this systemic response is caused by infection.

S. References

a. Tintinalli's: Chapters 25, 146

b. Rosen's: Chapters 6, 138

CASE 88: Altered mental status (Tiffany Truong, MD, MPH)

A. Chief complaint
a. 81-year-old male brought in by EMS from home with the complaint of altered mental status

B. Vital signs
a. BP: 150/56 HR: 130 RR: 22 T: 43°C Sat: 95% on RA FS: 176 (must ask)

C. What does the patient look like?
a. Patient is a disheveled, elderly male on stretcher mumbling incoherently, accompanied by daughter.

D. Primary survey
a. Airway: maintaining airway
b. Breathing: no apparent respiratory distress, no cyanosis
c. Circulation: warm and dry skin, normal capillary refill
d. Disability: no focal deficits, normal pupils
e. Exposure: undress the patient completely

E. Action
a. Oxygen via NC or nonrebreather mask
b. Two large-bore peripheral IV lines
c. Labs
  i. CBC, BMP, LFT, coagulation studies, blood type and cross-match
  ii. Lactate, blood cultures, UA, urine culture, troponin
d. 500 ml of cooled NS bolus
e. Monitor: BP: 155/61 HR: 132 RR: 22 Sat: 100% on O_2
f. EKG

F. History
a. HPI: an 81-year-old male with a history of hypertension, diabetes, and hypercholesterolemia brought in by EMS from home for altered mental status. EMS found the patient lying on the ground next to the bed in a very warm apartment. The daughter states that patient lives alone and at baseline is able to take care of himself. The patient mentioned to her a few days prior that his air conditioning had broken down. He had hoped that the landlord would fix it quickly as the summer temperature was rising outside. She has not seen him for 4 days and became concerned when he did not answer his phone the last few times she had called. This prompted her to call EMS.
b. PMHx: hypertension, diabetes, and hypercholesterolemia
c. PSHx: appendectomy over 30 years ago
d. Allergies: none
e. Meds: unknown
f. Social: lives alone, ex-smoker (quit 20 years ago), no drugs, not sexually active
g. FHx: not relevant
h. PMD: Dr Jagoda

G. Nurse
a. EKG (Figure 88.1)
b. If 500 ml NS given:
  i. BP: 140/66 HR: 125 RR: 20 T: 42.0°C Sat: 98% on 2 L NC O_2
c. If no fluids given, vital signs remain the same as triage

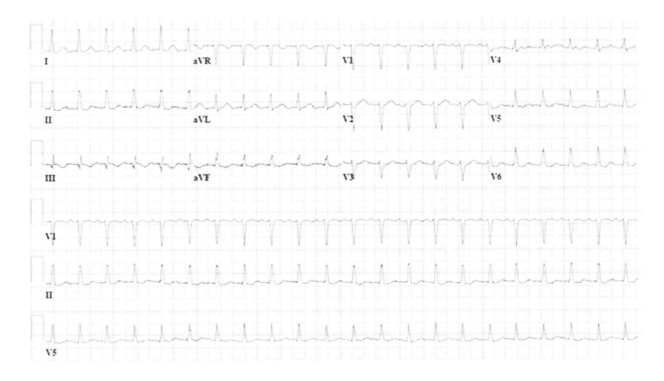

Figure 88.1

H. Secondary survey
  a. General: A & O × 0, cachetic elderly male, muttering incoherently, very warm to touch, not following commands, no apparent distress
  b. Head: normocephalic, atraumatic
  c. Eyes: mildly pale conjunctiva, extraocular movement intact, pupils equal, reactive to light
  d. Ears: normal tympanic membranes
  e. Nose: no discharge
  f. Neck: full range of motion, no jugular vein distension, no stridor
  g. Pharynx: dry mucous membranes, normal dentition, no lesions, no swelling
  h. Chest: nontender
  i. Lungs: clear bilaterally
  j. Heart: tachycardic rate, rhythm regular, no murmurs, rubs, or gallops
  k. Abdomen: normal bowel sounds, soft, nontender, nondistended
  l. Rectal: normal tone, brown stool, occult blood negative
  m. Urogenital: normal external genitalia
     i. Male: no discharge, normal testicular examination
  n. Extremities: full range of motion, no deformity, normal pulses
  o. Back: nontender
  p. Neuro: moves extremities equally spontaneously and withdraws to painful stimuli, uncooperative with rest of examination
  q. Skin: warm and dry, pale, no rashes, no edema, stage 1 ulcer on buttock, covered with stool and urine
  r. Lymph: no lymphadenopathy

I. Action
  a. Clean patient
  b. Hydration

     i. NS IVF 250 ml/hr
c. Cooling (evaporative or immersion)
     i. Evaporative cooling: position fans close to completely undressed patient and then spraying tepid water on the patient
     ii. Immersion cooling: place undressed patient into a tub of ice water to cover trunk and extremities
     iii. Adjuncts: ice pack to neck, axillae, and groin
d. Continuous core temperature monitor
     i. Insert electronic rectal probe thermometer
     ii. Discontinue cooling efforts if rectal temperature reaches 39°C to 40°C to avoid overshoot hypothermia
e. Monitor urine output
     i. Insert Foley catheter
f. Additional labs
     i. Myoglobin, TSH, toxicology screen, aspirin and acetaminophen levels
g. Meds
     i. Ceftriaxone IV
     ii. Vancomycin IV
     iii. Lorazepam IV (treat shivering)
h. Reassess
     i. Patient is now shivering from cooling
i. Imaging
     i. CXR
     ii. CT head
     iii. Lumbar puncture (after CT head)

J. Nurse
a. BP: 140/76 HR: 120 RR: 18 T: 41°C Sat: 98% on 2 L O$_2$ (after 1 L NS)
b. Patient: comfortable
c. CT head (Figure 88.2)
d. CXR (Figure 88.3)

Figure 88.2
A and B

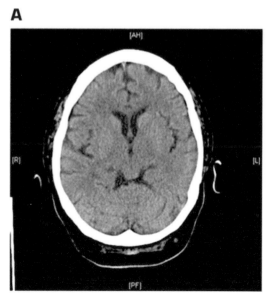 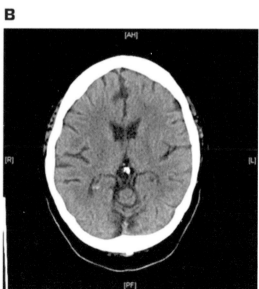

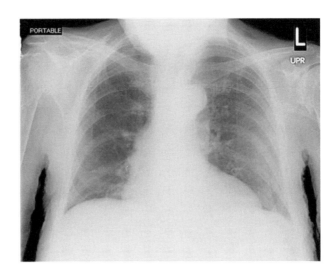

Figure 88.3

K. Results

Complete blood count:

WBC	$12.0 \times 10^3/uL$	T bili	1.0 mg/dL
Diff	56.6/8.4/1.8	D bili	0.3 mg/dL
Hct	36.5%	Amylase	50 U/L
Plt	$91 \times 10^3/uL$	Lipase	25 U/L
		Albumin	4.7 g/dL

Basic metabolic panel:

Na	155 mEq/L	**Urinalysis:**	
K	3.3 mEq/L	SG	1.010–1.030
Cl	121 mEq/L	pH	7
CO_2	19 mEq/L	Prot	Neg mg/dL
BUN	80 mEq/dL	Gluc	Neg mg/dL
Cr	2.1 mg/dL%	Ketones	Neg mg/dL
Gluc	202 mg/dL	Bili	Neg
		Blood	Neg
Coagulation panel:		LE	Neg
PT	12.6 sec	Nitrite	Neg
PTT	26.0 sec	Color	Yellow
INR	1.0		

Liver function panel:

		Arterial blood gas:	
AST	330 U/L	pH	7.4
ALT	230 U/L	PO_2	95 mmHg
Alk Phos	100 U/L	PCO_2	41 mmHg
		HCO_3	24 mmol/L

a. Lactate 1.8 mmol/L
b. Toxicology screen negative
c. PT/PTT 13.1/26 INR 1.2
d. Troponin normal, CPK 1580
e. Lumbar puncture clear, RBC 5, WBC 2 lymphocytes, glucose 66, protein 30, smear negative for organisms

L. Action

a. ICU consult

b. Discuss with family regarding advanced directives

c. Hydration: NS

M. Diagnosis

a. Heatstroke

N. Critical actions

▨ Check blood glucose

▨ Large-bore IV access and fluid bolus

▨ Immediate cooling

▨ Core temperature monitor

▨ CT head

▨ ICU admission

O. Examiner instructions

a. This is a case of classic heatstroke in an elderly patient who lives a sedentary lifestyle on medications for chronic illness. Heatstroke is a life-threatening condition in which the body loses its ability to regulate its temperature, causing dysfunction of multiple organ systems. It is caused by environmental heat exposure. The patient has been in a heated apartment with a broken air conditioner for days and presents with extremely high temperature. Important early actions include checking blood glucose, administering IV fluids, immediate cooling, continuous temperature monitor, and placement of Foley catheter to monitor urine output. In any patient presenting with altered mental status, it is paramount to rule out stroke and central nervous system infection; consider head CT head and lumbar puncture if warranted. It is also important to check for signs of end-organ and systemic injury (cardiac ischemia, pulmonary edema, elevated liver enzymes, renal failure, rhabdomyolysis, and coagulation disorders, for example). Patients who are intubated and hemodynamically labile require continued cooling and should be admitted to the ICU.

P. Pearls

a. The classic signs of heatstroke are CNS dysfunction, elevated temperature (usually above 40°C) and anhidrosis. This is a true medical emergency.

b. Anhidrosis (lack of sweating) may not be present for a variety of reasons, and is not considered an absolute diagnostic criteria.

c. Immediate, aggressive, rapid cooling down to 40°C. Morbidity is directly related to severity and duration of hyperthermia.

d. Supportive measures.

  i. Administer oxygen.

  ii. Those with classic heatstroke need IVF but do NOT rehydrate them aggressively (fluid requirements not large); rate 250 to 300 ml/hr.

  iii. Consider CVP monitoring to guide fluid therapy in the elderly or those with cerebral vascular disease.

   e. Meds

      i. Antipyretics (eg, acetaminophen, aspirin, ibuprofen) are not useful because anti-pyretics interrupt the change in the hypothalamic set point caused by pyrogens.

      ii. Control shivering with benzodiazepine or chlorpromazine as needed.

      iii. Dantrolene has not been demonstrated to be effective.

   f. Anticholinergic drugs are the most frequent cause of impaired sweating in classic heatstroke.

   g. Tachydysrhythmias are common and respond to cooling (do not cardioconvert).

   h. Management of encephalopathy is supportive, directed at minimizing cerebral edema by avoiding fluid overreplacement and assuring hemodynamic, thermal, and metabolic stability.

Q. References

a. Tintinalli's: Chapter 204

b. Rosen's: Chapter 141

CASE 89: Shortness of breath (Tiffany Truong, MD, MPH)

A. Chief complaint

a. 56-year-old male transferred from renal clinic by ambulance for hypotension, shortness of breath, and dizziness

B. Vital signs

a. BP: 86/40 HR: 128 RR: 22 T: 36.5°C Sat: 97% on RA FS: 178

C. What does the patient look like?

a. Cachectic male appears mildly short of breath, speaking in full sentences, and tachypneic.

D. Primary survey

a. Airway: speaking in full sentences

b. Breathing: rapid breathing; no apparent respiratory distress, no cyanosis

c. Circulation: pale and cool skin, normal capillary refill

E. Action

a. Oxygen via NC or nonrebreather mask

b. Two large-bore peripheral IV lines

c. Labs

      i. CBC, BMP, LFT, coagulation studies, blood type and screen.

      ii. Lactate, UA, troponin

d. 1 L NS bolus

e. Monitor: BP: 86/56 HR: 121 RR: 29 Sat: 96% on 2 L O_2

f. EKG

F. History

a. HPI: a 56-year-old male with past medical history of HIV, hypertension, and end-stage renal disease on hemodialysis sent from renal clinic after developing hypotension while receiving hemodialysis. Patient stated that his last hemodialysis was

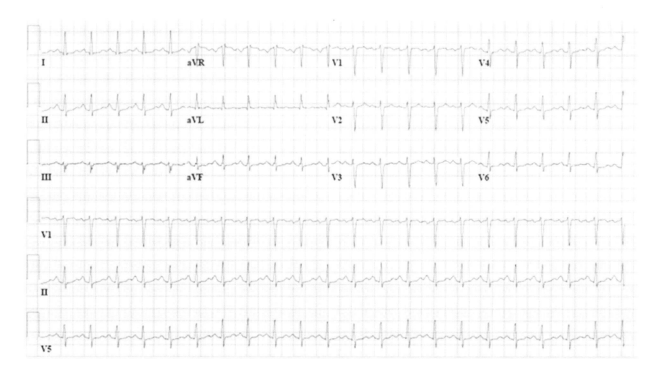

Figure 89.1

2 days ago and was told at that time his blood pressure was low. Today while receiving dialysis, he felt anxious then became short of breath, and was found to have low blood pressure. He completed most of his hemodialysis. He denies cough, fever, chills, nausea, vomiting, headache, chest pain, abdominal pain, urinary symptoms, lower extremity edema, or feeling ill.

b. PMHx: HIV+ (patient doesn't know his CD4 count), end-stage renal disease on hemodialysis, hypertension

c. PSHx: nephrectomy, right permacatheter placement

d. Allergies: none

e. Meds: does not remember, unable to locate transfer sheets

f. Social: lives in assisted-living facility, history of smoking and IV drug use in the past

g. FHx: not relevant

h. PMD: Dr Pepper

G. Nurse

a. EKG (Figure 89.1)

b. 1 L NS

i. BP: 103/73 HR: 108 RR: 22 Sat: 92% on 2 L O_2

c. No fluids

i. BP: 70/50 HR: 129 RR: 26 Sat: 92% on 2 L O_2

H. Secondary survey

a. General: A & O × 3, cachectic male, speaking in full sentences, rapid breathing, mild short of breath, + pulsus paradoxus

b. Head: normocephalic, atraumatic

c. Eyes: extraocular movement intact, pupils equal, reactive to light
d. Ears: normal tympanic membranes
e. Nose: no discharge
f. Neck: full range of motion, + jugular vein distension, no stridor
g. Pharynx: normal dentition, no lesions, no swelling
h. Chest: nontender
i. Lungs: tachypnea, good air entry, no crackles, wheezes, or rhonchi; trachea midline; right chest subclavian permacath in place with no surrounding erythema or drainage
j. Heart: diminished heart sounds, tachycardic rate, regular rhythm, no gallops or rubs, + pulsus paradoxus
k. Abdomen: normal bowel sounds, soft, nontender or distended, + hepatomegaly
l. Rectal: normal tone, brown stool, occult blood negative
m. Urogenital: normal external genitalia
    i. Male: no discharge, normal testicular examination
n. Extremities: full range of motion, no deformity, normal pulses, no edema
o. Back: nontender
p. Neuro: cranial nerves II to XII intact; normal sensation, strength; normal reflexes and gait
q. Skin: chronic venous stasis changes, no edema
r. Lymph: no lymphadenopathy

I. Action
a. Place patient on nonrebreather mask
b. Consultation
    i. Cardiology
    ii. Cardiothoracic surgery
c. Imaging
    i. CXR
    ii. Bedside ED cardiac sono (Figure 89.2)

J. Nurse
a. CXR (Figure 89.3)

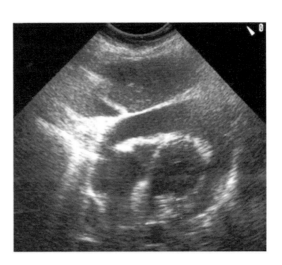

Figure 89.2

Figure 89.3

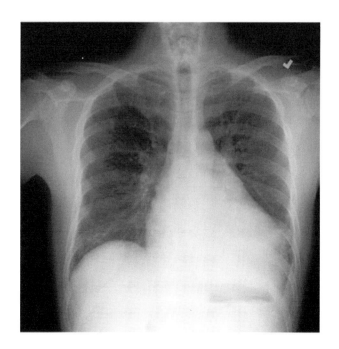

K. Results

Complete blood count:

WBC	4.6×10^3/uL	Alk Phos	42 U/L
Hct	32.7%	T bili	1.0 mg/dL
Plt	94×10^3/uL	D bili	0.3 mg/dL
		Amylase	50 U/L
Basic metabolic panel:		Lipase	25 U/L
Na	141 mEq/L	Albumin	4.7 g/dL
K	3.8 mEq/L		
Cl	101 mEq/L	**Urinalysis:**	
CO_2	22 mEq/L	SG	1.010–1.030
BUN	28 mEq/dL	pH	5–8
Cr	6.7 mg/dL%	Prot	Neg mg/dL
Gluc	94 mg/dL	Gluc	Neg mg/dL
		Ketones	Neg mg/dL
Coagulation panel:		Bili	Neg
PT	12.6 sec	Blood	Neg
PTT	26.0 sec	LE	Neg
INR	1.0	Nitrite	Neg
		Color	Yellow

Liver function panel:

AST	23 U/L
ALT	26 U/L

  a. Lactate 1.2 mmol/L
  b. Troponin normal

L. Action
  a. Consult
      i. Cardiothoracic surgery for emergent pericardial window

  b. Cardiology
     i. Confirms presence of cardiac tamponade
     ii. Recommends stat cardiothoracic surgery consult for pericardial window
  c. Admission
     i. OR

M. Diagnosis
a. Pericardial tamponade

N. Critical actions
▨ Large-bore IV access and fluid bolus
▨ CXR
▨ EKG
▨ Bedside cardiac echo
▨ Cardiothoracic surgery consult

O. Examiner instructions
a. This is a case of nontraumatic pericardial tamponade, a life-threatening condition caused by fluid accumulation around the heart which compresses the heart and prevents pumping. It is important to recognize that this is a medical emergency. His initial presentation of hypotension, tachycardia tachypnea, and shortness of breath should alert to the fact that he is an ill patient who may decompensate quickly. On examination, he presented with the classic signs of pericardial tamponade (Beck's triad): hypotension, + jugular venous distention, and diminished heart sounds. Although EKG, CXR, and echocardiography provide useful information, cardiac tamponade is a clinical diagnosis. Important early actions include administering IV fluids, consulting cardiothoracic surgery for pericardial window, keeping in mind that if the patient decompensated further, emergent ED pericardiocentesis may be necessary.

P. Pearls
a. Classic clinical findings: Beck's triad (hypotension, jugular venous distension, and distant heart sounds), narrow pulse pressure, dyspnea, tachycardia, pulsus paradoxus.
b. EKG: diminished amplitude, low voltage QRS, total electrical alternans.
c. Kussmaul's sign: rise in central venous pressure with spontaneous inspiration.
d. CXR: may not be used to exclude diagnosis since as little as 150 to 200 ml of effusion may result in cardiac tamponade in the acute setting. "Water bottle" shaped cardiac silhouette in chronic effusions is generally not seen in acute traumatic tamponade.
e. Echocardiography: gold standard for diagnosing perdicardial effusion and should be performed. Findings consistent with tamponade include the following:
     i. Diastolic collapse of right ventricle and right atrium
     ii. Echo-free space behind left ventricle and in front of right ventricle
     iii. Paradoxical septal motion
f. Temporizing measures include: IVF bolus and dobutamine or dopamine as needed for inotropic support.
g. In the settings of hemodynamic collapse pericardiocentesis should be performed emergently in the ED. Consider ultrasound guidance for this procedure.
h. Definitive therapy: pericardial window by cardiothoracic surgery.

Q. References

a. Tintinalli's: Chapter 259

b. Rosen's: Chapter 82

CASE 90: Stab to chest (Tiffany Truong, MD, MPH)

A. Chief complaint

a. 53-year-old female brought in by EMS for stab wound to chest and dyspnea

B. Vital signs

a. BP: 95/34 HR: 110 RR: 24 T: 37°C Sat: 95% on RA

C. What does the patient look like?

a. Anxious-appearing, middle-aged female, A & O × 3, appearing uncomfortable, tachypneic, and in moderate shortness of breath, speaking in short sentences.

D. Primary survey

a. Airway: speaking in short sentences

b. Breathing: moderate respiratory distress, no retractions or cyanosis; breath sounds diminished in right upper, middle, and lower chest; + right side jugular venous distention; unable to assess if there is tracheal deviation

c. Circulation: pink and warm skin, normal capillary refill

E. Action

a. Oxygen via NC or nonrebreather mask

b. Two large-bore peripheral IV lines

c. Labs

 i. CBC, chem 7, PT/PTT, type and cross-match two units

d. 1 L NS bolus

e. Monitor: BP: 95/34 HR: 110 RR: 24 T: 37°C Sat: 95% on RA

f. Decompression of pneumothorax using needle or tube thoracostomy (describe procedure to examiner)

g. Consult

 i. Surgery

F. Nurse

a. Decompression of pneumothorax

 i. BP: 110/56 HR: 84 RR: 18 Sat: 100% on O_2

 ii. Patient: breathing more comfortably, states she feels less short of breath

b. No decompression

 i. BP: 70/50 HR: 140 RR: 36 Sat: 92% on O_2

 ii. Patient: agitated, in severe respiratory distress

c. Consults

 i. Surgery/trauma

G. History

a. HPI: a 53-year-old female with history of breast cancer presents to the ED with the complaint of shortness of breath and stab to chest. Patient stated that while standing outside of a bar with her boyfriend she was stabbed once to the right anterior chest by an intoxicated male who ran away with her purse. She thought it looked like a small pocketknife. EMS stated that they found her sitting on the ground outside the bar complaining of difficulty in breathing. Patient denies any other injuries; no loss of consciousness.

b. PMHx: breast malignancy bilateral (ductal carcinoma in situ)
c. PSHx: hysterectomy 10 years ago, bilateral simple mastectomy with immediate reconstruction with tissue expanders followed by bilateral insertion of permanent saline breast implants
d. Allergies: none
e. Meds: none
f. Social: divorced, lives alone, 1 pack per day smoker since age 18, no drugs, not sexually active
g. FHx: noncontributory
h. PMD: Dr Deleon

H. Nurse
a. 1 L NS
   i. BP: 122/64 HR: 78 RR: 16 Sat: 100% on 2 L NC

I. Secondary survey
a. General: alert, oriented × 3, comfortable
b. Head: normocephalic, atraumatic
c. Eyes: extraocular movement intact, pupils equal, reactive to light
d. Ears: normal tympanic membranes
e. Nose: no discharge
f. Neck: full range of motion, no jugular vein distension (if chest tube in place), no stridor
g. Pharynx: normal dentition, no lesions, no swelling
h. Chest/lungs
   i. Needle decompression: breath sounds slightly diminished on right side, good air entry to left side, no wheezing or crackles, no ecchymosis, no crepitus, no bony tenderness
   ii. Chest tube: chest tube in right 4th intercostal space, midaxillary line, good air entry bilaterally, no wheezing or crackles, 2 cm linear wound to right 3 to 4 intercostal space in the mid axillary line above chest tube, no ecchymosis, crepitus, and bony tenderness
i. Heart: rate and rhythm regular, no murmurs, rubs, or gallops
j. Abdomen: normal bowel sounds, soft, nontender or distended
k. Rectal: normal tone, brown stool, occult blood negative
l. Urogenital: normal external genitalia
   i. Female: no blood or discharge, cervical os closed, no cervical motion tenderness, no adnexal tenderness
m. Extremities: full range of motion, no deformity, normal pulses
n. Back: nontender
o. Neuro: cranial nerves II to XII intact; normal sensation, strength; normal reflexes and gait
p. Skin: warm and dry, no other injuries noted except as described above
q. Lymph: no lymphadenopathy

J. Action

a. Bedside FAST examination (Figure 90.1)

b. Meds

    i. Morphine

    ii. Tetanus IM

c. Follow-up CXR (Figure 90.2) to assess tube positioning and lung reexpansion

Figure 90.1
A, B, C and D

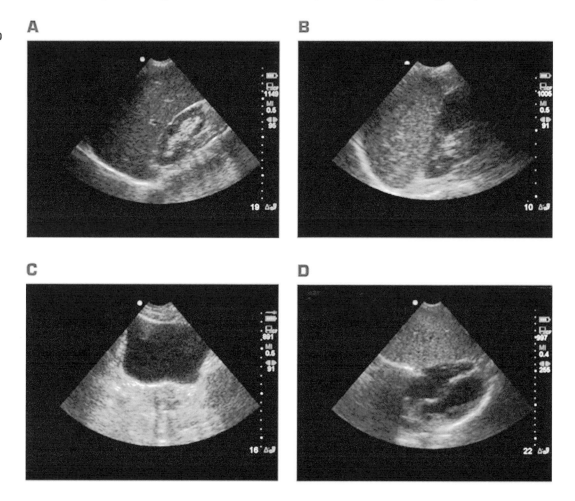

Figure 90.2

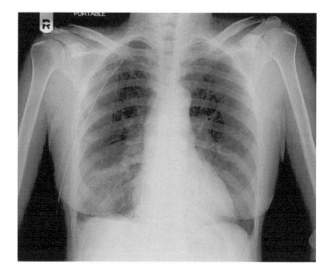

K. Nurse

a. BP: 125/79 HR: 88 RR: 16 Sat: 100% on 2 L O_2 (after 1 L)

b. Patient: feeling comfortable

L. Results

Complete blood count:

WBC	10.3×10^3/uL	D bili	0.3 mg/dL
Hct	39.1%	Amylase	50 U/L
Plt	142×10^3/uL	Lipase	25 U/L
		Albumin	4.7 g/dL

Basic metabolic panel:

Na	134 mEq/L	**Urinalysis:**	
K	4.3 mEq/L	SG	1.010–1.030
Cl	105 mEq/L	pH	5–8
CO_2	25 mEq/L	Prot	Neg mg/dL
BUN	12 mEq/dL	Gluc	Neg mg/dL
Cr	1.1 mg/dL%	Ketones	Neg mg/dL
Gluc	100 mg/dL	Bili	Neg
		Blood	Neg
		LE	Neg

Coagulation panel:

PT	12.6 sec	Nitrite	Neg
PTT	26.0 sec	Color	Yellow
INR	1.0		
		Arterial blood gas:	
		pH	7.4

Liver function panel:

AST	23 U/L	PO_2	95 mmHg
ALT	26 U/L	PCO_2	41 mmHg
Alk Phos	42 U/L	HCO_3	24 mmol/L
T bili	1.0 mg/dL		

M. Action

a. Consult

　i. Admitted to surgery

N. Diagnosis

a. Tension pneumothorax

O. Critical actions

▨ Emergent decompression of tension pneumothorax via tube thoracostomy, or needle decompression followed by immediate tube thoracostomy

▨ FAST examination (eFAST can be performed to support diagnosis of pneumothorax when in question)

▨ Pain management

▨ CXR to confirm chest tube placement

P. Examiner instructions

a. This is a case of a tension pneumothorax in a patient who suffered a stab wound to the chest. The condition is caused by a one-way air leak into the chest cavity secondary to a punctured lung which leads to air accumulation of air and compression of the heart. The patient presented with unstable vitals (hypotension, tachycardia, mild hypoxia, and tachypnea), moderate respiratory distress, and decreased breath sounds on the right side. Diagnosis of tension pneumothorax often requires a high level of suspicion in the presence of decreased or absent breath sounds on the affected side. The correct treatment is emergent needle decompression followed by thoracostomy tube. If the candidate asks for a CXR before needle decompression or chest tube, the patient will become more short of breath and the oxygen saturation will drop to 88%. If the patient's pneumothorax is still not decompressed, the patient will go into cardiac arrest.

Q. Pearls

a. Tension pneumothorax is a life-threatening condition that requires prompt management.

b. Tension pneumothorax is primarily a clinical diagnosis based on patient presentation. Do not delay delivery of treatment modalities while waiting for imaging or lab studies.

c. After needle decompression, immediately begin preparation to insert a thoracostomy tube. Then reassess the patient, as hemothorax is common with pneumothorax, especially in trauma. It may be necessary to place an additional thoracostomy tube.

d. Most common etiologies are trauma (blunt or penetrating) or iatrogenic, but pneumothorax has been seen in barotrauma secondary to positive-pressure ventilation, CPR, central venous catheter placement, or surgery.

e. Obtain a follow-up CXR to assess for lung reexpansion, thoracostomy tube positioning, and to correct any mediastinum deviation.

f. All patients with tension pneumothorax should be admitted.

R. References

a. Tintinalli's: Chapter 258

b. Rosen's: Chapter 45

CASE 91: Abdominal pain (Edward R. Melnick, MD, MHS)

A. Chief complaint

a. 50-year-old female brought in by EMS with the complaint of lower abdominal pain

B. Vital signs

a. BP: 135/83 HR: 98 RR: 18 T: 38.8°C Sat: 99% on RA FS: 94

C. What does the patient look like?

a. Patient appears stated age, in moderate distress due to pain.

D. Primary survey

a. Airway: speaking in full sentences

b. Breathing: no apparent respiratory distress, no cyanosis

c. Circulation: warm skin with mild diaphoresis, normal capillary refill

E. Action

a. Oxygen via NC or nonrebreather mask

b. Two large-bore peripheral IV lines

c. Labs
   i. CBC, BMP, LFT, coagulation studies, blood type and cross-match
   ii. UA, urine pregnancy test
d. 1 L NS bolus

F. History

a. HPI: a 50-year-old female with no past medical history was brought in by EMS with the complaint of lower abdominal pain. She describes the pain as sharp, constant, and progressively worsening for the last 36 hours with nausea and subjective fevers and chills. The pain does not radiate and has not migrated. She denies vomiting, back pain, urinary symptoms, and vaginal bleeding/discharge. She reports chronic constipation and denies diarrhea. Patient's last menstrual period was 3 weeks ago.
b. PMHx: hypertension and hypercholesterolemia
c. PSHx: none
d. Allergies: none
e. Meds: none
f. Social: denies alcohol use, smoking, or illicit drug use; lives with husband at home, sexually active and monogamous
g. FHx: not relevant
h. PMD: Dr Nelson

G. Secondary survey

a. General: alert, oriented × 3, moderate distress secondary to pain
b. Head: normocephalic, atraumatic
c. Eyes: extraocular movement intact, pupils equal, reactive to light
d. Ears: normal tympanic membranes
e. Nose: no discharge
f. Neck: full range of motion, no jugular vein distension, no stridor
g. Pharynx: normal dentition, no lesions, no swelling
h. Chest: nontender
i. Lungs: clear bilaterally
j. Heart: rate and rhythm regular, no murmurs, rubs, or gallops
k. Abdomen: normal active bowel sounds, soft with focal tenderness and voluntary guarding at LLQ, no masses, no hernias, nontender at McBurney's point, negative Murphy's sign, no rebound
l. Rectal: normal tone, brown stool, occult blood positive, nontender
m. Urogenital: normal external genitalia
   i. Female: no blood or discharge, cervical os closed, no cervical motion tenderness, no adnexal tenderness
n. Extremities: full range of motion, no deformity, normal pulses
o. Back: nontender, no CVA tenderness
p. Neuro: cranial nerves II to XII intact; normal sensation, strength; normal reflexes and gait
q. Skin: warm and dry
r. Lymph: no lymphadenopathy

H. Nurse

a. Patient: still with significant pain

b. Urine pregnancy test negative

I. Action

a. Meds

  i. Morphine

  ii. Acetaminophen

b. Reassess

  i. Patient still with significant discomfort, worsening until pain meds given, then discomfort improves

c. Consult

  i. Surgery

d. Imaging

  i. CT abdomen/pelvis with IV, PO, and rectal contrast

e. Diet

  i. NPO except PO contrast

J. Nurse

a. Vital signs

  i. With IV fluid

    1. BP: 135/83 HR: 86 RR: 18 Sat: 99% on RA

  ii. Without IV fluid

    1. BP: 135/83 HR: 108 RR: 18 Sat: 99% on RA

b. Patient: still with significant pain until pain meds given, then pain improved

K. Results

Complete blood count:	
WBC	16×10^3/uL
Diff	88.6/8.4/1.8
Hct	35.0%
Plt	327×10^3/uL

Basic metabolic panel:	
Na	138 mEq/L
K	4.3 mEq/L
Cl	105 mEq/L
CO_2	30 mEq/L
BUN	12 mEq/dL
Cr	1.1 mg/dL%
Gluc	100 mg/dL

Coagulation panel:	
PT	12.6 sec
PTT	26.0 sec
INR	1.0

Liver function panel:	
AST	23 U/L
ALT	26 U/L
Alk Phos	42 U/L
T bili	1.0 mg/dL
D bili	0.3 mg/dL
Amylase	50 U/L
Lipase	25 U/L
Albumin	4.7 g/dL

Urinalysis:	
SG	1.020
pH	7
Prot	Neg mg/dL
Gluc	Neg mg/dL
Ketones	Neg mg/dL
Bili	Neg
Blood	Neg
LE	Neg
Nitrite	Neg
Color	Yellow

a. CT abdomen/pelvis with IV and PO contrast – diverticulitis, without abscess (Figures 91.1–91.4)

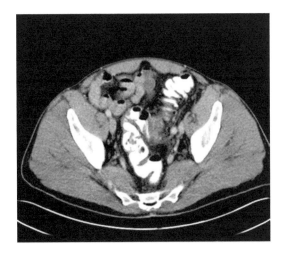

Figure 91.1

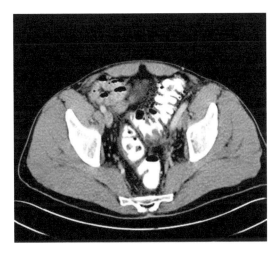

Figure 91.2

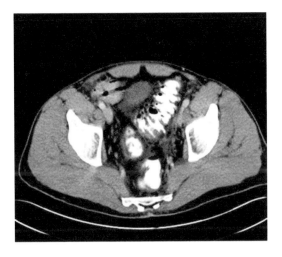

Figure 91.3

Figure 91.4

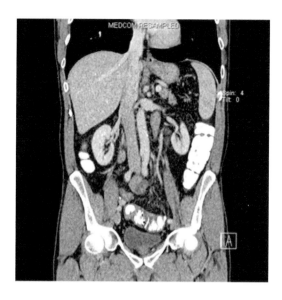

L. Action

a. Surgery consult

b. Discussion with family and PMD regarding need for admission, IV antibiotics, and bowel rest

c. Meds

   i. Gentamycin (or tobramycin) and metronidazole (or clindamycin), OR

   ii. Ticarcillin-clavulanic acid or imipenem, OR

   iii. If no antibiotics given, patient decompensates with worsening pain, low blood pressure, and high fever (sepsis)

d. NPO

e. Maintenance IV fluids

M. Diagnosis

a. Diverticulitis with fever

N. Critical actions

▪ Pelvic examination

▪ Urine pregnancy test

▪ Pain management

▪ CT abdomen/pelvis with IV and PO contrast

▪ Early surgery consult

▪ Antibiotics

O. Examiner instructions

a. This is a case of diverticulitis with fever, an infection in the large intestine that typically needs admission with IV antibiotics. Complications include perforation of bowel and abscess formation. The patient's symptoms of abdominal pain that is constant and localizing to the left lower quadrant are consistent with diverticulitis. Important early actions include administering IV fluids, evaluating for gynecologic diagnoses with a urine pregnancy test and pelvic examination. If fluids are not administered, the patient will become more tachycardic and eventually hypotensive. Her pain will continue to increase until an opioid medication (such as morphine) is administered. A CT abdomen/pelvis with IV and PO contrast is the diagnostic procedure of choice. Once the CT result is available the patient should be started on IV antibiotics, made NPO, and surgery consultation should be obtained. Without these actions, the patient will decompensate with a GI bleed or sepsis due to an intraabdominal abscess.

P. Pearls
a. The most common symptom of diverticulitis is pain.
b. One-third of Americans have diverticulosis by age 60 and two-thirds by age 85.
c. Diverticulitis is more common in men; however, frequency is increasing in women.
d. When younger patients develop diverticulitis, it tends to be more severe and require earlier surgical intervention.
e. Abdominal CT can show inflammation of pericolic fat, diverticuli, thickening of the bowel wall, or peridiverticular abscess.

Q. References
a. Tintinalli's: Chapter 85
b. Rosen's: Chapter 95

CASE 92: Seizure (Tiffany Truong, MD, MPH)

A. Chief complaint
a. 42-year-old female brought in by EMS from home accompanied by husband for "seizure"

B. Vital signs
a. BP: 190/100 HR: 100 RR: 16 T: 36°C Sat: 98% on RA FS: 110

C. What does the patient look like?
a. Patient appears stated age, lying on stretcher, comfortable, appears confused.

D. Primary survey
a. Airway: maintaining airway
b. Breathing: no apparent respiratory distress, no cyanosis
c. Circulation: pink and cool skin, normal capillary refill

E. Action
a. Oxygen via NC or nonrebreather mask
b. Two 16- or 18-gauge IV in antecubital fossa
c. Labs
   i. CBC, BMP, LFT, coagulation studies, blood type and cross-match
   ii. Lactate, urine pregnancy test, uric acid
d. Monitor: BP: 188/96 HR: 96 RR: 18 Sat: 100% on O_2 FS: 110

F. History
a. HPI: a 42-year-old female with a past medical history of hypertension brought into ED for seizures. G1P1A0, 7 days postpartum after an uncomplicated normal spontaneous vaginal delivery. She is brought in by EMS for possible seizure-like activity. Per husband, the patient has been "jerking her arms and legs" for about

2 to 3 minutes while sitting at the table after eating breakfast. Patient has been confused and sleepy ever since. The patient has no prior history of seizure. He states his wife was in her usual state of health except for complaint of headache and mild blurry vision in the past few days. She normally takes blood pressure medicine for her chronic hypertension but has forgotten to take them since her discharge from the hospital 6 days ago. She is currently breast-feeding. Husband denies fever, chills, vomiting, and abdominal pain.

b. PMHx: hypertension, breast cysts
c. PSHx: none
d. Allergies: PCN
e. Meds: none
f. Social: lives with husband at home, denies alcohol, smoking, drugs, not sexually active in the past 2 months
g. FHx: no family history of seizure
h. PMD: Dr Carpenter

G. Nurse
a. BP: 190/94 HR: 90 RR: 20 Sat: 98% on O_2
b. Patient: having another generalized tonic-clonic seizure; seizure stopped on its own after 2 minutes

H. Action
a. Meds
   i. Magnesium sulfate 4 to 6 g slowly over 15 minutes, then continuous IV infusion at 1 to 3 g/hr; place patient on cardiac monitor and have a Foley catheter placed; excretion is 100% renal so maintain the urine output at a rate >25 ml/hr
   ii. Lorazepam 2 mg IVP
b. Consults
   i. Emergency obstetric consultation

I. Secondary survey
a. General: appears postictal, confused, sleepy
b. Head: normocephalic, atraumatic
c. Eyes: extraocular movement intact, pupils 5mm equal, reactive to light
d. Ears: normal tympanic membranes
e. Nose: no discharge
f. Neck: full range of motion, no jugular vein distension, no stridor
g. Pharynx: normal dentition, no lesions, no swelling
h. Chest: nontender
i. Lungs: clear bilaterally
j. Heart: rate and rhythm regular, no murmurs, rubs, or gallops
k. Abdomen: no surgical scar, excess loose skin, midline striae, no masses, non-tender, + BS
l. Rectal: normal tone, brown stool, occult blood negative
m. Urogenital: normal external genitalia
   i. Female: no lochia, no vaginal bleeding, no signs of vaginal tear or episiotomy
n. Extremities: full range of motion, no deformity, normal pulses, 2+ bilateral pedal edema
o. Back: nontender

p. Neuro: grossly moving all four extremities, deep tendon reflexes 2+, appears postictal

q. Skin: warm and dry

r. Lymph: no lymphadenopathy

J. Nurse

a. BP: 180/86 HR: 90 RR: 16 Sat; 98% on O_2

b. Patient: resting comfortably in bed, no additional seizures, now more alert and answering questions, husband at bedside

K. Results

Complete blood count:

WBC	5.3×10^3/uL	Alk Phos	42 U/L
Hct	41.5%	T bili	1.0 mg/dL
Plt	350×10^3/uL	D bili	0.3 mg/dL
		Amylase	50 U/L
Basic metabolic panel:		Lipase	25 U/L
Na	138 mEq/L	Albumin	4.7 g/dL
K	4.3 mEq/L		
Cl	105 mEq/L	**Urinalysis:**	
CO2	30 mEq/L	SG	1.01
BUN	12 mEq/dL	pH	6.5
Cr	1.1 mg/dL%	Prot	large
Gluc	100 mg/dL	Gluc	Neg mg/dL
		Ketones	Neg mg/dL
Coagulation panel:		Bili	Neg
PT	12.6 sec	Blood	Neg
PTT	26.0 sec	LE	trace
INR	1.0	Nitrite	Neg
		Color	Yellow
Liver function panel:			
AST	23 U/L		
ALT	26 U/L		

a. Lactate 4.0 mmol/L

b. Uric acid pending

L. Action

a. Watch for signs of magnesium toxicity:

   i. Respiratory depression

   ii. Bradydysrhythmias

   iii. Loss of DTRs

b. Admitted to OB/GYN for observation

c. Meds

   i. Continue IV magnesium infusion

   ii. Labetolol IV

d. Imaging

   i. CT head (Figure 92.1)

e. Reassess

   i. Patient appears more alert and answering questions

Figure 92.1

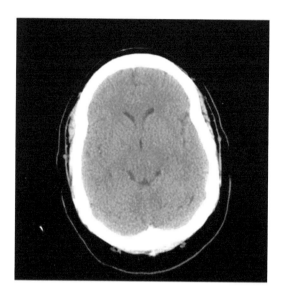

M. Diagnosis
a. Eclampsia

N. Critical actions
▪ Large-bore IV access
▪ Magnesium IV infusion
▪ CT head
▪ Emergency obstetric consultation
▪ UA

O. Examiner instructions
a. This is a case of eclampsia in a postpartum female. This is a condition that typically occurs during the last trimester of pregnancy associated with high blood pressure and seizures. The patient has a history of chronic hypertension and has been noncompliant with her medications in the past several days. She presented with several days of headache, blurry vision, new-onset seizure, and was found to have elevated blood pressure in the ED. She also has pedal edema and proteinuria. Important early actions include establishing IV access, administering magnesium sulfate for the seizure and antihypertensive medications as needed, and consulting obstetrics emergently.

P. Pearls
a. Eclampsia is the superimposition of generalized seizure on preeclampsia (hypertension, proteinuria, with or without edema).
b. Eclampsia can occur from the 20th week of gestation until up to 10 days postpartum (although it has been reported as late as 1 month postdelivery).
c. Eclampsia can occur without prior proteinuria.
d. Definitive treatment is delivery of the fetus. Get stat obstetrics consultation. Until that occurs or if the female is postpartum, give the following drug therapy:
   i. Magnesium sulfate
      1. Dose: 4 to 6 g IV over 5 to 15 minutes followed by 1 to 2 g/h
      2. Has both antiepileptic and antihypertension properties

3. Monitor for signs of toxicity: loss of DTR, respiratory depression, and bradydysrhythmias

ii. Hydralazine and labetolol are safe antihypertensive medications for eclamptic patients

e. All patients with sustained blood pressure of 140/90 mmHg or greater and any symptoms that may be related to the hypertensions should have stat obstetrics consultation and should be admitted.

f. Avoid ACE-inhibitor in pregnant females.

Q. References
a. Tintinalli's: Chapter 104
b. Rosen's: Chapter 178

CASE 93: Palpitations (Edward R. Melnick, MD, MHS)

A. Chief complaint
a. 59-year-old male brought in by EMS with the complaint of palpitations

B. Vital signs
a. BP: 101/73 HR: 162 RR: 22 T: 36.0°C Sat: 98% on RA FS: 167

C. What does the patient look like?
a. Patient appears older than stated age, pale, diaphoretic, and anxious.

D. Primary survey
a. Airway: speaking in full sentences
b. Breathing: no apparent respiratory distress, no cyanosis
c. Circulation: pale and warm skin, normal capillary refill

E. Action
a. Oxygen via NC or nonrebreather mask
b. Two large-bore peripheral IV lines
c. Place defibrillator/cardioverter pads on patient with defibrillator/cardioverter in case of deterioration.
d. Labs
    i. CBC, BMP, TSH, LFT, coagulation studies, blood type and cross-match
    ii. Troponin
e. 1 L NS bolus
f. Monitor: BP: 92/68 HR: 164 RR: 18 Sat: 100% on O_2, Rhythm strip (Figure 93.1)
g. EKG

F. History
a. HPI: a 59-year-old male with a history of coronary artery disease status post-myocardial infarction 2 years ago and hypertension brought in by EMS with the complaint of palpitations. He reports being awoken from sleep 30 minutes earlier at 5 am with palpitations, nausea, shortness of breath, and dizziness. EMS noted tachycardia on their monitor and gave the patient a bolus of amiodarone 150 mg.

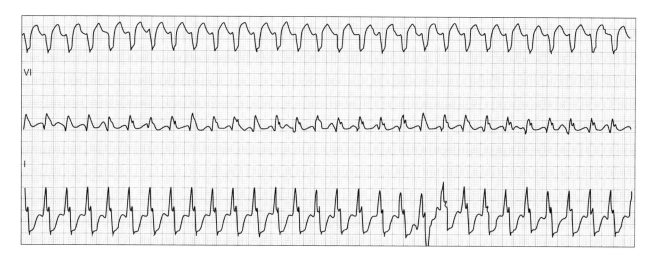

Figure 93.1

The patient's symptoms and rhythm strip failed to respond to this treatment. Patient denies chest pain, fever, cough, and syncope.

b. PMHx: coronary artery disease status postmyocardial infarction 2 years ago, hypertension, hypercholesterolemia

c. PSHx: coronary artery bypass graft 2 years ago

d. Allergies: none

e. Meds: hydrochlorothiazide, aspirin, losartan, atorvastatin

f. Social: lives with wife at home, quit smoking 20 years ago, denies alcohol or illicit drug use

g. FHx: father died of heart attack at age 53

h. PMD: Dr Bern

G. Nurse

a. EKG (Figure 93.2)

H. Action

a. Meds

   i. Amiodarone 150 mg IV bolus over 10 minutes

I. Secondary survey

a. General: alert, oriented × 3, pale, anxious

b. Head: normocephalic, atraumatic

c. Eyes: extraocular movement intact, pupils equal, reactive to light

d. Ears: normal tympanic membranes

e. Nose: no discharge

f. Neck: full range of motion, no jugular vein distension, no stridor

g. Pharynx: normal dentition, no lesions, no swelling

h. Chest: well-healed sternotomy scar, nontender

i. Lungs: clear bilaterally

j. Heart: tachycardic rate, rhythm regular, no murmurs, rubs, or gallops

k. Abdomen: normal bowel sounds, soft, nontender or distended

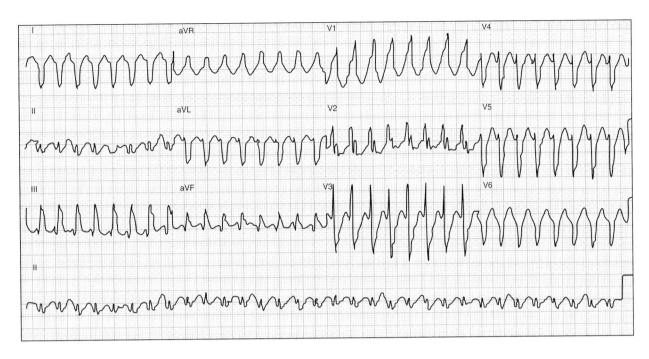

Figure 93.2

l. Rectal: normal tone, brown stool, occult blood negative

m. Urogenital: normal external genitalia
   i. Male: no discharge, normal testicular examination

n. Extremities: full range of motion, no deformity, normal pulses

o. Back: nontender

p. Neuro: cranial nerves II to XII intact; normal sensation, strength; normal reflexes
   and gait

q. Skin: warm and dry

r. Lymph: no lymphadenopathy

J. Action

a. Meds
   i. Amiodarone 150 mg IV bolus over 10 minutes

b. Reassess
   i. Rhythm strip unchanged from prior with or without amiodarone
   ii. BP: 106/71 HR: 161 RR: 20 Sat: 99% on O_2

c. Consult
   i. Cardiology

K. Nurse

a. Patient: complaining of chest pain

L. Action

a. Reassess
   i. Rhythm strip unchanged from prior with or without amiodarone
   ii. BP: 98/59 HR: 166 RR: 24 Sat: 99% on 2 L NC
   iii. Patient noted to be drowsy, cool, and diaphoretic

b. Synchronized cardioversion

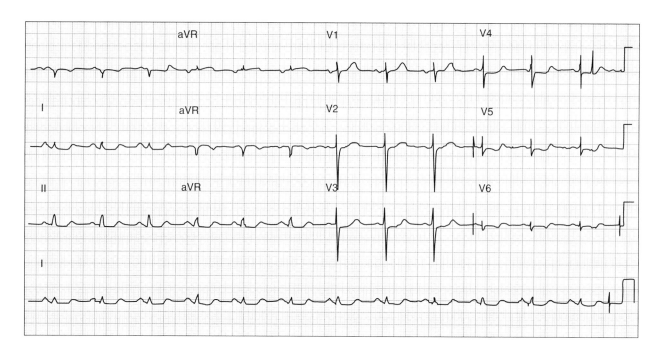

Figure 93.3

    i. Versed or equivalent for sedation (consider lower than usual moderate sedation dose due to low BP)

    ii. 100 J monophasic or equivalent biphasic

    iii. Rhythm strip converts to normal sinus rhythm after cardioversion

    iv. Order 12-lead EKG

M. Nurse

a. Patient

    i. If patient not cardioverted, patient noted to be pulseless and begin ACLS pulseless arrest algorithm

    ii. If patient cardioverted, chest pain improved, no longer feeling palpitations, nausea, and dizziness

b. EKG (Figure 93.3)

N. Results

Complete blood count:

WBC	6.4×10^3/uL
Hct	30.5%
Plt	250×10^3/uL

Basic metabolic panel:

Na	138 mEq/L
K	4.3 mEq/L
Cl	105 mEq/L
CO_2	30 mEq/L
BUN	12 mEq/dL
Cr	1.1 mg/dL%
Gluc	100 mg/dL

Coagulation panel:

PT	12.6 sec
PTT	26.0 sec
INR	1.0

Liver function panel:

AST	23 U/L
ALT	26 U/L
Alk Phos	42 U/L
T bili	1.0 mg/dL
D bili	0.3 mg/dL
Amylase	50 U/L
Lipase	25 U/L
Albumin	4.7 g/dL

Urinalysis:

SG	1.020	Nitrite	Neg
pH	7	Color	Yellow
Prot	Neg mg/dL		
Gluc	Neg mg/dL	**Arterial blood gas:**	
Ketones	Neg mg/dL	pH	7.4
Bili	Neg	PO_2	95 mmHg
Blood	Neg	PCO_2	41 mmHg
LE	Neg	HCO_3	24 mmol/L

a. Calcium 10.1, magnesium 2.2, phosphorous 3.8

b. Troponin I 0.6, CPK 308, CK-MB 19

O. Action

a. Cardiology consult

   i. CCU admission

b. Discussion with family regarding patient status and need for CCU admission

c. Med

   i. Amiodarone continuous drip 1 mg/min IV for 6 hours (360 mg), then 0.5 mg/min IV for 18 hours (540 mg)

P. Diagnosis

a. Ventricular tachycardia

Q. Critical actions

▨ 12-lead EKG

▨ Amiodarone boluses followed by drip while stable

▨ Synchronized cardioversion for instability, including hypotension, chest pain, or altered mental status

▨ Cardiology consult

R. Examiner instructions

a. This is a case of a ventricular tachycardia, likely from myocardial ischemia or infarction. Ventricular tachycardia is a life-threatening irregularity of the heart's conduction system, which is often caused by reduced blood flow to the heart. The patient's symptoms of palpitations, nausea, and dizziness occurred spontaneously, awaking him from sleep. Important early actions include obtaining a 12-lead EKG and administering amiodarone. This patient's ventricular tachycardia is refractory to amiodarone and will persist regardless of treatment (even treatment with lidocaine or procainamide). Eventually, the patient becomes unstable with chest pain, altered mental status, and hypotension. Without synchronized cardioversion (shock) at this point, the patient will become pulseless. After cardioversion, the patient will convert into normal sinus rhythm with a 12-lead EKG concerning for myocardial ischemia.

S. Pearls

a. Sudden cardiac death causes 460,000 deaths each year in the United States. Risk factors include age, male gender, coronary artery disease, left ventricular hypertrophy, congestive heart failure, and prolonged QT interval.

b. Myocardial ischemia decreases the homogeneity of left ventricular depolarization and repolarization that can cause reentry and sustained ventricular tachyarrhythmias.

c. Defibrillation and cardioversion simultaneously depolarize all cardiac tissue and terminate any sites of reentry causing all cardiac cells to be in the same depolarized state. This allows a dominant pacemaker – usually the sinus node – to pace the heart.

d. Wolff-Parkinson-White syndrome, Brugada and prolonged QT syndrome can also all cause fatal tachydysrhythmias.

T. References

a. Tintinalli's: Chapters 12, 22

b. Rosen's: Chapter 79

c. ACLS tachycardia with pulse algorithm (see Appendix E)

CASE 94: Seizure (Ram Parekh, MD)

A. Chief complaint

a. 28-year-old female brought in by her boyfriend who states the patient "had a seizure"

B. Vital signs

a. BP: 85/63 HR: 130 RR: 20 T: 36.2°C Sat: 98% on RA FS: 110 (must ask)

C. What does the patient look like?

a. Patient appears stated age, drowsy but arousable to painful stimuli, supine on stretcher, vomitus noted on clothes.

D. Primary survey

a. Airway: speaking in full sentences

b. Breathing: tachypneic but no apparent respiratory distress, no cyanosis

c. Circulation: dry and cool skin, normal capillary refill

E. Action

a. Oxygen via NC or nonrebreather mask

b. Two large-bore peripheral IV lines

c. Labs

   i. CBC, BMP, LFT, coagulation studies, blood type and cross-match, UA, urine pregnancy test

   ii. Blood cultures, lactate, alcohol level, acetaminophen level, salicylate level, urine toxicology screen

d. 1 L NS bolus

e. Monitor: BP: 92/68 HR: 112 RR: 18 Sat: 100% on O$_2$,

f. Rectal temperature

g. EKG

F. History

a. HPI: a 28-year-old female with a history of depression. According to the boyfriend, she has been taking amitriptyline for the past 6 months, and today admitted to

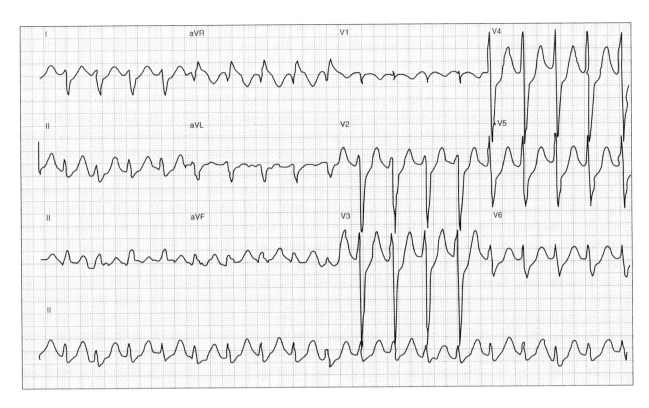

Figure 94.1

taking "a lot" of pills after a fight they had ~2 hours ago. Patient initially was nauseous, then vomited twice and then become "sleepy". Boyfriend admits to an argument taking place, states he left the patient in the bedroom after the argument but then was concerned when she did not come out after some time. He reports the patient was found lying in bed upon reentering bedroom, was able to arouse her briefly to ascertain what happened, at which time the patient developed a generalized tonic-clonic seizure lasting less than 1 minute. No prior suicidal attempts as per boyfriend. No known fevers, chills, headaches, rashes, abdominal pain, diarrhea, dysuria. Currently menstruating. In usual state of health before argument.
b. PMHx: depression
c. PSHx: none
d. Allergies: none
e. Meds: amitriptyline
f. Social: denies alcohol use, smoking, and illicit drug use; lives with boyfriend in apartment;
g. FHx: no relevant history
h. PMD: Dr Jung (psychiatrist)

G. Nurse
a. EKG (Figure 94.1)
b. 2 L NS
    i. BP: 98/59 HR: 115 RR: 18 Sat: 98% on O_2
c. Rectal temperature 100.6°F

H. Secondary survey

  a. General: drowsy but arousable, oriented to person

  b. Head: normocephalic, atraumatic

  c. Eyes: extraocular movement intact, 6 mm pupils, equal, sluggish to light

  d. Ears: normal tympanic membranes

  e. Nose: no discharge

  f. Neck: full range of motion, no jugular vein distension, no stridor

  g. Pharynx: normal dentition, no lesions, no swelling

  h. Chest: nontender

  i. Lungs: clear bilaterally

  j. Heart: tachycardic rate and rhythm regular, no murmurs, rubs, or gallops

  k. Abdomen: mildly tender in epigastrium, bowel sounds significantly decreased, no masses, no hernias, nontender at McBurney's, negative Murphy's sign, no rigidity

  l. Rectal: normal tone, brown stool, occult blood negative

  m. Extremities: full range of motion, no deformity, normal pulses

  n. Back: nontender

  o. Neuro: cranial nerves II to XII intact; normal sensation, strength; normal reflexes and gait

  p. Skin: warm and dry

  q. Lymph: no lymphadenopathy

I. Action

  a. Meds

    i. Sodium bicarbonate

    ii. Consider activated charcoal only if decision is made to intubate given risk for aspiration

  b. Consult

    i. Poison Control Center

    ii. Medical ICU

  c. Repeat EKG

J. Nurse

  a. 1 L NS

    i. BP: 98/59 HR: 125 RR: 18 Sat: 98% on O_2

  b. No fluids

    i. BP: 70/45 HR: 140 RR: 20 Sat: 98% on O_2

  c. Patient: still drowsy, has repeat generalized tonic-clonic seizure lasting 30 seconds

K. Action

  a. Meds

    i. Lorazepam IV

    ii. Sodium bicarbonate

L. Nurse

  a. Repeat EKG (Figure 94.2)

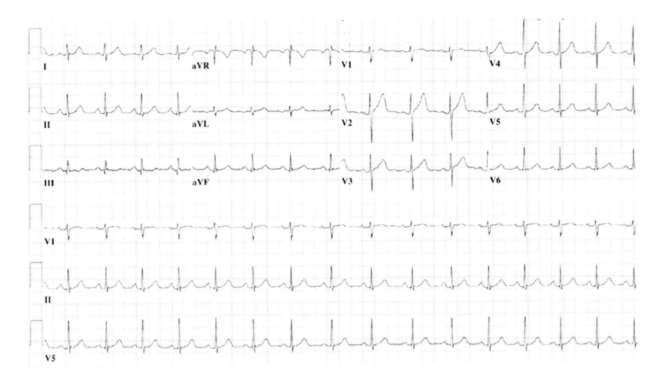

Figure 94.2

M. Results

Complete blood count:

WBC	$5.3 \times 10^3/uL$	ALT	26 U/L
Hct	41.5%	Alk Phos	42 U/L
Plt	$350 \times 10^3/uL$	T bili	1.0 mg/dL
		D bili	0.3 mg/dL
Basic metabolic panel:		Amylase	50 U/L
Na	138 mEq/L	Lipase	25 U/L
K	4.3 mEq/L	Albumin	4.7 g/dL
Cl	105 mEq/L		
CO_2	18.9 mEq/L	**Urinalysis:**	
BUN	22 mEq/dL	SG	1.015
Cr	1.1 mg/dL%	pH	6
Gluc	100 mg/dL	Prot	Neg mg/dL
		Gluc	Neg mg/dL
Coagulation panel:		Ketones	Neg mg/dL
PT	12.6 sec	Bili	Neg
PTT	26.0 sec	Blood	Neg
INR	1.0	LE	Neg
		Nitrite	Neg
Liver function panel:		Color	Yellow
AST	23 U/L		

a. Lactate 2.2 mmol/L

b. Urine pregnancy test negative

c. Urine tox screen pending

d. Serum tox screen

i. EtOH 6
ii. Acetaminophen <5
iii. Salicylate <5

N. Action
a. Admit to medical ICU

O. Diagnosis
a. Tricyclic antidepressant toxicity

P. Critical actions
▓ Large-bore peripheral IV access
▓ Fluid bolus
▓ EKG
▓ Repeat EKG after treatment
▓ Sodium bicarbonate
▓ Medical ICU

Q. Examiner instructions
a. This is a case of intentional tricyclic antidepressant (TCA) in a suicidal attempt. Taking large doses of TCA is a medical emergency that can lead to life-threatening abnormalities in heart rhythm, seizures, and death if untreated. In this patient, the symptoms of nausea, vomiting, mental status changes, and seizures began within 2 hours of amitryptyline ingestion signifying a large dose or co-ingestion of another drug. Important early actions include administering IV fluids, preferably NS for hypotension, obtaining an EKG, alkalizing the serum for increased excretion and sodium loading to reduce risk of cardiac dysrhythmias, and management of TCA-induced seizures. If an EKG is not obtained early in the course of management, the patient should seize.

R. Pearls
a. Most poison control directors in the United States use a QRS of 100 msec or greater as the cutoff for IV sodium bicarbonate.
b. The greatest risk of seizures and arrhythmias occurs within the first 6 to 8 hours of TCA ingestion.
c. Normal saline IV fluids are indicated for TCA-induced hypotension. For hypotension refractory to IV saline, vasopressors such as phenylephrine or norepinephrine, with α-agonist effect, may be used.
d. Once the patient is stabilized, activated charcoal can be considered for gastrointestinal decontamination.
e. The treatment of choice for prolonged or recurrent seizures in TCA toxicity is a benzodiazepine though most are self-limited.

S. References
a. Tintinalli's: Chapter 171
b. Rosen's: Chapter 151

CASE 95: Fever (Ram Parekh, MD)

A. Chief complaint
a. 66-year-old male presents to the ED with fever to 101.2°F and abdominal pain in setting of recent liver transplantation

B. Vital signs
a. BP: 110/63 HR: 114 RR: 22 T: 101.2°F Sat: 98% on RA FS: 120 (must ask)

C. What does the patient look like?
a. Patient appears stated age and in no acute distress.

D. Primary survey
a. Airway: speaking in full sentences
b. Breathing: tachypneic but in no apparent respiratory distress, no cyanosis
c. Circulation: warm to touch, well perfused

E. Action
a. Oxygen via NC or nonrebreather mask
b. Two large-bore peripheral IV lines
c. Labs
  i. CBC, BMP, LFT, coagulation studies, blood type and cross-match
  ii. Blood cultures, UA, urine culture, lactate, immunosuppressant levels
d. 1 L NS bolus
e. Monitor: BP: 118/69 HR: 108 RR: 22 Sat: 100% on O_2
f. EKG
g. CXR
h. Meds
  i. Acetaminophen

F. History
a. HPI: a 66-year-old male with a history of hepatitis B cirrhosis, status post-liver transplantation 3 weeks ago, presents to the ED with fever to 101°F each day for the past 4 days associated with diffuse abdominal pain and distension. Other than mild generalized malaise, he denies any other symptoms such as nausea, vomiting, diarrhea, dysuria, frequency, headaches, cough, rhinorrhea, vision complaints, or neurological symptoms.
b. PMHx: hepatitis B cirrhosis
c. PSHx: orthotopic liver transplantation 3 weeks ago
d. Allergies: none
e. Meds: cyclosporine, azathioprine, prednisone
f. Social: married with 2 children, denies alcohol, smoking, or recreational drugs
g. FHx: not relevant

G. Nurse
a. EKG (Figure 95.1)
b. 500 cc NS bolus
c. Acetaminophen PO
  i. BP: 115/75 HR: 102 RR: 20 T: 37.6°C Sat: 100% on O_2

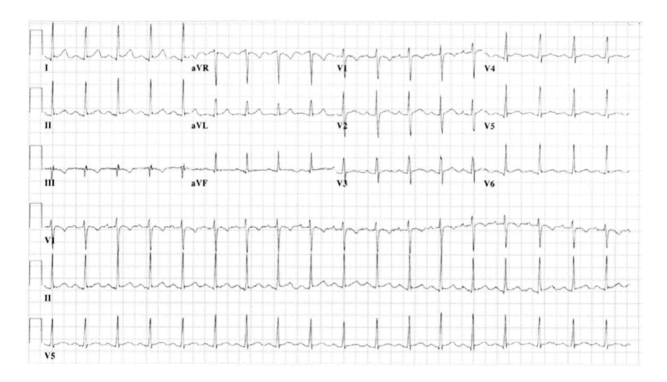

Figure 95.1

H. Secondary survey

a. General: alert, oriented × 3, comfortable
b. Head: normocephalic, atraumatic
c. Eyes: extraocular movement intact, pupils equal, reactive to light, icteric sclera
d. Ears: normal tympanic membranes
e. Nose: no discharge
f. Neck: full range of motion, no jugular vein distension, no stridor
g. Pharynx: normal dentition, no lesions, no swelling
h. Chest: nontender
i. Lungs: clear bilaterally
j. Heart: tachycardic rate, rhythm regular, no murmurs, rubs, or gallops
k. Abdomen: surgical incision well-healed, moderate diffuse tenderness, ascites present with distension. No guarding or rebound tenderness
l. Rectal: deferred due to concern for neutropenia
m. Urogenital: normal external genitalia
   i. Male: no discharge, normal testicular examination
n. Extremities: full range of motion, no deformity, normal pulses
o. Back: nontender
p. Neuro: cranial nerves II to XII intact; normal sensation, strength; normal reflexes and gait
q. Skin: hot to touch, jaundice to lower extremities, peripherally flushed
r. Lymph: no lymphadenopathy

I. Action

a. Ultrasound-guided abdominal paracentesis: cell count with differential, glucose, protein, Gram stain, and culture

Figure 95.2

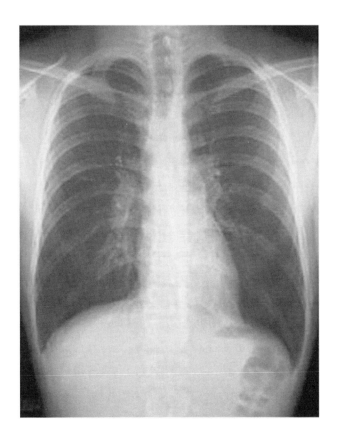

b. Meds
    i. Piperacillin and tazobactam
    ii. Vancomycin
    iii. Fluconazole
c. Reassess
d. Consult
    i. Liver transplant doctor

J. Nurse
a. CXR (Figure 95.2)
b. BP: 89/59 HR: 128 RR: 22 Sat: 98% on O_2 (after 500 cc bolus)
c. Patient: still complaining of abdominal pain

K. Action
a. Continue IV hydration with NS
b. Obtain central access using aseptic technique
c. Reassess
d. Morphine IV

L. Nurse
a. BP: 119/70 HR: 98 RR: 22 Sat: 98% on O_2 (after 1 L)

M. Action
a. Imaging
    i. Abdominal US

N. Results

Complete blood count:

WBC	$1.1 \times 10^3/uL$
Diff	45/9.4/1.2
Hct	41.5%
Plt	$350 \times 10^3/uL$

Basic metabolic panel:

Na	138 mEq/L
K	4.3 mEq/L
Cl	105 mEq/L
CO_2	30 mEq/L
BUN	12 mEq/dL
Cr	1.1 mg/dL%
Gluc	100 mg/dL

Coagulation panel:

PT	14 sec
PTT	26.0 sec
INR	1.3

Liver function panel:

AST	23 U/L
ALT	26 U/L
Alk Phos	42 U/L
T bili	9.0 mg/dL
D bili	4.1 mg/dL
Amylase	50 U/L
Lipase	25 U/L
Albumin	3.3 g/dL

Urinalysis:

SG	1.020
pH	6
Prot	Neg mg/dL
Gluc	Neg mg/dL
Ketones	Neg mg/dL
Bili	large
Blood	Neg
LE	Neg
Nitrite	Neg
Color	Yellow

a. Lactate 4.2 mmol/L
b. Peritoneal fluid: 274 polymorphonuclear cells, Gram negative
c. US abdomen: (Figure 95.3): 3.4 cm by 4.5 cm fluid collection concerning for hepatic abscess with hepatic artery thrombosis and ascites
d. Patient: return from radiology
e. BP: 103/54 HR: 112 RR: 22 Sat: 98% on O_2

O. Action

a. Discussion with liver transplant team
    i. Admit for IV antibiotics and possible abscess drainage
    ii. Reverse isolation hospital bed/ICU
b. Discussion with family and PMD regarding need for hospitalization to rule out infection/rejection

Figure 95.3

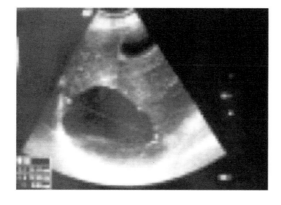

P. Diagnosis
a. Postliver transplant fever

Q. Critical actions
▨ IV access and fluid bolus
▨ Cultures before antibiotics
▨ Paracentesis with peritoneal fluid analysis/culture
▨ Broad-spectrum antibiotics
▨ Pain medication
▨ Contacting appropriate consultant

R. Examiner instructions
a. This is a case of a fever in a post-transplant patient, which is a serious concern because these patients are on multiple medications to suppress their immunity and are at high risk for serious infections. The patient's symptoms of fevers, abdominal pain, ascites, and malaise began 4 days before evaluation. Important early actions include administering IV fluids, preferably isotonic fluids (NS or lactated ringers) for hypotension, obtaining cultures of blood, urine, and peritoneal fluid via ultrasound-guided paracentesis, early antibiotics, contacting the appropriate consultant (in this case the liver transplant team), and appropriate disposition to the ICU given high risk and signs of ongoing SIRS or sepsis once cell count results are obtained. If CT ordered, may substitute for US but report the radiologist states the "scanner is full" and may take a while to obtain study.

S. Pearls
a. Fever in most transplant recipients should be considered an emergency.
b. Bacterial infection is most common in the first month post-transplant. Although gram-negative organisms predominate (especially *Pseudomonas aeruginosa*), gram-positive and anaerobic organisms are not uncommon.
c. During the first postoperative month, intra-abdominal infections including cholangitis, peritonitis, and liver predominate.
d. Fungi are also common within the first month post-transplantation.
e. Although there is large regional variability, the incidence of tuberculosis in solid organ transplant recipients is 20 to 74 times the general population with a mortality rate approaching 30%.
f. US and CT are appropriate in the work-up of post-liver transplant patients with fever, ascites, jaundice, and abdominal pain.

T. References
a. Tintinalli's: Chapter 90
b. Rosen's: Chapter 184

CASE 96: Abdominal trauma (Ram Parekh, MD)

A. Chief complaint
a. 46-year-old male brought in by EMS on backboard and cervical collar in full spinal precautions after being involved in a high-speed motor vehicle collision

B. Vital signs

a. BP: 95/63 HR: 120 RR: 20 T: 36.2°C Sat: 98% on RA FS: 110

C. What does the patient look like?

a. Patient appears stated age, immobilized, moaning and complaining of abdominal pain.

D. Primary survey

a. Airway: speaking in full sentences

b. Breathing: no apparent respiratory distress, no cyanosis

c. Circulation: diaphoretic and cool skin, normal capillary refill

E. Action

a. Oxygen via NC or nonrebreather mask

b. Two large-bore peripheral IV lines

c. Labs

   i. CBC, BMP, LFT, coagulation studies, blood type and cross-match 2 units

   ii. Lactate, alcohol level

d. 1 L NS bolus

e. Monitor: BP: 98/69 HR: 112 RR: 22 Sat: 100% on O_2

F. History

a. HPI: a 46-year-old male with a history of hypertension was the unrestrained driver in a 30- to 40-mph motor vehicle collision, car versus tree, with significant front car damage with intrusion and bent steering wheel. Airbag was deployed. The patient was extricated by EMS, noted to have a GCS 15 and not ambulatory on scene. The patient denies loss of consciousness and denies alcohol ingestion; complains mainly of significant abdominal pain; denies head injury, headache, nausea, vomiting, neck pain, numbness, tingling, shortness of breath, dizziness, or chest pain.

b. PMHx: hypertension

c. PSHx: none

d. Allergies: none

e. Social: married with 2 children, social EtOH, denies smoking, drugs

f. FHx: no relevant history

G. Nurse

a. 1 to 2 L NS

   i. BP: 105/75 HR: 102 RR: 18 Sat: 100% on O_2

b. No fluid

   i. BP: 80/45 HR: 120 RR: 24 Sat: 98% on O_2

H. Secondary survey (must include use of logroll technique with spinal immobilization)

a. General: alert, oriented × 3, spinal immobilization, complaining of abdominal pain

b. Head: normocephalic, atraumatic

c. Eyes: extraocular movement intact, pupils equal, reactive to light

d. Ears: normal tympanic membranes

e. Nose: no discharge

  f. Neck: cervical collar, no gross deformity or abrasion

  g. Pharynx: normal dentition, no lesions, no swelling

  h. Chest: nontender

  i. Lungs: clear bilaterally

  j. Heart: rate and rhythm regular, no murmurs, rubs, or gallops

  k. Abdomen: horizontal abrasion to epigastrium, diffuse tenderness, moderately distended, left flank ecchymosis, bowel sounds mildly decreased, no masses, no hernias, no rebound, no rigidity

  l. Pelvis: stable

  m. Rectal: normal tone, brown stool, occult blood negative, normal prostate

  n. Urogenital: normal external genitalia

    i. Male: no discharge, normal testicular examination

  o. Extremities: full range of motion, no deformity, normal pulses

  p. Back: nontender

  q. Neuro: cranial nerves II to XII intact; normal sensation, strength; normal reflexes and gait

  r. Skin: warm and dry

  s. Lymph: no lymphadenopathy

I. Action

  a. Foley placement

  b. Meds

    i. Morphine

  c. Reassess

    i. Patient still with significant pain

  d. Consult

    i. Trauma surgery or general surgery

  e. Imaging

    i. CXR

    ii. Pelvic x-ray

    iii. FAST examination (Figure 96.1)

  f. EKG

J. Nurse

  a. CXR (Figure 96.2)

  b. Pelvic x-ray (Figure 96.3)

  c. EKG (Figure 96.4)

  d. BP: 89/59 HR: 128 RR: 22 Sat: 98% on O_2 (after 1 L)

  e. Patient: still complaining of abdominal pain, abdominal distension worsening

K. Action

  a. Infuse O + packed red blood cells 1 unit; awaiting 2 units cross-matched

  b. Imaging

    i. Repeat FAST (Figure 96.1)

L. Nurse

  a. Blood

    i. BP: 119/70 HR: 98 RR: 22 Sat: 98% on O_2 (after 1 L NS, 1U PRBC)

Figure 96.1
A, B, C and D

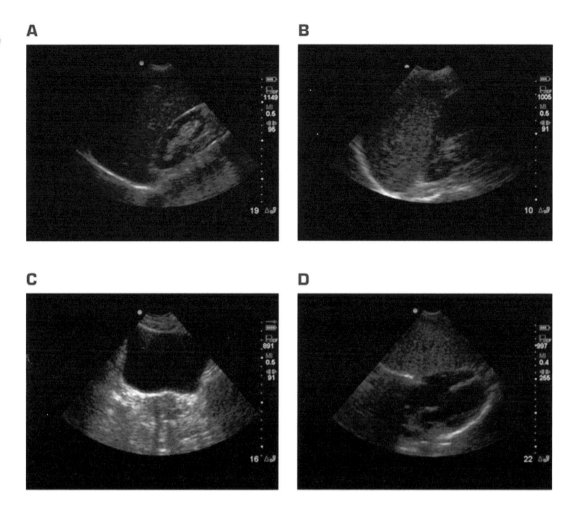

Figure 96.2

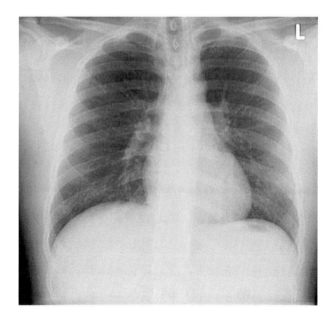

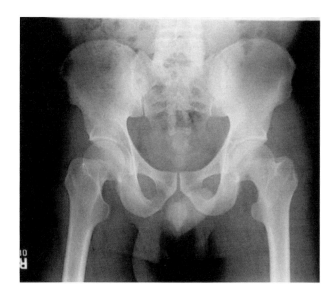

Figure 96.3

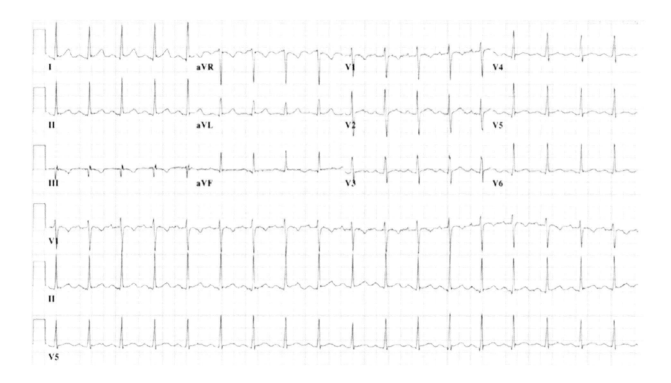

Figure 96.4

b. No blood or less than 2 L NS
   i. BP: 70/30 HR: 130 RR: 28 Sat: 96% on O_2

M. Action

a. Imaging
   i. CT head
   ii. CT cervical spine
   iii. CT chest/thoracic spine
   iv. CT abdomen/pelvis/lumbar spine

N. Results

Complete blood count:

WBC	5.3×10^3/uL
Hct	37.5%
Plt	350×10^3/uL

Basic metabolic panel:

Na	138 mEq/L
K	4.3 mEq/L
Cl	105 mEq/L
CO_2	30 mEq/L
BUN	12 mEq/dL
Cr	1.1 mg/dL%
Gluc	100 mg/dL

Coagulation panel:

PT	12.6 sec
PTT	26.0 sec
INR	1.0

Liver function panel:

AST	23 U/L
ALT	26 U/L
Alk Phos	42 U/L
T bili	1.0 mg/dL
D bili	0.3 mg/dL
Amylase	50 U/L
Lipase	25 U/L
Albumin	4.7 g/dL

Urinalysis:

SG	1.020
pH	7
Prot	Neg mg/dL
Gluc	Neg mg/dL
Ketones	Neg mg/dL
Bili	Neg
Blood	Neg
LE	Neg
Nitrite	Neg
Color	Yellow

a. Lactate 4.2 mmol/L
b. CT head – (Figure 96.5)
c. CT cervical spine – (Figure 96.6) negative
d. CT chest/thoracic spine – (Figure 96.7) negative
e. CT abdomen/pelvis/lumbar spine (Figure 96.8)
  i. Grade IV splenic laceration with rupture and retroperitoneal hemorrhage
f. Patient: Returns from radiology
g. BP: 83/54 HR: 132 RR: 22 Sat: 98% on O_2

Figure 96.5

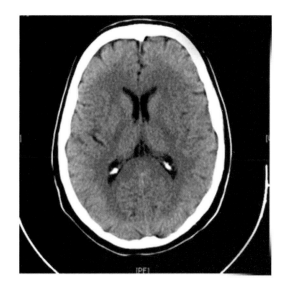

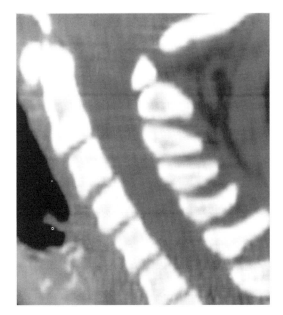

Figure 96.6

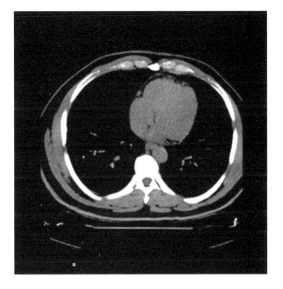

Figure 96.7

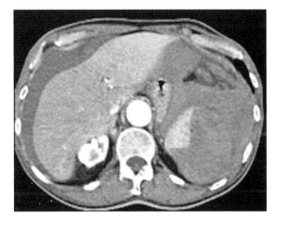

Figure 96.8

O. Action

a. Discussion with trauma surgeon

   i. To operating room for laparotomy (surgeon initially reluctant)

b. Discussion with family and PMD regarding need for emergent OR for hemostasis and splenectomy

P. Diagnosis

a. Blunt abdominal trauma – splenic rupture

Q. Critical actions

▧ Large-bore IV access and fluid bolus

▧ Blood type and cross-match

▧ Pain control

▧ Trauma surgery or general surgery

▧ FAST examination

▧ Early PRBC infusion with destabilization of vital signs

▧ Advocate for laparotomy once the patient decompensates and diagnosis of splenic rupture made on CT

R. Examiner instructions

a. This is a case of splenic rupture from blunt abdominal trauma, an injury which can lead to significant bleeding when severe. The patient's symptoms of abdominal pain, distention, hypotension, and tachycardia in the setting of a high-speed MVC point to intraabdominal injury with hemorrhage when other sources of bleeding (brain, chest, extremity) have been ruled out. Important early actions include obtaining large-bore IV line access, administering initial IV fluid challenge, preferably NS for hypotension, performing a FAST examination including thoracic views, early PRBC infusion once hemorrhage recognized, early trauma surgery involvement, pain control, and advocating for laparotomy given the patient decompensated twice with CT findings of splenic rupture. If IV access is not obtained in a timely fashion, resuscitation will be slowed. If pain is not controlled, full evaluation of the patient's injuries will be difficult.

S. Pearls

a. Although protected under the bony ribcage, the spleen remains the most commonly affected organ in blunt injury to the abdomen in all age groups.

b. The spleen is a highly vascular organ that filters an estimated 10% to 15% of total blood volume every minute.

c. CT scanning has made conservative management more practical and safer for victims of splenic injury; however, unstable patients with presumed intra-abdominal injury and clinical signs of hemorrhagic shock including abdominal distension, peritoneal signs, and hypotension require emergent operative intervention for hemostasis especially in high-risk patients such as those on anticoagulation.

d. The lethal triad of hypothermia, coagulopathy, and acidosis must be avoided with proper resuscitation to offer the patient the best chance of survival and minimal morbidity.

T. References

a. Tintinalli's: Chapter 260

b. Rosen's: Chapter 46

CASE 97: Hematochezia (Ram Parekh, MD)

A. Chief complaint

a. 20-day-old male infant brought in by parents for poor feeding and blood in diaper

B. Vital signs

a. BP: 68/43 HR: 162 RR: 50 T: 36.2°C Sat: 98% on RA FS: 110

C. What does the patient look like?

a. Patient is listless appearing neonate with sunken eyes, intermittently crying without tear formation.

D. Primary survey

a. Airway: intermittently crying

b. Breathing: no apparent respiratory distress, no cyanosis

c. Circulation: mucous membranes dry, no tears, thready brachial pulse, poor skin turgor, tachycardic

E. Action

a. Oxygen supplementation (blow-by oxygen)

b. Peripheral IV access, largest caliber possible

c. Labs

    i. CBC, BMP, LFT, coagulation studies, blood type and cross-match

    ii. Lactate, blood cultures

d. 20 cc/kg NS bolus

e. Monitor: BP: 66/38 HR: 166 RR: 45 Sat: 100% on O_2 T: 37.8°C

F. History

a. HPI: a 20-day-old male neonate status post normal spontaneous vaginal delivery at 29 weeks' gestational age, with birth weight 975g, is brought in by mom because he has not been feeding well over the past 2 days. He had an unremarkable postnatal course in the neonatal intensive care unit, formula fed since 7 days of age. Mother notes the baby has been crying incessantly and noted bright red blood in the diaper with the last bowel movement 4 hours before arrival. There have been no fevers or vomiting. He has not taken any feeds since last night, but has made wet diapers today.

b. PMHx: 29-week preterm infant

c. PSHx: none

d. Allergies: none

e. Social: lives at home with mom and dad; no tobacco exposure

f. FHx: unremarkable

G. Nurse

a. 20 cc/kg NS bolus

    i. BP: 74/49 HR: 140 RR: 55 Sat: 98% on O_2

b. No IV fluids

    i. BP: 59/30 HR: 170 RR: 75 Sat: 98% on O_2

H. Secondary survey

a. General: awake, crying but lethargic, current weight 2175g

b. HEENT: dry oral mucosa, sunken anterior fontanelle, sunken eyes

c. Neck: normal

d. Chest: deep, rapid breathing

e. Heart: tachycardic, no murmurs

f. Abdomen: + distension, diffusely tender, bowel sounds decreased, no masses, no hernias

g. Rectal: no anal fissures appreciated, positive for gross blood, yellow stool, hemoccult positive

h. Urogenital: normal, descended testes

i. Extremities: normal, radial pulse rapid and weak, capillary refill 2 seconds

j. Back: normal

k. Neuro: normal

l. Skin: normal, delayed retraction on pinch

I. Action

a. Spinal tap, urine catherization for culture, urinalysis

b. Meds
    i. Vancomycin IV
    ii. Cefotaxime IV
    iii. Clindamycin IV

c. Reassess
    i. Neonate still crying inconsolably

d. Consult
    i. Pediatric surgery

e. Imaging
    i. Upright and left lateral decubitus abdominal x-ray

J. Nurse

a. BP: 72/49 HR: 40 RR: 55 Sat: 98% on O_2 (after 20 cc/kg bolus)

b. Patient: had brief period of bradycardia to 40 beats/minute

K. Results

Complete blood count:

WBC	12.1×10^3/uL
Diff	88.6/8.4/1.8
Hct	39.5%
Plt	253×10^3/uL

Basic metabolic panel:

Na	138 mEq/L
K	4.3 mEq/L
Cl	105 mEq/L
CO_2	30 mEq/L
BUN	22 mEq/dL
Cr	0.8 mg/dL%
Gluc	100 mg/dL

Coagulation panel:

PT	12.6 sec
PTT	26.0 sec
INR	1.0

Liver function panel:

AST	23 U/L
ALT	26 U/L
Alk Phos	42 U/L
T bili	1.0 mg/dL
D bili	0.3 mg/dL
Amylase	50 U/L
Lipase	25 U/L
Albumin	4.7 g/dL

Urinalysis:

SG	1.020
pH	7
Prot	Neg mg/dL
Gluc	Neg mg/dL
Ketones	Positive
Bili	Neg
Blood	Neg
LE	Neg
Nitrite	Neg
Color	Yellow

Figure 97.1

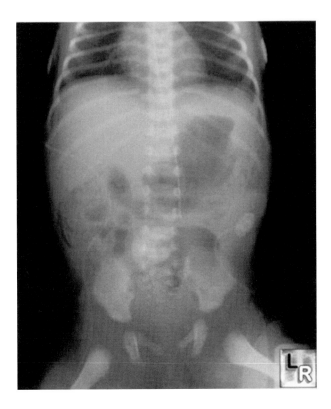

a. Lactate 3.2 mmol/L

b. Abdominal x-ray (Figure 97.1)

L. Action

a. Pediatric surgery consult

    i. To admit for IV antibiotics and possible OR

b. Discussion with family and PMD regarding need for admission for parenteral antibiotics and feeding and possible need for operative intervention

M. Diagnosis

a. Necrotizing enterocolitis

N. Critical actions

■ IV access and fluid bolus

■ Abdominal x-ray +/− US (if suspicion high and inconclusive x-ray)

■ Cultures/antibiotics to rule out sepsis, NOS

■ Pediatric surgery consult

O. Examiner instructions

a. This is a case of necrotizing enterocolitis, a serious condition that can occur in neonates causing inflammation and resulting injury to the intestine and often leading to intestinal rupture. The patient's symptoms of poor feeding, irritability, abdominal distension with tenderness, and blood in stools began fairly indolently and progressively worsened over a period of hours. Important early actions include administering IV fluids, sending blood, urine, and CSF cultures, consulting pediatric surgery, starting antibiotics, obtaining an abdominal x-ray +/− US if x-ray inconclusive. If fluids are not administered, the patient's blood pressure will begin to drop due to worsening dehydration. An abdominal and left lateral decubitus x-ray can be readily obtained; if an US is ordered, note that the radiologist is busy, and it will "be a while" before the test can be performed. Note the patient has a clinical picture consistent with moderate dehydration.

P. Pearls

a. Blood in the diaper or stool can be a difficult complaint to evaluate in the ED. After the first few days of life, coagulopathies, necrotizing enterocolitis, anal fissures, allergic or infectious colitis, and congenital defects should be considered.

b. Necrotizing enterocolitis remains incompletely understood, but is thought to be multifactorial. It is the result of inflammation or injury to the bowel wall that has been associated with infectious causes and hypoxic-ischemic insults.

c. Anterior-posterior (AP) abdominal and left lateral decubitus x-ray are the mainstay of diagnostic imaging for pediatric abdominal complaints. The classic x-ray finding is pneumatosis intestinalis.

d. Free air may be seen and is a surgical emergency. Consider early antibiotics, fluids, and surgical consultation.

Q. References

a. Tintinalli's: Chapter 124
b. Rosen's: Chapter 172

CASE 98: Abdominal pain (Anita Vashi, MD)

A. Chief complaint

a. 68-year-old male brought in by son with the complaint of worsening abdominal pain for the past 2 days

B. Vital signs

a. BP: 90/68 HR: 98 RR: 18 T: 39.2°C Sat: 98% on RA FS: 80

C. What does the patient look like?

a. Patient appearing uncomfortable secondary to pain in mild distress, lying still supine on stretcher.

D. Primary survey

a. Airway: speaking in full sentences
b. Breathing: no apparent respiratory distress, no cyanosis
c. Circulation: pale and cool skin, normal capillary refill

E. Action

a. Oxygen via NC or nonrebreather mask
b. Two large-bore peripheral IV lines
c. Labs
   i. CBC, BMP, LFT, coagulation studies, blood type and cross-match
   ii. Lactate, UA, blood cultures, urine culture
d. 1 L NS bolus
e. Monitor: BP: 91/68 HR: 99 RR: 18 Sat: 100% on O_2
f. EKG

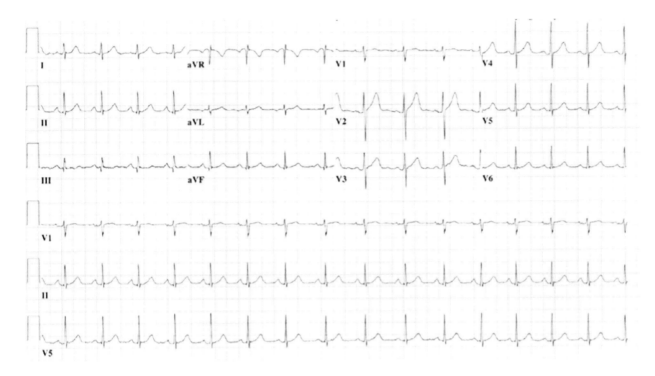

Figure 98.1

F. History

a. HPI: a 68-year-old male with history of cirrhosis secondary to hepatitis C, esophageal varices, hypertension, and chronic renal insufficiency with the complaint of worsening abdominal pain over the past 2 days. Pain is constant, diffuse, and worse with movement. Symptoms are associated with fever and chills; denies nausea, vomiting, diarrhea, chest pain, or shortness of breath. Son notes patient seems more tired and slow to answer today compared to baseline.

b. PMHx: cirrhosis, hepatitis C, esophageal varicies, hypertension, chronic renal insufficiency; denies any history of spontaneous bacterial peritonitis; has had paracentesis in past, last several months ago

c. PSHx: esophageal banding following an episode of upper gastrointestinal bleed several years ago

d. Allergies: none

e. Meds: noncompliant

f. Social: lives at home alone, alcohol use in the past (quit 10 years ago), ex-smoker (quit 5 years ago), remote history of IV drug use (1 year ago), not sexually active

g. FHx: no relevant history

h. PMD: Dr Manoogian

G. Nurse

a. EKG (Figure 98.1)

b. 1 L NS

  i. BP: 98/59 HR: 90 RR: 18 Sat: 98% on O_2

c. No fluids

  i. BP: 90/97 HR: 101 RR: 20 Sat: 98% on O_2

Figure 98.2
A and B

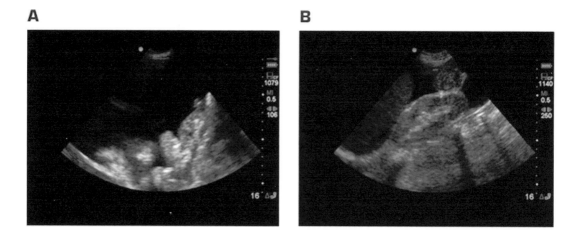

H. Secondary survey
  a. General: alert, oriented × 3, comfortable
  b. Head: mildly icteric conjunctivae, normocephalic, atraumatic
  c. Eyes: extraocular movement intact, pupils equal, reactive to light
  d. Ears: normal tympanic membranes
  e. Nose: no discharge
  f. Neck: full range of motion, no jugular vein distension, no stridor
  g. Pharynx: normal dentition, no lesions, no swelling
  h. Chest: nontender
  i. Lungs: clear bilaterally
  j. Heart: tachycardic rate, rhythm regular, no murmurs, rubs, or gallops
  k. Abdomen: soft, + distension, diffusely tender, − rebound, − guarding, + large ascites, + hepatosplenomegaly, no pulsatile masses, no hernias, bowel sounds normal
  l. Rectal: normal tone, brown stool, occult blood negative
  m. Urogenital: normal external genitalia
      i. Male: no discharge, normal testicular examination
  n. Extremities: full range of motion, no deformity, normal pulses, 2+ pitting edema to knees
  o. Back: nontender
  p. Neuro: cranial nerves II to XII intact; normal sensation, strength; normal reflexes and gait, mild asterixis
  q. Skin: warm and dry, slightly jaundiced
  r. Lymph: no lymphadenopathy

I. Action
a. Procedures
    i. Bedside abdominal US (Figure 98.2A and 98.2B)
    ii. Paracentesis
        1. Must send fluid for cell count, Gram stain, culture
        2. Also helpful to check fluid protein, glucose, and LDH levels
b. Meds
    i. Cefotaxime
    ii. Morphine

c. Reassess
  i. Patient still with moderate discomfort

J. Nurse

a. BP: 98/59 HR: 90 RR: 18 Sat: 98% on O_2 (after 1L fluids)

b. Patient: still with significant pain

K. Results

Complete blood count:

WBC	16.1×10^3/uL	Alk Phos	153 U/L
Diff	89.2/7.4/1.9	T bili	4.3 mg/dL
Hct	41.5%	D bili	3.1 mg/dL
Plt	350×10^3/uL	Amylase	50 U/L
		Lipase	25 U/L
Basic metabolic panel:		Albumin	2.2 g/dL
Na	138 mEq/L		
K	4.3 mEq/L	**Urinalysis:**	
Cl	105 mEq/L	SG	1.020
CO_2	30 mEq/L	pH	7
BUN	47 mEq/dL	Prot	Neg mg/dL
Cr	2.6 mg/dL%	Gluc	Neg mg/dL
Gluc	100 mg/dL	Ketones	Neg mg/dL
		Bili	positive
Coagulation panel:		Blood	Neg
PT	16.6 sec	LE	Neg
PTT	26.0 sec	Nitrite	Neg
INR	1.7	Color	Yellow

Liver function panel:

AST	93 U/L
ALT	150 U/L

a. Lactate 2.2 mmol/L

b. Urine culture in progress

c. Ascitic fluid: cloudy
  i. Cell count: 425 WBC, 90% PMNs
  ii. Albumin 0.5
  iii. Total protein 0.7
  iv. Gram stain/culture: pending

d. Blood culture in progress

e. CXR (Figure 98.3)

L. Action

a. Admit

b. Meds
  i. Morphine
  ii. Lactulose

Figure 98 3

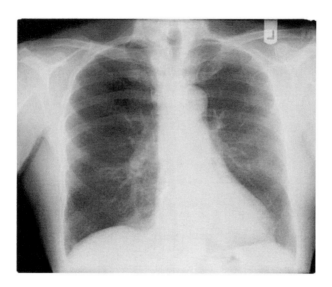

M. Diagnosis
a. Spontaneous bacterial peritonitis

N. Critical actions
- IV access and fluid bolus
- Early paracentesis
- Early antibiotics
- Pain management

O. Examiner instructions
a. This is a case of spontaneous bacterial peritonitis (SBP) in a patient with cirrhosis. SBP is an isolated spontaneous infection of the abdominal fluid collection that often occurs in patients with end-stage liver disease. Critical early actions include initial resuscitation with IV fluids, pan culturing, and most important, early antibiotics. If fluids and antibiotics are not given early, patient's clinical course will deteriorate with a drop in blood pressure.

P. Pearls
a. Diagnosis of SBP requires paracentesis with a fluid polymorphonucleocyte count of greater than 250 cells/mm^3. However, when suspicion is high (unexplained fever, abdominal pain, or change in mental status) antibiotics should be started immediately after paracentesis without waiting for results.
b. Fever is the most common presentation.
c. Findings of shock before antibiotic administration is an ominous sign.
d. The most frequent organism isolated in SBP is *Escherichia coli*, followed by streptococcal species.
e. Spontaneous peritonitis should be distinguished from secondary peritonitis.

Q. References
a. Tintinalli's: Chapter 83
b. Rosen's: Chapter 90

CASE 99: Cough (Anita Vashi, MD)

A. Chief complaint

a. 42-year-old male brought in by EMS with the complaint of worsening cough and shortness of breath for the past 8 hours

B. Vital signs

a. BP: 90/50 HR: 107 RR: 28 T: 37.2°C Sat: 92% on RA FS: 90

C. What does the patient look like?

a. Patient appears stated age, diaphoretic, uncomfortable-appearing secondary to moderate respiratory distress.

D. Primary survey

a. Airway: speaking in full sentences

b. Breathing: tachypneic, mildly cyanotic

c. Circulation: pale and cool skin, normal capillary refill

E. Action

a. Oxygen via nonrebreather mask

b. Two large-bore peripheral IV lines

c. Labs
   i. CBC, BMP, LFT, coagulation studies, VBG and lactate, blood type and cross-match
   ii. Blood cultures

d. 1 L NS bolus

e. Monitor: BP: 105/70 HR: 96 RR: 26 Sat: 96% on nonrebreather mask

f. EKG

F. History

a. HPI: a 42-year-old farmer with no past medical history states he has been suffering from 2 days of flu-like symptoms including fever, nonproductive cough, malaise, myalgias. Today, however, symptoms worsened with additional shortness of breath and difficulty breathing; denies any chest pain, nausea, vomiting, or diarrhea; no sick contacts; no recent travel.

b. PMHx: none

c. PSHx: none

d. Allergies: none

e. Social: lives with wife at home, occupation consists of farming with animals including an alpaca wool business (must inquire about nature of occupation), denies EtOH, smoking, drugs

f. FHx: no relevant history

g. PMD: Dr Nicklaus

G. Nurse

a. EKG (Figure 99.1)

H. Secondary survey

a. General: alert, oriented × 3, moderate distress secondary to tachypnea

b. Head: normocephalic, atraumatic

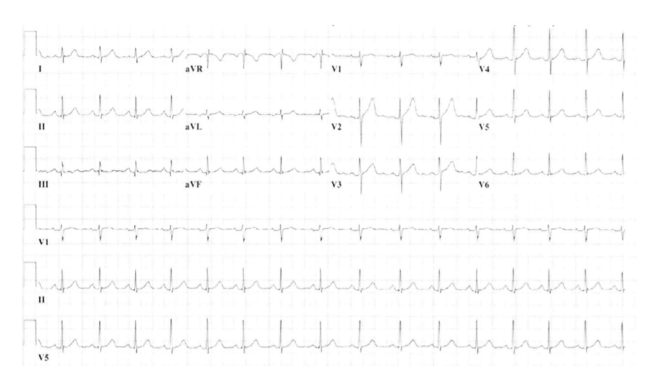

Figure 99.1

c. Eyes: extraocular movement intact, pupils equal, reactive to light
d. Ears: normal tympanic membranes
e. Nose: no discharge
f. Neck: full range of motion, no jugular vein distension, no stridor
g. Pharynx: normal dentition, no lesions, no swelling
h. Chest: nontender
i. Lungs: scattered crackles at bilateral bases
j. Heart: tachycardic, no murmurs, rubs, or gallops
k. Abdomen: normal bowel sounds, soft, nontender or distended
l. Rectal: normal tone, brown stool, occult blood negative
m. Urogenital: normal external genitalia
    i. Male: no discharge, normal testicular examination
n. Extremities: full range of motion, no deformity, normal pulses
o. Back: nontender
p. Neuro: cranial nerves II to XII intact; normal sensation, strength; normal reflexes and gait
q. Skin: pale, diaphoretic, no rashes, no edema, no lesions, no cellulitis
r. Lymph: no lymphadenopathy

I. Action
a. Reassess
    i. Patient with worsening respiratory distress and tachypnea
b. Imaging
    i. CXR

J. Nurse

a. BP: 110/79 HR: 120 RR: 38 Sat: 92% on O_2 (after 1 L)

b. Patient: with increasing moderate to severe respiratory distress

K. Results

Complete blood count:

WBC	13.0×10^3/uL	D bili	0.3 mg/dL
Hct	41.5%	Amylase	50 U/L
Plt	350×10^3/uL	Lipase	25 U/L
		Albumin	4.7 g/dL

Basic metabolic panel:

		Urinalysis:	
Na	138 mEq/L		
K	4.3 mEq/L	SG	1.0.20
Cl	105 mEq/L	pH	7
CO_2	30 mEq/L	Prot	Neg mg/dL
BUN	12 mEq/dL	Gluc	Neg mg/dL
Cr	1.1 mg/dL%	Ketones	Neg mg/dL
Gluc	100 mg/dL	Bili	Neg
		Blood	Neg
Coagulation panel:		LE	Neg
PT	12.6 sec	Nitrite	Neg
PTT	26.0 sec	Color	Yellow
INR	1.0		

Arterial blood gas:

Liver function panel:		pH	7.42
AST	23 U/L	PO_2	66 mmHg
ALT	26 U/L	PCO_2	25 mmHg
Alk Phos	42 U/L	HCO_3	24 mmol/L
T bili	1.0 mg/dL		

a. Lactate 4.5 mmol/L

b. Portable CXR (Figure 99.2)

c. Troponin negative

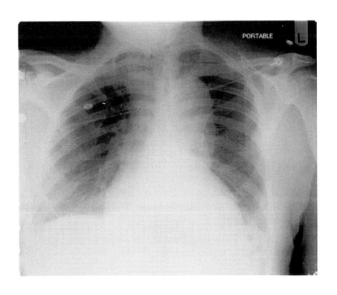

Figure 99.2

L. Action

a. Isolation

    i. Contact Centers for Disease Control

b. Intubation with rapid sequence intubation techniques

c. Admit to MICU for medical management

d. Antibiotic coverage for both community-acquired pneumonia and anthrax (acceptable regiments include ceftriaxone + doxycyline, ceftriaxone + azithromycin, ciprofloxacin ± vancomycin)

e. Provision of ciprofloxacin to exposed healthcare providers and family members

M. Diagnosis

a. Pulmonary inhalation anthrax

N. Critical actions

▨ Intubation

▨ CXR

▨ Early antibiotics

▨ MICU admission

▨ Isolation

▨ Contact Centers for Disease Control

▨ Prophylaxis for healthcare workers and family

O. Examiner instructions

a. This is a case of a pulmonary anthrax resulting from exposure to spores on animal hide in this patient who is a farmer and sells alpaca wool. Pulmonary anthrax is a fatal condition resulting in a severe hemorrhagic pneumonia. Important early actions include careful history, securing a definitive airway, obtaining blood cultures, recognizing pathognomonic CXR findings (see below), administering appropriate antibiotics, isolation of the patient, and medical ICU admission. If fluids are not administered, the patient's blood pressure will begin to drop. If airway is not secured, respiratory distress will worsen. A CXR can be readily obtained; if a CT scan is ordered, note that the scanner is busy, and it will "be a while" before the test can be performed. Once the diagnosis is realized by the candidate, they should isolate the patient with airborne precautions, give prophylaxis to healthcare workers and family, and contact the CDC.

P. Pearls

a. Manifestations of anthrax vary from cutaneous disease, pulmonary disease from inhalation of spores, and GI disease.

b. The course of inhalational anthrax can progress from initial nonspecific influenza-like symptoms to severe respiratory distress, hypotension, and hemorrhage within days of exposure.

c. Pathognomonic CXR findings include mediastinal widening and pleural effusions that are reflective of hemorrhagic effusions. CXR will not show interstitial infiltrates that is common in pneumonia. When diagnosis is suspected, CT of the chest is the test of choice.

d. Anthrax is highly susceptible to penicillin, amoxicillin, chloramphenicol, doxycycline, erythromycin, streptomycin, and ciprofloxacin. Anthrax is resistant to third-generation cephalosporins.

   e. ICU monitoring and care is necessary as inhalation anthrax progresses to sepsis and/or hemorrhagic shock.

Q. References
a. Tintinalli's: Chapter 155
b. Rosen's: Chapter 194

CASE 100: Headache (Anita Vashi, MD)

A. Chief complaint
a. 56-year-old male brought in by ambulance with severe, throbbing headache for the past 6 hours

B. Vital signs
a. BP: 235/128 HR: 76 RR: 18 T: 36.3°C Sat: 99% on RA FS: 89

C. What does the patient look like?
a. Patient appears stated age, uncomfortable, lying on stretcher with eyes closed, but arousable.

D. Primary survey
a. Airway: speaking in full sentences
b. Breathing: no apparent respiratory distress, no cyanosis
c. Circulation: skin warm and dry, normal capillary refill

E. Action
a. Oxygen via NC or nonrebreather mask
b. Two large-bore peripheral IV lines
c. Labs
    i. CBC, BMP, LFT, coagulation studies, blood type and cross-match
    ii. Troponin, UA
d. Monitor: repeat vitals: BP: 240/125 HR: 73 RR: 18 T: 36.3°C Sat: 99%
e. EKG

F. History
a. HPI: a 56-year-old male with a history of hypertension and hypercholesterolemia states he has had a severe headache that started this morning which has gradually worsened. Headache is frontal and constant, severe, and sudden onset. States he feels nauseous and sleepy. Denies fever, chills, and sweats; no neck pain, photophobia, change in vision or speech, numbness or tingling, chest pain, shortness of breath, vomiting, diarrhea, recent history of trauma, or history of similar headaches.
b. PMHx: hypertension and hypercholesterolemia
c. PSHx: none
d. Allergies: none
e. Meds: metoprolol, hydrochlorothiazide, clonidine; unknown doses; patient states he has not been taking his medications for the past week because he ran out of his pills

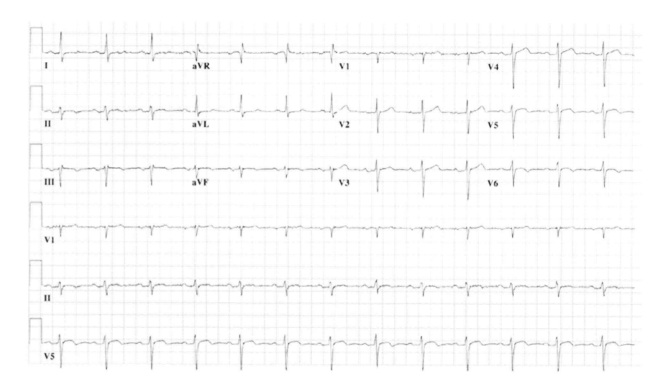

Figure 100.1

f. Social: lives alone, denies alcohol, smoking, or drug use, not sexually active
g. FHx: no relevant history
h. PMD: Dr Gill

G. Nurse
a. EKG (Figure 100.1)
b. Patient: complaining of headache and nausea; vomited × 1

H. Secondary survey
a. General: A & O × 2 (person, place), thinks it is 1998, uncomfortable-appearing
b. Head: normocephalic, atraumatic
c. Eyes: extraocular movement intact, pupils equal, reactive to light, unable to visualize fundus
d. Ears: normal tympanic membranes
e. Nose: no discharge
f. Neck: full range of motion, no jugular vein distension, no stridor
g. Pharynx: normal dentition, no lesions, no swelling
h. Chest: nontender
i. Lungs: clear bilaterally
j. Heart: rate and rhythm regular, no murmurs, rubs, or gallops
k. Abdomen: normal bowel sounds, soft, nontender; nondistended
l. Rectal: normal tone, brown stool, occult blood negative
    i. Male: no discharge, normal testicular examination
m. Extremities: full range of motion, no deformity, normal pulses
n. Back: nontender

   o. Neuro: cranial nerves II to XII intact; normal sensation, strength; normal reflexes and gait

   p. Skin: warm and dry

   q. Lymph: no lymphadenopathy

I. Action

a. Frequent BP checks

b. Lumbar puncture

c. Meds

   i. Antihypertensive: goal is for slow titratable decline in BP (i.e. labetalol IV). Nurse asks "what is goal of BP control?" 25% reduction of MAP.

   ii. Pain control with IV narcotics (i.e. fentanyl)

   iii. Antiemetic

d. Imaging

   i. CXR (Figure 100.2)

   ii. CT brain, noncontrast (Figure 100.3)

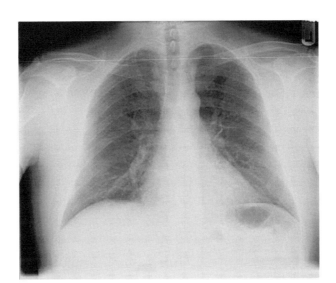

Figure 100.2

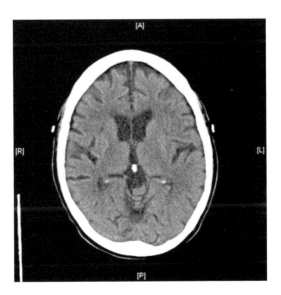

Figure 100.3

J. Nurse

a. BP: 188/98 (after 45 minutes)

b. Patient: moderate improvement of symptoms

c. If IV antihypertensive not given, BP remains elevated and patient has sudden worsening in mental status, becomes confused, and responsive only to painful stimuli

K. Results

Complete blood count:

WBC	8.6×10^3/uL	Alk Phos	42 U/L
Hct	41.5%	T bili	1.0 mg/dL
Plt	350×10^3/uL	D bili	0.3 mg/dL
		Amylase	50 U/L
Basic metabolic panel:		Lipase	25 U/L
Na	138 mEq/L	Albumin	4.7 g/dL
K	4.3 mEq/L		
Cl	105 mEq/L	**Urinalysis:**	
CO₂	30 mEq/L	SG	1.0.20
BUN	37 mEq/dL	pH	7
Cr	2.4 mg/dL%	Prot	3 +
Gluc	88 mg/dL	Gluc	Neg mg/dL
		Ketones	Neg mg/dL
Coagulation panel:		Bili	Neg
PT	12.6 sec	Blood	trace
PTT	26.0 sec	LE	Neg
INR	1.0	Nitrite	Neg
		Color	Yellow
Liver function panel:			
AST	23 U/L		
ALT	26 U/L		

a. CXR (Figure 100.2)

b. CT head (Figure 100.3)

c. Lumbar puncture: RBC 0, WBC 0, Glucose 45, Protein 30, negative xanthrochromia

L. Action

a. Admission to monitored medical bed

M. Diagnosis

a. Hypertensive emergency

N. Critical actions

▨ IV antihypertensive medication

▨ Pain control

▨ CT brain

▨ Lumbar puncture

▨ Admission with telemetry

O. Examiner instructions

a. This is a case of hypertensive emergency with evidence of end-organ insult to the brain and kidneys in setting of abrupt cessation of antihypertensive medications in a patient with chronic hypertension. Patient presents early after start of symptoms.

Important early actions include frequent blood pressure monitoring, administering IV antihypertensive medication, EKG, CXR, labs, UA, and brain CT. If IV medication is not given early, blood pressure will increase and patient will have an acute change in mental status. The patient should have a lumbar puncture as subarachnoid or intracerebral hemorrhage are still within the differential.

P. Pearls

a. Treatment goal is to reduce mean arterial pressure by 20% to 25% in the first 1 to 2 hours, followed by eventual BP reduction to 160/100 mmHg over next 6 to 12 hours.

b. If patient presents with symptoms consistent with ischemic stroke, it is recommended to only treat BP if it exceeds 220/120 mmHg with a goal to reduce BP by 10% to 15%.

c. Aggressive reduction in blood pressure can lead to coronary, cerebral, or renal hypoperfusion.

d. Hypertensive emergency warrants medical admission with telemetry.

e. Pharmacologic therapy should be used to provide a predictable, dose-dependent, transient effect. Commonly used medications include IV nitroprusside, labetalol, and nitroglycerin.

f. Management of hypertensive urgency differs from that of hypertensive emergency. The blood pressure can be equally high; however, the patient does not have any evidence of end-organ failure in hypertensive urgency. In such cases, the goal is to reduce BP over 24 to 48 hours. Patients with reliable follow-up can often be discharged home without any pharmacological intervention. If medication is used, oral antihypertensive medications often are sufficient.

Q. References

a. Tintinalli's: Chapter 61
b. Rosen's: Chapter 82

CASE 101: Drowning (Anita Vashi, MD)

A. Chief complaint

a. 15-year-old female brought in by EMS after falling into a lake that was only partially frozen over. Required CPR on scene with return to spontaneous circulation. Patient on backboard with C-collar

B. Vital signs

a. BP: 83/62 HR: 56 RR: 18 T: 33.5°C Sat: 94% on RA FS: 70

C. What does the patient look like?

a. Patient appears wet, cold; not shivering; arousable to sternal rub.

D. Primary survey

a. Airway: occasional groaning
b. Breathing: mild respiratory distress, no cyanosis
c. Circulation: pale and cold skin, delayed capillary refill
d. Disability: pupils 6 mm bilaterally and sluggish, no spontaneous movement
e. Exposure: removal of all clothes

E. Action

a. Intubation for airway protection using RSI and inline immobilization, warm humidified oxygen

b. Two large-bore peripheral IV lines

c. Warm blankets, external warmer (ie. Bair hugger)

d. Labs

   i. Point of care glucose, VBG with lactate

   ii. CBC, BMP, LFT, coagulation studies, blood type and cross-match, alcohol level, acetaminophen level, salicylate level, urine toxicology screen and pregnancy test.

e. 2 L warm NS bolus

f. Monitor: BP: 92/68 HR: 96 RR: 18 Sat: 100% on O_2

g. Rectal temperature: 30°C

h. Temperature sensing Foley catheter (or temperature sensing esophageal probe or rectal probe that reads temperatures <30°C)

i. EKG

j. Initial imaging

k. CXR

l. Cautious handling of patient to minimize movements

F. History

a. HPI: a 15-year-old female with no past medical history was playing on partially frozen ice when she suddenly fell through the ice and into the water. She remained submerged for ~10 minutes while friend summoned help. EMS was then called. On arrival to scene, the patient had no detectable pulses. Compressions were started, pulse was quickly regained and patient was brought to ED with minimal transport time. Patient grimacing but not speaking or spontaneously moving extremities.

b. PMHx: none

c. PSHx: none

d. Allergies: none

e. Meds: none

f. Social: lives with family at home, denies EtOH, smoking, or drug use, not sexually active

g. FHx: not relevant

h. PMD: Dr Silverstein

G. Nurse

a. EKG (Figure 101.1)

b. After intubation

   i. BP: 98/59 HR: 60 RR: 18 Sat: 98% on mechanical ventilation

c. If not intubated

   i. BP: 90/55 HR: 38 RR: 10 Sat: 85% on O_2

   ii. Will need intubation

d. CXR (Figure 101.2)

H. Secondary survey

a. General: A & O × 0, intubated, no spontaneous movement

b. Head: normocephalic, atraumatic

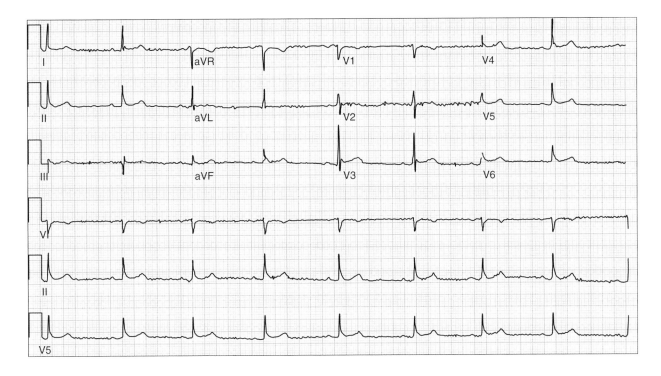

Figure 101.1

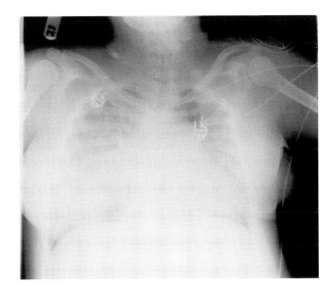

Figure 101.2

c. Eyes: extraocular movement intact, pupils 6 mm bilaterally and sluggish
d. Ears: normal tympanic membranes
e. Nose: no discharge
f. Neck: C-collar in place, no obvious signs of trauma
g. Pharynx: normal dentition, no lesions, no swelling
h. Chest: nontender
i. Lungs: bilateral coarse breath sounds
j. Heart: bradycardic rate, rhythm regular, no murmurs, rubs, or gallops
k. Abdomen: normal bowel sounds, soft, nontender or distended

l. Rectal: diminished tone, brown stool, occult blood negative

m. Extremities: full range of passive motion, no deformity, normal pulses, peripheral cyanosis

n. Back: nontender

o. Neuro: no spontaneous movements

p. Skin: pale, cool

q. Lymph: no lymphadenopathy

I. Action

a. Rewarming intervention

    i. Rewarming device (ie. Bair hugger), warm IV fluids, warm humidified oxygen. Focus on rewarming the core, avoid rewarming the extremities while leaving the trunk exposed and cold when doing procedures or exam

    ii. Nasogastric tube and urinary catheter placement with infusion of warmed saline

    iii. Consider warm pleural or peritoneal lavage

    iv. If dialysis or cardiopulmonary bypass requested, unavailable at this time

b. Reassess

    i. If warming intervention taken, temperature improves to 33°C (by internal sensing device)

    ii. If some form of warming intervention not taken, patient's cardiac rhythm changes to ventricular fibrillation that does not respond to medications and/or defibrillation

c. Pediatric ICU admission

d. Imaging

    i. C-spine x-ray or CT c-spine (Figure 101.3)

    ii. Head CT (Figure 101.4)

J. Nurse

a. BP: 98/59 HR: 90 RR: 18 Sat: 98% on mechanical ventilation

b. Patient: intubated, no spontaneous movement

Figure 101.3

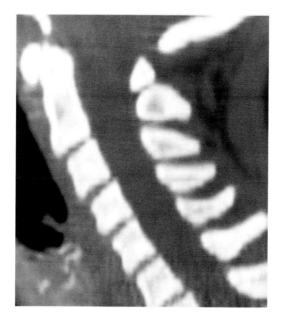

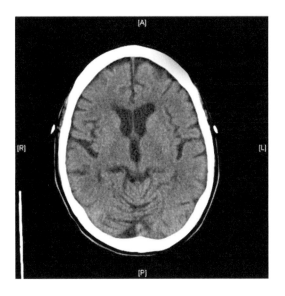

Figure 101.4

K Results

Complete blood count:

WBC	5.3×10^3/uL	D bili	0.3 mg/dL
Hct	41.5%	Amylase	50 U/L
Plt	350×10^3/uL	Lipase	25 U/L
		Albumin	4.7 g/dL

Basic metabolic panel:

		Urinalysis:	
Na	138 mEq/L		
K	4.3 mEq/L	SG	1.0.20
Cl	105 mEq/L	pH	7
CO_2	20 mEq/L	Prot	Neg mg/dL
BUN	12 mEq/dL	Gluc	Neg mg/dL
Cr	1.1 mg/dL%	Ketones	Neg mg/dL
Gluc	100 mg/dL	Bili	Neg
		Blood	Neg
Coagulation panel:		LE	Neg
PT	12.6 sec	Nitrite	Neg
PTT	26.0 sec	Color	Yellow
INR	1.0		

Arterial blood gas (pre-intubation):

Liver function panel:

AST	23 U/L	pH	7.24
ALT	26 U/L	pO_2	62
Alk Phos	42 U/L	pCO_2	48
T bili	1.0 mg/dL	HCO_3	22

a. Lactate 5.2 mmol/L

b. CT head (Figure 101.4)

c. CT c-spine (Figure 101.3)

d. EtOH, aspirin, and acetaminophen levels, urine toxicology, urine pregnancy negative

L. Action
a. Continue rewarming

M. Diagnosis
a. Hypothermia secondary to cold-water immersion

N. Critical actions
■ Airway management
■ Undressing patient and assessing for any signs of trauma
■ Temperature monitoring via internal probe (esophageal, Foley, or rectal)
■ Point of care glucose
■ Aggressive rewarming
■ PICU admission

O. Examiner instructions
a. This is a case of hypothermia secondary to cold-water immersion. The patient initially was found in cardiac arrest because of either the extremely cold water or lack of oxygen supply to the brain but was revived with CPR. Aggressive rewarming is necessary as well as early intubation for airway protection. It is critical to recognize the potential for hypothermia in cold-water immersion cases. Critical early actions include airway management, complete undressing of patient, placement of internal temperature sensing device for constant temperature monitoring, and aggressive rewarming techniques. Because the circumstances are unclear, the candidate should consider potential head and neck injury.

P. Pearls
a. In hypothermic patients, axillary and tympanic temperatures are often unreliable. Internal temperature sensing devices should be used for constant and accurate temperature monitoring in these patients.
b. Moderate hypothermia (between 30°C and 34°C) can present with loss of the shivering reflex, mild alteration in consciousness, bradycardia, and atrial fibrillation.
c. Patients with severe hypothermia (at temperatures below 30°C) can present with fixed, dilated pupils, diminished reflexes, coma, ventricular fibrillation, asystole. The patient should be carefully handled to minimize movements that may lead to lethal arrhythmias.
d. Remember, no one is dead until they are "warm and dead."
e. An Osborne wave, or up-slurring of the QRS-ST junction, is the classic EKG finding for hypothermia (usually temperatures <32°C).
f. Attempts at defibrillation are usually unsuccessful at temperatures less than 30°C.
g. Rapid rewarming can cause lethal arrhythmias in hypothermic patients. Core rewarming (dialysis, cardiopulmonary bypass, thoracic and peritoneal cavity lavage) should be reserved for patients with severe cardiovascular instability (cardiac arrest, ventricular fibrillation). In milder cases of hypothermia, warm blankets, forced air blankets (such as Bair Hugger), warm humidified oxygen, and warm fluids are usually sufficient to safely rewarm the patient.
h. Initial CXR may grossly underestimate extent of pulmonary damage in near-drowning cases.
i. Antibiotics can be given on a case-by-case basis. Consider coverage if submersion occurs in grossly contaminated water or if aspiration is a concern.

Q. References

a. Tintinalli's: Chapters 203, 209

b. Rosen's: Chapters 139, 140, 145

CASE 102: Cyanosis (Evelyn Chow, MD)

A. Chief complaint

a. 12-day-old male brought in by his mother for an episode of turning blue in the face

B. Vital signs

a. BP: 110/81 HR 185 RR: 100 T: 37.1°C Sat: 90% on RA

C. What does the patient look like?

a. Patient tachypneic, awake, and alert.

D. Primary survey

a. Airway: patent

b. Breathing: tachypneic, no apparent respiratory distress, no cyanosis

c. Circulation: upper extremities warm and well perfused, lower extremities with slightly delayed capillary refill bilaterally

E. Action

a. Oxygen supplementation (blow-by oxygen)

b. Peripheral IV line placement

c. Labs: CBC, CMP, venous blood gas, coagulation studies, type and screen, urinalysis

d. Check BP in all four extremities

e. Cardiac monitor and EKG

F. History

a. HPI: a 12-day-old male, full term, normal spontaneous vaginal delivery without complications presents with an episode of turning blue and diaphoretic while feeding; no fever, cough, or other URI symptoms; no vomiting or diarrhea; no change in urine output.

b. PMHx: normal spontaneous vaginal delivery at 39 weeks, no complications

c. PSHx: none

d. Allergies: none

e. Meds: none

f. Social: lives at home with family

g. FHx: noncontributory

h. PMD: Dr Han

G. Nurse

a. Oxygen supplementation

   i. HR: 176 RR: 83 Sat: 94% on O_2

b. No supplemental oxygen

   i. HR: 192 RR: 105 Sat: 90% on RA

c. BP: Left upper extremity 110/81, right upper extremity 114/82, left lower extremity unable to obtain, right lower extremity unable to obtain

d. EKG (Figure 102.1)

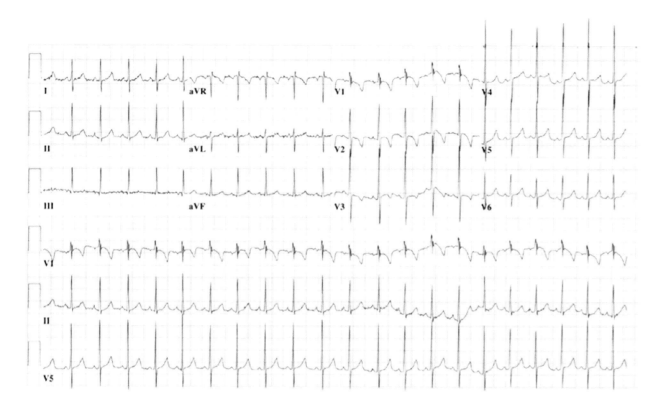

Figure 102.1

H. Secondary survey
a. General: awake and alert, tachypneic
b. Head: anterior fontanelle flat, atraumatic
c. Eyes: extraocular movement intact, pupils equal, reactive to light
d. Ears: normal tympanic membranes
e. Nose: no discharge
f. Neck: full range of motion, no stridor
g. Pharynx: no lesions, no swelling
h. Chest: nontender
i. Lungs: tachypneic, clear bilaterally
j. Heart: tachycardic rate, rhythm regular, systolic murmur heard best posteriorly over t-spine
k. Abdomen: normal bowel sounds, soft, nontender or distended
l. Rectal: normal tone, brown stool, occult blood negative
m. Urogenital: normal external genitalia
    i. Male: no discharge, normal testicular examination
n. Extremities: 2+ radial pulses bilaterally, femoral pulses not palpable, bilateral upper extremities warm and well perfused, bilateral lower extremities warm with slightly delayed capillary refill
o. Back: nontender
p. Neuro: awake and alert, appropriate for age
q. Skin: warm and dry
r. Lymph: no lymphadenopathy

I. Action

a. Meds

  i. Prostaglandin E1 IV infusion

b. Reassess

  i. Patient starts to improve a few minutes after starting prostaglandin E1

c. Consult

  i. Pediatric cardiology

d. Imaging

  i. CXR (Figure 102.2)

J. Nurse

a. Prostaglandin E1 started

  i. HR: 141 RR: 48 Sat: 97% 2 L

b. No prostaglandin E1 started

  i. HR: 196 RR: 110 Sat: 88% 2 L, patient turns cyanotic

K. Results

Complete blood count:

WBC	9.5×10^3/uL	D bili	0.3 mg/dL
Hct	52.2%	Amylase	50 U/L
Plt	131×10^3/uL	Lipase	25 U/L
		Albumin	4.7 g/dL

Basic metabolic panel:

Na	138 mEq/L	**Urinalysis:**	
K	4.3 mEq/L	SG	1.0.20
Cl	100 mEq/L	pH	7
CO_2	35 mEq/L	Prot	Neg mg/dL
BUN	9 mEq/dL	Gluc	Neg mg/dL
Cr	0.5 mg/dL%	Ketones	Neg mg/dL
Gluc	116 mg/dL	Bili	Neg
		Blood	Neg

Coagulation panel:

		LE	Neg
PT	12.6 sec	Nitrite	Neg
PTT	26.0 sec	Color	Yellow
INR	1.0		

Liver function panel:

		Arterial blood gas:	
		pH	7.54
AST	23 U/L	PO_2	146
ALT	26 U/L	PCO_2	46
Alk Phos	42 U/L	HCO_3	35
T bili	1.0 mg/dL		

a. CXR (Figure 102.2)

L. Action

a. Pediatric cardiology performs bedside echo which confirms coarctation of the aorta

b. Consult cardiothoracic surgery

c. Discussion with parents regarding need for admission and surgical correction of the coarctation

Figure 102.2

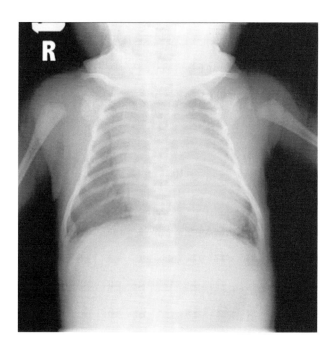

M. Diagnosis

a. Aortic coarctation

N. Critical actions

▨ Supplemental oxygen
▨ Listen to anterior chest and back for murmurs
▨ CXR
▨ Prostaglandin E1
▨ Discuss condition with family
▨ Cardiology consult

O. Examiner instructions

a. This is a case of congenital coarctation of the aorta. This is a condition where there is an abnormal development of the aorta which results in decreased blood flow to the lower body. In this patient, the symptoms have become more prominent in the second week of life as the ductus arteriosus closes. Stress, such as feeding, exacerbates the symptoms. Important early actions include supplemental oxygen, checking the blood pressure in all extremities, EKG, CXR, cardiology consult, and prostaglandin E1. The EKG is obtained to assess the axis of the heart and chamber sizes. The CXR shows significant cardiomegaly, which is another indication of congenital heart disease. Prostaglandin E1 is given to maintain patency of the ductus arteriosus. If prostaglandin E1 is not given, the patient will deteriorate. Labs generally are not helpful in the diagnosis of aortic coarctation, but can be used to rule out sepsis and to see if the patient is acidotic. An echocardiogram should be obtained to definitively diagnose the coarctation. If an MRI is ordered, note that it is busy and is unlikely to become available.

P. Pearls

a. Cyanosis, dyspnea, or diaphoresis during feeding can be a sign of a congenital heart defect.

b. Classic clinical findings in aortic coarctation are hypertension in the upper extremities (normally the BP is 10 mmHg higher in the lower extremities) and diminished pulses in the lower extremities. Any child with hypertension needs to be ruled out for aortic coarctation.

c. Prostaglandin E1 prevents closure of a patent ductus arteriosus, which can help stabilize an infant with a cyanotic heart defect.

Q. References
a. Tintinalli's: Chapter 122
b. Rosen's: Chapter 169

CASE 103: Diarrhea (Meika Close, MD)

A. Chief complaint
a. 33-year-old male with bloody diarrhea for the past 2 days

B. Vital signs
a. BP: 110/68 HR: 96 RR: 12 T: 37.5°C Sat: 100%

C. What does the patient look like?
a. Patient appears comfortable, lying supine on stretcher.

D. Primary survey
a. Airway: speaking in full sentences
b. Breathing: no respiratory distress, no cyanosis
c. Circulation: warm skin, normal capillary refill

E. Action
a. Oxygen via NC or nonrebreather mask
b. Two large-bore peripheral IV lines
c. Labs
   i. CBC, CMP, coagulation studies, urinalysis
d. Monitor: BP: 120/66 HR: 96 RR: 12 Sat: 100%

F. History
a. HPI: a 33-year-old male with no past medical history complaining of diarrhea for the past 2 days. He notes eight to ten episodes per day, first watery, now bloody, and associated with mild lower abdominal pain and cramping, fever, chills, and malaise. Patient denies nausea, vomiting, hematuria; denies recent travel or antibiotic use. Patient lives alone, no known sick contacts.
b. PMHx: none
c. PSHx: appendectomy
d. Allergies: none
e. Meds: none
f. Social: lives alone, denies alcohol, smoking, or drug use, not sexually active for 5 years
g. FHx: not relevant
h. PMD: none

G. Nurse

a. 1 L NS

    i. BP: 120/74 HR: 88 RR: 12 Sat: 100%

H. Secondary survey

a. General: alert, oriented × 3, comfortable

b. Head: normocephalic, atraumatic

c. Eyes: extraocular movement intact, pupils equal, reactive to light

d. Ears: normal tympanic membranes

e. Nose: no discharge

f. Neck: full range of motion, no jugular vein distension, no stridor

g. Pharynx: normal dentition, no lesions, no swelling

h. Chest: nontender

i. Lungs: clear bilaterally

j. Heart: rate and rhythm regular, no murmurs, rubs, or gallops

k. Abdomen: hyperactive bowel sounds, nontender, no masses or organomegaly, no rebound or guarding

l. Rectal: tenderness, grossly bloody stool in rectum

m. Urogenital: normal external genitalia

    i. Male: no discharge, normal testicular examination

n. Extremities: full range of motion, no deformity, normal pulses

o. Back: nontender

p. Neuro: cranial nerves II to XII intact; normal sensation, strength; normal reflexes and gait

q. Skin: decreased skin turgor

r. Lymph: no lymphadenopathy

I. Action

a. Meds

    i. Repeat 1 L NS IV bolus

b. Reassess

    i. Patient has one episode of bloody diarrhea in ED

c. Labs

    i. Stool culture

J. Nurse

a. BP: 122/72 HR: 82 RR: 12 Sat: 100%

b. Patient: stable, comfortable

K. Results

Complete blood count:

WBC	10.8×10^3/uL	BUN	12 mEq/dL
Hct	41.8%	Cr	1.1 mg/dL%
Plt	280×10^3/uL	Gluc	110 mg/dL

Basic metabolic panel:

		Coagulation panel:	
Na	138 mEq/L	PT	12.6 sec
K	3.3 mEq/L	PTT	26.0 sec
Cl	105 mEq/L	INR	1.0
CO_2	22 mEq/L		

Liver function panel:		Urinalysis:	
AST	23 U/L	SG	1.0.20
ALT	26 U/L	pH	7
Alk Phos	42 U/L	Prot	Neg mg/dL
T bili	1.0 mg/dL	Gluc	Neg mg/dL
D bili	0.3 mg/dL	Ketones	Neg mg/dL
Amylase	50 U/L	Bili	Neg
Lipase	25 U/L	Blood	Neg
Albumin	4.7 g/dL	LE	Neg
		Nitrite	Neg
		Color	Yellow

a. Stool culture pending

L. Action
a. Meds
　i. Ciprofloxacin
　ii. Potassium chloride

M. Nurse
a. Patient: feeling significantly better

N. Action
a. Disposition
　i. Discharge from ED with prescription for ciprofloxacin and outpatient follow-up after rehydration with IVF
b. Patient education regarding diarrhea
c. Discussion about diet

O. Diagnosis
a. Enteroinvasive diarrhea

P. Critical actions
▨ Rehydration
▨ Repletion of electrolytes
▨ Antibiotics

Q. Examiner instructions
a. This is a case of enteroinvasive diarrhea from a bacterial infection. Viruses most commonly cause gastroenteritis leading to diarrhea. However, the bloody diarrhea in this case is suggestive of an invasive bacterial etiology. History of travel, antibiotic use, known sick contacts, or ingestion of contaminated food or water during an outbreak are also suggestive of bacterial infection. Key actions in this case are rehydration and repletion of electrolytes.

R. Pearls
a. Infectious diarrhea is usually self-limiting and does not require antimicrobial therapy except in severe cases, including fevers, bloody diarrhea, or duration greater than 3 days.

b. Culture should be sent in children, toxic patients, immunocompromised patients, or patients with history of travel. Culture for ova and parasites should be sent for high-risk patients.

c. Typical viruses causing diarrhea are rotavirus, adenovirus, calicivirus, astro-virus, and Norwalk virus. Viruses typically affect the small intestine and do not present with bloody diarrhea.

d. Bloody diarrhea is suggestive of an invasive bacterial etiology. Bacteria causing bloody diarrhea include:
     i. Enterohemorrhagic *Escherichia coli* (*E coli* 0157:H7)
     ii. Enteroinvasive *E. coli*
     iii. *Shigella* species
     iv. *Salmonella* species
     v. *Campylobacter* species
     vi. *Yersinia* species
     vii. *Aeromonas* species
     viii. *Plesiomonas* species

e. Thrombotic-thrombocytopenic purpura and hemolytic-urenic syndrome is a complication of infectious diarrhea, usually caused by *E. coli* 0157:H7, and should be considered in children presenting with grossly bloody stool and oliguria or anuria.

f. In the setting of recent antibiotic use, stool specimen should be tested for the *Clostridium difficile* toxin and metronidazole should be administered by the PO route.

g. In a patient presenting with bloody diarrhea, other conditions that should be considered include diverticulitis, mesenteric ischemia, gastrointestinal hemorrhage, and inflammatory bowel disease.

S. References
a. Tintinalli's: Chapter 76
b. Rosen's: Chapter 171

CASE 104: Cough (Meika Close, MD)

A. Chief complaint
a. 59-year-old male brought in by EMS from prison with the complaint of productive cough and shortness of breath

B. Vital signs
a. BP: 110/68 HR: 125 RR: 26 T: 38.2°C Sat: 87% on RA FS: 110

C. What does the patient look like?
a. Patient cachectic, appears older than stated age, moderate respiratory distress, sitting up in stretcher.

D. Primary survey
a. Airway: speaking in full sentences
b. Breathing: moderate respiratory distress, + cyanosis
c. Circulation: warm skin, normal capillary refill

E. Action

  a. Airborne isolation

  b. Oxygen supplementation via nonrebreather mask

  c. Two large-bore peripheral IV lines

  d. Labs

    i. CBC, BMP, LFT, coagulation studies, blood type and cross-match

    ii. VBG or ABG with lactate, blood cultures, UA, urine culture, LDH

  e. 1 L NS bolus

  f. Antipyretic (i.e. acetaminophen)

  g. Monitor: BP: 108/68 HR: 118 RR: 20 Sat: 94% on NRB

F. History

  a. HPI: a 59-year-old male with a history of AIDS, non-complaint with antiretroviral medications complaining of cough for the past 5 days with production of yellow sputum, and shortness of breath for the past 2 days, associated with low-grade fevers and chest tightness. Patient denies headache, neck stiffness, abdominal pain, nausea, vomiting, diarrhea, or urinary symptoms.

  b. PMHx: AIDS, noncompliant on antiretroviral medications, last CD4 count 94, history of PCP and HIV lymphoma

  c. PSHx: none

  d. Allergies: none

  e. Meds: only remembers Bactrim

  f. Social: incarcerated × 5 months; denies alcohol use or illicit drug use. Half to one pack per day smoker for 40 years

  g. FHx: no relevant history

  h. PMD: corrections facility clinic

G. Nurse

  a. EKG (Figure 104.1)

  b. Fluids

    i. BP: 112/70 HR: 106 RR: 18 Sat: 93% on NRB

  c. No fluids

    i. BP: 100/65 HR: 124 RR: 20 Sat: 93% on NRB

H. Secondary survey

  a. General: alert, oriented × 3, cachectic, appears in mild respiratory distress

  b. Head: normocephalic, atraumatic

  c. Eyes: extraocular movement intact, pupils equal, reactive to light

  d. Ears: normal tympanic membranes

  e. Nose: no discharge

  f. Neck: full range of motion, no jugular vein distension, no stridor

  g. Pharynx: normal dentition, no lesions, no swelling, + thrush

  h. Chest: nontender

  i. Lungs: tachypneic, diffuse crackles bilaterally

  j. Heart: tachycardic, no murmurs, rubs, or gallops

  k. Abdomen: normal bowel sounds, soft, nontender or distended

  l. Rectal: normal tone, brown stool, occult blood negative

  m. Urogenital: normal external genitalia

    i. Male: no discharge, normal testicular examination

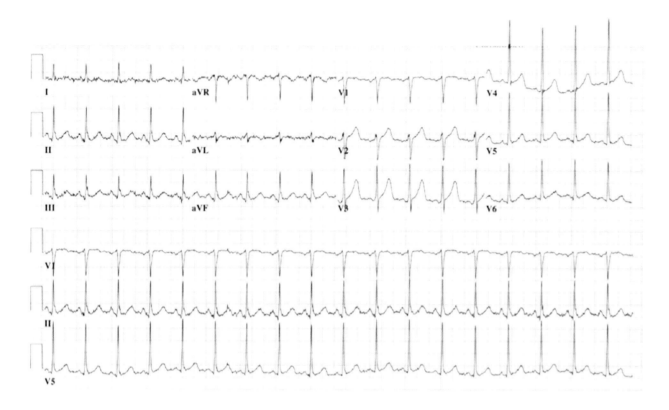

Figure 104.1

n. Extremities: full range of motion, no deformity, normal pulses
o. Back: nontender
p. Neuro: cranial nerves II to XII intact; normal sensation, strength; normal reflexes and gait
q. Skin: warm and dry
r. Lymph: no lymphadenopathy

I. Action
a. Meds
   i. Ceftriaxone
   ii. Azithromycin
   iii. Bactrim DS
   iv. Prednisone
   v. Consider therapy for TB
b. Reassess
   i. Patient still tachypneic with mild respiratory distress, improving
c. Consult
   i. MICU
d. Imaging
   i. CXR (Figure 104.2)

J. Nurse
a. BP: 118/76 HR: 106 RR: 18 Sat: 94% on NRB
b. Patient: respiratory distress, improving

K. Results

Complete blood count:

WBC	5.9×10^3/uL	D bili	0.3 mg/dL
Hct	36.5%	Amylase	50 U/L
Plt	110×10^3/uL	Lipase	25 U/L
		Albumin	2.7 g/dL

Basic metabolic panel:

Na	138 mEq/L	**Urinalysis:**	
K	4.3 mEq/L	SG	1.0.20
Cl	105 mEq/L	pH	7
CO_2	20 mEq/L	Prot	Neg mg/dL
BUN	22 mEq/dL	Gluc	Neg mg/dL
Cr	0.9 mg/dL%	Ketones	Neg mg/dL
Gluc	100 mg/dL	Bili	Neg
		Blood	Neg
		LE	Neg
Coagulation panel:		Nitrite	Neg
PT	12.6 sec	Color	Yellow
PTT	26.0 sec		
INR	1.0		
		Arterial blood gas:	
		pH	7.36
Liver function panel:		PO_2	58 mmHg on RA
AST	23 U/L	PCO_2	30 mmHg
ALT	26 U/L	HCO_3	18 mmol/L
Alk Phos	42 U/L		
T bili	1.0 mg/dL		

a. Lactate 1.6 mmol/L

b. LDH 360

c. CXR (Figure 104.2)

L. Action

a. Admit patient to MICU

b. Discussion with patient regarding goals of care and patient's current condition with possibility of respiratory failure requiring endotracheal intubation

M. Diagnosis

a. Pneumocystis pneumonia (PCP)

N. Critical actions

▦ CXR

▦ Airway management – oxygen

▦ Antibiotics for community-acquired pneumonia and PCP

▦ Corticosteroids

▦ Airborne isolation

▦ MICU admission

O. Examiner instructions

a. This is a case of pneumonia in a patient with history of acquired immunodeficiency syndrome (AIDS), likely due to *Pneumocystis jiroveci* (formerly known as *Pneumocystis carinii*). This is a type of pneumonia seen in patients with severely reduced immune systems. Patients with AIDS have helper T-cell counts below 200 that

A   **B**

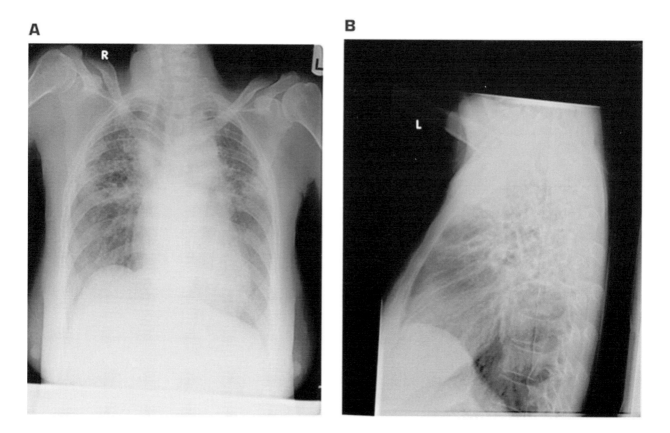

Figure 104.2 A and B

significantly increase their risk for opportunistic infections such as PCP pneumonia. In our patient, key actions are obtaining a CXR, administration of antibiotics to treat community-acquired pneumonia (CAP) and pneumocystis pneumonia (PCP), corticosteroid administration, and oxygen administration. The patient should also be placed in airborne isolation for possible concurrent tuberculosis.

P. Pearls

a. Bacterial infection is the most common cause of pneumonia in HIV patients; *Streptococcus pneumoniae* is the most common cause of bacterial pneumonia.

b. CD4 count is suggestive of etiology; however, coverage for bacterial pneumonia should be included in treatment regimen at any CD4 count.

   i. CD4 >800: bacterial pneumonia is most common.

   ii. CD4 250 to 500: *Mycobacterium tuberculosis, Cryptococcus neoformans,* and *Histoplasma capsulatum* are common causes.

   iii. CD4 <200: PCP is common.

c. Typical presentation of PCP is with nonproductive cough, fatigue, exertional dyspnea, pleuritic chest pain, and fever.

d. Corticosteroids are indicated in PCP for the following criteria, based on RA ABG:

   i. PaO_2 <70 mmHg

   ii. Alveolar-arterial gradient >35 mmHg

e. Patients meeting corticosteroid criteria or with otherwise tenuous respiratory status or predicted poor compliance should be hospitalized. ICU admission should be considered, as respiratory status often worsens after 2 to 3 days of antipneumocystis therapy.

f. Serum LDH is nonspecific and variable. If radiologic evidence of PCP is present, initial LDH may be of little utility. However, baseline LDH may be important in the hospitalized patient, as it has prognostic value.

Q. References
a. Tintinalli's: Chapter 149
b. Rosen's: Chapter 75

CASE 105: Altered mental status (Meika Close, MD)

A. Chief complaint
a. 63-year-old homeless male brought in by EMS after being found on the floor in the shelter by a friend

B. Vital signs
a. BP: 168/97 HR: 112 RR: 20 T: 37.1°C Sat: 96% on RA FS: 110 (must ask)

C. What does the patient look like?
a. Patient disheveled, appears older than stated age, mumbling incoherently, vomitus around mouth.

D. Primary survey
a. Airway: mumbling words
b. Breathing: no respiratory distress, no cyanosis
c. Circulation: warm skin, normal capillary refill

E. Action
a. Oxygen via NC or nonrebreather mask
b. Monitor: BP: 164/93 HR: 110 RR: 20 Sat: 99% on 2 L NC
c. EKG (Figure 105.1)
d. Two large-bore peripheral IV lines
e. Labs
   i. VBG or ABG with lactate, point of care glucose
   ii. CBC, BMP, LFT, coagulation studies, blood type, and cross-match alcohol level, acetaminophen level, salicylate level, urine toxicology screen.

F. History
a. HPI: a 63-year-old homeless male brought in by EMS after being found down on the bathroom floor of the homeless shelter. Per friend accompanying patient, patient had been vomiting for the past hour, and then became confused with incoherent speech. Patient has a history of positive PPD 3 months ago and has been taking isoniazid (must ask) with questionable compliance. Per friend, patient smokes one pack of cigarettes per day but does not drink alcohol, or use illicit drugs. Patient had been feeling increasingly depressed about living conditions over the past week but otherwise had no complaints.
b. PMHx: positive PPD
c. PSHx: unknown
d. Allergies: none

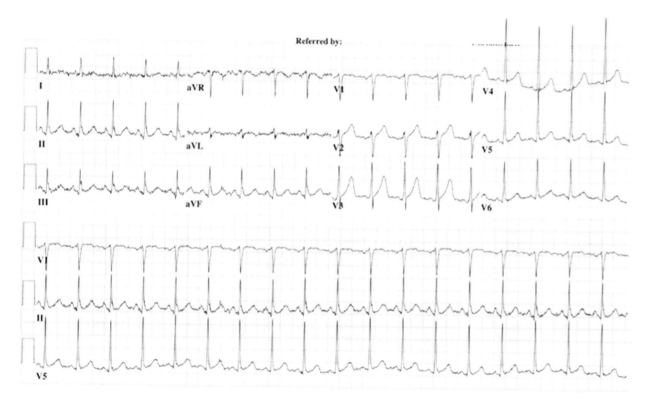

Figure 105.1

e. Meds: isoniazid (must ask)
f. Social: homeless, smokes one pack per day
g. FHx: no relevant history
h. PMD: unknown

G. Nurse
a. EKG (Figure 105.1)
b. NS 1 L IV bolus
    i. BP: 170/94 HR: 102 RR: 20 Sat: 99% on O_2
c. Patient is having a generalized tonic-clonic seizure

H. Action
a. If lorazepam given (no improvement of seizures)
    i. Total dose over 10 mg
        1. Continued seizures
        2. BP: 152/84 HR: 112 RR: 8 Sat: 88% on O_2
        3. Intubation for airway protection and hypoxia
    ii. Less than 8 mg
        1. Continued seizures
        2. BP: 160/94 HR: 110 RR: 14 Sat: 94% on O_2
b. Seizures will continue until pyridoxine IV is given

I. Secondary survey (unable to do until pyridoxine given)
a. General: confused, disoriented, and disheveled
b. Head: normocephalic, atraumatic

c. Eyes: extraocular movement intact, pupils 5 mm equal, reactive to light
d. Ears: normal tympanic membranes
e. Nose: no discharge
f. Neck: full range of motion, no jugular vein distension, no stridor
g. Pharynx: normal dentition, no lesions, no swelling
h. Chest: nontender
i. Lungs: clear bilaterally
j. Heart: tachycardic, no murmurs, rubs, or gallops
k. Abdomen: normal bowel sounds, soft, nontender or distended
l. Rectal: normal tone, brown stool, occult blood negative
m. Urogenital: normal external genitalia
   i. Male: no discharge, normal testicular examination
n. Extremities: full range of motion, no deformity, normal pulses
o. Back: nontender
p. Neuro: opens eyes spontaneously, mumbling incoherently, moves all extremities, withdraws from painful stimuli, DTRs 2+ bilaterally, no clonus
q. Skin: warm and dry
r. Lymph: no lymphadenopathy

J. Action
a. Meds
   i. Repeat NS 1 L IV bolus
b. Imaging
   i. CXR
   ii. CT head

K. Nurse
a. BP: 160/94 HR: 82 RR: 12 Sat: 100% on O_2
b. Imaging
   i. If intubated, portable CXR (Figure 105.2)
   ii. Not intubated, portable CXR (Figure 105.3)
c. Patient: sedated, no seizure activity
d. Noncontrast brain CT head (Figure 105.4)

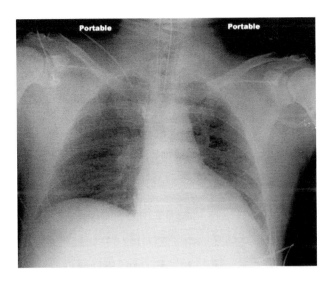

Figure 105.2

Figure 105.3

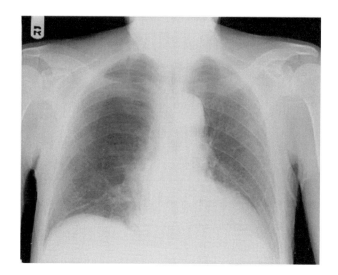

Figure 105.4

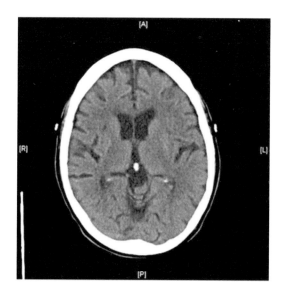

L. Results

Complete blood count:

WBC	14.1×10^3/uL
Hct	41.5%
Plt	150×10^3/uL

Basic metabolic panel:

Na	138 mEq/L
K	4.3 mEq/L
Cl	105 mEq/L
CO_2	15 mEq/L
BUN	12 mEq/dL
Cr	1.1 mg/dL%
Gluc	100 mg/dL

Coagulation panel:

PT	12.6 sec
PTT	26.0 sec
INR	1.0

Liver function panel:

AST	23 U/L
ALT	26 U/L
Alk Phos	42 U/L
T bili	1.0 mg/dL
D bili	0.3 mg/dL
Amylase	50 U/L
Lipase	25 U/L
Albumin	4.7 g/dL

Urinalysis:

SG	1.0.20	Nitrite	Neg
pH	7	Color	Yellow
Prot	Neg mg/dL		
Gluc	Neg mg/dL	**Arterial blood gas:**	
Ketones	Neg mg/dL	pH	7.28
Bili	Neg	PO_2	89 mmHg
Blood	Neg	PCO_2	28 mmHg
LE	Neg	HCO_3	17 mmol/L

a. Lactate 8.2 mmol/L
b. Urine tox negative
c. Aspirin negative
d. Acetaminophen negative
e. Alcohol negative

M. Action

a. Consults
    i. Toxicology
    ii. Neurology
    iii. Medical ICU

N. Diagnosis

a. INH overdose

O. Critical actions

▨ Airway management
▨ Point of care blood glucose
▨ Pyridoxine administration
▨ Serum toxicology for aspirin and acetaminophen
▨ Noncontrast brain CT

P. Examiner instructions

a. This is a case of INH toxicity, either due to INH overdose or noncompliance with pyridoxine. INH is a medication used for the treatment of tuberculosis which when taken in excess can lead to central nervous system changes including seizure. This presentation is a typical one, with nausea, vomiting, and mental status changes, and in the case of severe toxicity, progression to seizure, metabolic acidosis and even death. Key actions in this case are airway management and pyridoxine administration, as seizures caused by INH toxicity may be refractory to standard anticonvulsants, such as benzodiazepines and barbiturates. The seizures in this patient will not stop until pyridoxine is given. If a large dose of lorazepam is given, the patient should desaturate and require intubation.

Q. Pearls

a. At therapeutic doses (5 mg/kg), INH carries a high risk of side effects, including neurotoxicity and hepatotoxicity.
b. In acute overdose, typical presentation is with nausea, mental status changes, and ataxia, which may progress to seizure, coma, and metabolic acidosis if more than 20 to 40 mg/kg are ingested.

c. Toxicity is due to depletion of pyridoxine (Vitamin B_6), which leads to impaired synthesis of inhibitory neurotransmitter GABA.

d. Pyridoxine is given to prevent and/or treat seizures caused by INH toxicity. IV dosing of pyridoxine is based on amount of INH ingested, at a gram-to-gram equivalent. If amount is unknown, the recommended starting dose is 5 g.

e. Activated charcoal may be administered to decrease absorption of INH, if given within 1 hour of ingestion.

f. Metabolic acidosis may occur in severe overdose with seizure activity, due to production of lactic acid. Sodium bicarbonate is not recommended in treatment of acidosis. Hemodialysis may be required to correct acidemia and to remove INH from blood.

g. Most toxicity is manifested within 2 hours of ingestion. Patients who remain asymptomatic after 6 hours may be medically cleared for discharge from the ED.

R. References
a. Tintinalli's: Chapter 200
b. Rosen's: Chapter 122

CASE 106: Weakness (Meika Close, MD)

A. Chief complaint
a. 92-year-old male brought in by EMS after being found by neighbor in bed, covered in urine and feces

B. Vital signs
a. BP: 118/66 HR: 110 RR: 12 T: 36.7°C Sat: 98% on RA FS: 84

C. What does the patient look like?
a. Patient appears cachectic, disheveled, with poor hygiene, and covered in urine and feces.

D. Primary survey
a. Airway: A & O × 3, speaking in full sentences
b. Breathing: no respiratory distress, no cyanosis
c. Circulation: warm skin, normal capillary refill

E. Action
a. Oxygen via NC or nonrebreather mask
b. Two large-bore peripheral IV lines
c. Labs
   i. Point of care glucose
   ii. CBC, BMP, LFT, coagulation studies, blood type and cross-match, lactate, troponin, total CPK, UA
d. Monitor: BP: 118/64 HR: 108 RR: 12 Sat: 98% on RA FS: 80
e. EKG

F. History
a. HPI: a 92-year-old male was brought in by EMS after being found by neighbor, who had entered apartment after not hearing from patient for 2 days. Patient found lying

in bed covered in urine and feces. Patient reports that his son is his caretaker but has not come by in several days. Patient states he was too weak to get out of bed. He reports no PO intake or ambulation since caretaker's last visit. He complains of mild headache, hunger, decreased urination, and no BMs for the past few weeks. ROS otherwise negative.

b. PMHx: none
c. PSHx: none
d. Allergies: none
e. Meds: unknown
f. Social: lives alone in apartment, son is caretaker
g. FHx: not relevant
h. PMD: none

G. Nurse
a. EKG (Figure 106.1)
b. 1 L NS
   i. BP: 124/72 HR: 98 RR: 12 Sat: 98% on RA

H. Secondary survey
a. General: alert, oriented × 3, cachectic, disheveled, poor dentition and hygiene, covered in urine and feces
b. Head: normocephalic, atraumatic
c. Eyes: sunken eyes, extraocular movement intact, pupils equal, reactive to light
d. Ears: normal tympanic membranes

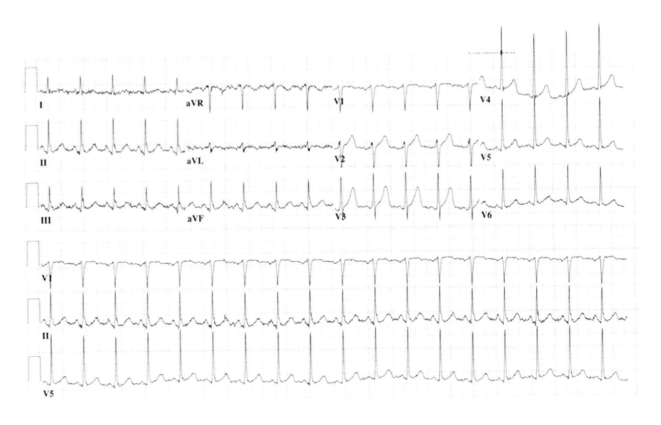

Figure 106.1

e. Nose: no discharge

f. Neck: full range of motion, no jugular vein distension, no stridor

g. Pharynx: dry mucous membranes, normal dentition, no lesions, no swelling

h. Chest: nontender

i. Lungs: bibasilar crackles

j. Heart: tachycardic, no murmurs, rubs, or gallops

k. Abdomen: normal bowel sounds, soft, nontender or distended

l. Rectal: normal tone, brown stool, occult blood negative

m. Urogenital: normal external genitalia

   i. Male: no discharge, normal testicular examination

n. Extremities: full range of motion, no deformity, normal pulses, ecchymosis around right arm

o. Back: nontender

p. Neuro: cranial nerves II to XII intact; normal sensation, strength; normal reflexes, unable to ambulate secondary to weakness

q. Skin: decreased skin turgor; sacral stage III decubitus ulcers ×2

r. Lymph: no lymphadenopathy

I. Action

a. Foley catheter placement

b. Skin and wound care – clean off skin for full exam, dressing applied to decubiti

c. Meds

   i. IVF – NS at maintenance rate

  ii. PO nourishment

d. Reassess

   i. Patient reports feeling better after IV fluids and PO nourishment

e. Consult – social work

f. Imaging

   i. CXR (Figure 106.2)

J. Nurse

a. BP: 130/78 HR: 82 RR: 12 Sat: 98%

b. Patient: stable, no urine output

Figure 106.2

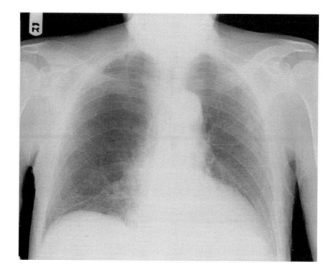

K. Results

Complete blood count:

WBC	5.3×10^3/uL
Hct	41.5%
Plt	350×10^3/uL

Basic metabolic panel:

Na	148 mEq/L
K	4.6 mEq/L
Cl	105 mEq/L
CO_2	23 mEq/L
BUN	48 mEq/dL
Cr	1.9 mg/dL%
Gluc	100 mg/dL

Coagulation panel:

PT	12.6 sec
PTT	26.0 sec
INR	1.0

Liver function panel:

AST	23 U/L
ALT	26 U/L

Alk Phos	42 U/L
T bili	1.0 mg/dL
D bili	0.3 mg/dL
Amylase	50 U/L
Lipase	25 U/L
Albumin	3.7 g/dL

Urinalysis:

SG	>1.030
pH	7.0
Prot	+1 mg/dL
Gluc	Neg mg/dL
Ketones	positive
Bili	Neg
Blood	Neg
LE	Neg
Nitrite	Neg
Color	Dark yellow

a. Lactate 1.0 mmol/L
b. Portable CXR (Figure 106.2)
c. CPK 30
d. Troponin negative

L. Action
a. Admit patient to medicine
b. Report case of elder abuse to proper authorities as mandated by state

M. Diagnosis
a. Elder abuse
b. Dehydration

N. Critical actions
▧ Reporting of case as mandated for elder abuse
▧ Social work involvement
▧ IV hydration
▧ Check CPK for rhabdomyolysis
▧ EKG
▧ Work-up for infection including UA and CXR

O. Examiner instructions
a. This is a case of elder abuse in the form of neglect. The patient is in acute renal failure secondary to dehydration and has sacral decubitus ulcers from being left lying in bed unattended. Complete exposure and thorough physical examination is key in exposing any signs of abuse or neglect. Ecchymoses encircling the upper extremities would be suggestive of the patient being grabbed or shaken; if found on

the lower extremities, sexual abuse should be suspected. The candidate should look not only for signs of physical abuse, but sexual abuse and neglect as well. This patient is unsafe to return home and should be admitted for assessment of renal failure and social service assessment.

P. Pearls

a. The diagnosis of elder abuse rests on a clinician's awareness of the problem, recognition of risk factors and red flags in a patient's history, and a thorough physical examination.

b. There are three basic categories of elder abuse: domestic abuse (occurring in the home), institutional abuse, and self-abuse or self-neglect.

c. Elder abuse may present in the following forms (as defined by the National Center on Elder Abuse):

    i. Physical abuse

    ii. Sexual abuse

    iii. Emotional or psychological abuse

    iv. Financial or material exploitation

    v. Neglect

    vi. Abandonment

    vii. Self-neglect

d. Elder abuse should be reported by the clinician to the appropriate hospital staff and to the proper authorities as mandated by the state.

Q. References

a. Tintinalli's: Chapter 293

b. Rosen's: Chapter 66

CASE 107: Foot pain (Meika Close, MD)

A. Chief complaint

a. 43-year-old male complaining of severe right foot pain and swelling for the past 4 hours

B. Vital signs

a. BP: 142/94 HR: 98 RR: 16 T: 36.5°C Sat: 100%

C. What does the patient look like?

a. Patient appears in moderate distress secondary to pain.

D. Primary survey

a. Airway: speaking in full sentences

b. Breathing: no respiratory distress, no cyanosis

c. Circulation: warm skin, normal capillary refill

E. Action

a. One large-bore peripheral IV line

b. Labs

    i. CBC, BMP, uric acid

c. Monitor: BP: 148/93 HR: 96 RR: 16 Sat: 100%

F. History

a. HPI: a 43-year-old male with no significant PMHx presenting to ED with the complaint of right foot pain since waking this morning, about 4 hours ago. Pain is rated at 10/10 and does not radiate. Patient has taken acetaminophen with no relief. He is able to ambulate, but with pain. He denies trauma or prior episodes. He denies fever or other systemic symptoms.

b. PMHx: none

c. PSHx: none

d. Allergies: none

e. Meds: none

f. Social: not sexually active; drinks alcohol several times per week

g. FHx: diabetes, hypertension

h. PMD: none

G. Nurse

a. BP: 146/92 HR: 96 RR: 14 Sat: 98% on RA

b. Patient: reports 10/10 pain

H. Secondary survey

a. General: alert, oriented × 3

b. Head: normocephalic, atraumatic

c. Eyes: extraocular movement intact, pupils equal, reactive to light

d. Ears: normal tympanic membranes

e. Nose: no discharge

f. Neck: full range of motion, no jugular vein distension, no stridor

g. Pharynx: normal dentition, no lesions, no swelling

h. Chest: nontender

i. Lungs: clear bilaterally

j. Heart: rate and rhythm regular, no murmurs, rubs, or gallops

k. Abdomen: normal bowel sounds, soft, nontender or distended

l. Rectal: deferred

m. Urogenital: deferred

n. Extremities: warmth, erythema, swelling, and tenderness of right 1st metatarsal-phalangeal (MTP) joint, with decreased ROM secondary to pain, able to bear weight

o. Back: nontender

p. Neuro: cranial nerves II to XII intact; normal sensation, strength; normal reflexes and gait

q. Skin: warm and dry

r. Lymph: no lymphadenopathy

I. Action

a. Procedure

   i. Arthrocentesis of right 1st MTP joint to send fluid for studies (cell count, crystals, and gram stain/culture)

b. Meds

   i. NSAIDs

   ii. +/-Opioids

Figure 107.1

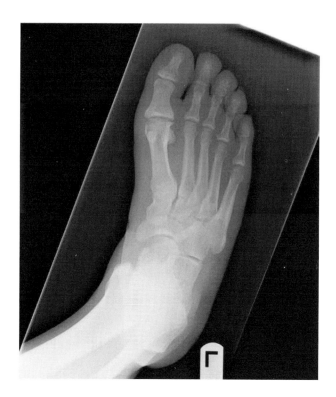

c. Reassess
  i. Patient continues to report 10/10 pain
d. Imaging
  i. X-ray right foot

J. Nurse

a. X-ray right foot (Figure 107.1)
b. BP: 142/74 HR: 92 RR: 12 Sat: 99%
c. Patient:
  i. No pain meds: continues to have pain
  ii. Pain meds given: pain is now moderately reduced, 4/10

K. Results

Complete blood count:

WBC	8.9×10^3/uL
Hct	41.5%
Plt	380×10^3/uL

Basic metabolic panel:

Na	138 mEq/L
K	4.3 mEq/L
Cl	105 mEq/L
CO_2	24 mEq/L
BUN	12 mEq/dL
Cr	1.1 mg/dL%
Gluc	100 mg/dL

Coagulation panel:

PT	12.6 sec
PTT	26.0 sec
INR	1.0

Liver function panel:

AST	23 U/L
ALT	26 U/L
Alk Phos	42 U/L
T bili	1.0 mg/dL
D bili	0.3 mg/dL
Amylase	50 U/L
Lipase	25 U/L
Albumin	4.7 g/dL

Urinalysis:

SG	1.0.20	Bili	Neg
pH	7	Blood	Neg
Prot	Neg mg/dL	LE	Neg
Gluc	Neg mg/dL	Nitrite	Neg
Ketones	Neg mg/dL	Color	Yellow

i. Serum uric acid: 9.0 mg/dL
ii. Joint aspirate
    1. Cell count: WBC 22,000/µL
    2. Microscopy: negatively birefringent needle-shaped crystals present
    3. Gram stain: no organisms

L. Action
a. Meds
    i. Colchicine prescription
b. Disposition
    i. Discharge home with instructions regarding gout
    ii. NSAID and colchicine prescription

M. Diagnosis
a. Acute gout

N. Critical actions
▨ Aspiration of joint to rule out septic arthritis
▨ Pain management
▨ Counseling on alcohol reduction

O. Examiner instructions
a. This is a case of acute gout in a patient with no prior history. Gout is an inflammatory reaction in the joint, most commonly the big toe, which is not infectious in origin and caused by uric acid crystal formation. This is a typical presentation of gout, with acute pain evolving over hours, which may or may not be triggered by trauma, surgery, illness, or heavy protein load. In a patient presenting with pain and inflammation of a joint, it is critical to rule out septic arthritis. Patients with crystal-induced arthritis may present with low-grade fever and normal serum uric acid levels, further complicating the picture and making joint aspiration crucial. Disposition is contingent on exclusion of a septic joint and adequate analgesia. Patient should be counseled on alcohol cessation given it is likely worsening his gout.

P. Pearls
a. Gout typically occurs in male patients in their forties. The majority of patients initially present with monoarticular disease, typically in the lower extremity. Polyarticular disease is more common in recurrences.
b. Acute attacks may be triggered by trauma, surgery, malnutrition, or overconsumption of meat, fish, and/or alcohol.
c. Microscopy of joint aspirate is the key to diagnosis of gout or pseudogout. In both conditions, crystals are present; however, uric acid crystals in gout are needle-

shaped and negatively birefringent, whereas the calcium pyrophosphate crystals of pseudogout are rhomboid-shaped and positively birefringent.

d. Serum uric acid levels are of low utility in the diagnosis of gout, as levels may be normal in many patients. Erythrocyte sedimentation rate is also low-yield in differentiating between crystal-induced arthropathy and septic arthritis, as levels may be elevated in both conditions.

e. Indomethacin is first-line therapy for gout.

f. With pain refractory to NSAID therapy, colchicine may be administered at 0.6 mg/hr until adequate analgesia is achieved or intolerable side effects (vomiting or diarrhea) manifest.

g. If diagnosis is unclear, antibiotics should be started in ED until results of joint aspirate are available.

h. If adequate analgesia is not achieved in ED, or diagnosis of septic arthritis is not excluded, patient requires inpatient management. If discharged from ED, patient should have outpatient follow-up, as long-term therapy with allopurinol or probenicid may be necessary to prevent further attacks. Patient should also receive counseling regarding diet and lifestyle changes to reduce the chance of gout recurrence.

Q. References
a. Tintinalli's: Chapter 281
b. Rosen's: Chapter 114

CASE 108: Neck pain (Evelyn Chow, MD)

A. Chief complaint
a. 37-year-old female presents with headache, neck pain, and visual changes

B. Vital signs
a. BP: 114/62 HR: 84 RR: 18 T: 36.5°C Sat: 99% on RA

C. What does the patient look like?
a. Patient appears stated age, uncomfortable-appearing secondary to pain, holding head, in mild distress, lying still supine on stretcher.

D. Primary survey
a. Airway: speaking in full sentences
b. Breathing: no apparent respiratory distress, no cyanosis
c. Circulation: dry and cool skin, normal capillary refill

E. Action
a. Oxygen via NC or nonrebreather mask
b. Two large-bore peripheral IV lines
c. Labs
   i. CBC, BMP, LFT, coagulation studies, blood type and cross-match, urine hcg
d. Monitor: BP: 114/62 HR: 84 RR: 18 Sat: 99% on RA
e. EKG

F. History

a. HPI: a 37-year-old female status postmotor vehicle accident 2 days ago presents with persistent right-sided headache and neck pain since the accident. Today she had an episode of darkening of the vision in her right eye, lasting 10 minutes. Her vision is now back to baseline. Two days ago the patient was a restrained passenger in a vehicle that rear-ended another. She was seen at an outside hospital at that time and had a normal head CT. Patient denies slurred speech, weakness, numbness, nausea, vomiting, bowel or bladder changes, photophobia, or fever.

b. PMHx: none

c. PSHx: none

d. Allergies: NKDA

e. Meds: none

f. Social: occasional alcohol use, denies tobacco or drugs

g. FHx: noncontributory

h. PMD: none

G. Nurse

a. EKG (Figure 108.1)

b. Urine pregnancy test negative

H. Physical examination

a. General: alert, oriented × 3, holding head, in mild distress

b. Head: normocephalic, atraumatic

c. Eyes: mild right ptosis, right pupil 3 mm, left pupil 5 mm, extraocular movements intact, visual acuity normal, normal sweating on both sides of face.

d. Ears: normal tympanic membranes

e. Nose: no discharge

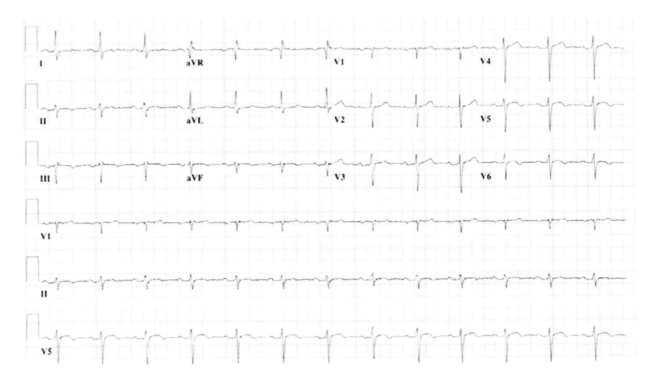

Figure 108.1

    f. Neck: right paraspinal neck tenderness, right carotid bruit (must ask), no mid-line C-spine tenderness

    g. Pharynx: normal dentition, no lesions, no swelling

    h. Chest: nontender

    i. Lungs: clear bilaterally

    j. Heart: rate and rhythm regular, no murmurs, rubs, or gallops

    k. Abdomen: normal bowel sounds, soft, nontender or distended

    l. Rectal: normal tone, brown stool, occult blood negative

    m. Urogenital: deferred

    n. Extremities: full range of motion, no deformity, normal pulses

    o. Back: nontender

    p. Neuro: alert and oriented × 3, mild right ptosis, right pupil 3 mm, left pupil 5 mm, extraocular movements intact, no facial droop, sensation intact, 5/5 motor in all extremities, no cerebellar findings, normal DTRs, downgoing toes and gait

    q. Skin: warm and dry

    r. Lymph: no lymphadenopathy

I. Action

    a. Meds

        i. Narcotic analgesia (Fentanyl, Morphine, Dilaudid, or oxycodone)

    b. Consult neurology

    c. Imaging

        i. CT noncontrast of brain

        ii. CT C-spine

        iii. CT neck with angiography OR MRA neck

J. Nurse

    a. Patient: pain improves with pain medications

K. Results

Complete blood count:

WBC	6.5×10^3/uL	Alk Phos	42 U/L
Hct	41.5%	T bili	1.0 mg/dL
Plt	350×10^3/uL	D bili	0.3 mg/dL
		Amylase	50 U/L
Basic metabolic panel:		Lipase	25 U/L
Na	138 mEq/L	Albumin	4.7 g/dL
K	4.3 mEq/L		
Cl	105 mEq/L	**Urinalysis:**	
CO_2	30 mEq/L	SG	1.0.20
BUN	12 mEq/dL	pH	7
Cr	1.1 mg/dL%	Prot	Neg mg/dL
Gluc	100 mg/dL	Gluc	Neg mg/dL
		Ketones	Neg mg/dL
Coagulation panel:		Bili	Neg
PT	12.6 sec	Blood	Neg
PTT	26.0 sec	LE	Neg
INR	1.0	Nitrite	Neg
		Color	Yellow
Liver function panel:			
AST	23 U/L		
ALT	26 U/L		

Figure 108.2

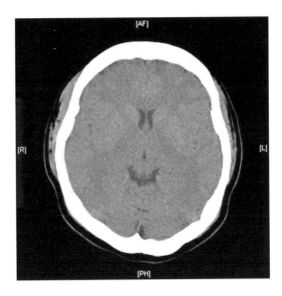

a. CT brain (Figure 108.2)
b. X-ray C-spine (Figure 108.3)
c. CT C-spine – negative for fracture
d. MRA of the neck – + dissection of carotid artery on right side

L. Action
a. Neurology consult evaluates patient and admits her to the stroke unit
b. Heparin

M. Diagnosis
a. Carotid artery dissection on right

N. Critical actions
▨ Pain control
▨ CT head without IV contrast
▨ CT neck angiography or MRA
▨ Neurology consult
▨ Heparin

O. Examiner instructions
a. This is a case of carotid artery dissection secondary to injury from a recent motor vehicle accident. In our patient, the recent neck injury caused a tearing in the wall of the carotid artery that led to a stroke presenting with visual changes. Important actions in this case include imaging of the brain and of the carotid artery. If carotid artery dissection is not considered in the differential and the patient is not started on anticoagulation, the patient should develop signs of an acute stroke in the distribution of the right middle cerebral artery, with left-sided hemiparesis and slurred speech.

P. Pearls
a. Carotid artery dissection is rare, but it is a common cause of stroke in patients younger than 50 years old.

A

B

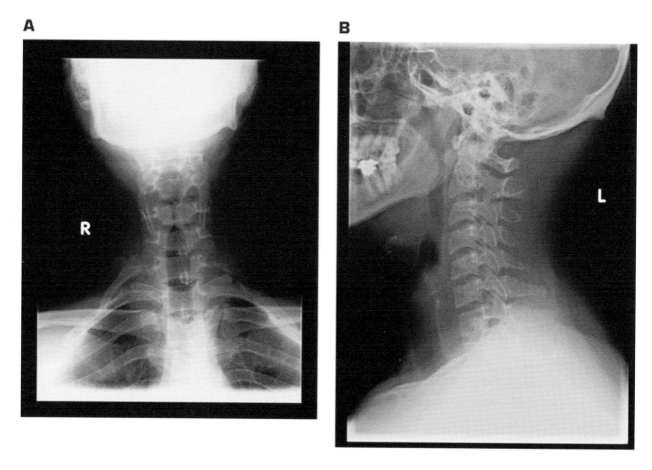

C

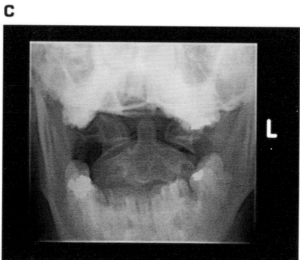

Figure 108.3 A, B and C

    b. They can occur spontaneously or secondary to minor trauma, such as chiropractic manipulation, talking on the phone for long periods of time, coughing, and motor vehicle accidents.

    c. Patients can present with headache, neck pain, facial pain, hypoageusia (decreased taste), or focal neurologic complaints. Some patients have a partial Horner syndrome on examination (ptosis, miosis, without anhidrosis).

d. If the dissection is extracranial, then treatment involves anticoagulation with heparin to prevent thromboembolic events.

e. Do not give heparin if there is an intracranial dissection as this can lead to a subarachnoid hemorrhage. In this case an antiplatelet agent should be started.

Q. References
a. Tintinalli's: Chapter 161
b. Rosen's: Chapter 99

CASE 109: Abdominal pain (Evelyn Chow, MD)

A. Chief complaint
a. 78-year-old male sent from nursing home for abdominal pain

B. Vital signs
a. BP: 137/78 HR: 88 RR: 20 T: 36.9°C Sat: 96% on RA

C. What does the patient look like?
a. Patient is an elderly male, awake and alert, uncomfortable-appearing secondary to pain.

D. Action
a. Oxygen via NC or nonrebreather mask
b. Two large-bore peripheral IV lines
c. Labs
    i. CBC, BMP, LFT, coagulation studies, blood type and cross-match, urinalysis
    ii. Lactate–preferably as part of blood gas results since the results are quickly available. Serum lactate must be obtained if not available as part of the blood gas.
d. 1 L NS bolus
e. Monitor: BP: 137/78 HR: 88 RR: 20 Sat: 96% on RA
f. EKG

E. Primary survey
a. Airway: speaking in full sentences
b. Breathing: no respiratory distress
c. Circulation: warm skin, normal capillary refill

F. History
a. HPI: a 78-year-old male with a history of Parkinson's and hypertension sent from nursing home for increasing abdominal pain and distension for 1 week. Patient complains of nausea, but has not vomited. Patient has chronic constipation at baseline. Last bowel movement was several days ago; no fevers or chills; no diarrhea, urinary symptoms; worse with eating.
b. PMHx: Parkinson's, hypertension
c. PSHx: none
d. Allergies: none

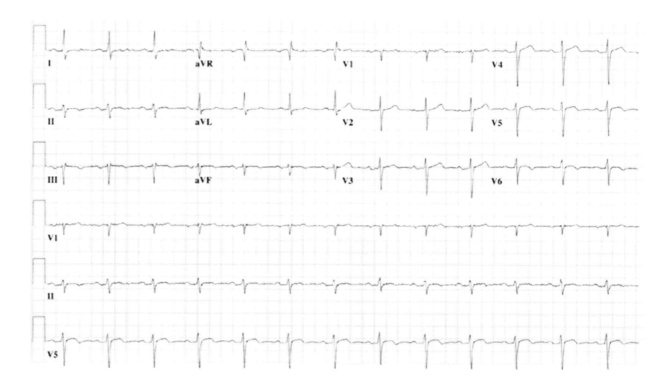

Figure 109.1

e. Meds: carbidopa-levidopa, metoprolol, colace, senna
f. Social: lives in a nursing home
g. FHx: no relevant history
h. PMD: nursing home doctor

G. Nurse
a. EKG (Figure 109.1)

H. Physical examination
a. General: alert, oriented × 2 (baseline),
b. Head: normocephalic, atraumatic
c. Eyes: extraocular movement intact, pupils equal, reactive to light
d. Ears: normal tympanic membranes
e. Nose: no discharge
f. Neck: full range of motion, no jugular vein distension, no stridor
g. Pharynx: mucous membranes dry, normal dentition, no lesions, no swelling
h. Chest: nontender
i. Lungs: clear bilaterally
j. Heart: rate and rhythm regular, no murmurs, rubs, or gallops
k. Abdomen: hypoactive bowel sounds, soft, moderate diffuse tenderness, no rebound or guarding, distended, tympanic
l. Rectal: normal tone, minimal hard stool, occult blood negative
m. Urogenital: normal external genitalia
    i. Male: no discharge, normal testicular examination

n. Extremities: full range of motion, no deformity, normal pulses
o. Back: nontender
p. Neuro: cranial nerves II to XII intact; normal sensation, strength; normal reflexes and gait, bilateral hands with resting tremor
q. Skin: warm and dry
r. Lymph: no lymphadenopathy

I. Action
a. Meds
   i. Narcotic analgesia (i.e. fentanyl for short-acting pain control during work-up)
b. Imaging: obstructive series (if CT abdomen/pelvis ordered, there is a delay in scanner)

J. Nurse
a. BP: 132/74 HR: 72 RR: 18 Sat: 96%
b. Abdominal series XR (Figure 109.2)

K. Action
a. Consult
   i. Gastroenterology
   ii. Surgery
b. Nasogastric tube

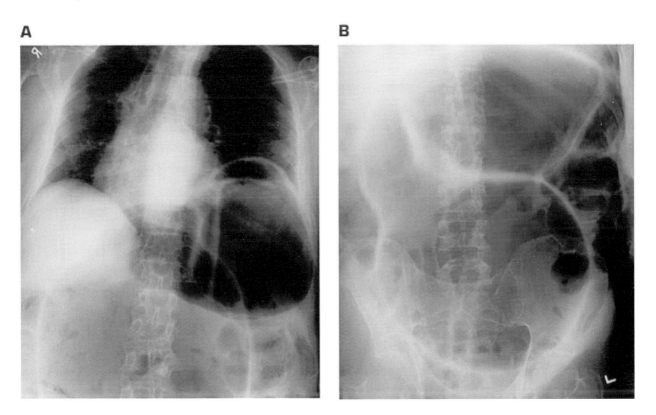

Figure 109.2 A and B

L. Results

Complete blood count:

WBC	16.2×10^3/uL	Alk Phos	42 U/L
Hct	40.5%	T bili	1.0 mg/dL
Plt	230×10^3/uL	D bili	0.3 mg/dL
		Amylase	50 U/L
Basic metabolic panel:		Lipase	25 U/L
Na	141 mEq/L	Albumin	4.7 g/dL
K	4.3 mEq/L		
Cl	105 mEq/L	**Urinalysis:**	
CO$_2$	30 mEq/L	SG	1.0.20
BUN	25 mEq/dL	pH	7
Cr	1.2 mg/dL%	Prot	Neg mg/dL
Gluc	70 mg/dL	Gluc	Neg mg/dL
		Ketones	Neg mg/dL
Coagulation panel:		Bili	Neg
PT	12.6 sec	Blood	Neg
PTT	26.0 sec	LE	trace
INR	1.0	Nitrite	Neg
		Color	Yellow
Liver function panel:			
AST	23 U/L		
ALT	26 U/L		

a. Lactate 2.8 mmol/L

M. Action

a. Antibiotics (acceptable regimens include ciprofloxacin/metronidazole or pipercillin/tazobactam)

b. Gastroenterology performs sigmoidoscopy and decompresses volvulus with rectal tube.

c. Patient is admitted for monitoring and surgical intervention to prevent recurrence.

N. Diagnosis

a. Sigmoid volvulus

O. Critical actions

▪ Pain control

▪ IV line placement

▪ Obstructive series

▪ Nasogastric tube

▪ Consult gastroenterology and surgery

P. Examiner instructions

a. This is a case of sigmoid volvulus in a nursing home patient with chronic constipation. Volvulus is a twisting of the intestine, commonly occurring in the sigmoid colon, which leads to severe pain and distension of the stomach and ultimately perforation of the intestine if not treated. Important early actions include an obstructive series, nasogastric tube placement, gastroenterology consult, and/or surgery consult. If a CT scan is ordered, note that the scan is delayed. By the time the CT is done, the patient starts to exhibit peritoneal signs on examination suggestive of bowel necrosis, in which case a sigmoidoscopy would be contraindicated. Patient would then have to go straight to the operating room.

Q. Pearls

a. Sigmoid volvulus often occurs in elderly patients who are debilitated or in patients with psychiatric or neurologic disorders.

b. Chronic constipation is a risk factor for sigmoid volvulus.

c. The "bent innertube" or "coffee bean" sign is classically seen on x-ray.

d. There is a high rate of recurrence with sigmoid volvulus. Even if the volvulus is decompressed with a rectal tube, patients usually go for definitive treatment in the OR.

e. If there is any sign of bowel necrosis (i.e., peritoneal signs on examination, signs of shock, WBC >20,000, high lactate) then rectal tube decompression is contraindicated. Patient must go directly to the OR.

R. References

a. Tintinalli's: Chapter 86

b. Rosen's: Chapter 93

CASE 110: Shortness of breath (Tarlan Hedayati, MD)

A. Chief complaint

a. 68-year-old man with shortness of breath

B. Vital signs

a. BP: 52/34 (MAP 40) HR: 110 RR: 26 T: 98°F pulse oximetry: 86% on room air

C. What does the patient look like?

a. The patient is a thin man, pale, diaphoretic, and sitting on a gurney. His left ventricular assist device (LVAD) device is alarming

D. Primary survey

a. Airway: speaking in full sentences

b. Breathing: tachypneic, in mild respiratory distress

c. Circulation: diaphoretic, cool, pale skin

E. Action

a. Oxygen via nonrebreather mask

b. Two large-bore peripheral IV lines

c. Labs

   i. CBC, BMP, LFT, coagulation studies, blood type and cross-match

   ii. Troponin

   iii. BNP

d. Monitor: MAP: 40 HR: 110 RR: 26 T: 98°F

e. Order electrocardiogram

   f. Order chest radiograph

   g. Request bedside echocardiogram

F. History

  a. HPI: a 68-year-old man presents with shortness of breath, lightheadedness, and generalized fatigue for the last 6 hours. He has associated diaphoresis. He denies nausea, vomiting, fevers, chills. He admits to a non-productive cough for the same amount of time. He has noticed that his LVAD parameters have changed in the last 6 hours, with higher power readings and lower flow rates. He states he has been taking all his medications as prescribed.

  b. PMHx: congestive heart failure, coronary artery disease, hyperlipidemia

  c. PSHx: Left ventricular assist device implanted 2 years ago; drug eluting stents placed 3 years ago to the LVAD and left circumflex arteries

  d. Allergies: none

  e. Meds: carvedilol, furosemide, enalapril, simvastatin, aspirin, warfarin

  f. Social: denies drug or alcohol use; quit tobacco 3 years ago

  g. FHx: Father died of MI at age 60; Mother died of MI at 55

  h. Cardiologist: Dr Shah

G. Secondary survey

  a. General: alert, oriented x 3, diaphoretic, in mild respiratory distress

  b. Head: normocephalic, atraumatic

  c. Eyes: extraocular movement intact, pupils equal and reactive to light

  d. Ears: normal tympanic membranes

  e. Pharynx: noerythema or exudates

  f. Neck: soft, supple, jugular venous distension to angle of the jaw

  g. Chest: nontender to palpation, well-healed sternotomy scar

  h. Lungs: crackles at bilateral bases to mid-lung fields

  i. Heart: muffled heart sounds

  j. Abdomen: soft, nontender to palpation, LVAD catheter exiting at RUQ is clean, dry, and secure

  k. Extremities: full range of motion, no deformity, thready pulses, 2+ pitting edema to the thighs bilaterally

  l. Neuro: cranial nerves II-XII intact; normal sensation and strength, normal reflexes, normal but slow gait

  m. Skin: cool and diaphoretic, no rashes

  n. Lymph: no lymphadenopathy

H. Action

  a. Electrocardiogram (Figure 110.1. Courtesy of Atman P. Shah, MD)

  b. Chest radiograph (Figure 110.2. Courtesy of Atman P. Shah, MD)

  c. Meds:

     i. Heparin drip

  d. Consult

     i. VAD coordinator

     ii. Cardiothoracic surgery, cardiology, or heart failure service

ORDER MD:

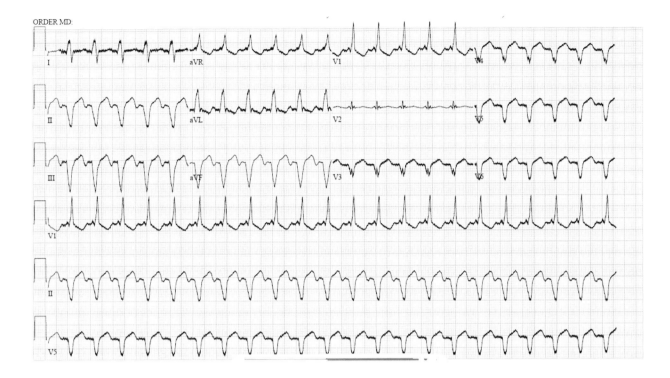

Figure 110.1

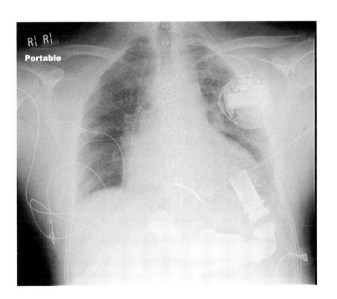

Figure 110.2

I. Results

Complete blood count:

WBC	11.1×10^3/uL	Cl	104 mEq/L
Hct	30%	CO_2	24 mEq/L
Plt	186×10^3/uL	BUN	20 mEq/dL
		Cr	1.7 mg/dL
Basic metabolic panel:		Glucose	96 mg/dL
Na	134 mEq/L		
K	3.5 mEq/L	**Coagulation panel:**	
		INR	1.7

Liver function panel:

LDH	3880 U/L	ALT	38 U/L
Albumin	3.8 g/dL	Alkaline phosphatase	106 U/L
Direct bilirubin	0.5 mg/dL		
Indirect bilirubin	2.5 mg/dL	**Urinalysis:**	normal
AST	35 U/L		

a. Troponin-I 0.143 ng/mL
b. BNP 977 pg/mL
c. Portable echocardiogram demonstrates ejection fraction less than 15%, small pericardial effusion

J. Diagnosis
a. Heart failure due to LVAD failure caused by pump thrombosis

K. Critical actions
a. Electrocardiogram
b. Bedside echocardiogram
c. Heparin drip
d. VAD coordinator or CT surgery consult or Cardiology consult

L. Examiner instructions
a. This is a case of heart failure caused by LVAD failure due to thrombosis in the device pump. The candidate should recognize signs of heart failure on the physical examination and look for causes of this failure as related to the LVAD. The presence of a palpable pulse and LV contraction on bedside echocardiogram implies failure of the continuous flow of the LVAD. The subtherapeutic INR puts the patients at risk for LVAD thrombosis and device failure. The candidate should also recognize laboratory findings consistent with hemolysis are a sign of pump thrombosis. Once recognized, anticoagulation with heparin and consult CT surgery, the VAD coordinator, heart failure service, or cardiology in an attempt to lyse and/or aspirate the clot.

M. Pearls
a. Patients with LVAD are at risk for thrombosis
   i. Anticoagulated patients with therapeutic INR are still at risk for thrombosis
   ii. Patients with pump failure will present with signs of heart failure
   iii. Pump thrombosis may elicit elevated troponins and elevated BNP as well as laboratory findings consistent with hemolysis including elevated LDH and indirect bilirubin
   iv. Patients with VAD thrombosis will see an increase in device power readings but decreased flow readings on their device console

N. References
a. Tintinalli's Chapter 295. The Transplant Patient
b. Rosen Chapter 80. Implantable Cardiac Devices

CASE 111: Arm pain (Yuemi An-Grogan, MD)

A. Chief complaint
  a. 4-year-old male with right arm pain

B. Vital signs
  a. BP: 84/46 HR: 125 RR: 26 T: 37.6°C Wt: 16 kg

C. What does the patient look like?
  a. Child is not in acute distress, but is crying

D. Primary survey
  a. Airway: crying
  b. Breathing: no apparent respiratory distress, no cyanosis
  c. Circulation: peripheral pulses equal (including left radial pulse)

E. History
  a. A 4-year-old boy presents with right arm pain that started just prior to arrival, per mom. She states they were just at the playground with her older son and all of a sudden the patient started crying and screaming. This morning, mom states that the patient was in his usual state of health. No sick contacts. No obvious trauma witnessed by mom. Mom denies any fevers and any recent illnesses.
  b. PMHx: full term, NSVD, eczema
  c. PSHx: none
  d. Meds: cortisone cream as needed, otherwise no regular medications
  e. Allergies: Amoxicillin
  f. Social: lives with parents and his older sibling – brother
  g. FHx: no sick contacts
  h. Immunizations: up-to-date

F. Secondary survey
  a. General: awake, crying, appropriate for age
  b. HEENT: pupils equal, round, reactive; moist mucous membranes, oropharynx clear, tympanic membranes with minimal erythema bilaterally, but clear, no hemotympanum, no evidence of external trauma
  c. Neck: no cervical lymphadenopathy, trachea midline, no midline cervical spine tenderness
  d. Chest: no rashes, no chest wall tenderness, equal chest rise
  e. Heart: normal heart sounds, no murmurs
  f. Abdomen: no tenderness, no distention, no bruising
  g. Rectal: deferred
  h. GU: deferred
  i. Extremities: patient is holding his right arm in 20 degree flexion. No obvious bony deformity, no obvious tenderness over the left shoulder or wrist, but patient screams when you try to touch his right elbow. No effusion present, left arm and bilateral legs normal, full range of motion of other extremities, no deformity, normal pulses, <2 second capillary refill in all extremities
  j. Back: normal, no midline tenderness

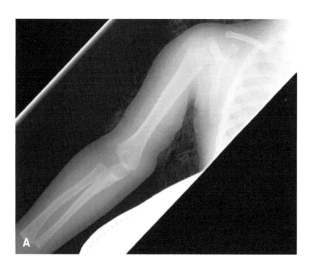 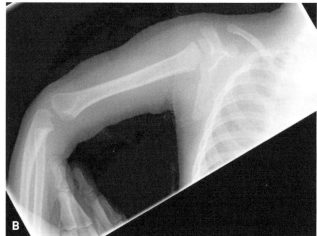

Figure 111.1

    k. Neuro: appropriate for age. Sensation to light touch intact bilateral upper extremities including finger grip strength left hand normal; patient will not grasp anything in right hand.
    l. Skin: no obvious rashes or lesions
   m. Lymph: normal

G. Action
    a. First attempted reduction: unsuccessful
    b. Imaging
      i. Right elbow x-ray (Figure 111.1. Reproduced with permission from Clinical Emergency Radiology (J. Christian Fox) Figure 7.22, page 126)

H. Results
    a. Labs: none

I. Action
    a. Second attempted reduction: successful if correct method
      i. Hyperpronation: with finger on radial head and in 90 degree flexion
      ii. Supination–flexion: with finger on radial head and in 90 degree flexion

J. Diagnosis
    a. Radial head subluxation, also known as "nursemaids elbow"

K. Critical actions
    a. Attempted manual reduction
    b. Reassessment of range of motion, vascular integrity, and tenderness after reduction

L. Examiner instructions
    a. The child has a nursemaid's elbow, which most commonly occurs in children from 2 to 3 years of age, but can occur from 6 months to 7 years of age. It is more common in girls and on the left side, since most providers or parents are right-handed. The mechanism of injury is commonly a sudden longitudinal traction or

axial traction on a pronated forearm and extended elbow, such as in a "pulling" motion. Other mechanisms include fall, direct blow, or twisting motions.

b. When prompted or asked what mom was doing, mom states she was talking to her friend and that her older son was playing with the patient. Mom then states that the brother mentioned he was playing with the patient by swinging him side to side by his wrists and then all of a sudden the patient started crying.

M. Pearls
a. Radial head subluxation is a clinical diagnosis.
b. Imaging is only needed if the mechanism of injury is other than minor direct injury or pulling or if focal tenderness and/or swelling is present.
c. Children will often hold the affected arm close to the body with the elbow slightly flexed and there may be mild tenderness over the anterolateral aspect of the radial head.
d. Reduction is most successful using hyperpronation or supination–flexion methods.

N. References
a. Tintinalli's: Chapter 143C. Pediatric Procedures: Nursemaid's Elbow Reduction
b. Rosen: Chapter 52. Humerus and Elbow.

CASE 112: Altered mental status (Raashee Kedia, MD)

A. Chief complaint
a. 88-year-old female with altered mental status

B. Vital signs
a. BP: 88/56 HR: 118 RR: 20 T 101.6°F O_2 Sat: 99% on RA

C. What does the patient look like?
a. Patient is a frail elderly female, eyes closed and not speaking

D. Primary survey
a. Airway: able to state her name and answer yes/no to questions
b. Breathing: no apparent respiratory distress, no cyanosis
c. Circulation: warm and diaphoretic skin, delayed capillary refill, equal peripheral pulses

E. History
a. HPI: 88-year-old bed-bound female from nursing home with decreased verbal responsiveness for 2 days. Decreased oral intake. Patient usually is talkative and able to feed herself.
b. PMHx: hypertension
c. PSHx: recent non-operable left hip fracture 6 months earlier.
d. Meds: Lisinopril (held for last 2 days due to low blood pressure).
e. Allergies: none

f. Social: denies drug, alcohol, or tobacco use. Good family support system.

g. FH: noncontributory

h. PMD: Dr. Marks

F. Secondary survey

a. General: lying with eyes closed, opens eyes to verbal stimulation, responds yes/no appropriately to questions

b. HEENT: atraumatic, no facial droop

c. Eyes: pupils equal, round, and reactive; sunken eyes. Extraocular movement intact, fundi sharp, no papilledema

d. Ears: normal tympanic membranes

e. Nose: no discharge

f. Neck: full range of motion, supple, no jugular vein distension, no stridor

g. Pharynx: normal dentition, no lesions, no tonsillar swelling

h. Chest: nontender, no crepitus

i. Lungs: clear bilaterally

j. Heart: tachycardic, regular rhythm, no murmurs, rubs, or gallops

k. Abdomen: normal bowel sounds, soft, nontender, nondistended

l. Rectal: normal tone, brown stool, occult blood negative

m. Back: stage 4 decubitus ulcer with purulent drainage and surrounding erythema

n. Extremities: Left leg slightly shorter than right leg. Full range of motion of upper and right lower extremities. Equal strength in upper extremities. Unable to move left hip but able to move left ankle and wiggle toes. Mild tenderness over left hip, no overlying skin changes. Pulses equal in all extremities

o. Neuro: cranial nerves II to XII intact; normal sensation

p. Skin: warm and diaphoretic

q. Lymph: no lymphadenopathy

G. Action

a. Two large-bore peripheral IV lines

b. Labs

   i. CBC, BMP, lactate, venous blood gas, PT/PTT/INR, blood culture, urinalysis, urine culture

c. Monitor: BP: 88/56 HR: 118 RR: 20

d. Normal saline 2L bolus

e. Imaging

   i. CXR (Fig 112.1)

   ii. X-ray left hip

   iii. CT head (patient too unstable to go to radiology)

f. Meds

   i. Vancomycin 1g IV

   ii. Tylenol 650mg PO

H. Nurse

a. EKG (Fig 112.2)

b. Foley catheter

c. Rectal temperature: 103.5°F

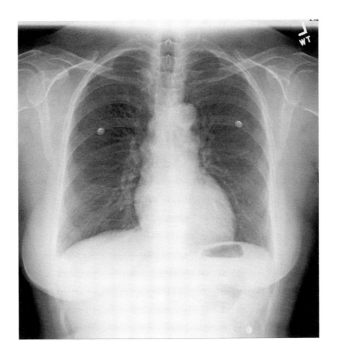

Figure 112.1

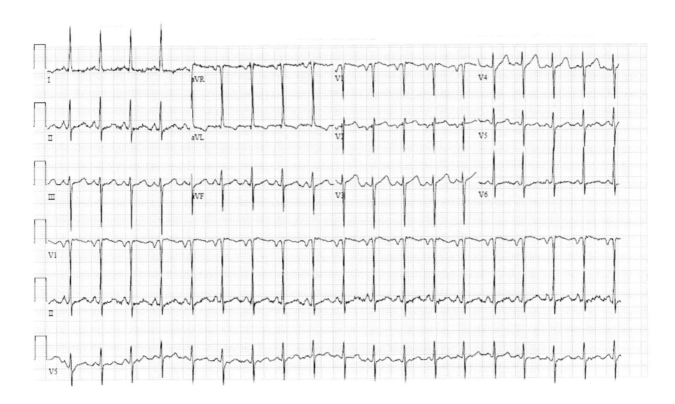

Figure 112.2

I. Results

Complete blood count:

WBC	15.3 x 10^3/uL
Hgb	8
Hct	24.1%
Plt	45 x 10^3/uL

Basic metabolic panel:

Na	138 mEq/L
K	3.8 mEq/L
Cl	100 mEq/L
CO_2	21 mEq/L
BUN	38 mEq/dL
Cr	2.0 mg/dL
Gluc	128 mg/dL

Coagulation panel:

PT	34 sec	(10–12 sec)
PTT	72 sec	(30–45 sec)
INR	1.3	

Blood gas:

pH	7.30
pCO_2	44 mmHg
pO_2	40 mmHg

HCO_3	21 mEq/L
Lactate	6 mmol/L

Urinalysis:

SG	1.025
pH	6
Prot	Neg
Gluc	Neg
Ketones	Neg
Bili	Neg
Blood	Moderate
LE	Neg
Nitrite	Neg
Color	Yellow

a. Hip X-ray: old left intertrochanteric fracture, no acute fracture

J. Action

a. Labs
   i. Recheck PT/PTT/INR, add fibrinogen, D-dimer
b. Reassess vitals
   i. If no IVF given: BP: 70/48 HR 128 RR: 20
   ii. If 1L IVF given: BP: 100/72 HR: 103 RR: 20
   iii. If 2L IVF given: BP: 122/78 HR: 96 RR: 20
c. Recheck lactate
   i. If no IVF given: Lactate = 6.5 mmol/L
   ii. If 1L IVF given: Lactate = 4.0 mmol/L
   iii. If 2L IVF given: Lactate = 2.5 mmol/L
d. Recheck mental status
   i. If no IVF given: patient more lethargic with decreased responsiveness
   ii. If IVF given: patient more alert and talkative

K. Results

Coagulation panel:

PT	34 sec	(10–12 sec)
PTT	72 sec	(30–45 sec)
INR	1.3	

D-dimer:	>500 mmol/L
Fibrinogen:	<100 mmol/L

L. Action
a. Administer 1U platelets, 2U FFP
b. Administer Vitamin K 10mg subq and folate 1 mg IV
c. Admit to ICU

M. Diagnosis
a. Sepsis from decubitus ulcer causing disseminated intravascular coagulation (DIC)

N. Critical actions
a. Fluid resuscitation
b. Finding source of sepsis as decubitus ulcer
c. Antibiotic administration
d. Re-check lactate
e. Recognize DIC

O. Examiner instructions
a. This patient has an overwhelming systemic infection (sepsis) due to a skin infection on her back (decubitus ulcer). The ulcer developed from continued pressure on her skin from being immobile due to her hip fracture 6 months ago. This patient arrives already decompensated; she is tachycardic, febrile, hypotensive, and has altered mental status. She needs immediate care including fluid and antibiotic administration.

P. Pearls
a. If there is no improvement in blood pressure after fluid administration (up to 4–6 L of crystalloid), dopamine should be titrated to appropriate blood pressure response.
b. In persistent hypotension, adrenal insufficiency should be suspected and glucocorticoid should be administered (hydrocortisone 100 mg IV).
c. When the source of sepsis is unknown, empiric antibiotic therapy against gram-positive and gram-negative organisms should be started.
d. Persistent severe acidosis can be treated with sodium bicarbonate 1 mEq/kg IV.
e. DIC is a possible complication of severe sepsis. DIC should be treated with fresh-frozen plasma and platelets, keep PT 1.5 to 2 times normal and platelet counts to at least 50,000/microL.

Q. References
a. Tintinalli's: Chapter 146. Septic Shock
b. Rosen: Chapter 6. Shock

CASE 113: Cardiac arrest (Benjamin H. Slovis MD)

A. Chief complaint
a. 56-year-old male is brought in by EMS after cardiac arrest.

B. Vital signs
a. BP: 95/50 HR: 65 on monitor RR: Intubated, bagged at 8 breaths per minute T: 36.7°C

C. What does the patient look like?
a. Middle-aged male, intubated, pale, and unresponsive to painful stimuli.

D. Primary survey
a. Airway: ET tube in place at 23 cm. Otherwise patent.
b. Breathing: No spontaneous breaths, respirations at 8 breaths per minute by EMS.
c. Circulation: palpable radial and carotid pulses.

E. Action
a. Place patient on ventilator. Confirm tube placement with $ETCO_2$.
b. Place patient on cardiac monitor.
    i. BP: 95/50, HR: 65, RR: now 12 on vent, T: 36.7°C, O_2 Sat: 99% on 100% FiO_2
c. Finger stick blood glucose
d. Two large-bore IVs if not already established by EMS.
e. EKG
f. X-ray
g. Labs
    i. CBC, BMP, coagulation studies, LFTs
    ii. Troponin
    iii. Blood gas, lctate

F. History
a. HPI: 56-year-old male presenting after cardiac arrest. According to EMS, patient was eating dinner with wife at restaurant, collapsed at table. Bystanders promptly initiated CPR. Upon EMS arrival, patient found to be pulseless. Shockable rhythm on monitor with single shock delivered with return of spontaneous circulation to sinus bradycardia. Single dose of atropine 0.5 mg given and patient intubated for airway stabilization with confirmation by continuous end-tidal capnography. Transferred to ED in under 15 minutes.
b. PMHx: Hypertension, diabetes, coronary artery disease with stents 10 years ago
c. PSHx: Cholecystectomy 15 years ago
d. Meds: Clopidogrel, simvastatin, metformin
e. Allergies: ACE inhibitors
f. Social: Lives with wife. Ex-smoker, 20 pack year history. Social drinker. No illicit drug use.
g. FHx: CAD and DM in both parents. Father died of MI at 62.

G. Paramedic
a. Rhythm strip (Figure 113.1)

H. Secondary survey
a. General: intubated, not responsive to painful stimuli.
b. HEENT: NCAT. Pupils equal, reactive to light. No tracking noted. Normal sclera.
c. Neck: trachea midline, no bruit. No jugular venous distension.
d. Chest: bilateral chest rise with rescue breaths. No signs of trauma.
e. Lungs: clear to auscultation bilaterally. No wheezes, rhonchi, or rales.
f. Heart: regular rate and rhythm, normal S1, S2 with S3 present. No clicks or rubs.
g. Abdomen: normal bowel sounds, soft, not distended.

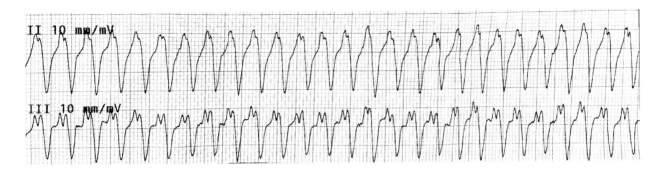

Figure 113.1

h. Extremities: full range of motion, no deformities. Palpable pulses throughout. No spontaneous movement.

i. Neuro: eyes do not open spontaneously. Pupils react to light bilaterally. Pupillary reflex intact. Does not withdraw from pain. No posturing.

j. Skin: cool and pale

I. Action

a. Airway
  i. End-tidal CO_2 monitoring
  ii. Ventilator set up
  iii. CXR

b. Finger stick blood glucose

c. Establish central venous access

d. Establish arterial line

e. Rectal temperature

f. Aspirin

g. CCU / ICU consult

h. Chill patient to 36°C between 2 and 8 hours
  i. Ice packs
  ii. 1–2 L 4°C chilled saline over 30 minutes
  iii. Cooling blankets
  iv. Commercial cooling devices
  v. Sedation and shivering inhibition
    1. Consider meperidine
    2. Consider buspirone
  vi. Esophageal or bladder temperature probe

i. Heparin

j. GI prophylaxis

J. Nurse

a. If no sedation during therapeutic hypothermia
  i. Patient is at 37 degrees and shivering

b. If patient is sedated with therapeutic hypothermia
  i. Patient is at 36 degrees and comfortable

K. Results
a. EKG (Figure 113.2)

Complete blood count:

WBC	9.2×10^3/uL
Hb / Hct	13.1 / 43.2%
Plt	157×10^3/uL

Basic metabolic panel:

Na	139 mEq/L
K	4.9 mEq/L
Cl	91 mEq/L
CO_2	21 mEq/L
BUN	12 mEq/L
Cr	1.1 mEq/dL
Gluc	138 mEq/dL

Coagulation panel:

PT	15.0 sec (10–12 sec)
PTT	29.8 sec (30–45 sec)
INR	1.4

Liver function panel:

AST	21 U/L
ALT	45 U/L
Alk Phos	104 U/L
T Bili	6.5 mg/d/L
D Bili	0.1 mg/d/L
Amylase	56 U/L
Lipase	100 U/L
Albumin	3.6 g/dL

Arterial blood gas:

pH	7.12
PCO_2	52 mmHg
PO_2	96 mmHg
HCO_3	21 mEq/L
Lactate	2.9 mmol/L

Troponin	negative

a. End-tidal CO_2 at 40 mmHg

L. Action
a. Maintain hypothermia for 12–24 hours with rewarming over 12–24 hours.
b. Repeat labs q4 hours
   i. Watch for hypokalemia / hypomagnesemia / hypophosphatemia

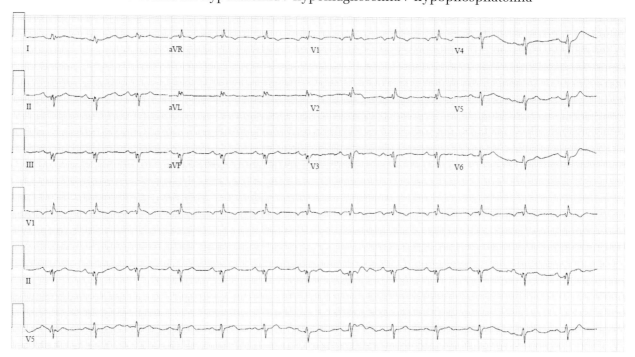

Figure 113.2

 c. Nursing phase of care
  i. Eye lubrication
  ii. Glycemic control
  iii. NPO
  iv. Core temp monitoring

M. Diagnosis
a. Pulseless ventricular tachycardia – cardiac arrest

N. Critical actions
a. Confirmation of airway
b. Cardiac monitoring
c. Recognizing pulseless VT arrest with ROSC
d. Neurologic examination
e. Therapeutic hypothermia
f. Appropriate sedation

O. Examiner instructions
a. In this case there is an episode of pulseless ventricular tachycardia with return of spontaneous circulation in the field. The candidate should be capable of post-arrest management, including recognition of non-perfusing and perfusing rhythms on EKG, as well as confirmation of endotracheal tube placement. Once stable a neurologic examination should be completed and therapeutic hypothermia should be initiated if the patient meets inclusion criteria.

P. Pearls
a. Therapeutic hypothermia has been shown to improve outcomes in neurologically compromised patients after cardiac arrest.
b. Therapeutic hypothermia must be maintained at 36 °C for 12–24 hours.
c. Management of shivering and other thermoregulatory mechanisms is required for adequate hypothermia. Meperidine and buspirone have been shown to be effective in reducing shivering.
d. Electrolyte abnormalities are a common side effect of cooling, and labs should be monitored and electrolytes repleted as needed.
e. Hypothermia should not delay other necessary interventions in the setting of cardiac arrest such as emergent catheterization for ST-elevation myocardial infarction but can be performed in conjunction with such procedures.

Q. References
a. Tintinalli's: Chapter 18. Cerebral Resuscitation and Therapeutic Hypothermia.
b. Rosen: Chapter 8. Brain Resuscitation.
c. Nielsen et al. Targeted temperature management at 33°C versus 36°C after cardiac arrest *NEJM* 2013

CASE 114: Leg pain (Sunil Aradhya, MD)

A. Chief complaint
a. 45-year-old female with right leg pain

B. Vital signs

a. BP: 136/77, HR: 90, RR: 18, T: 37.3°C, Wt: 80kg

C. What does the patient look like?

a. Patient appears stated age, obviously uncomfortable; massaging right leg while on stretcher

D. Primary survey

a. Airway: speaking in full sentences, phonating well
b. Breathing: no apparent respiratory distress, no cyanosis
c. Circulation: peripheral pulses equal

E. Action

a. Place on continuous telemetry monitor, including pulse oximetry
b. Large-bore peripheral IV lines
c. EKG

F. History

a. HPI: A 45-year-old female presents with one-day history of right lower extremity pain and swelling. Patient reports she began noticing pain shortly after awakening when she walked down her driveway this morning to check her mail. She reports subjective fever, but otherwise denies any headache, chest pain, shortness of breath, nausea, vomiting, or abdominal pain.
b. PMHx: diabetes mellitus (type 2), hypertension, and hypothyroidism
c. PSHx: perforated diverticulitis requiring bowel resection (3 weeks prior), cholecystectomy and hysterectomy (at age 40)
d. Meds: metformin, losartan, levothyroxine
e. Allergies: none
f. Social: Married with 2 children. Denies alcohol, drug use. Smokes ½ pack of cigarettes per day (25 pack-year history)
g. FHx: no pertinent history

G. Secondary survey

a. General: awake, alert, oriented
b. HEENT: pupils equal, round, reactive; oropharynx clear, mucous membranes moist.
c. Neck: no appreciated lymphadenopathy or JVD.
d. Heart: Regular rate and rhythm, without murmurs/rubs/gallops
e: Lungs: Clear to auscultation, bilaterally
f. Abdomen: soft, nondistended, with normal bowel sounds. Appropriately tender to palpation over well-healing surgical wound site without guarding or rebound tenderness.
g. Extremities: right lower leg appears enlarged when compared to left. There is pain at rest that is augmented by palpation of extremity. Dorsalis pedis and posterior tibialis pulses are 2+ bilaterally.
h. Neuro: no focal neurological findings
i. Skin: right lower extremity with mild diffuse erythema. No other abnormal skin findings.

H. Action

a. Right lower extremity venous ultrasound/Doppler

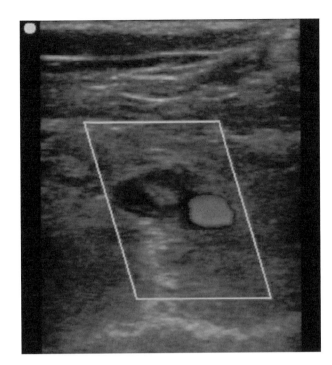

Figure 114.1
See color plate section (in some formats this figure will only appear in black and white).

b. Labs
   i. CBC with differential, BMP, PT/PTT/INR

I. Results

Complete blood count:
WBC 12.3×10^3/uL
Hgb   13.1 g/dL
Hct   39.3%
Plt 400×10^9/L

Basic metabolic panel:
Na   142 mEq/L
K   4.1 mEq/L
Cl   101 mEq/L
CO_2 18 mEq/L

BUN   20 mEq/dL
Cr   0.8 mg/dL
Gluc   129 mg/dL

Coagulation panel:
PT   12.3 sec
PTT   30 sec
INR   1.1

D-Dimer: 2,250 ng/mL (normal < 500 ng/mL)

a. US right lower extremity (Figures 114.1, 114.2) shows proximal common femoral vein is non-compressible with poor augmentation of flow. Highly suspicious for deep vein thrombosis (DVT).

J. Action
a. Begin Lovenox
b. Chest x-ray
c. Warfarin
d. If patient responsible, has reliable follow-up with PCP, may discharge home with INR to be re-checked in 5 days.

K. Diagnosis
a. DVT after surgery

Figure 114.2
See color plate
section (in some
formats this figure
will only appear in
black and white).

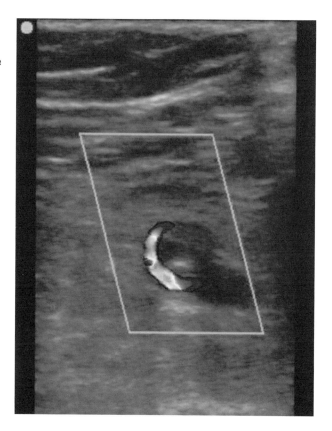

L. Critical actions

a. Ultrasound

b. Anticoagulation with enoxaparin bridge for initiation of oral warfarin anticoagulation therapy

c. Pain management

M. Examiner instructions

a. This patient is suffering from a DVT after surgery, likely a combination of a procoagulable state post-surgery and prolonged immobilization. Common symptoms include pain and swelling of the affected extremity, which is most often a lower extremity. Compression ultrasonography is the key to diagnosis. The patient's recent history of surgery is a significant risk factor.

N. Pearls

a. Risk factors for DVTs include malignancy, recent surgery, history of DVT/PE, genetic predisposition to a hypercoagulable state, hospitalization, OCP/hormone replacement, pregnancy, and prolonged immobilization

b. Symptoms include erythema, swelling, and pain of affected extremity with increased calf diameter in lower extremity DVTs increasing likelihood of its presence.

c. Differential diagnosis includes, but is not limited to, cellulitis, musculoskeletal injury, Baker's cyst, lymphangitis, chronic venous stasis without evidence of DVT.

d. D-Dimer is useful to rule out DVT in those with low suspicion, but has limited utility if suspicion is moderate to high

e. Compression ultrasonography is the most reliable diagnostic exam

f. Patients who present with signs/symptoms concerning for PE (SOB, hypoxia, tachypnea, tachycardia) require further imaging such as CT scan or V/Q study.

Presence of PE does not change treatment, though hospitalization may be warranted if PE present

g. LMWH (enoxaparin) or unfractionated heparin followed by warfarin is standard treatment, though novel anticoagulants such as rivaroxaban, dabigatran, ximelagatran, and apixaban are increasingly being used.

O. References

a. Tintinalli Chapter 60. Thromboembolism.

b. Rosen Chapter 88. Pulmonary Embolism and Deep Vein Thrombosis.

CASE 115: Shortness of breath and swelling (Bashar A. Ismail, MD)

A. Chief complaint

a. 60-year-old female complaining of shortness of breath with exertion and associated neck swelling for the last 3 weeks.

B. Vital signs

a. BP: 100/90 HR 107 RR 22 T: 37.1°C Wt: 70 kg

C. What does the patient look like?

a. Patient appears stated age, uncomfortable, but not in distress; dyspneic with grossly obvious superficial vascular distention of neck veins.

D. Primary survey

a. Airway: patent airway, speaking in full sentences, no stridor.

b. Breathing: No apparent respiratory distress, and no cyanosis.

c. Circulation: warm, flushed skin, peripheral pulses equal.

E. Action

a. Place on telemetry monitor with pulse oximetry (94% on RA) and begin supplemental O_2 by NC

b. EKG

c. Large-bore peripheral IV line (contralateral to swelling)

F. History

a. HPI: 60-year-old female with known history of small cell lung cancer, currently undergoing chemotherapy. Reports her last treatment was more than 8 weeks prior to her presentation, and presented to the emergency department complaining of dyspnea on exertion that started 3 weeks ago. Dyspnea associated with facial and neck swelling which is more evident during early morning hours and seems to subside by mid-morning. She also reports decreased appetite and weight loss. No history of chest pain, no syncope, no fever or chills. Denies recent travel or sick contacts.

b. PMHx: small cell carcinoma of the lungs diagnosed 10 months ago.

c. PSHx: none

d. Meds: none

e. Allergy: none

f. Social history: Cigarette smoking since she was 16 years old, stopped last month. Lives with her husband

g. FHx: None

G. Secondary survey
  a. General: mildly obese, awake and alert; not in pain or distress
  b. HEENT: pupils equal, round, reactive. Facial and neck swelling are evident, no stridor or papilledema
  c. Neck: swollen with obviously distended superficial veins
  d. Chest: dilated superficial veins over upper chest. No rash or deformity
  e. Lungs: Clear to auscultation bilaterally, good air movement
  f. Heart: tachycardic, no murmurs
  g. Abdomen: no distension, no tenderness, no guarding or rebound tenderness. Normal bowel sounds
  h. Rectal: normal
  i. Urogenital: normal
  j. Extremities: normal
  k. Back: normal, no CVA tenderness
  l. Neuro: normal
  m. Skin: distended superficial veins of the neck and upper chest. No ulcers
  n. Lymph: normal

H. Action
  a. Elevate the head of bed 45 degrees
  b. Labs
      i. CBC, BMP, LFT, PT/PTT, blood type and cross-match
  c. Reassess oxygenation (100% on 2L by NC)
  d. Imaging
      i. CXR (Figure 115.1)
      ii. CT chest (unavailable due to scanner malfunction)

I. Nurse
  a. Repeat VS – BP: 100/90 HR: 101 RR: 18 T: 37.1°C

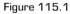 Figure 115.1

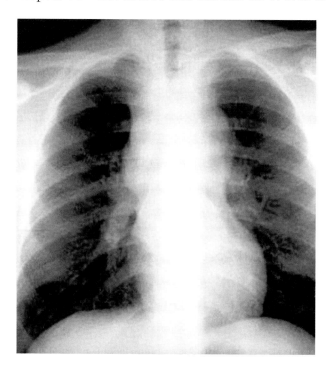

J. Results

Complete blood count:

WBC	9×10^9/L
Hb	15 g/dL
Hct	40%
Plt	350×10^9/L

Basic metabolic panel:

Na	135 mEq/L
K	3.5 mEq/L
Cl	100 mEq/L
BUN	15 mEq/L
Cr	1.0 mEq/L
Mg	1.5 mEq/L
Glucose	110 mg/dL

Arterial blood gas:

pH	7.45
pCO_2	46 mmHg
pO_2	95 mmHg

Liver function panel:

AST	20 U/L
ALT	15 U/L
Alk	20 U/L
D.Bili	0.1 mg/dL
Albumin	3.9 g/dL

Coagulation panel:

PT	10–12 sec
INR	1
PTT	30–45 sec

K. Action

a. Oncology consult: admission to ICU and arrange for tissue biopsy

b. Consult Interventional radiologist for emergent percutaneous stent placement to SVC for symptomatic relief

c. Medications: Lasix

L. Diagnosis

a. Superior vena cava syndrome

M. Critical actions

a. Clinical identification of the diagnosis

b. Elevate the head and give diuretics

c. Start supplemental oxygen and monitor closely

d. Consult Oncology and Interventional Radiology

N. Examiner instructions

a. This patient is suffering from superior vena cava syndrome (SVCS), which can be an acute or sub-acute condition resulting from obstruction of the blood flow through the superior vena cava (SVC). This can be a result of direct compression, infiltration, or thrombosis. Malignancy, specifically lung cancer, is the most common cause of SVCS. Early signs of SVCS can include periorbital edema and facial swelling, classically described as worse in the early morning hours with noted improvement throughout the day. Dyspnea and facial swelling are most commonly reported symptoms of SVCS. SVCS is not usually an immediately life-threatening oncological emergency, but careful and thorough work-up of potential etiology is warranted in all cases.

O. Pearls

a. Elevation of the head of bed has been shown to be an effective and immediate therapeutic measure. Diuretics may also provide transient relief of symptoms, but should be used judiciously due to resulting hypovolemia. Steroids have shown limited effectiveness, but are occasionally used as part of standard therapy in patients presenting with respiratory compromise. More definitive management options include percutaneous transluminal stent placement or bypass surgery.

The prognosis for treated patients varies by underlying tumor type, and overall survival is ~25% at 1 year.

b. Venography is relatively contraindicated due to associated bleeding complications, but other invasive procedures (bronchoscopy, mediastinoscopy, biopsy) are often required to establish diagnosis and underlying disease progression. Venous access is preferable on the contralateral side of the obstruction.

c. Emergency radiotherapy is recommended in patients with stridor due to central airway obstruction or severe laryngeal edema.

P. References

a. Tintinalli's: Chapter 235. Emergency Complications of Malignancy.

b. Rosen: Chapter 123. Selected Oncologic Emergencies.

CASE 116: Finger pain (Alisa Wray, MD, and Jeffrey R. Suchard, MD)

A. Chief complaint

a. 35-year-old male with severe pain to right index finger for 4 hours

B. Vital signs

a. BP: 142/90 HR: 114 RR: 16 T: 37.1°C Wt: 75kg

C. What does the patient look like?

a. Patient appears in moderate distress secondary to right index finger pain.

D. Primary survey

a. Airway: speaking in full sentences

b. Breathing: no apparent respiratory distress, no cyanosis

c. Circulation: peripheral pulses equal in bilateral upper and lower extremities

E. History

a. HPI: 35-year-old male presents with complaint of right index finger pain that is progressive, throbbing, and burning, over the last 4 hours. The pain started at approximately 3pm while the patient was at work. He went home and the pain progressed to where he could not tolerate it any longer and he came to the ED at 7pm. The patient doesn't recall hitting his finger against anything.
  i. When questioned the patient should state that he works as a glass etcher.
  ii. When questioned about chemicals, patient should state that he works with hydrofluoric acid, but wears gloves and eye protection, but he is concerned that maybe there was a hole in his glove.

b. PMHx: none

c. PSHx: appendectomy

d. Allergies: none

e. Social: lives with wife, drinks 1–2 beers per week, denies smoking or drug use

f. FHx: adopted, unknown family history

F. Action

a. Copious irrigation of the affected area

b. IV line placement

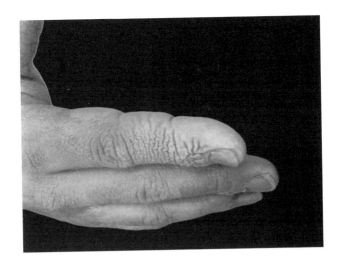

Figure 116.1
See color
plate section
(in some
formats this
figure will
only appear
in black and
white).

c. Labs: CBC, BMP, calcium, magnesium

d. EKG

G. Secondary survey

a. General: Moderate distress, complaining of right hand pain

b. HEENT: Normocephalic, atraumatic, pupils equal, reactive to light, normal tympanic membranes, no nasal discharge

c. NECK: full range of motion

d. Chest: heart regular rate and rhythm, lungs clear bilaterally

e. Abdomen: soft, nontender, nondistended, normal bowel sounds

f. Extremities: right index finger with edematous, grayish and blistered skin from the DIP joint to the tip of finger, including fingernail and cuticle. He has pain out of proportion to examination, has a full range of motion and normal strength. All other extremities within normal limits (Figure 116.1, compliments of Dr. Watchorn)

g. Back: nontender

h. Neuro: normal sensation and strength, normal gait, CN II-XII intact

i. Skin: warm, well perfused, no skin changes

j. Lymph: no lymphadenopathy

H. Meds

a. Calcium: Application by any means: Topical calcium gel application, 3.5 g of calcium gluconate powder in 150 ml of sterile water soluble lubricant OR 10% calcium gluconate in 75 ml of sterile water soluble lubricant OR intradermal injection of 5% calcium gluconate OR IV calcium gluconate OR intra-arterial calcium gluconate

b. Pain control with IV or oral analgesics

I. Results

a. EKG: normal sinus rhythm

b. BMP: Na 141, K 4.0, Cl 95, CO_2 22, BUN 9, Cr 0.9, Ca 8.0

c. iCa: 4.0

d. Mg: 1.9

e. Patient reports no significant pain relief with topical, intradermal, or IV calcium therapy. Only intra-arterial calcium therapy will reduce pain if initiated in ED

J. Consult:

a. Burn specialist or toxicologist

K. Diagnosis

a. Hydrofluoric acid exposure

L. Critical actions

a. Diagnose HF burn

b. Check EKG for dysrhythmia

c. Attempt calcium therapy (by any means possible)

d. Administer analgesics

e. Consult a toxicologist or burn specialist

f. Admit patient (when calcium therapy fails)

g. Check labs, including calcium level and potassium level

M. Examiner instructions

a. This patient is suffering from dermal exposure to hydrofluoric acid, a chemical commonly used in glass etching. It is important that the examinee makes the connection between glass etching and HF exposure.

N. Pearls

a. Treatment of HF acid burns depends on the exposure (ingestion, dermal, inhalation) and the strength of concentration of the HF acid (higher concentrations have worse outcomes). HF acid dissociates to H+ and fluoride ions, which then bind Ca and Mg, leading to hypocalcemia, hypomagnesemia, and hyperkalemia (via efflux of intracellular K); this can cause cardiotoxicity via prolonged QT.

b. Dermal exposures: HF acid concentrations of 50% and greater cause immediate pain and visible damage, household products are typically 6–10% and cause delayed pain. Exposure to >2% of BSA with high concentration can cause life-threatening systemic toxicity. Treatment for dermal exposure is calcium gluconate gel or intradermal calcium gluconate injection. For serious exposures, intra-arterial calcium gluconate is indicated.

c. Inhalation exposures: Typically present with complaints of shortness of breath and throat burning. Treatment consists of nebulized calcium gluconate, typically 4 ml of 2.5% to a 5% solution.

d. Gastrointestinal exposures: Ingestion of concentrated HF causes significant gastritis, altered mental status, nausea, vomiting, airway compromise, severe hypocalcemia, and hyperkalemia. Management includes ABC's and resuscitation. NG tubes can be placed to drain the stomach (this should be done under great care) and oral or NG tube calcium or magnesium salts can be given. Ingestions of HF acid can be fatal.

e. Ophthalmic exposures: Typically occurs from splashes or exposure to hydrogen fluoride gas. This can cause corneal edema, conjunctival ischemia, sloughing and chemosis. Treatment includes irrigation with 1L Ringer's lactate or normal saline and 1% calcium eye drops. Limited data suggest that prolonged irrigation can cause worse outcomes.

O. References

a. Tintinalli's: Chapter 211. Chemical Burns.

b. Rosen: Chapter 64. Chemical Injuries.

CASE 117: Dizziness (Maxwell Jen, MD, and Bharath Chakravarthy, MD, MPH)

A. Chief complaint
  a. 61-year-old male with dizziness since this morning

B. Vital signs
  a. BP: 92/51 HR: 51 RR: 16 T: 37.4°C Wt: 85 kg

C. What does the patient look like?
  a. Patient is lying on the bed quietly in no apparent distress

D. Primary survey
  a. Airway: speaking full sentences
  b. Breathing: no apparent respiratory distress, no cyanosis
  c. Circulation: peripheral pulses equal

E. History
  a. HPI: a 61-year-old male presents with dizziness since this morning. He has had intermittent dizziness over past week, but worse this morning. He describes his dizziness as "lightheadedness." He also endorses feeling "weak all over," but denies chest pain, shortness of breath, nausea, or vomiting. Denies headache.
  b. PMHx: cannot recall his medical issues
  c. PSHx: none
  d. Meds: none since he lost his health insurance; cannot recall what meds were
  e. Allergies: penicillin – rash
  f. Social: Lives alone, no tobacco, alcohol, drugs
  g. FHx: father with myocardial infarction at age 55

F. Secondary survey
  a. General: awake, alert, appropriate for age, appears fatigued
  b. HEENT: pupils equal, round, reactive, no papilledema
  c. Neck: no cervical adenopathy, no meningismus
  d. Chest: clear to auscultation bilaterally, pacemaker to L chest (only given if a good skin exam is performed)
  e. Heart: bradycardic, regular rhythm
  f. Abdomen: soft, nontender, nondistended
  g. Rectal: hemoccult negative
  h. GU: no testicular masses or tenderness, no penile discharge
  i. Extremities: normal
  j. Back: tenderness to L-spine and paralumbar regions bilaterally, no CVA tenderness
  k. Neuro: normal
  l. Skin: normal
  m. Lymph: normal

G. Action
  a. Two large-bore peripheral IV lines
  b. Note pacemaker to left chest wall

    c. Cardiac monitor: BP: 85/49, HR: 45, RR: 18, O_2 Sat: 98% on RA

    d. EKG: Sinus bradycardia, rate 33

    e. Meds

        i. Atropine 0.5mg IV

    f. Apply transcutaneous pacing pads, pace, and ensure mechanical capture

    g. Imaging: CXR (to ensure the pacemaker wires are not fractured)

    h. Labs: CBC, BMP, troponin, BNP

    i. Consult

        i. Cardiology

        ii. Pacemaker interrogation

H. Results

Complete blood count:

WBC	8.3 x 10³/uL
Hct	36.1%
Plt	310 x 10³/uL

Basic metabolic panel

Na	139 mEq/L
K	3.7 mEq/L
Cl	105 mEq/L
CO_2	27 mEq/L
BUN	19 mEq/dL
Cr	1.7 mg/dL
Gluc	130 mg/dL

Coagulation panel

PT	14 sec
PTT	34 sec
INR	0.8

Liver function panel

AST	18 U/L
ALT	21 U/L
Total bilirubin	0.9 mg/dL
Direct bilirubin	0.2 mg/dL
Albumin	3.9 g/dL

Cardiac enzymes

Troponin	<0.04
BNP	99

I. Diagnosis

a. Malfunctioning pacemaker

J. Critical actions

a. Note pacemaker to left chest on physical exam

b. Obtain EKG

c. Atropine 0.5mg IV

d. Apply transcutaneous pacemaker pads; ensure mechanical capture

e. Apply magnet over pacemaker

f. Consult cardiology and/or device manufacturer

K. Examiner instructions

a. This is a case of a malfunctioning pacemaker in which the set rate is too slow, resulting in decreased cerebral perfusion and dizziness. Specifically, the candidate should note on physical exam that the patient has had a pacemaker implanted (confirmed on CXR), even though the patient has neglected to volunteer this information in the past medical history. The candidate should address this issue in several ways: medically treat the bradycardia with atropine per ACLS, apply transcutaneous pacemaker pads and ensure mechanical capture, return the pacemaker to its default settings with a magnet.

L. Pearls
a. Patients are often unaware of their own medical history, especially those who have been out of medical care.
b. Transcutaneous pacing can be initiated over an existing pacemaker.
c. Applying a magnet over a pacemaker will revert the pacemaker settings to an asynchronous, pre-set rate (the rate depends on the manufacturer). If this is unsuccessful, the pacemaker battery may be depleted or the device may be programmed to ignore the magnet. Alternative management, such as transcutaneous pacing, will then be required.

M. References
a. Tintinalli's: Chapter 35. Cardiac Pacing.
b. Rosen: Chapter 80. Implantable Cardiac Devices.

CASE 118: Intoxication (Desmond Fitzpatrick, MD and Lars K. Beattie, MD)

A. Chief complaint
a. 47-year-old confused male found stumbling in a pile of beer cans by police, brought in by EMS.

B. Vital signs
a. BP: 136/83 HR: 92 RR: 18 T: 37.1°C Wt: 72 kg

C. What does the patient look like?
a. Patient appears older than stated age, disheveled

D. Primary survey
a. Airway: nonsensical speech, airway patent
b. Breathing: no apparent respiratory distress, no cyanosis
c. Circulation: pale, peripheral pulses equal

E. Action
a. Oxygen via NC or nonrebreather mask
b. Two large-bore peripheral IV lines
    i. CBC, BMP, LFT, coagulation studies, blood type and cross-match
    ii. Alcohol level, acetaminophen level, salicylate level, urine toxicology screen
c. Monitor: BP: 152/78 HR: 86 RR: 16 Sat: 100% on NC
d. Thiamine 100 mg IV
e. Dextrose 50% AMP (25g) IV push
f. Narcan 0.4mg IV push

F. History
a. HPI: a 47-year-old male with a history of alcohol abuse known to EMS and triage nurse. The patient does not contribute to the history, and only stares at you upon questioning. The triage nurse states he is familiar with the patient and says "all he does is drink beer." EMS states they were called because of police concern about his mental status after they witnessed the patient shaking violently. There was no

trauma, as the patient had already been placed in the police vehicle when the shaking started.

b. PMHx: Alcoholism

c. Social: Alcohol abuse, transient lifestyle

d. PSHx-Meds-Allergies-FHx: Unknown

G. Secondary survey

a. General: lethargic, alert to self, urine-soaked pants

b. Head: normocephalic, atraumatic

c. Eyes: pupils equal, normal conjunctiva

d. Ears: normal

e. Mouth: tongue bite mark

f. Neck: supple, full ROM

g. Chest: no rashes

h. Heart: regular rate and rhythm, no murmurs

i. Abdomen: nontender, normal bowel sounds

j. Rectal: hemoccult negative

k. Urogenital: normal external genitalia

l. Extremities: full range of motion

m. Back: normal, no CVA tenderness

n. Neuro: alert to self, does not follow commands, no focal weakness, no tremors, no tongue fasciculations

o. Skin: ruddy, scattered abrasions

p. Lymph: no lymphadenopathy

H. Nurse

a. O_2, thiamine, naloxone, D50, IV push

    i. BP: 121/78 HR: 84 RR: 16 Sat: 100% on NC

    ii. No change in mental status

b. Labs drawn

I. Action

a. EKG, CXR

b. Noncontrast CT head

J. Results

Complete blood count:

WBC	5.9×10^3/uL
Hct	39.1%
Plt	190×10^3/uL

Basic metabolic panel:

Na	113 mEq/L
K	2.9 mEq/L
Cl	79 mEq/L
CO_2	26 mEq/L
BUN	15 mEq/dL
Cr	0.9 mg/dL
Gluc	71 mg/dL

Coagulation panel:

PT	13 sec
PTT	25 sec
INR	1.0

Liver function panel:

AST	80 U/L
ALT	53 U/L
Alk Phos	179 U/L
T bili	1.3 mg/dL
D bili	0.2 mg/dL
Amylase	61 U/L
Lipase	80 U/L
Albumin	3.9 g/dL
NH_4	30

Urinalysis:

SG	1.003	LE	Neg
pH	5–8	Nitrite	Neg
Prot	Neg mg/dL	Color	Yellow
Gluc	Neg mg/dL		
Ketones	Neg mg/dL	**Additional labs**	
Bili	Neg	EtOH level	122 mg/dL
Blood	Neg		

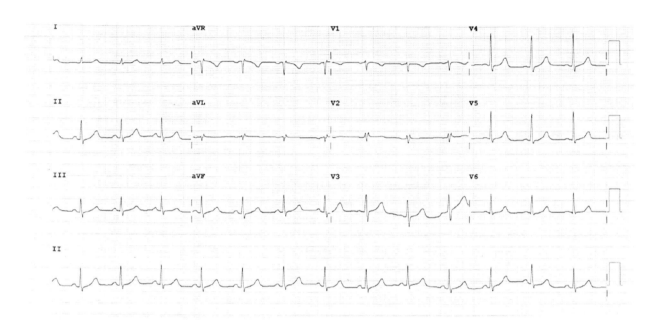

Figure 118.1

a. EKG (Figure 118.1)
b. CXR (Figure 118.2)
c. Noncontrast CT head (Figure 118.3)

K. Action
a. 100cc 3% hypertonic saline over 1 hour
b. Serum osmolality
c. Urine osmolality

L. Nurse
a. Serum osmolality = 260 mOsm/kg
b. Urine osmolality = 59 mOsm/kg

M. Action
a. Serial BMP
b. Admission to ICU

N. Diagnosis
a. Hypo-osmolar hyponatremia with cerebral edema, secondary to beer potomania

Figure 118.2

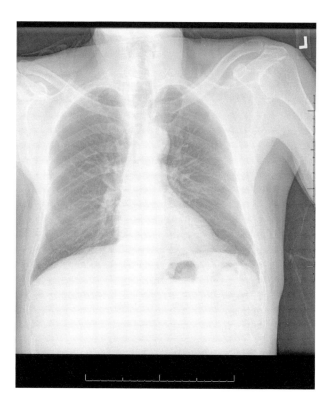

Figure 118.3

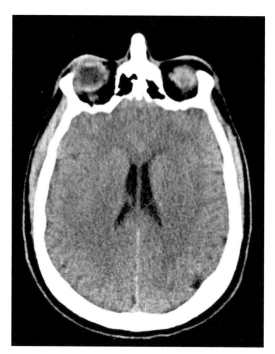

O. Critical actions
a. Initial treatment of altered mental status (assess glucose, ABCs, give naloxone)
b. Recognition of altered mental status out of proportion to patient's alcohol level
c. Recognition of severe hyponatremia with neurologic findings
d. Up to 100cc 3% hypertonic saline bolus over 1 hour

e. Slow sodium correction on monitor

f. Admission to ICU

P. Examiner instructions

a. This is a case of altered mental status and seizure secondary to hyponatremia. The patient has a hypo-osmolar hyponatremia with cerebral edema secondary to beer potomania. There are many potential causes for this patient's altered mental status and seizure. However, with normal vital signs, absent response to dextrose-oxygen-narcan-thiamine, absence of tremor/tongue fasciculations, and ultimately when labs show a low alcohol level should prompt the examinee to search for other causes. With the dangerously low serum sodium level on BMP, the etiology of the altered mental status and seizure should become clear. Failure to recognize and treat severe hyponatremia will result in a declining mental status and seizures, requiring intubation and treatment for status epilepticus. The goal of the case is to have the examinee work through an undifferentiated altered mental status case with seizure, then treat severe hyponatremia with cerebral edema.

Q. Pearls

a. Patients with sodium levels less than 120 mEq/L are more likely to exhibit symptoms of nausea, vomiting, anorexia, muscle cramps, confusion, and lethargy.

b. Altered mental status, seizures, and coma are serious sequelae of hyponatremia, caused by cerebral edema.

c. The rate of sodium repletion should be no greater than 0.5 to 1.0 mEq/L/hour in chronic severe hyponatremia, but may be increased to 1–2 mEq/L in the setting of acute severe hyponatremia. (No more than 10 mEq/L in 24 hours.)

d. In patients with severe neurologic symptoms (seizures, altered mental status), up to 100cc of 3% hypertonic saline bolus can be administered over an hour, raising serum sodium by 2–3 mEq/L.

e. Patient are at risk for *central pontine myelinolysis* if serum sodium is too rapidly replaced.

f. Hyponatremia due to "beer potomania" can occur in any patient with a very low intake of dietary solutes. Classically, this occurs in alcoholics whose sole nutrient is beer, hence the diagnostic label "beer potomania." Beer has low protein and salt content (1–2 mmol Na+ per liter). Reduced body solutes limit urinary water excretion and hyponatremia can ensue even after modest polydipsia.

R. References

a. Tintinalli's: Chapter 21. Fluids and Electrolytes

b. Rosen: Chapter 125. Electrolyte Disorders

CASE 119: Altered mental status (Lars K. Beattie, MD and Matthew Ryan, MD, PhD)

A. Chief complaint

a. 64-year-old male with confusion

B. Vital signs

a. BP: 162/88 HR: 58 RR: 18 T: 98.6°F

C. What does the patient look like?

a. Patient is a thin man who is tugging at the room curtains.

D. Primary survey

a. Airway: patient speaking full sentences

b. Breathing: no apparent respiratory distress, no cyanosis

c. Circulation: warm and dry skin, normal capillary refill

E. Action

a. Oxygen via NC or nonrebreather mask

b. Two large-bore peripheral IV lines

c. Labs

   i. CBC, BMP, LFT, coagulation studies, blood type and cross-match

   ii. Finger stick

d. Monitor: BP: 165/80 HR: 62 RR: 18 T: 98.6°F O$_2$Sat: 95%

e. CXR, EKG

F. History

a. HPI: a 64-year-old man who presents with confusion worsening over the last week. He has associated weakness. EMS states family lives in a cabin in "the sticks" (the deep woods). Per family, the patient has been having increasing weakness, itching, and abdominal cramps over the last week. He has also been exhibiting increasing confusion over the last 2 days. Today the patient was too weak to get out of bed, and started speaking to dead relatives. History is per EMS discussion with family.

b. PMHx: COPD

c. PSHx: none

d. Allergies: none

e. Meds: none

f. Social: 2.5 packs per day for 30 years, no drug or alcohol use

g. FHx: none

h. PMD: none

G. Nurse

a. EKG (Figure 119.1)

H. Secondary survey

a. General: cachectic disheveled man, oriented to self, grasping at room curtains

b. Head: normocephalic, atraumatic

c. Eyes: extraocular movement intact, pupils equal, reactive to light

d. Ears: cerumen, normal tympanic membranes

e. Nose: no discharge

f. Neck: full range of motion, no jugular vein distension, no stridor

g. Pharynx: edentulous, no lesions, no swelling

h. Chest: cachectic chest, nontender

i. Lungs: distant breath sounds, clear bilaterally

j. Heart: rate and rhythm regular, no murmurs, rubs, or gallops

k. Abdomen: normal bowel sounds, soft, (+)tender diffusely, no rebound

l. Rectal: normal tone, brown stool, occult blood negative

m. Extremities: full range of motion, no deformity, normal pulses

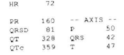

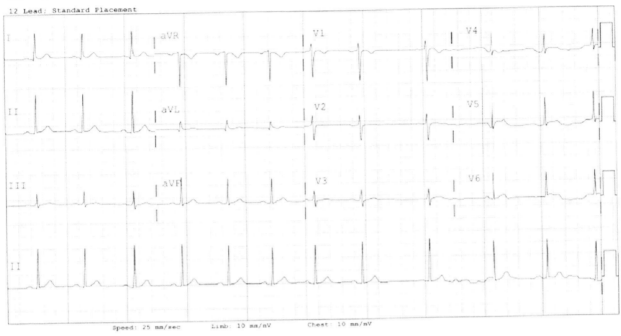

Figure 119.1

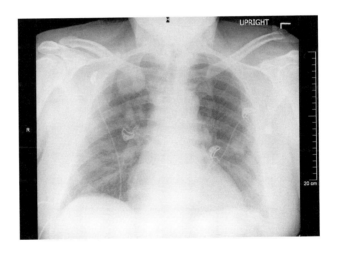

Figure 119.2

n. Back: nontender
o. Neuro: cranial nerves II-XII intact; normal sensation, strength; normal reflexes and gait
p. Skin: warm and dry
q. Lymph: no lymphadenopathy

I. Nurse

a. CXR (Figure 119.2)

J. Action
a. Lipase
b. ABG
c. Ca, iCa, Mg

K. Results

Complete blood count:

WBC	7.3×10^3/uL	D bili	0.3 mg/dL
Hct	36.5%	Amylase	50 U/L
Plt	330×10^3/uL	Lipase	25 U/L
		Albumin	3.2 g/dL

Basic metabolic panel:

Na	141 mEq/L	**ABG**	
K	2.9 mEq/L	pH	7.38
Cl	105 mEq/L	PaO_2	98 mmHg
CO_2	24 mEq/L	$PaCO_2$	36 mmHg
BUN	29 mEq/dL	HCO_3	23 mEq/L
Cr	2.2 mg/dL	O_2Sat	99%
Gluc	89 mg/dL		

Coagulation panel:

		Urinalysis:	
PT	12.6 sec	SG	1.010–1.030
PTT	26 sec	pH	5–8
INR	1.0	Prot	Neg mg/dL
		Gluc	Neg mg/dL
		Ketones	Neg mg/dL

Liver function panel:

AST	23 U/L	Bili	Neg
ALT	26 U/L	Blood	Neg
Alk Phos	42 U/L	LE	Neg
T bili	1.0 mg/dL	Nitrite	Neg
		Color	Yellow

L. Nurse
a. Results
   i. Ca 14.5 mg/dL
   ii. iCa 3.9 mmol/L
   iii. Mg 0.7 mg/dL

M. Action
a. 1L NS bolus, then 200–300 cc/hour to urine output of 100–150 cc/h
b. Bisphosphonate
   i. Palmidronate 90 mg IV over 2h
OR
   ii. Zoledronic acid 4 mg IV over 15min
c. Calcitonin 4 IU SQ
d. Electrolyte replacement
e. Admission to ICU

N. Diagnosis
a. Hypercalcemia from squamous cell lung cancer

Figure 119.3

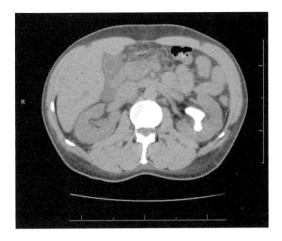

O. Critical actions

a. IVF

b. EKG – Identification of short QTc

c. CXR – Identification of pulmonary nodules

d. Identification of clinical hypercalcemia presentation

e. Ca, iCa levels

f. Bisphosphonate

g. ICU admission

P. Examiner instructions

a. This is a case of hypercalcemia secondary to squamous cell lung cancer. Cancer-induced hypercalcemia is a paraneoplastic syndrome caused by direct destruction of bone by tumor, and by tumor secretion of parathyroid hormone. The patient presents with moans (altered mental status and psychiatric complaints), groans (constipation and abdominal pain) in the setting of an EKG showing hypercalcemic changes (shortened QTc intervals), and a chest x-ray showing multiple pulmonary nodules. If an abdominal CT is obtained during the case, an incidental non-obstructing kidney stone will be present in the renal calyx in an otherwise normal CT (Figure 119.3). Other findings consistent with hypercalcemia are hypertension, hypokalemia, hypomagnesemia, and renal insufficiency. Hypercalcemia is a common complication of many cancers, and is an oncologic emergency. The lung nodules seen on CXR should prompt the examinee to order calcium levels. If the examinee does not identify the clinical presentation of hypercalcemia, the patient will develop increasing lethargy that will progress to a comatose state, requiring intubation.

Q. Pearls

a. Patients with hypercalcemia present with stones (renal calculi), bones (osteolysis), moans (altered mental status and psychiatric disorders), and groans (peptic ulcer disease, pancreatitis, or constipation).

b. 20–40% of cancer patients develop hypercalcemia, and it is the most common life-threatening metabolic disorder in these patients.

c. The majority of patients presenting with hypercalcemia (90%) have associated malignancy or hyperparathyroidism.

d. EKG findings include short QTc intervals, short ST segments, depressed ST segments, and widened T waves. Bradyarrhythmias with bundle branch patterns can occur, and may progress to second-degree block, complete heart block, and even cardiac arrest.

e. Treatment consists primarily of fluid resuscitation followed by medically lowering calcium levels. Patients with severe symptomatic hypercalcemia should be admitted to the ICU until symptoms resolve and calcium levels return to normal levels.

R. References

a. Tintinalli's: Chapter 21. Fluids and Electrolytes.

b. Rosen: Chapter 125. Electrolyte Disorders.

CASE 120: Patient with fatigue, weight gain, and bruising (Mason Shieh, MD, MBA, and Thomas Nguyen, MD)

A. Chief complaint:

a. 38-year-old female with weight gain and fatigue over the last few months

B. Vital signs:

a. T: 98.6°F HR: 88 BP: 136/90 RR: 18 O$_2$: 99% FS: 256 Wt: 100 kg

C. What does the patient look like?

a. Patient appears comfortable

D. Primary survey

a. Airway: speaking in full sentences

b. Breathing: spontaneous, non-labored breathing

c. Circulation: peripheral pulses equal

E. History

a. HPI: 38-year-old female presents with weight gain, amenorrhea, and generalized decrease in energy over the past 3 months. She also noticed easy bruising on her body. She denies any blood thinner use, increased sun exposure, new medications, recent illness, or recent trauma.

b. PMHx: none

c. PSHx: none

d. Meds: none

e. Allergies: no known drug allergies

f. Social: lives alone in apartment

g. FHx: family history of diabetes

F. Secondary survey (Figure 120.1)

a. General: awake, alert, no distress

b. HEENT: pupils equal, round, reactive to light, slight puffiness around eyes, round cheeks

c. Neck: obese with moderate fat padding on posterior of neck

d. Chest: no rashes

e. Heart: regular rate, rhythm, no murmurs

f. Abdomen: obese, soft, no tenderness, no fluid wave, normal bowel sounds

g. Rectal: deferred

h. GU: normal

i. Extremities: no swelling

j. Back: no deformities, no CVA tenderness

k. Neuro: normal

l. Skin: purple striae noted in abdomen, thighs, axillae, and buttocks. Old bruises seen on the arm and leg.

m. Lymph: normal

G. Action

a. IV

    i. 20-gauge peripheral IV

b. Labs

    i. CBC, BMP, PT/PTT, urine pregnancy

c. Fluids

    i. Not required, optional

d. Monitor

    i. Not required

e. Consult

    i. Endocrinology

f. Medicines

    i. None

g. Additional labs

    i. Orders a random cortisol level.

    ii. (if admitted) Orders a 24 hour cortisol urine, serum cortisol, serum ACTH, dexamethasone suppression test

h. Imaging

    i. CT abdomen/pelvis (Can be ordered if there is a concern for primary adrenal tumor, based on exam and laboratory findings. This is more likely done as outpatient work-up or during hospital admission. If the examinee requests, radiologist states, "what are you looking for? ")

H. Results

Basic metabolic panel			
Na	138 mEq/L	Hct	42.7%
K	3.3 mEq/L	Plt	280 x 10^3/uL
Cl	102 mEq/L		
CO_2	25 mEq/L	Coagulation panel	
BUN	16 mEq/dL	PT	12.3 sec
Cr	0.81 mg/dL	PTT	31.2 sec
Glucose	270 mg/dL	INR	0.9
		Pregnancy test	Negative
Complete blood count			
WBC	9.2 d 10^3/uL		
Hgb	14.3		

a. Random serum cortisol – 54 µg/dL (normal range 5–20 µg/dL)

b. If ordered, CT abdomen/pelvis – demonstrates adrenal tumor/ hyperplasia

c. If admitted, follow up labs show 24-hour free urinary cortisol – 318 μg/24 h (normal range 10–150 μg/24 h), serum ACTH – <4 pg/mL (normal range 10–60 pg/mL), dexamethasone suppression test – there is no drop in levels of blood cortisol following administration of dexamethasone.

I. Action

a. Referral to Endocrine and surgery for adrenal removal
b. Refer to primary care doctor for management of possible diabetes and hypertension

J. Diagnosis

a. Cushing syndrome from a cortisol-secreting adrenal mass

K. Critical actions

a. Pregnancy test
b. CBC to check platelets and coagulation profile
c. Recognizes potential Cushing syndrome/endocrine etiology of the case presentation
d. Endocrine consult or referral
e. Orders random cortisol level

L. Examiner instructions

a. The patient is suffering from Cushing syndrome, or hypercortisolism, due to excess secretion of cortisol (steroid hormone) from an adrenal gland tumor. She is

Figure 120.1
See color plate section (in some formats this figure will only appear in black and white).

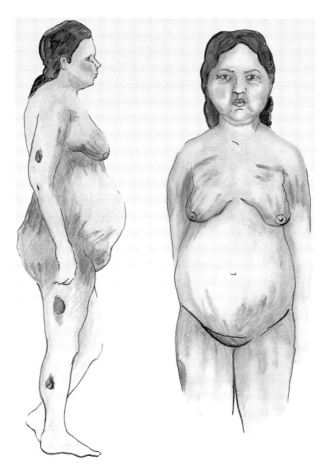

presenting with very nonspecific complaints that could easily be missed in the ED setting. The key to the work-up is to ensure the examinee checks for non-immediate life-threatening etiologies, and ensures appropriate follow up for work-up. Cushing syndrome can occur via any mechanism that increases cortisol levels in the body. This includes a cortisol-secreting adrenal tumor, an ACTH-secreting pituitary mass, an ectopic ACTH-secreting mass such as a lung cancer, or endogenous chronic steroid use such as prednisone for rheumatoid arthritis.

b. Patients with suspected Cushing syndrome should get endocrine follow-up and/or consult. They may be discharged for out patient work-up if stable.

M. Pearls

a. The most specific lab test is the 24-hour free urinary cortisol, which should be elevated. Cortisol is released in spurts throughout the day, making random cortisol levels less reliable.

b. Specific findings include easy bruising, purple striae, psychological changes, proximal myopathy, and fat deposition in the face and neck.

c. Common nonspecific findings include central obesity, hypertension, osteoporosis, acne, hirsutism, amenorrhea, and diabetes mellitus.

d. Lung tumors account for over 50% of ectopic ACTH-secreting tumors, with small cell being the most common type.

e. Dexamethasone suppression test and CRH stimulation test will help differentiate between pituitary ACTH-secreting adenoma, ectopic ACTH secretion, and cortisol-secreting adrenal tumors. Determining the type of tumor will dictate where to perform imaging studies as well as management.

f. Complications – if Cushing syndrome is left untreated, can have high morbidity and even death. Patients may suffer complications from hypertension, diabetes mellitus, and osteoporosis.

g. Polycystic Ovarian Syndrome can mimic Cushing syndrome in females.

N. References

a. Harrison's Principles of Internal Medicine.18th ed. / Longo, Dan L. McGraw-Hill, 2011. Chapter 342.

b. Current Medical Diagnosis and Treatment 2013. 52th ed. / Papadakis, Maxine. McGraw-Hill Medical Publishing Division, 2012. Chapter 26.

CASE 121: Rash and bilateral leg pain (Daniel Goldstein, MD, and Thomas Nguyen, MD)

A. Chief complaint
a. 14-year-old male with bilateral leg pain

B. Vital signs
a. BP: 100/65 HR: 125 RR: 22 T: 100.5°F Sat: 98%

C. What does the patient look like?
a. Patient is sitting in bed, uncomfortable; complaining of pain.

D. Primary survey

a. Airway: speaking in full sentences

b. Breathing: no apparent respiratory distress; no cyanosis

c. Circulation: bounding peripheral pulses, equal bilaterally.

E. History

a. HPI: 14-year-old male with 3 days of fever, sore throat, and rhinorrhea, after attending his cousin's birthday party. Yesterday, he noted the development of a red rash on his face and today, became concerned upon developing bilateral lower extremity arthralgias, and feeling too exhausted to leave bed. He denies cough, shortness of breath, vomiting, diarrhea, abdominal pain, focal bone pain, recent travel, neck stiffness, headache, dysuria, recent antibiotic use.

b. PMHx: sickle-cell disease

c. PSHx: none

d. Meds: Oxycodone

e. Social: denies drugs, smoking, and alcohol

f. FHx: father with MI at 52, mother passed away in 30s from complications of sickle-cell disease.

F. Action

a. Oxygen via NC or nonrebreather mask

b. Two large-bore peripheral IV lines

c. Labs:

   i. CBC, blood cultures, BMP, LFT, reticulocyte count, Group A strep rapid and culture, type & cross, lactic acid

d. Monitor: BP: 95/65 HR: 130 RR: 22

e. 1 L NS Bolus

f. CXR

G. Secondary survey

a. General: awake, alert, oriented x3, diaphoretic, uncomfortable

b. HEENT: normocephalic, atraumatic, jaundiced, conjunctival pallor, erythema of posterior oropharynx, no tonsillar exudate or petechiae, uvula midline, +rhinorrhea

c. Neck: bilateral, tender, anterior cervical lymphadenopathy, supple

d. Chest: nontender

e. Heart: tachycardic, no murmurs, rubs, or gallops

f. Abdomen: normal bowel sounds, soft, nontender, no distention

g. Rectal: normal

h. GU: normal

i. Extremities: full passive and active range of motion, pain with movement of knees and ankles bilaterally, no erythema or swelling, no focal bony tenderness

j. Back: nontender

k. Neuro: cranial nerves II–XII intact, normal sensation, strength, reflexes, and gait

l. Skin: maculopapular, fiery red rash along cheeks, no involvement of bridge of nose or forehead, no petechiae or purpura

m. Lymph: anterior cervical lymphadenopathy

H. CXR (Figure 121.1)

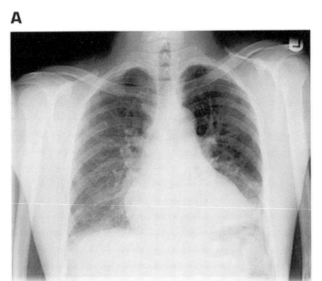

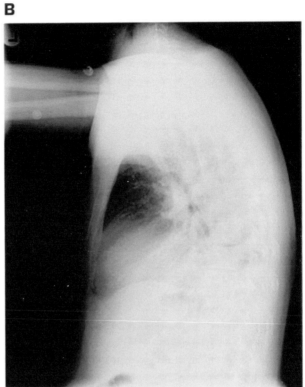

Figure 121.1 A and B

I. Results

a. Rapid Group A Strep negative

Complete blood count:

WBC	2.2 x10³/uL
Hct	17%
Plt	60 x10³/uL
PMN:	35%
Lymphs:	60%
Monos:	5%

Reticulocyte count:

Retic	2%

Basic metabolic panel:

Na	138 mEq/L
K	5.0 mEq/L
Cl	104 mEq/L
CO_2	21 mEq/L
BUN	19 mEq/dL
Cr	0.9 mg/dL%
Gluc	122 mg/dL

Coagulation panel:

PT	13 sec
PTT	27 sec
INR	1.0

Liver function panel:

AST	42 U/L
ALT	36 U/L
Alk Phos	145 U/L
T bili	4.0 mg/dL
D bili	0.3 mg/dL
Amylase	76 U/L
Lipase	140 U/L
Albumin	3.7 g/dL
Lactic Acid	1.5 mmol/L

Urinalysis:

SG	1.010–1.030
pH	5–8
Prot	Neg
Gluc	Neg
Ketones	Neg
Bili	Trace
Blood	Neg
LE	Neg
Nitrite	Neg
Color	Yellow

J. Action

a. Meds

   i. IV morphine or dilaudid

   ii. Vancomycin and Cefepime or Imipenem

   iii. Antipyretic

b. Consultation

   i. Hematology

c. Transfuse 2 units PRBC and repeat CBC

K. Nurse

a. Transfusion of PRBC

   i. BP: 110/82 HR: 100 RR: 18

b. No transfusion of PRBC

   i. BP: 90/62 HR: 134 RR: 30

   ii. Nurse states patient now says he is becoming short of breath.

L. Action

a. Admission to monitored setting

b. Repeat CBC

M. Diagnosis

a. Aplastic anemia

N. Critical actions

a. CBC, reticulocyte count, blood cultures

b. Transfusion

c. CXR

d. Pain control

e. Admit

O. Examiner instructions

a. This is a case of a child with aplastic anemia, when the bone marrow shuts down and does not produce blood cells. In this case, the aplastic anemia is likely due to a viral infection caused by Parvovirus B19, which can present with fever, runny nose, headache, facial rash, joint pain. Other causes of infection should be ruled out, and patient started on broad-spectrum antibiotic coverage. Joint pain should be treated with appropriate pain medications. The most important initial treatment is transfusion and admission for hematology consultation and further monitoring of CBC.

P. Pearls

a. Aplastic anemia is a disease in which the bone marrow is unable to produce a sufficient number of new blood cells.
   See Figure 121.2: Bone marrow biopsy shows paucity of stem precursor cells with a predominance of fatty infiltrates.

b. Aplastic anemia can be caused by medications such as chloramphenicol, anticonvulsants, solvents, benzene.

c. Other causes of aplastic anemia include Parvovirus B19, viral hepatitis, ionizing radiation, autoimmune disorders, and genetics.

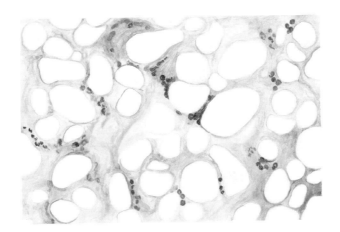

Figure 121.2 See color plate section (in some formats this figure will only appear in black and white).

d. Parvovirus B19 can cause aplastic anemia in sickle-cell and pregnant patients, with a drop in the red cells, white cells, and platelets.

e. In most cases, Parvovirus B19 causes only a drop in the red cell line. This may go clinically unnoticed, as a short-lived aplastic episode may not cause a significant drop in red blood cells, which, on average, live for 120 days; however, in individuals with sickle-cell disease, where a red blood cell only lives, on average, for 10–20 days, this can cause a profound drop in Hgb, leading to symptoms including pale skin or mucosa, fatigue, shortness of breath, fever, fast heart rate, weakness, headache, or agitation.

f. In the case of a patient with sickle-cell disease, a transfusion can be lifesaving, as these individuals are unable to compensate for the temporary bone marrow suppression, which commonly lasts 5 to 10 days. The WBC and platelets are generally not affected.

g. Remember to calculate the Reticulocyte Index for all patients, as the Reticulocyte Count can be misleading in anemic patients. A value of 45% is used as the '"Normal Hematocrit."

ReticIndex=ReticCount x (Hematocrit/Normal Hematocrit)

h. With anemia, a Reticulocyte Index:
  i. Values <2 indicates loss of RBCs and a decreased production of new RBCs (an inadequate response to correct the anemia)
  ii. Values >3 indicate the appropriate response, with an increased compensatory production of RBCs to replace lost RBCs.

Q. References
a. *Tintinalli's Emergency Medicine: A Comprehensive Study Guide.* 7th edition / Tintinalli, Judith E. McGraw-Hill, 2011. Chapter 231
b. *Rosen's Emergency Medicine: Concepts and Clinical Practice*, 7th ed. / Rosen, Peter. Elsevier/Saunders, 2011. Chapter 121

CASE 122: Arm pain (Michael A. Cole, MD)

A. Chief complaint:
a. 28-year-old male who comes to the ED with arm pain.

B. Vital signs
a. BP: 90/65 HR: 125 RR: 16 T: 102°F

C. What does the patient look like?

a. Patient is a well-built man, diaphoretic and anxious but in no apparent distress.

D. Primary survey

a. Airway: speaking in full sentences
b. Breathing: no apparent respiratory distress, no cyanosis
c. Circulation: warm, diaphoretic skin; diminished peripheral pulses with slightly delayed capillary refill (2–3 second)

E. Action

a. Two large-bore peripheral IV lines
b. Monitor: BP: 90/65 HR: 125 RR: 18 T: 102°F
c. Labs
d. CBC, BMP, LFTs, CK, urinalysis
e. Optional: troponin, CK-MB, coagulation studies, blood type & screen
f. 1 L NS bolus
g. EKG

F. History

a. HPI: This is a 28-year-old man who presents with pain that started in left arm 8 hours ago and has now spread to both arms as well as chest. The pain is currently starting in both of his legs. The pain is achy and he rates it as an 8 out of 10. The pain is worse with movement. He has had associated fever, nausea, and darker urine. He went to the gym yesterday and had a workout that lasted longer than usual. He went to work this morning as a demolition specialist in 95-degree F weather but left early because of the pain.
b. PMHx: occasional back pain from work
c. PSHx: none
d. Allergies: none
e. Meds: ibuprofen 1200mg PRN for back pain, he has been taking "a lot" recently (4–5 doses a day for last 3 days for back pain)
f. Social: uses cocaine "occasionally" last used yesterday, smokes tobacco–one pack per day for 10 years, no alcohol use. Works as demolition specialist.
g. FHx: father with MI at 50-years-old; mother with a stroke at 72-years-old
h. PMD: Dr. Steinberg

G. Secondary survey

a. General: alert, oriented × 3, uncomfortable, diaphoretic
b. Head: normocephalic, atraumatic
c. Eyes: extraocular movements intact, pupils equal and reactive to light
d. Ears: normal ear canals and tympanic membranes
e. Nose: no discharge
f. Neck: full range of motion, no jugular vein distention, no stridor
g. Pharynx: normal dentition, no lesions, no swelling, no erythema
h. Chest: nontender
i. Lungs: clear and equal bilaterally
j. Heart: tachycardic, rhythm regular, no murmurs, rubs, or gallops
k. Abdomen: normal bowel sounds, soft, nontender, nondistended
l. Rectal: normal tone, brown stool, occult blood negative

m. Extremities: mild tenderness on palpation of extremities but no joint findings, full range of motion, no deformity, diminished pulses

n. Back: nontender, no deformity

o. Neuro: cranial nerves II to XII intact; normal sensation, strength; normal reflexes, stable gait, negative cerebellar testing

p. Skin: warm and diaphoretic, no rashes or ecchymosis

q. Heme: no lymphadenopathy

H. Action

a. 2nd L NS IV bolus

b. Meds:

  i. Morphine or hydromorphone (NSAIDs should be avoided due to renal damage from rhabdomyolysis and dehydration)

c. Cool patient with ice packs or cooling device.

d. Bicarbonate therapy (not vital to patient's care)

e. Mannitol therapy (not vital to patient's care)

I. Nurse

a. EKG (Figure 122.1)

b. Fluid resuscitation

  i. 2 L IV fluids given

    1. BP: 110/80 HR: 95

  ii. Less than 2L IV fluids given

    1. BP: 90/65 HR: 130

c. Analgesics

  i) Pain improves to 3/10 and patient appears more comfortable

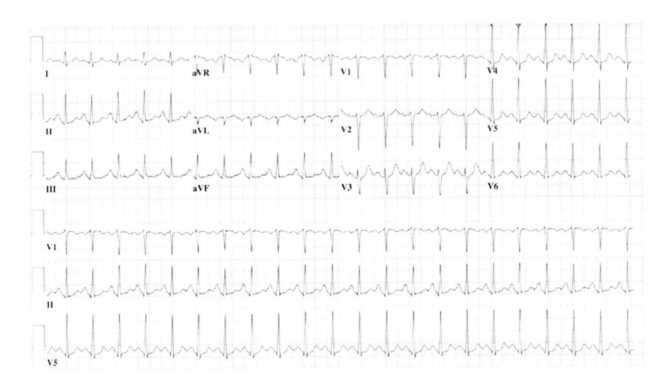

Figure 122.1

    d. Cooling with ice packs

        i) Temperature improves to 100.5°F

    e. Bicarbonate and/or mannitol therapy

        i) No effect on patient

J. Results

Complete blood count:

WBC	9×10^3/uL
Hct	47%
Plt	150×10^3/uL

Basic metabolic panel:

Na	132 mEq/L
K	4.9 mEq/L
Cl	99 mEq/L
CO_2	17 mEq/L
BUN	85 mEq/dL
Cr	4.8 mg/dL%
Glu	110 mg/dL

Liver function panel:

AST	32 U/L
ALT	38 U/L
Alk Phos	98 U/L
T bili	0.7 mg/dL
D bili	0.1 mg/dL
Albumin	5.5 g/dL
Total protein	7.4 g/dL

Creatinine kinase	12000 U/L
Lactate	2.4 mmol/L

Blood gas:

pH	7.32
pCO_2	35 mmHg
HCO_3	15 mEq/L

Urinalysis:

SG	1.015
pH	6.2
Prot	Trace
Gluc	Neg
Ketones	Present
Bili	Neg
Blood	Pos
LE	Neg
Nitrite	Neg
Color	Tea-colored
RBCs	0
WBCs	0
Casts	Pigmented, brown

K. Diagnosis

a. Primary: rhabdomyolysis

b. Secondary:

    i. Heat exhaustion

    ii. Acute kidney injury due combination of:

        1. Dehydration/heat exhaustion

        2. Rhabdomyolysis (myoglobin effect on kidney)

        3. High-dose ibuprofen use (decreases GFR)

L. Critical actions

a. Cardiac monitoring

b. IV fluid administration

c. EKG within 10 minutes of arrival (due to chest pain and cocaine)

d. Pain control with opiates or other appropriate analgesic

e. Obtain cardiac history and/or ROS (no need to do cardiac work-up)

f. Consult Renal for potential dialysis

g. Admit the patient to the ICU.

M. Examiner instructions

a. This is a case of rhabdomyolysis, a breakdown of muscle tissue, which in this patient was caused by cocaine use and heavy workout. Rhabdomyolysis is defined as a CK level 5–10 times normal. The rhabdomyloysis, coupled with heat exhaustion, dehydration, and high-dose ibuprofen use, ultimately led to the patient's acute kidney damage, exacerbating the patient's condition.

b. The candidate should recognize the pathology that the patient has and aggressively hydrate him. Hyperthermia should also be treated. The candidate should obtain renal consultation for possible dialysis. Intravenous bicarbonate therapy may be considered as it may provide benefit in severe cases. Mannitol therapy has been suggested but the data on its use in the treatment of rhabdomyolysis is not conclusive but may be considered to maintain urine output.

N. Pearls

a. Dehydration causes a pre-renal/volume depleted state, creating clinically significant rhabdomyolysis with early renal dysfunction at lower CK levels.

b. Aggressive IV hydration improves the glomerular filtration rate (GFR), which reduces renal injury and improves outcomes in patients with rhabdomyolysis.

c. A significant complication of rhabdomyolysis is electrolyte abnormalities due to acute kidney injury as well as skeletal muscle damage.

d. NSAIDs can cause renal artery vasoconstriction (via prostaglandin inhibition), which reduces GFR, and makes patients more prone to renal injury from rhabdomyolysis.

O. References

a. LJ Bontempo and AH Kaji. Rhabdomyolysis. In: Marx J, Hockberger R, Walls RM eds. *Rosen's Emergency Medicine: Concepts and Clinical Practice.* Philadelphia: Mosby Elsevier; 2010; 1650–7.

b. Scharman EJ, Troutman WG. Prevention of kidney injury following rhabdomyolysis: a systematic review. *Ann Pharmacother.* 2013;47(1):90–105. doi:10.1345/aph.1R215.

CASE 123: Headache (Elisabeth Lessenich, MD, MPH)

A. Chief complaint

a. 26-year-old female with headache, worsening since this afternoon.

B. Vital signs

a. T: 36.0°C, HR: 69, BP: 131/76, RR: 16, O_2 Sat: 100% on RA

C. What does the patient look like?

a. Patient appears stated age, appears uncomfortable, resting her head on the stretcher with her eyes closed.

D. Primary survey

a. Airway: speaking quietly, but in full sentences

b. Breathing: no apparent respiratory distress, good air entry bilaterally

c. Circulation: intact peripheral pulses bilaterally, capillary refill normal

E. History

a. HPI: This is a 26-year-old female who presents with a throbbing headache, rated 8/10 and worse on the right side, which started this morning. She has associated nausea but has not vomited. She feels the pain is worsened by sunlight or room lights. She took acetaminophen and ibuprofen, which usually helps her by lunchtime, but the headache has progressed. She denies fevers, recent travel, fall or head trauma, neck or back pain, speech changes, visual changes, focal weakness, numbness, or trouble walking. She reports a history of 1–2 migraine episodes per month, which typically respond to over-the-counter medication and rest. Over the past 2 weeks, she has had increased stress and workload at her job and has not been sleeping well.

b. PMHx: paroxysmal SVT; migraines
c. PSHx: S/p SVT ablation 4 months prior
d. Medications: oral contraceptive pill daily; acetaminophen and ibuprofen prn
e. Allergies: none
f. Social Hx: denies smoking or illicit drug use; 3–4 alcoholic drinks per week. She lives with roommates and works in the music industry doing concert promotion.
g. FHx: mother has a history of migraines; brother also has a history of undifferentiated headaches.

F. Action

a. Large peripheral IV
b. 1 liter NS bolus intravenously
c. Urine pregnancy test
d. EKG (candidate may request given the history of SVT although not required)

G. Secondary survey

a. General: obese, uncomfortable, resting with eyes closed, holding her head
b. Head: normocephalic, atraumatic
c. Eyes: extraocular movements intact without nystagmus, fundi unremarkable, pupils equal and reactive to light
d. Ears: normal ear canals and tympanic membranes
e. Nose: no discharge
f. Neck: full range of motion, no jugular vein distention, no stridor
g. Pharynx: clear without exudates or erythema
h. Neck: supple with full range of motion
i. Cardiovascular: regular rate and rhythm, no murmurs or rubs
j. Lungs: clear to auscultation bilaterally, no wheezing or crackles
k. Abdomen: bowel sounds present, soft, nondistended, nontender
l. Back: nontender, normal range of motion
m. GU: deferred
n. Extremities: no edema, 2+ radial and DP pulses bilaterally
o. Neuro: alert and oriented x 3, intact concentration and short-term memory, cranial nerves II-XII intact, visual fields full, speech fluent, 5/5 strength in all extremities with normal tone and bulk, light touch sense intact bilaterally, no pronator drift, 2 + reflexes in upper and lower extremities, finger-to-nose and heel-to-shin intact without dysmetria, Romberg negative, normal gait
p. Skin: warm, dry, well-perfused, without rashes
q. Lymph: no cervical or axillary lymphadenopathy

H. Results

a. Negative urine pregnancy test
b. EKG (Figure 123.1)

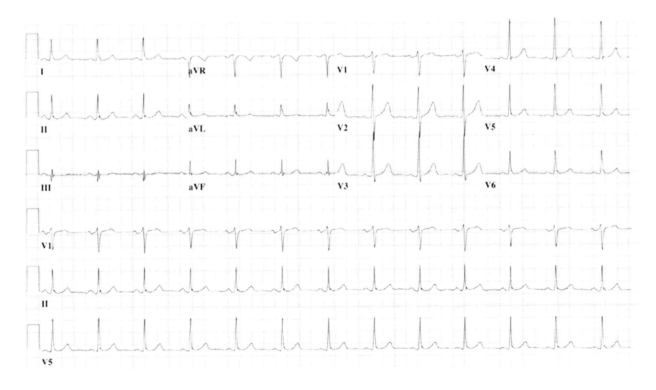

Figure 123.1

I. Action
a. Medications
    i. Prochlorperazine 10mg IV (or IM)
    ii. Benadryl 25mg IV – may give with prochlorperazine
    iii. Sumatriptan 6mg SC (or IM)

J. Nurse
a. Headache now minimal (should not improve sufficiently until sumatriptan given), patient feels improved and ready to go home

K. Action
a. Arrange Neurology outpatient follow-up for patient, to discuss possible prophylactic migraine therapy if episodes remain severe or become more frequent

L. Diagnosis
a. Migraine without aura ("common migraine")

M. Critical actions
a. Full neurological exam
b. Fluids and medication administration for migraine management
c. Consideration of neuroimaging if the patient has abnormalities / deficits on neurologic examination, or if headaches were more sudden in onset

N. Examiner instructions
a. This is a case of a patient suffering from a migraine headache without aura, or common migraine, which accounts for about 80% of migraine cases. Migraine is a

chronic neurovascular disorder that manifests with severe headache episodes and, in the case of "classic migraine", is also associated with auras of particular neurologic symptoms like visual scotomas, photopsias, or transient motor deficits. Migraines have been noted to be triggered or exacerbated by such elements as stress, disturbances of sleep pattern, menstrual cycles in women, and weather – some of which could be elicited in this patient's history.

b. Given that the patient has already tried over-the-counter medications unsuccessfully at home, she should be treated with IV medications. She should not improve sufficiently until the candidate administers, or at least considers, a triptan medication such as sumatriptan. The candidate should demonstrate consideration of other neurological entities by questions asked to obtain patient history.

O. Pearls

a. In the evaluation of patients with headache in the emergency department, the provider must first distinguish between primary headache entities (such as migraines, tension headaches, and cluster headaches) and secondary headaches (where the headache is a manifestation of another insult or underlying abnormality, such as hemorrhage, infection, or malignancy).

b. Migraine treatment involves acute or abortive therapies as well as preventive or prophylactic regimens.

c. For a patient presenting with a mild migrainous headache, common analgesics such as NSAIDs or combinations of acetaminophen, aspirin, and caffeine have been shown to be effective – if the patient has not already tried them prior to arrival.

d. For more severe migraine pain, neuroleptics such as prochlorperazine, and/or triptans, which act specifically on the 5-HT1 serotonin receptors, have been recommended. Triptans may diminish migraine pain by constricting dilated cerebral vessels and can be given subcutaneously or intranasally (or orally, if the patient has no associated nausea or vomiting). They are contraindicated in patients with coronary artery disease, peripheral vascular disease, pregnancy, or recent use of ergotamine-type medications.

e. Because frequent severe migraine attacks can have a negative effect on patients' quality of life and productivity, patients with multiple episodes that do not respond to their usual analgesic regimen, or that require emergency room treatment, should be referred to a neurologist for discussion of the risks and benefits of prophylactic medication for their migraines (such as beta-blockers, TCAs, or antiepileptics).

P. References

a. Rosen's: Chapter 103

b. Edlow JA, Panagos PD, Godwin SA, Thomas TL, Decker WW, for the American College of Emergency Physicians Clinical Policies Subcommittee. Clinical policy: Critical issues in the evaluation and management of adult patients presenting to the Emergency Department With acute headache. *Annals of Emergency Medicine*. 2008 Oct; 52(4): 407–436.

CASE 124: Dizziness (Anne Chipman, MD, MS)

A: Chief complaint
a. 72-year-old female with dizziness

B: Vital signs
a. BP: 180/105 HR: 62 RR: 16 SaO_2: 98% on RA T: 37.4°C

C: What does the patient look like?
a. The patient appears her stated age, lying in bed in no acute distress.

D: Primary survey
a. Airway: patent
b. Breathing: breathing comfortably
c. Circulation: normal capillary refill

E: Action
a. Oxygen via nasal cannula
b. Two large-bore peripheral IVs
c. Labs:
  i. Bedside glucose 175 (must ask)
  ii. CBC, BMP, LFTs, coagulation studies, troponin
d. Monitor EKG

F: History
a. The patient reports that 2 days prior she awoke from sleep and felt dizzy, as though the room was swaying and the dizziness has persisted since then. She's too unsteady to walk without assistance. Dizziness is constant and not affected by change in position. Her left arm has been shaking. She reports a mild headache and nausea. She denies other symptoms of vision or hearing changes, fevers, chills, confusion, chest pain, or palpitations. She has been diagnosed with "vertigo" in the past by her PMD who prescribed meclizine. She tried meclizine today but it had no effect on her symptoms.
b. PMHx: Type II DM, HTN
c. PSH: none
d. Allergies: penicillin
e. Medications: Metformin, hydrochlorothiazide lisinopril
f. Social: lives alone. Does not smoke, drink or use drugs.
g. FHx: mother with CVA at age 65, father with MI at 70.
h. PMD: Dr. White

G: Nurse
a. EKG (Figure 124.1)
b. BP: 195/110 HR: 65 RR: 18 Sat: 100% on 2L NC

H: Secondary survey
a. General: NAD, lying in bed with eyes closed.
b. Head: NCAT

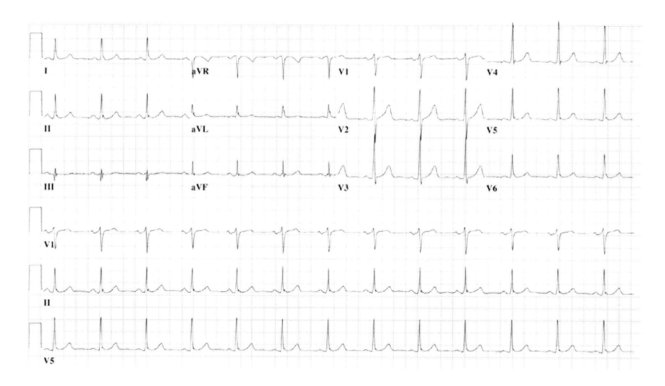

Figure 124.1

   c. Eyes: pupils equal, round, and reactive to light; extraocular movements intact with vertical nystagmus present on movement and at rest; visual acuity normal
   d. Ears: normal tympanic membranes
   e. Nose: no nasal discharge
   f. Neck: supple, with full range of motion. No carotid bruits
   g. Pharynx: normal dentition, no lesions, no swelling
   h. Lungs: clear bilaterally
   i. Heart: rate and rhythm regular, no murmurs, rubs, or gallops
   j. Abdomen: soft, nontender, nondistended, normal bowel sounds
   k. Rectal: normal rectal tone
   l. Extremities: no deformity, normal pulses
  m. Back: nontender
   n. Neuro: alert and oriented x 3; CNs intact. Speech is clear. Left upper extremity has severe intention tremor and dysmetria and dysdiadochokinesia with testing. Significant truncal ataxia. Gait is wide-based and unsteady. Strength difficult to assess in the left upper extremity due to intention tremor, but is otherwise intact. Sensation intact throughout the upper and lower extremities
   o. Skin: warm and dry

I: Action
  a. Imaging
     i: Stroke protocol MRI/MRA of the brain
     ii: Head CT without contrast (optional – if ordered will be negative)
  b. Meds:
     i. Aspirin should not be given until after negative MRI/CT

  ii. Antiemetic (patient will vomit if not given)
 c. Additional testing:
    i. Dix-Hallpike maneuver is not indicated. However, if done, should produce no
       change in nystagmus or experience of vertigo.

J: Nurse

 a. BP: 232/130 HR: 80 RR: 17 Sat: 100% on 2L NC
 b. Patient continues to appear comfortable

K: Results

Complete blood count:

WBC	6.4×10^3/uL
Hct	40.5%
Plt	400×10^3/uL

Coagulation panel:

PT	12.5 sec
PTT	26.0 sec
INR	1.0

Basic metabolic panel:

Na	137 mEq/L
K	4.5 mEq/L
Cl	105 mEq/L
CO_2	30 mEq/L
BUN	15 mEq/dL
Cr	1.2 mg/dL%
Gluc	170 mg/dL

Liver function panel:

AST	24 U/L
ALT	26 U/L
Alk Phos	45 U/L
T bili	1.0 mg/dL
D bili	0.3 mg/dL
Amylase	40 U/L
Lipase	20 U/L
Albumin	4.3 g/dL

Urinalysis:

SG	1.010 – 1.030
pH	5 – 8
Prot	Neg mg/dL
Gluc	Neg mg/dL
Ketones	Neg mg/dL
Bili	Neg mg/dL
Blood	Neg mg/dL
LE	Neg
Nitrate	Neg
Color	Yellow

Arterial blood gas:

pH	7.4
pO_2	95 mmHg
pCO_2	40 mmHg
HCO_3	25 mmol/L

 a. Troponin < 0.1
 b. MRI/MRA brain (Figure 124.2A,B,C): area of abnormal signal intensity in the L superior
    cerebellum. No hydrocephalus or brain herniation. Left vertebral artery occlusion.

L: Actions

 a. Consults:
    i.) Neurology consult: admission
    ii.) Neurosurgery consult: consultation for possibility of progression of edema and
        herniation
 b. Discussion with patient about findings
 c. Meds
    i.) Aspirin PO
    ii.) Blood pressure control: indicated now given sBP >220 and dBP>120. Easily
         titratable IV options (labetalol, esmolol, nitroprusside) are preferred given risk
         of hypotension and decreased cerebral perfusion pressure.

Figure 124.2
A, B and C

A

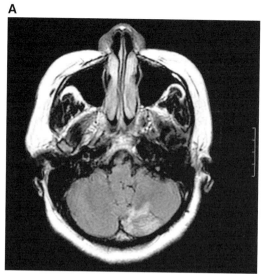

B

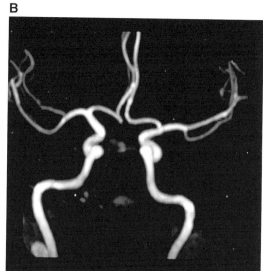

C

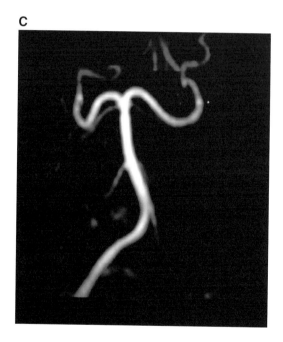

M: Diagnosis

a. Acute cerebellar stroke

N: Critical actions

▪ Establishing time of onset of symptoms
▪ Detailed neurological examination
▪ MRI/MRA brain
▪ Neurology and neurosurgery consultation
▪ BP control with IV agents
▪ Aspirin within 24 hours

O: Examiner instructions

a. This is a case of an acute cerebellar infarction. The clinical features can be subtle and may include vertigo, gait instability, limb ataxia, headache, nausea, vomiting, dysarthria, and cranial nerve abnormalities.[1] Early critical actions include the assessing for central causes of vertigo with a thorough history and neurologic exam, establishing time of onset, obtaining IV access and hemodynamic monitoring, ordering an MRI/MRA of the brain, and obtaining immediate neurology and neurosurgery consultations. Blood pressure management with the goal of permissive hypertension is important throughout the case. Once the determination of an ischemic infarction has been made, antiplatelet therapy with aspirin should be initiated.

P: Pearls

a. Cerebellar infarction tends to present with vague symptoms including vertigo, ataxia, headache, nausea, and vomiting.[1]

b. It is imperative to determine whether vertigo has features of a central etiology (as in this case) or a peripheral etiology. Peripheral causes of vertigo are often relatively benign, although the symptoms are distressing. In contrast, central causes of vertigo typically have more serious consequences. Peripheral vertigo is often intermittent provoked by position changes, reproducible, and fatigable. Central vertigo tends to be more constant, and relatively unaffected by positional changes. Nystagmus present in peripheral vertigo may be vertical-rotary or horizontal, usually suppresses with visual fixation and eventually fatigues. In contrast, nystagmus associated with central vertigo is usually sustained and not suppressible with visual fixation. Vertical nystagmus almost invariably implies a central etiology. Finally, any abnormal neurologic exam findings must always raise concern for a central cause of vertigo.[1,2]

c. MRI/MRA is the best imaging to assess cerebellar and posterior circulation pathology. CT is inadequate due to the artifact from posterior fossa bone.[1]

d. Cerebellar infarction may result in cerebellar edema, followed by herniation and rapid clinical deterioration. Therefore all patients with cerebellar infarction must have frequent neurologic exams and early neurosurgical consultation.[1]

e. For management of all ischemic strokes, blood pressure must be continuously monitored. This patient is not a candidate for tPA given the onset of symptoms well over 4 hours from presentation. Current guidelines call for permissive hypertension with no blood pressure control indicated unless the systolic BP rises above 220 or the diastolic blood pressure, above 120. [1]

Q. References

1.) Tintinalli's: Chapters 161, 164

2.) J.S. Olshaker. Dizziness and vertigo. In Marx JA, Hockberger RS, Walls RM, et al, eds. *Rosen's Emergency Medicine: Concepts and Clinical Practice* 7th ed. Philadelphia, Mosby Elsevier, 2010; 93–101.

CASE 125: Weakness (Bonnie Lau, MD)

A. Chief complaint

a. 29-year-old female with weakness

B. Vital signs

a. BP: 117/70 HR: 85 RR: 14 T: 37°C Sat: 92% RA

C. What does the patient look like?

a. Patient appears stated age, sitting up

D. Primary survey

a. Airway: speaking in full sentences
b. Breathing: no apparent distress, no cyanosis
c. Circulation: dry and warm skin, normal capillary refill

E. Action

a. Oxygen via 2L NC or nonrebreather mask
b. Two peripheral IV lines
c. Monitor: BP: 117/70 HR: 85 RR: 14 T: 37°C Sat: 98% on O_2
d. EKG

F. History

a. HPI: 29-year-old female with one week of generalized weakness worse over the past day. She is having difficulty studying, due to double vision and feeling like her eyelids droop, especially at night. Denies HA, fevers/chills, cough, chest pain, abdominal pain, NVD, urinary symptoms, numbness. Reports occasional shortness of breath.
b. PMHx: denies
c. Allergies: none
d. Meds: none
e. Social: denies tobacco, illicit drug use. Social EtOH. Pharmacy student.
f. FHx: denies
g. PMD: Dr. Bond

G. Secondary survey

a. General: alert, oriented x 3, appears fatigued
b. Head: normocephalic, atraumatic
c. Eyes: pupils equal, reactive to light, bilateral ptosis, weak CN III, IV, VI, end-gaze nystagmus, diplopia
d. Ears: normal tympanic membranes
e. Nose: no discharge
f. Neck: full range of motion, no jugular vein distension, no stridor
g. Pharynx: normal dentition, no lesions, no swelling
h. Lungs: clear bilaterally
i. Heart: rate and rhythm regular, no murmurs, rubs, or gallops
j. Abdomen: normal bowel sounds, soft, nontender
k. Rectal: normal tone, brown stool, occult blood negative
l. Extremities: no deformity, normal pulses
m. Back: nontender
n. Neuro: bilateral ptosis, end-gaze nystagmus, diplopia, weak CN III, IV, VI; other CNs intact, 4/5 proximal strength of bilateral upper extremities (UEs) and lower extremities (LEs), 5/5 distal strength UEs and LEs; normal sensation, reflexes, cerebellar testing
o. Skin: warm and dry
p. Lymph: no lymphadenopathy

H. Action

a. Labs

    i. CBC, BMP, LFT, coagulation studies, TSH

    ii. Urinalysis, urine hCG, urine toxicology screen

b. Imaging:

    i. CXR

    ii. Noncontrast brain CT

c. Neurology consult

I. Results

Complete blood count:

WBC	5.0×10^3/uL
Hct	40.5%
Plt	350×10^3/uL

Basic metabolic panel:

Na	137 mEq/L
K	3.9 mEq/L
Cl	101 mEq/L
CO_2	25 mEq/L
BUN	15 mEq/dL
Cr	0.9 mg/dL%
Gluc	129 mg/dL

Coagulation panel:

PT	11.8 sec
PTT	29.0 sec
INR	1.1

Liver function panel:

AST	22 U/L
ALT	27 U/L
Alk Phos	88 U/L
T Bili	1.0 mg/dL
D Bili	0.2 mg/dL
Lipase	21 U/L
Albumin	4.9 g/dL

Urinalysis:

SG	1.020
pH	7
Prot	Neg mg/dL
Gluc	Neg mg/dL
Ketones	Neg mg/dL
Bili	Neg
Blood	Neg
LE	Neg
Nitrite	Neg
Color	Yellow

a. TSH normal

b. Urine toxicology and urine pregnancy test negative

c. EKG (Figure 125.1)

d. CXR (Figure 125.2)

e. Brain CT (Figure 125.3)

J. Action

a. Neurology consultant plans to administer edrophonium at the bedside.

    i. Examinee should verbalize the need to be present with airway preparation due to the potential need for ventilatory support/intubation during edrophonium testing.

    ii. Examinee should be prompted to prepare airway support and verbalize intubation medications and doses.

b. Edrophonium testing confirms diagnosis of myasthenia gravis

c. Meds:

    i. Acetylcholinesterase inhibitor (ie. pyridostigmine or neostigmine)

    ii. Consider corticosteroids, plasma exchange, or IVIG

d. Admission to ICU

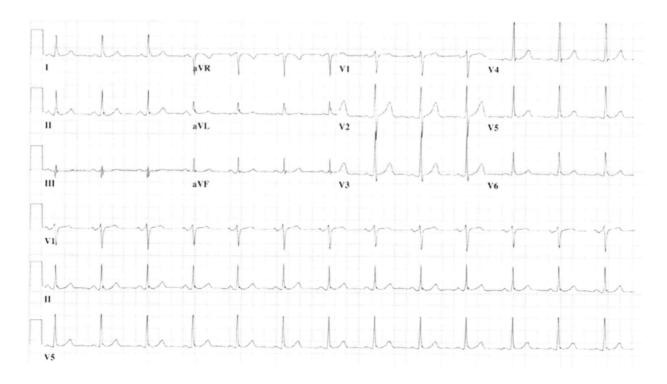

Figure 125.1

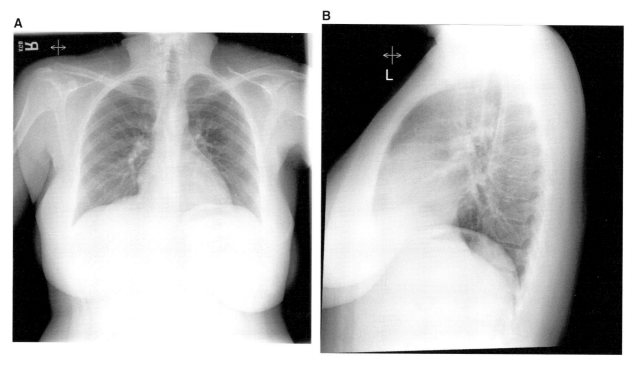

Figure 125.2 A and B

K. Diagnosis
a. Myasthenia gravis

L. Critical actions
a. Obtain detailed history and examination

Figure 125.3

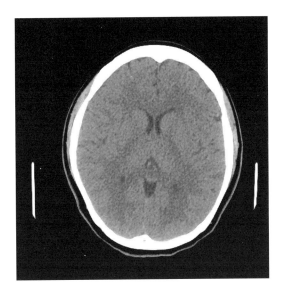

b. Consult neurology

c. Preparation for airway support during neurology testing

d. Avoid or reduce the use of depolarizing or nondepolarizing agents

e. Admit to ICU

M. Examiner instructions

a. This is a case of newly diagnosed myasthenia gravis (MG). MG is an autoimmune disease characterized by muscle weakness and fatigue, especially of proximal extremity, facial, and bulbar muscles. A detailed history and physical examination are key in making the clinical diagnosis. The diagnosis is confirmed with bedside edrophonium testing. The examinee must recognize that edrophonium testing may potentially cause profound respiratory weakness, and must be prepared to provide ventilatory support. Depolarizing and nondepolarizing agents should be avoided since MG patients are extremely sensitive to these. MG treatment involves administration of acetylcholinesterase inhibitors (ie. pyridostigmine or neostigmine).

N. Pearls

a. In MG, there is a marked decrease in the number and function of muscle fiber acetylcholine receptors (AChRs). Decreased response to acetylcholine stimulation causes decreased muscle strength, including the diaphragm.

b. MG is called the "great imitator" since it may mimic the symptoms of many other chronic neurologic disorders. Ptosis and diplopia are the most common presenting symptoms. Other MG findings may include: limb weakness, oropharyngeal symptoms (such as dysphagia and dysarthria, dysphonia), cranial nerve III, IV, or VI weakness, gaze palsies, internuclear ophthalmoplegia, end-gaze nystagmus, and dyspnea. There is usually no deficit in sensory, reflex, or cerebellar functioning.

c. Symptoms fluctuate throughout the day, usually worsening later in the day or with prolonged muscle group use (ie. prolonged reading or prolonged chewing).

d. Myasthenic crisis may be seen prior to the diagnosis of MG or as a result of inadequate drug therapy. It is characterized by respiratory failure due to extreme weakness in the muscles of respiration.

e. Depolarizing or nondepolarizing paralytic agents should be avoided in MG patients because the paralytic effects may persist two to three times longer than in normal patients. If paralytic agents are necessary, some support using half the dose, although no clinical studies support this practice.

f. The diagnosis of MG requires strong clinical suspicion and confirmation through the administration of edrophonium chloride (an acetylcholinesterase inhibitor).

g. In the presence of abnormal neuromuscular transmission, edrophonium is expected to improve muscle strength in weak limbs, ocular, and pharyngeal muscles. However, edrophonium can also cause profound weakness if given to other disorders that impair neuromuscular transmission. Therefore, one must be prepared to provide ventilatory support during edrophonium testing.

h. Treatment of MG involves administration of acetylcholinesterase inhibitors (i.e. pyridostigmine or neostigmine). Severe symptoms may require high dose corticosteroids, plasma exchange, or IV immunoglobulin.

O. References

a. Tintinalli's: Chapter 167
b. Rosen's: Chapter 108

CASE 126: "Found drunk" (Michael Cassara, DO)

A. Chief complaint

a. 35-year-old man "found drunk," with signs of acute intoxication

B. Vital signs

a. BP: 120/60 HR: 102 RR: 30 T: 97°F (36.5°C) SaO$_2$: 96%

C. What does the patient look like?

a. Thin, disheveled man with poor personal hygiene; moaning (incomprehensible words); abrasions to face and head

D. Primary survey

a. Airway: patent airway; gag reflex present; no pooling of secretions; no drooling; no stridor

b. Breathing: tachypnea and hyperpnea

c. Circulation: tachycardia

d. Disability: lethargy and obtundation; opens eyes only to painful stimuli; withdraws to painful stimuli; no posturing; no focal weakness; moaning and slurring of "speech"(incomprehensible words/sounds in response to name and other verbal/painful stimuli)

e. Exposure: no rashes, no lesions, no "track marks," no evidence of trauma

E. Action

a. Apply cervical collar (if candidate expresses concern over occult traumatic injury)

b. Administer supplemental oxygen with nonrebreather mask

c. Place two large-bore peripheral IV lines

    i. Administer NS fluid bolus (two liters)

    ii. Order laboratory tests

        1. Point of care testing: ABG, serum glucose

2. CBC, CMP, hepatic function tests, PT/INR/PTT, UA, serum toxicology panel (acetaminophen, salicylate, ethanol)

3. Serum osmolarity

4. At faculty discretion, allow ordering ethylene glycol and methanol

d. Place on continuous cardiac monitoring and obtain 12-lead ECG

   i. BP: 120/60 HR: 102 RR: 30 T: 97°F (36.5°C)

e. Place on continuous pulse oximetry and end-tidal capnography/capnometry

   i. SaO$_2$: 100% (with supplemental oxygen); ETCO$_2$: 22 mmHg

f. Consider administration of thiamine and naloxone

F. History (item a is provided only if the candidate requests that EMS or police "stay" at the beginning of the case; if candidate requests access to an old medical record, items b-e should be provided by examiner as necessary; otherwise, any other attempts to obtain this information should be answered with "unknown" or "unable")

a. HPI: 35-year-old man presents with altered mental status and clinical intoxication. He was "found drunk" by police on one of the benches in the village park in the center of town. He had been seen earlier in the evening at a local bar, where he was seen to drink an unknown amount of alcohol, but was "thrown out following an argument with his girlfriend." He is known to the ED staff as a "frequent flier." The patient is unable to provide any HPI or any past medical/surgical history because of his altered mental status and current level of intoxication.

b. PMHx: chronic alcoholism (medical records demonstrate greater than 15 separate ED visits for "intoxication"); depression (medical records demonstrate two admissions for "depression/suicidal ideation")

c. PSHx: appendicitis (22 years ago)

d. Allergies: none

e. Meds: none

   i. Social: excessive ethanol use; regular tobacco use (one pack per day for 18 years); occasional marijuana use

f. FHx: mother (deceased) with breast cancer at 54; father (deceased) with cirrhosis at 62

g. PMD: Dr. Brewer (non-compliant with visits to the local medicine clinic)

G. Nurse

a. 12-lead ECG (Figure 126.1)

b. Oxygen / IV fluid

   a. No change in vital signs

c. Thiamine / naloxone

   i. No change in altered mental status if ordered

H. Secondary survey

a. General: disheveled, thin, male, with a somnolent, lethargic, obtunded mental status; disoriented (only "moans" in response to name, and to other verbal/painful stimuli)

b. Head: normocephalic; atraumatic

c. Eyes: pupils equal, sluggishly reactive to light; extraocular muscles intact; horizontal nystagmus; optic disk margins normal

d. Ears: normal

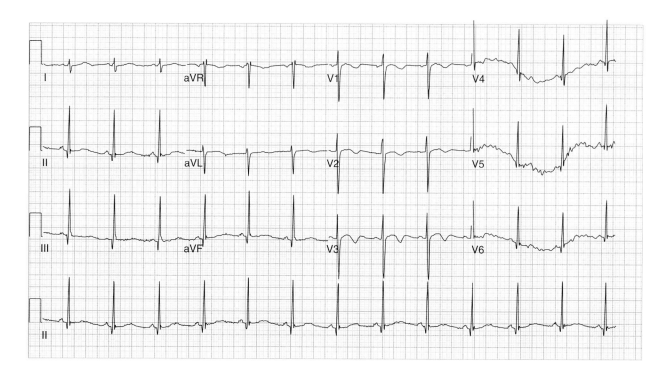

Figure 126.1

    e. Nose: normal

    f. Neck: full range of motion, no jugular vein distension; no stridor; midline trachea

    g. Pharynx: dry mucous membranes, lips, and tongue; no drooling; intact gag reflexes

    h. Chest: nontender to palpation

    i. Lungs: clear bilaterally; no wheezing; tachypnea and hyperpnea (Kussmaul respirations)

    j. Heart: rate and rhythm regular; no murmurs, rubs, or gallops

    k. Abdomen: normal bowel sounds, soft, nontender, nondistended

    l. Rectal: normal tone, brown stool, occult blood negative

    m. Extremities: full range of motion, no deformities or evidence of trauma; normal pulses

    n. Back: nontender to palpation

    o. Neuro: cranial nerves II to XII intact; horizontal nystagmus; normal reflexes; ataxia, unsteadiness (cannot stand/walk), and inability to comply with neurologic exam because of intoxication; disoriented; slurring of incomprehensible words/sounds

    p. Skin: cool, dry skin; no rashes, lesions, petechiae, purpura, or "track marks"

    q. Lymph: no lymphadenopathy

I. Action

a. Order CT brain

J. Results

Complete blood count:

WBC	10.3×10^3/uL
Hct	35.7%
Plt	150×10^3/uL

Basic metabolic panel:

Na	148 mEq/L
K	4.9 mEq/L
Cl	108 mEq/L

CO_2	5 mEq/L
BUN	10 mEq/dL
Cr	1.1 mg/dL
Gluc	146 mg/dL
Ca	7 mEq/L

Coagulation panel:

PT	12.6 sec
PTT	26.0 sec
INR	1.0

Liver function panel:

AST	23 U/L
ALT	26 U/L
Alk Phos	42 U/L
T bili	1.0 mg/dL
D bili	0.3 mg/dL
Amylase	50 U/L
Lipase	25 U/L
Albumin	4.7 g/dL

Urinalysis:

SG	1.010
pH	5
Prot	Trace 1+
Gluc	Neg
Ketones	1+
Bili	Neg
Blood	Trace 1+

LE	Neg
Nitrite	Neg
Color	Yellow; calcium oxalate crystals; fluorescence with Wood's lamp

Arterial blood gas:

pH	6.99
PO_2	600 mmHg
PCO_2	21 mmHg
HCO_3	5 mmol/L

Other tests:

Serum lactate	16 mmol/L (normal < 2mmol/L)
Anion gap	Anion gap 35 (elevated), normal <12)
Serum osmolarity (calculated)	311 mOsm/kg H_2O (normal is 285–295 mOsm/kg H_2O)
Serum osmolarity (measured)	350 mOsm/kg H_2O
Osmolal gap:	39 mOsm/kg H_2O (elevated; normal is -14 to +10)
Acetaminophen	undetectable
Salicylate	undetectable
Ethanol	14 mg/dL
Methanol	undetectable
Ethylene glycol	170 mg/dL

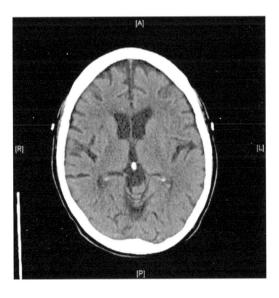

Figure 126.2

a. CT brain (Figure 126.2)

K. Action
a. Meds
    i. Fomepizole or equivalent antidote (e.g ethanol)

    ii. Pyridoxine

    iii. Calcium chloride or calcium gluconate, to correct hypocalcemia

b. Consult renal for hemodialysis

c. Admit to ICU

L. Diagnosis

a. Ethylene glycol poisoning

b. Hypocalcemia causing prolonged QT

M. Critical actions

a. Obtain EKG

b. Order bedside serum glucose testing

c. Administer sodium bicarbonate (bolus and/or continuous infusion)

d. Correct hypocalcemia

e. Administer fomepizole or equivalent antidote (e.g. ethanol)

f. Arrange for hemodialysis

g. Admit to the ICU

N. Examiner instructions

a. This is a case of ethylene glycol toxicity. The patient intentionally ingested antifreeze after getting intoxicated at a local bar, arguing with his girlfriend (he got "dumped"), and getting "thrown out." The candidate should perform the primary survey and recognize the metabolic acidosis by observing the patient's altered mental status, Kussmaul respirations, and ABG results. The candidate should then perform a diligent search for the causes (MUDPILES) while attempting to stabilize the patient. Stabilization measures include reversal of acidosis, electrolyte correction, blockade of alcohol dehydrogenase (toxin production), and elimination of ethylene glycol with hemodialysis.

O. Pearls

a. Toxic alcohol poisoning should be considered in any patient with altered mental status, evidence of acute intoxication, an elevated anion gap metabolic acidosis, and an elevated measured serum osmolarity with a significant osmolal gap. Toxic alcohol poisoning should definitely be suspected when other causes for the findings above (e.g. diabetic ketoacidosis with hyperglycemia) are absent.

b. Administration of fomepizole and ethanol works by (competitively) inhibiting alcohol dehydrogenase and preventing the metabolism of ethylene glycol into multiple toxic metabolites (glycoaldehyde, glycolate, glyoxalate, and oxalate). These toxic metabolites cause direct tissue destruction, hypocalcemia, and elevated anion gap metabolic acidosis. If ethanol is used, the target serum ethanol level to reach is 100–150 mg/dL.

c. Hemodialysis is the definitive management. There is no role for gastrointestinal decontamination in this patient.

d. Sodium bicarbonate, pyridoxine, thiamine, and calcium administration may be helpful. Sodium bicarbonate may enhance toxic metabolite excretion with acidosis correction, but may complicate hypocalcemia. Pyridoxine may inhibit the metabolism of glycolate to oxalate. Thiamine may promote the conversion of glyoxalate to alpha-hydroxy-beta-ketoadipate. Calcium correction will correct ECG abnormalities related to hypocalcemia (long QT), but may result in calcium oxalate crystal precipitation.

e. A dangerous commission during this case is to perform endotracheal intubation with sedation without recognizing and acknowledging the compensatory respiratory alkalosis (e.g. Kussmaul respirations) inherent in this situation. If the decision is made to intubate the patient, the candidate must order mechanical ventilation settings that maintain the patient's pre-intubation level of hyperventilation. The acidosis will rapidly worsen, and the patient will arrest if this is not done.

P. References

a. Rosens: Chapter 155

b. Tintinalli's: Chapter 179

c. Davis DP, Bramwell KJ, Hamilton RS, Williams SR. Ethylene glycol poisoning: a case report of a record-high level and a review. *J Emerg Med*. 15(5): 653–667.

d. Meng QH, Adeli K, Zello GA, Porter WH, Krahn J. Elevated lactate in ethylene glycol poisoning: True or false? *Clinica Chimica Acta* 411 (2010): 601–604.

The chest pain patient: Five life-threatening causes and critical actions

Luke Hermann, MD

The Approach to the Chest Pain Patient

Place every patient on a cardiac monitor and establish IV access.

Symptom descriptors and what differentials they suggest are as follows:

1. Abrupt onset, severe intensity, ripping or tearing, radiation to back: aortic dissection or esophageal rupture
2. Pleuritic pain with dyspnea: pulmonary embolism or spontaneous pneumothorax
3. Gradual onset, pressure-like: myocardial infarction

Essential examination features and what they suggest are as follows:

1. Look
   a. Significant tachypnea or respiratory distress: pulmonary embolism or spontaneous pneumothorax
2. Listen
   a. Unilateral breath sounds: spontaneous pneumothorax
   b. Diastolic murmur: aortic dissection
3. Examine
   a. Subcutaneous emphysema: ruptured esophagus
   b. Pulse deficit, BP differential >20 mmHg, or neuro deficit: aortic dissection
   c. Unilateral leg swelling, palpable cord: pulmonary embolus

Essential EKG findings and what they suggest are as follows:

1. ST elevations: myocardial infarction or (rarely) aortic dissection
2. Right heart strain (prominent S wave in lead I): pulmonary embolus

Essential CXR findings and what they suggest are as follows:

1. Widened mediastinum: aortic dissection
2. Pleural edge: spontaneous pneumothorax

1. MYOCARDIAL INFARCTION (ST SEGMENT ELEVATION)

High-yield risk factors: Diabetes, hypertension, smoking, family history

High-yield history: Substernal pain, gradual onset, pressure sensation

Essential work-up

EKG: ST elevations/new left bundle branch block (LBBB), if inferior leads involved, obtained right-sided EKG

CXR: Typically nonspecific, obtain to evaluate for widened mediastinum

BIOMARKERS: Send but rarely helpful with initial diagnosis

TREATMENT
1. Antiplatelet
    a. Aspirin
    b. Clopidogrel if allergic to aspirin
2. Anti-ischemic
    a. beta blockers no longer recommended as part of initial management of STEMI
    b. nitroglycerine (avoid if right ventricular infarct)
3. Anticoagulation
    a. heparin or low molecular weight heparin
4. Reperfusion
    a. Cardiac catheterization if available (thrombolytics as alternative)

2. PULMONARY EMBOLISM

High-yield risk factors: Cancer, recent surgery, long trip, history of deep vein thrombus (DVT)

High-yield history: Dyspnea, cough, pleuritic pain

High-yield examination: Tachypnea, tachycardia, clear lungs, signs of DVT

Essential work-up

EKG: Typically nonspecific, look for right axis deviation (prominent S in lead I)

CXR: Typically nonspecific, primary purpose to evaluate for pneumothorax

D-DIMER: Can use for rule out in low-risk patients

CT ANGIOGRAM: Preferred modality for definitive testing

VQ SCAN: Alternative to CT when IV contrast contraindicated (allergy, renal insufficiency, etc.)

TREATMENT
1. Anticoagulation: low molecular weight heparin or unfractionated heparin

3. AORTIC DISSECTION

High-yield risk factors: Marfan syndrome or other connective tissue disease, family history of dissection, aortic instrumentation (i.e., cardiac catheterization or valve surgery)

High-yield history: Pain that is abrupt in onset, severe intensity, ripping or tearing

High-yield examination: Pulse deficit, focal neurologic deficit, new diastolic murmur

Essential work-up

EKG: Typically nonspecific, look for concomitant STEMI

CXR: Often nonspecific, look for widened mediastinum

CT ANGIOGRAM: Most commonly used study

BEDSIDE TRANSESOPHAGEAL ECHOCARDIOGRAPHY: Preferred if patient unstable

TREATMENT
1. Initiate rate control with ß-blocker – titrate to pulse <60
2. Initiate pain control with IV morphine
3. If systolic BP still >120 mmHg add nitroprusside
4. Stat surgical evaluation for operative intervention

4. SPONTANEOUS PNEUMOTHORAX

High-yield risk factors: Tall, thin, young patients, history of Marfan syndrome

High-yield history: Sudden onset pleuritic pain with dyspnea

High-yield examination: Decreased or absent breath sounds on affected side (not always)

Essential work-up

CXR: If difficulty visualizing pleural edge, get end expiratory film

TREATMENT
1. Stable patient with small pneumothorax (< 3 cm between lung and chest wall)
   a. Supplemental O_2 and repeat film in 6 hours
2. Stable patient with larger pneumothorax
   a. Tube thoracostomy
3. Unstable patient
   a. Immediate decompression with 14-gauge angiocatheter, second intercostal space, followed by tube thoracostomy

5. RUPTURED ESOPHAGUS

High-yield risk factors: Alcohol abuse, caustic ingestion

High-yield history: Retrosternal pain following vomiting or retching

High-yield examination: Typically not helpful, check for subcutaneous air in chest wall

Essential work-up

CXR: Screen for pneumomediastinum or pneumoperitoneum

CT OF CHEST OR GASTROGRAFFIN SWALLOW STUDY: To confirm diagnosis

TREATMENT
1. Broad-spectrum antibiotics
2. Surgical consult

The confused patient: Ten most common causes and critical actions

Denise Nassisi, MD, FACEP

Altered Mental Status

▓ Common ED presentation with extensive possible underlying etiologies
▓ Recognition
　▶ May present as decreased responsiveness with obvious coma or more subtle lethargy or confusion
　▶ Alternatively may present hyperactively with agitation or combativeness
　▶ Subtle presentations must not be missed as delirium is associated with high morbidity and mortality
▓ Need for expedient targeted evaluation for serious and potentially life-threatening etiology

Immediate Actions and Stabilization for Altered Mental Status

Must rapidly identify and intervene to reverse immediately life-threatening etiologies

▓ Assess ABCs and initiate resuscitation with CPR and ACLS/ATLS as needed
　▶ Airway: protect and secure airway
　▶ Breathing: check oxygenation and adequacy of ventilation
　▶ Circulation: check blood pressure and pulse, fluid and pressor support as needed
▓ Check VITAL SIGNS, place on cardiac and pulse oxygen monitors, evaluate pupillary response
▓ Check finger stick glucose and consider "coma cocktail" (glucose, naloxone, thiamine) administration

Key History for Altered Mental Status

Obtain a thorough history from all available sources to uncover the likely etiology

▓ Recent symptoms and complaints
▓ Recent trauma
▓ Substance abuse and toxin exposures
▓ Medications
▓ Underlying medical conditions
▓ Baseline mental status

▨ Check for medic alert tag, EMS and bystander history, information from family or caregiver, medication list and contact information in wallet, check for old chart, and/or prior visits

Key Physical Assessment and Tests for Altered Mental Status

Physical examination and targeted work-up should search for evidence of medical or surgical causes including trauma, infection, or focal neurologic deficits.

▨ Vital signs including accurate temperature measurement
▨ Oxygen saturation
▨ Rapid glucose determination
▨ Physical examination with thorough neurologic examination
▨ Chemistry including electrolytes, renal function, liver function panels
▨ Complete blood count
▨ Urinalysis
▨ Chest x-ray
▨ Electrocardiogram
▨ Target work-up dependent upon the clinical scenario, consider: head CT, lumbar puncture, blood cultures, toxicology screening, thyroid function
▨ Head CT: obtain when scenario suggests CNS etiology but also obtain if no other etiology for the altered mental status is uncovered

Differential Diagnosis of Altered Mental Status

There are many possible etiologies for altered mental status and the differential diagnosis is extensive.

O_2/CO_2

Hypoxemia
▨ Pneumonia, pneumothorax, pulmonary embolism, asthma or COPD exacerbation, congestive heart failure
▨ Monitor with pulse O_2
▨ Provide supplemental O_2

Hypercarbia
▨ Acute rise may cause lethargy and coma
▨ May occur in COPD patient placed on supplemental oxygen with loss of hypoxic drive
▨ Hypoventilation from any cause
▨ Measure with bedside capnography or ABG
▨ Provide ventilatory support when needed

Glucose

Hypoglycemia
▨ May present with confusion, agitation, or focal neurologic deficit, if untreated severe coma or seizures may ensue
▨ Immediate treatment with glucose IV bolus

Hyperglycemia
- Both diabetic ketoacidosis and hyperosmolar nonketotic state can present with altered mental status, lethargy, and coma
- May or may not have prior diabetes history
- Often with polyuria and polydipsia
- Search for an underlying precipitant or stressor, especially infection
- Treat with IV fluids and insulin

Fluid/electrolyte disturbance

Hypoperfusion/hypotension
- Volume loss, for example from severe gastroenteritis
- Acute hemorrhage
- Shock from any cause including sepsis
- Treat with fluids, transfusion, pressors as needed

Dehydration
- More likely etiology in elderly and debilitated patients

Hypernatremia
- Usually due to inadequate thirst mechanism or inability to respond to thirst
- May also be due to diabetes insipidus (urine concentrating defect)
- Chronic hypernatremia, if corrected too rapidly, can lead to cerebral edema or myelinolysis

Hyponatremia
- Degree of mental status change related to absolute degree and also the rate of reduction, sudden decrease is more likely to induce seizures
- Syndrome of Inappropriate Antidiuretic Hormone (SIADH) – consider in patient with malignancy, more common with lung cancer, brain metastases
- Hypertonic (3%) saline is administered in severe cases (obtundation, seizures); if corrected too rapidly can lead to central pontine myelinolysis

Hypercalcemia
- Malignancy
- Hyperparathyroidism
- Renal failure
- Associated symptoms include nausea, vomiting, abdominal pain, joint pain, polyuria, and constipation
- Treat initially with IV fluids and furosemide, additional adjunct therapies may be necessary

Infection/sepsis

- Pneumonia
- Urinary tract infection
- Meningitis
- Encephalitis
- Intraabdominal infection
- Skin / soft tissue infection

■ Sepsis
■ Common cause of mental status change, particularly in the elderly
■ Start empiric antibiotic therapy as quickly as possible to cover likely pathogens, especially for meningitis
■ Treat severe sepsis with early goal directed therapy (EGDT)

Drugs/toxins

Alcohol and drug toxicity
■ Acute intoxication with alcohol or drugs
■ Wernicke-Korsakoff syndrome: deficiency of thiamine (Vitamin B_1), found in malnourished patients, chronic alcoholics; check for ataxia and ophthalmoplegia
■ Administer thiamine with glucose if suspected, to prevent precipitating Wernicke-Korsakoff syndrome

Alcohol and drug withdrawal
■ Alcohol and benzodiazepine withdrawal can cause delirium and may cause seizures
■ Delirium tremens from alcohol withdrawal – classical findings of tachycardia, elevated blood pressure, tremor, and mydriasis
■ Must be treated with benzodiazepines

Medication
■ The elderly are particularly susceptible to polypharmacy and adverse drug effects
■ Medications with sedative and anticholinergic properties are common culprits

Poisoning/toxins
■ Evaluate for potential toxidrome
■ Consider accidental poisoning particularly in young children
■ Opiate: pinpoint pupils and respiratory depression
■ Anticholinergic: mydriasis, hyperthermia, anhydrosis, hyperemia
■ Sympathomimetics and hallucinogens: increased heart rate and blood pressure; possible increased temperature, agitation, diaphoresis
■ Carbon monoxide: flu-like symptoms, headache; if possible exposure check carboxyhemoglobin (COHgB) level
■ Pesticides
■ Cyanide
■ Methemoglobinemia
■ Poisonous envenomations
■ Occupational exposures

CNS pathology

Head trauma
■ Altered mental status from diffuse axonal injury or intracranial bleed (subdural hematoma, epidural hematoma, traumatic subarachnoid hemorrhage)
■ Elevated ICP, evaluate for Cushing's triad of bradycardia, HTN, irregular breathing
■ Obtain stat head CT and neurosurgical consultation
■ Protect airway and perform rapid sequence intubation with CNS protection

Nontraumatic CNS causes
- Cerebrovascular accident (CVA) – check for focal neurologic signs
- Subarachnoid hemorrhage (SAH) – headache, nuchal rigidity
- Lumbar puncture needed if CT negative
- Meningitis
  - ▶ Lumbar puncture for diagnosis, early empiric antibiotics
- Encephalitis
  - ▶ High index of suspicion in HIV/immunocompromised host for uncommon infections (e.g., toxoplasmosis, cryptococcal meningitis)
- Brain tumor

Seizure or postictal state
- History of seizures, witnessed seizure activity
- Postictal state following a generalized seizure should resolve in a few hours
- Absence seizures – brief altered mental status without motor activity, more common in children
- Nonconvulsive status epilepticus – may present with confusion, personality changes, hallucinations, delusions, nonfocal examination
  - ▶ EEG is needed

Endocrinopathies

Thyroid
- Hypothyroid – gradual alteration in mental status, lethargy, bradycardia, hypotension. Severe = myxedema coma
- Hyperthyroid – agitated and tremulous, tachycardia, fever. Severe = thyroid storm
- Check serum TSH level, supportive care, β-blocker for thyroid storm

Adrenal
- Adrenal insufficiency
- Cushing syndrome

Encephalopathies and organ failure/damage

Hypertensive encephalopathy
- Elevated blood pressure
- Check for evidence of end-organ damage (e.g., heart failure, kidney failure)

Liver disease/hepatic encephalopathy
- History of liver disease, physical stigmata of chronic liver disease and specifically history of prior hepatic encephalopathy
- Treat with lactulose
- Search for underlying precipitant particularly spontaneous bacterial peritonitis (SBP) or GI bleeding

Renal disease/uremia
- Inquire about dialysis schedule and compliance

Cardiac disease
- Arrhythmia
- Myocardial infarction
- Congestive heart failure, cardiogenic shock

Acute abdomen
- Ischemic bowel
- GI obstruction, incarceration, or perforation
- Infection (appendicitis, diverticulitis, cholecystitis)

Extremes of temperature

Hyperthermia
- Temperature greater than 40°C
- Confusion, tachycardia, tachypnea
- Immediately initiate cooling interventions; evaporative cooling with water mist and fan is most effective

Hypothermia
- Temperature less than 35°C
- Apathy, slurred speech
- When severe loss of shivering ensues
- Immediately begin rewarming with blankets, warming blanket, warm IV fluids

Psychiatric

- Exacerbations of a psychiatric disorder or the first presentation of psychiatric illness may present with altered mental status
- This should be a diagnosis of exclusion; psychiatric etiology is more likely in younger patients with prior psychiatric history
- Exclude medical and reversible causes of altered mental status before transferring patient to a psychiatrist

Dementia

- Do not assume that altered mental status in an elderly patient is just chronic dementia. Delirium must not be missed and should be ruled out.
- Search for a reversible medical etiology in all patients with abnormal mental status
- Ascertain what the patient's usual baseline mental status is

Mnemonic for altered mental status: AEIOU TIPS

A Alcohol
E Electrolytes, Endocrine, Encephalopathy
I Insulin (glucose)
O Oxygen, Opiates, Overdose
U Uremia
T Trauma, Temperature, Toxin
I Infection, Intracranial process
P Pharmacology, Poisoning, Psychiatric
S Seizure, Stroke, Subdural, Shock

Sedation of Severely Agitated and Uncooperative Patients

Sedation may be necessary for agitated patients to proceed with necessary stabilization, evaluation, and treatment.

▓ Try to reassure and verbally de-escalate whenever possible
▓ Pharmacologic sedation is needed for agitated patients if there is a potential for patient to harm himself or others or if agitation is impeding medical evaluation and treatment
▓ Use an antipsychotic such as haloperidol or a benzodiazepine such as lorazepam
  ▶ With benzodiazepines monitor for respiratory depression, particularly in elderly or debilitated patients
  ▶ With antipsychotics beware of potential for QT prolongation (may rarely result in torsades de pointes), extrapyramidal side effects (e.g., dystonic reaction), potential lowering of seizure threshold

The poisoned patient: Most common toxidromes and treatments

Ruben Olmedo, MD

Stabilization

The clinical management of the overdosed or poisoned patient is underscored by the basic principle of treating the patient and not the poison. In following this clinical tenet, the critically ill poisoned patient is rapidly stabilized during the primary survey, emphasizing the ABCs to correct airway, breathing, and circulatory problems. Abnormalities in the patient's vital signs (heart rate, blood pressure, temperature, respiratory rate, pulse oximetry, and finger stick glucose) are also corrected at this time.

History

As with other patients, a key element in the approach to the poisoned patient is in obtaining a history of present illness. The presentation of the overdosed/poisoned patient will depend on both the patient and the toxin. Therefore it is important to ask about the patient's general medical condition, medications and allergies, and the circumstances surrounding the overdose/poisoning. It is also important to inquire about what toxin(s) the patient may have access to, the dose, route, and time of overdose/poisoning. When inquiring about the circumstances surrounding the event, it is important to ask what signs and symptoms were experienced, their onset, and if anything has been done about them.

As there are many toxins, there are many toxidromes to be identified. This undertaking may seem daunting. However, it is simplified by classifying the toxidromes into categories that correspond to large pharmacological classes of agents (i.e., opioids, sympathomimetics, cholinergics, etc.). This is important since a specific agent may give you most but not all the signs and symptoms of that particular class of toxin. However, this information may be enough to suggest the correct agent implicated.

The physical examination is one of the most important tools that a physician has during the medical assessment since it provides supporting information in making the correct diagnosis. This fact is especially important in toxicology. The name given to the constellation of signs and symptoms that a patient may have after an exposure to a specific toxin (or class of toxin) is called toxidrome. The finding of a specific toxidrome during a focused physical examination gives a clue to the type of toxin ingested.

It is important to note that many patients may ingest more than one toxin. As such, the physical examination will manifest mixed signs and symptoms of the agents involved. In a mixed overdose, therefore, the toxidromes may be obscured.

The toxicological physical examination begins with careful evaluation of the vital signs. These include pulse, blood pressure, respiratory rate, temperature, and pulse oximetry. Since normal vital signs are influenced by age and general state of health, attention should be paid to these parameters during the clinical assessment. Vital signs should be monitored for further clues to temporal changes of end-organ manifestations since this may be relevant to a specific toxin. Abnormalities of vital signs detected during a physical examination may also point to specific toxins involved (Table C.1).

To quickly identify common toxidromes, the physical examination in toxicology is simplified. Conducting an assessment of the mental status first is important, especially in toxins that cause mental disturbances. For ease of its determination, this assessment may be described as normal, depressed (lethargy or comatose), or agitated (hyperdynamic). In the following part of the physical assessment, the size and reactivity of the pupils should be noted. The abdominal examination should note presence or absence of bowel sounds, including hyperactivity. The bladder should be percussed for urinary retention. The skin examination should similarly be noted for whether it is dry, normal, or wet. Lastly, a neurological examination is performed to assess for any focal deficits.

Table C.2 describes the physical examination findings of some of the most common toxidromes encountered in an overdose. It is also important to note that the sudden discontinuation of a medication/toxin may produce clinical manifestations that may be opposite to those manifested during an acute ingestion. In such a case, the constellation of signs and symptoms will be categorized as a withdrawal toxidrome (Table C.3). Table C.4 gives examples of agents that cause common toxidromes.

TABLE C.1. TOXIN-ASSOCIATED VITAL SIGN ABNORMALITIES

Temperature: Hypothermia
Ethanol
Sedative hypnotics
Barbiturates
Oral hypoglycemics
Opioids
General anesthetics
Carbon monoxide
β-blockers
α-blockers

Temperature: Hyperthermia
Cocaine
Amphetamines
Neuroleptics
Anticholinergics
Salicylates
PCP

Respiratory rate: Hyperventilation
Sympathomimetics
Anticholinergics
Caffeine
Seizuregenic agents (i.e., INH, gyromitra)
Agents causing AG (i.e., salicylates, electron transport inhibitors [CO, cyanide], toxic alcohols)
Cocaine
Amphetamines
Neuroleptics
Anticholinergics
Salicylates
Dinitrophenol

Respiratory rate: Hypoventilation
Barbiturates
Neuromuscular blockers (botulism, nicotine, organophosphates, elapid envenomation)
Opioids, clonidine
Tetrodotoxin
Poison hemlock
Strychnine
Colchicine

Blood pressure: Hypertension
Sympathomimetics
Cocaine
PCP
Lead
MAOI overdose
MAOI interaction

Blood pressure: Hypotension
Calcium channel blockers (CCBs)
β-blockers (BBs)
Antihypertensives
TCAs
Barbiturates

Pulse: Tachycardia
Anticholinergics
Sympathomimetics
Cocaine
TCAs
Theophylline
Iron
Diuretics

Pulse: Bradycardia
CCBs
BBs
Digoxin
Clonidine
Opioids (Ops)

Abbreviations: AG, anion gap; CO, carbon monoxide; MAOI, monoamine oxidase inhibitor; PCP, pentachlorophenol; TCA, tricyclic antidepressant.

TABLE C.2. COMMON TOXIDROMES

Toxidromes	Vital signs				Physical examination			
	BP	HR	RR	T	MS	Pupils	Abdomen (BS)	Skin
Sympathomimetic	↑	↑	↑	↑	Agitated	Dilated	↑	Wet
Cholinergic (nicotinic)	↔	↑	↑	↔	Agitated	↔	↑	No change
Cholinergic (muscarinic)	↔	↔	No change	No change	Agitated	↔	↑	Wet
Anticholinergic	↔	↑	↔	↑	Agitated	Dilated	↓	Dry

Abbreviations: BP, blood pressure; BS, bowel sounds; HR, heart rate; MS, mental status; RR, respiratory rate; T, temperature.

TABLE C.3. COMMON TOXIDROMES AND THEIR RESPECTIVE WITHDRAWAL TOXIDROMES

Toxidromes	Vital signs				Physical examination			
	BP	HR	RR	T	MS	Pupils	Abdomen (BS)	Skin
Sedative hypnotic (SH)	↓	↓	↓	↓	Depressed	Dilated	No change	No change
SH withdrawal	↑	↑	↑	↑	Agitated	No change	No change	Wet
Opioid	↓	↓	↓	↓	Depressed	Pinpoint	↓	No change
Opioid withdrawal	↑	↑	No change	No change	Anxious	Dilated	↑	Wet

Abbreviations: BP, blood pressure; BS, bowel sounds; HR, heart rate; MS, mental status; RR, respiratory rate; T, temperature.

TABLE C.4. EXAMPLES OF TOXINS THAT CAUSE COMMON TOXIDROMES

Sympathomimetics	Cholinergics (nicotinic)	Cholinergic (muscarinic)	Anticholinergic
Cocaine	Organophosphates	Organophosphates	Antihistamines
Amphetamines	Nicotine	Carbamates	Antipsychotics
Theophylline		Physostigmine	Selective serotonin reuptake inhibitors (SSRIs)
Epinephrine		Pyridostigmine	Tricyclic antidepressants (TCAs)
Norepinephrine		Neostigmine	Atropine
Levothyroxine			Hyoscyamine
Albuterol			Scopolamine
Ephedra			Glycopyrrolate
Caffeine			Benztropine
Guarana			Glutethimide
Yohimbine			
Adderall (dextroamphetamine)			
Atomoxetine			
methylphenidate			
Phentermine			
Terbutaline			

TABLE C.4. Cont'd.

Sedative hypnotics	Sedative hypnotic withdrawal	Opioid	Opioid withdrawal
Benzodiazepines	Benzodiazepine withdrawal	Heroin	In opioid-dependent person:
Barbiturates	Barbiturate withdrawal	Codeine	Opioid antagonists
Ethanol	Ethanol withdrawal	Hydromorphone	
Alcohols		Oxycodone	
Carisoprodol		Methadone	
Flexeril	In sedative-hypnotic-dependent person:	Fentanyl	
Chloral hydrate	Flumazenil	Hydrocodone	
Buspirone		Propoxyphene	
Propofol		Clonidine	
Zolpidem			
Zaleplon			
Ethchlorvynol			
Meprobamate			
Glutethimide			
Bromides			
Kava kava			

The trauma patient: The approach and important principles

David Cherkas, MD

Questions to ask for EVERY trauma victim:

"When I walk into the room what do I see?"

"Is there any more information from EMS about the scene or mechanism?" If the answer seems long or they have lists of the patient's medications or past medical history, ask them to stay and get back to them later.

ABCDE: "I would like to assess the patient's airway, breathing and circulation, have the patient exposed and placed on a monitor, have 2 large-bore IVs placed, and see the patient's vital signs."

The initial assessment will drive the first BIG decisions:

Intubation: GCS <8, combative, airway protection, injury with likelihood of airway compromise later (burns, neck or facial trauma). Use rapid sequence intubation (RSI) unless difficulty is predicted and then be prepared for surgical airway and consider awake or fiberoptic intubation. The simplest approach is to use etomidate as an induction agent and succinylcholine or rocuronium as a paralytic for all traumatic RSI cases – deviation from the standard may cause unnecessary extra questions. Don't forget to consider lidocaine and fentanyl for patients with head injury.

Tube thoracostomy: Decreased breath sounds on initial evaluation, asymmetrical chest movement (flail segment). Unless you are asked to describe the procedure, keep it simple.

Next do a FAST or e-FAST exam if you are comfortable describing the later. Take other obvious steps – stanch arterial bleeding, assess the abdomen and pelvis, and wrap the pelvis if unstable.

For tachycardic or hypotensive patients you will want to start 1–2 L of crystalloid resuscitation at this point.

Order basic trauma labs and studies – CBC, chemistry, alcohol, coagulation studies, type and cross-match for two units, C spine (cross-table if high suspicion for injury, otherwise defer to CT scan), chest and pelvis x-ray.

While those are pending, verbalize your *complete* secondary survey including FAST examination and *complete* medical history including *allergies*.

Now ask for the trauma team to be activated or the trauma surgeon to be notified and for the repeat vital signs after initial resuscitation.

Now you will come to the next BIG decisions:

Transfusion: ABEM would like you to transfuse all patients that are hypotensive after appropriate initial resuscitation. If you are going to use a permissive hypotension strategy, verbalize this clearly.

Central access: Is of less value than most people think in initial resuscitation in the real world and unlikely to win you any points – stick with multiple large-bore peripheral IVs unless the patient has multiple limb injuries or if the examiner describes a problem in obtaining peripheral IV access.

Invasive monitoring: Unlike the place where you work, the monitoring devices at ABEM General "work flawlessly." Don't worry about invasive monitoring unless you are specifically told there is an issue with monitoring.

Next, fully define the patient's injuries and begin to order appropriate subspecialty consultations:

"Pan scan" may be en vogue with some emergency physicians, including those seeking greater security in their clinical practice at the expense of greater radiation exposure. The oral boards are not the place to debate the relative merits of this approach. Simply order the tests which are appropriate for the patient's suspected injuries.

Pitfalls

- Expecting someone to help you – that is, thinking the case will likely end when the surgeon, neurosurgeon, or other consultant shows up.
- Expecting anesthesia to assist with the intubation – again, at ABEM General you are expected to handle all the EM procedures yourself.
- Attempting to skip to sophisticated intermediate resuscitation before the appropriciate initial evaluation steps have been taken. For example, attempting to push the patient to the operating room or admission before a reasonable primary and secondary survey has been completed or appropriate diagnostic tests and ED therapy had been initiated.

Addressing variations in the standard of care: There are areas of clinical controversy that remain and they will likely not be heavily weighted in your evaluation but they can hinder your thought process and rhythm in the heat of a case.
For example:

- Is it your responsibility to give phenytoin to every patient with a head injury?
- Should you administer high-dose steroids to patients with spinal cord injury?

One way around this is to ask/tell your consultant what your plan is and ask if they have any specific objections or suggestions.

For example:

> "Jane Doe has a moderate right subdural hematoma with shift, her initial GCS was 7 and she was intubated on arrival for airway protection. Since arrival, her left pupil has become fixed and dilated. I was planning on initiating dilantin and mannitol (or hypertonic saline). Do you have any objections or other suggestions? It is imperative that you evaluate the patient soon. Thank you."

Advanced cardiac life support review

Thomas Nguyen, MD; Uyen Nguyen, MD

I. CPR: Emphasis on High-Quality CPR

- Always find your landmarks (lower half of sternum)
- Push hard (adequately compress the chest **at least** 2 inches)
- Push fast (**at least** 100 compressions per minute)
- Allow chest to recoil after each compression
- Compression to ventilation ratio is 30:2 (1 cycle) for one and two rescuers for adult CPR
- Ventilations should be given over about 1 second; sufficient just to cause the chest to rise
- Continuous compressions: providers must minimize interruptions in chest compressions for rhythm check, shock delivery, advanced airway insertion, or vascular access

II. Sequence for CPR

Call for help and defibrillator immediately

- CAB is the New ABC: The sequence of Basic Life Support has changed: "CAB" Chest Compressions, Airway, Breathing has replaced "ABC" Airway, Breathing, Chest Compressions
- CPR (five cycles or 2 minutes) or until defibrillator or automatic external defibrillator (AED) arrives
- For AED, turn power on first, and then attach pads
- No CPR during analyze mode of AED
- Shock if indicated
- Continue CPR (2 minutes) then do pulse check
- Repeat sequence as needed

III. Sequence to Activate EMS In Out of Hospital Cardiac Arrest

- Call first: Activate emergency response system for adult victims found unresponsive
- If asphyxial arrest (drowning, choking) is likely, call after five cycles (or 2 minutes) of CPR

- Call for an AED or defibrillator as soon as possible
- If with another person, send that person for help and make sure they come back to assist

IV. Defibrillation Plus CPR

- Whenever defibrillator or AED is available, it should be used as soon as possible when indicated
- For out of hospital UNWITNESSED arrests, providers/EMS should give five cycles of CPR in about 2 minutes before checking ECG and defibrillator (especially if wait time is greater than 4–5 minutes)
- Charge for all shockable pulseless VF/VT
- One shock only
- Energy level 360 J for monophasic and whatever is recommended by manufacturer with biphasic (200 J is default if unknown)
- The one shock is followed immediately with 2 minutes of CPR (five cycles) beginning with chest compressions; start thinking about pushing meds
- If an organized rhythm is apparent during rhythm checks after 2 minutes (five cycles) of CPR, the provider checks a pulse; if still in VF/pulseless VT, shock again at 360 J or biphasic equivalent and continue with CPR sequence

V. Airway and Ventilation

- Avoid prolonged interruptions of CPR when inserting an advanced airway device
- Once airway device is in place, deliver 1 breath every 6 to 8 seconds (8–10 breaths per minute)
- The breaths are given asynchronously while compressions are being done continuously at a rate of at least 100 per minute
- Insertion of an advanced airway device should not take precedence over good-quality CPR
- Use of endotracheal intubation is limited to providers with adequate training and opportunities to practice or perform intubations
- No Cricoid Pressure: not recommended as an aide to ventilation

VI. Other Points to Remember

- Pacing: considered for symptomatic bradycardia with a pulse; NOT recommended for asystolic cardiac arrest
- Vascular access: IV or IO (intraosseous) PREFERRED to endotracheal. ETT dose is 2 times the IV/IO dose
- There is an increased emphasis on physiologic monitoring to optimize CPR quality and detect ROSC. (e.g., $ETCO_2$, if <10 mmHg attempt to improve CPR quality)
- Drugs: timing of drug delivery less important than the need to minimize interruptions in chest compressions. Give drug during CPR immediately following rhythm check; that is, have drugs prepared before rhythm check
- Vasopressin: may be used as alternative to epinephrine, one dose of 40 units to replace either the first or second dose of epinephrine in all types of cardiac arrests

(VF/pulseless VT and PEA/asystole). For persistent VF/VT pulseless arrests, either epinephrine or vasopressin can be given as soon as possible after the rhythm check either during the CPR that precedes (until the defibrillator is charged) or after the shock

I. Pulseless Arrest

Call for help, perform CPR until defibrillator/monitor arrives

- **Shockable** rhythm (VF/pulseless VT)
  - ▶ Give 1 shock (360 J monophasic or 200 J biphasic or manufacturer's recommended dose)
  - ▶ Resume CPR (no pulse check) five cycles of CPR or 2 minutes
  - ▶ Monitor check and pulse check
  - ▶ Give another shock (if no pulse); if pulse is present begin postresuscitation care
- Give drugs
  - ▶ Epinephrine 1 mg IV/IO (each round) or
  - ▶ Vasopressin 40 units (just one time) then consider
  - ▶ Amiodarone 300 mg IV/IO once over 2 minutes then consider additional 150 mg IV/IO next round or
  - ▶ Lidocaine 1 to 1.5 mg/kg, IV/IO may repeat × 3 up to total 3 mg/kg
- Repeat from the top starting with CPR
- **Not shockable** (asystole/PEA)
  - ▶ CPR for five cycles or 2 minutes
  - ▶ Vasopressin 40 units (just one time) IV/IO or
  - ▶ Epinephrine 1 mg IV/IO (may repeat each round)
  - ▶ Check for pulses/rhythm
  - ▶ Repeat cycle
    - ▷ Look for reversible causes
      - • **H**ypovolemia
      - • **H**ypoxia
      - • **H**ydrogen ion (acidosis)
      - • **H**ypo/hyperkalemia
      - • **H**ypothermia
      - • **T**ension pneumothorax
      - • **T**amponade, cardiac
      - • **T**oxins
      - • **T**hrombosis – pulmonary and coronary

II. Bradycardia

- Maintain airway, give oxygen
- Monitor rhythm, blood pressure, oximetry
- Signs of adequate perfusion (good mentation, no chest pain, no hypotension, no signs of shock, no CHF)
  - ▶ Observe/monitor
- Signs of poor perfusion (altered mental status, chest pain, hypotension, no signs of shock, no CHF)

▷ Prepare for transcutaneous pacing
▷ Consider atropine 0.5 mg IV (may repeat to a total of 3 mg)
▷ Consider epinephrine drip (2–10 mcg/min) or dopamine drip (2–10 mcg/kg/min)
▷ Consider transvenous pacing

III. Tachycardia (with pulse)

▣ Monitor, support ABCs, give oxygen
▣ Is patient stable or unstable?
▣ **Unstable**
  ▷ Perform synchronized cardioversion
    ▷ Atrial fibrillation: 120 to 200 J biphasic or monophasic
    ▷ Atrial flutter / SVT: 50 to 100 J biphasic or monophasic
    ▷ Stable monomorphic VT: 100 J biphasic or monophasic
  ▷ Consider sedation if patient is conscious
▣ **Stable**
  ▷ Is QRS narrow or wide?
    ▷ **Narrow** QRS
      a. Regular narrow (SVT, atrial flutter, junctional rhythm)
        Attempt vagal maneuvers
        Adenosine 6 mg IVP (may repeat 12 mg IVP × 2)
        Consider rate control with calcium channel blocker or β-blockers IV
      b. Irregular narrow (rapid atrial fibrillation, multifocal atrial tachycardia)
        Rate control with calcium channel blocker or β-blockers IV
    ▷ **Wide** QRS
      a. Regular wide: VT, SVT with aberrancy
        VT: Give amiodarone 150 mg IV over 10 minutes (repeat up to 2.2 g/24 hr) or
          procainamide 20–50 mg/min (max 17mg/kg) or sotalol 1.5mg/kg IV over
          5 mins, or lidocaine 1 to 1.5mg/kg IV (repeat 0.5 to 0.75 mg/kg IV every
          5–10 mins max total 3 mg/kg)
        SVT with aberrancy: Give adenosine 6 mg IVP (may repeat 12 mg × 2).
          Consider β-blocker, diltiazem, amiodarone, digoxin
      b. Irregular wide QRS: AFib w. aberrancy, WPW, polymorphic VT, Torsades
        AFib w. aberrancy: Rate control w. diltiazem or β-blocker
        WPW – consider amiodarine 150 mg IV 10 minutes (avoid AV node blockers
          adenosine, diltiazem, digoxin)
        Polymorphic VT: Seek expert consultation. Consider amiodarone 150 mg
          IV or
        magnesium 1 to 2 g IV
        Torsades de pointes: Shock immediately (see pulseless section above).
        Magnesium 1 to 2 g over 5 to 6 minutes, then infusion

ACLS DRUG LIST – ANTIARRHYTHMICS

Adenosine

Action: Briefly suppresses AV and sinus node activity

Use in ACLS: Drug of choice for stable, narrow-complex regular tachycardias (AV nodal or sinus nodal reentrant tachycardias) or wide-complex regular tachycardias confirmed as supraventricular

Dose: 6 mg IV push rapidly over 1 to 3 seconds, followed by a 20 ml saline flush. May give 12 mg if does not convert within 1 to 2 minutes. A second 12-mg bolus can be given if does not convert after the first 12-mg bolus

Adverse effects: Transient flushing, dyspnea, chest pain; risk of acceleration of accessory conduction

Amiodarone

Action: Class II antiarrhythmic; acts on blocking sodium, potassium, and calcium channels; also has α- and β-adrenergic blockade properties

Use in ACLS

1. Narrow complex tachycardias originating from a reentry mechanism if uncontrolled by adenosine, vagal maneuvers, and AV nodal blockade in patients with preserved or impaired ventricular function
2. In cardiac arrest with VT or VF after defibrillation and epinephrine
3. Control of hemodynamically stable VT, polymorphic VT, and wide-complex tachycardia of uncertain origin
4. Control of rapid ventricular rate due to accessory pathway conduction in pre-exited atrial arrhythmias

Dose*

- For pulseless VT or VF: can give 300 mg. Take two 10 ml syringes. Draw up 150 mg of amiodarone and 7 ml NS into each syringe for a total of 300 mg amiodarone. Give each over 1 minute if refractory or recurrent VT. Initial dose of 300 mg may be followed by one dose of 150 mg IV/IO.
- For VT with a pulse: can give 150 mg IV over 10 minutes which can be repeated if ineffective. Maintenance infusion: 1 mg/min infusion × 6 hours. Then, 0.5 mg/min infusion × 18 hours.

Adverse effects: Hypotension and bradycardia

Lidocaine

Action: Class Ib antiarrhythmic; sodium channel blocker

Use in ACLS: May be considered but not the treatment of choice for:

1. Stable monomorphic VT with preserved heart function
2. Polymorphic VT with normal baseline QT interval

---

* Note that bolus doses can be given without using a glass bottle. A glass bottle and an in-line filter should be used for infusions. The amiodarone infusion is best given in a central line but a peripheral line can be used until a central line is available in an emergency.

3. Polymorphic VT with prolonged QT interval that suggests torsades
4. Alternative treatment to amiodarone in VF/pulseless VT cardiac arrest

Dose

- 1 to 1.5 mg/kg IV push in VT/VF cardiac arrest; 1.5 mg/kg preferable in adults. Additional 0.5 to 0.75 mg/kg for refractory VT/VF at 5 to 10 minutes intervals to a maximum dose of 3 mg/kg
- REDUCE DOSE or use amiodarone in low cardiac output states, such as in AMI with hypotension or shock, CHF, >70 years, or hepatic dysfunction

Adverse effects: Hypotension; CNS effects

Procainamide

Action: Class Ia antiarrhythmic; sodium channel blocker

Use in ACLS

1. One of several drugs for stable monomorphic VT with preserved heart function
2. One of several drugs that may be used to restore sinus rhythm for atrial fibrillation or atrial flutter in patients with preserved ventricular function
3. One of several drugs that can be used for acute control to restore normal sinus rhythm in atrial fibrillation or atrial flutter in patients with known WPW and preserved heart function
4. One of several drugs that can be used for AV reentrant, narrow-complex tachycardias such as reentry SVT if rhythm is uncontrolled by adenosine and vagal maneuvers in patients with preserved heart function

Dose

- 20 mg/min infusion until arrhythmia suppressed, hypotension, prolonged QRS by 50% from its original duration or total of 17 mg/kg; maintenance infusion is 1 to 4 mg/min
- In refractory VF/VT or urgent situation, infusion rate can be increased up to 50 mg/min to a total of 17 mg/kg

Adverse effect: Hypotension

Magnesium

Action: Corrects magnesium deficiency, which is associated with arrhythmias, cardiac insufficiency, and cardiac death

Use in ACLS

1. Torsades de pointes
2. Magnesium deficiency

Dose

- Torsades with pulses: 1 to 2 g in 50–100 D_5W over 5 to 60 minutes, followed by infusion of 0.5 to 1 g over 5 to 60 minutes

▧ Torsades with VF/pulseless VT cardiac arrest: defibrillate, then, give magnesium 1 to 2 g diluted in 10 ml D_5W

Adverse effects: If given too rapidly, hypotension or asystole

Calcium Channel Blocker: Diltiazem or Verapamil

Action: Slows conduction and increases refractoriness in the AV node

Use in ACLS

1. Stable, narrow-complex, reentry mechanism tachycardias (reentry SVT) if uncontrolled or unconverted by adenosine or vagal maneuvers
2. Stable, narrow-complex, automaticity mechanism tachycardias (junctional, ectopic, multifocal) if rhythm not controlled or converted by adenosine or vagal maneuvers
3. Control rate of ventricular response in patients with atrial fib or flutter; may be harmful in patients with WPW or similar syndrome

Dose

▧ Diltiazem: 0.25 mg/kg followed by second dose of 0.35 mg/kg if no response in 10 to 15 minutes; maintenance of 5 to 15 mg/hr to control ventricular rate in AF or atrial flutter

▧ Verapamil: 2.5 to 5 mg IV given over 2 minutes; can give repeated doses of 5 to 10 mg every 15 to 30 minutes to a total dose of 20 mg

Adverse effects: May decrease myocardial contractility and exacerbate CHF in patients with severe LV dysfunction; hypotension, bradycardia

β-Adrenergic Blockers

Use in ACLS

1. All patients with suspected AMI and high-risk unstable angina in the absence of contraindications (acute CHF, bradycardia or heart block, active asthma/COPD)
2. Narrow complex tachycardias from reentry mechanism, for example, reentry SVT or automatic focus (junctional, ectopic, or multifocal tachycardia) uncontrolled by vagal maneuvers and adenosine in the patient with preserved ventricular function
3. Rate control in atrial fibrillation and atrial flutter in patients with preserved ventricular function

Dose

▧ Atenolol: 5 mg slow IV push over 5 minutes; wait 10 minutes and if tolerated, second dose of 5 mg slow IV over 5 minutes

▧ Metaprolol: 5 mg slow IV push at 5-minute intervals to a total of 15 mg

▧ Propranolol: 0.1 mg/kg slow IV push divided into three equal doses at 2 to 3 minutes intervals with rate not to exceed 1 mg/min

▧ Esmolol: 500 mcg/kg over 1 minute followed by maintenance infusion of 50 mcg/kg/min for 4 minutes; if inadequate, second bolus of 500 mcg/kg over 1 minute with maintenance of 100 mcg/kg/min for 4 minutes, bolus 500 mcg/kg and titration of infusion (addition of 50 mcg/kg/min) can be repeated up to maximum maintenance infusion of 300 mcg/kg/min

Adverse effects: Bradycardias, AV conduction delays, hypotension; contraindicated in second- or third-degree heart block, hypotension, severe CHF, and lung disease with bronchospasm; caution with preexisting sinus bradycardia and sick sinus syndrome; may be harmful for patients with atrial fibrillation or atrial flutter associated with known WPW

Atropine

Action: Reverses cholinergic-mediated decreases in heart rate, systemic vascular resistance, and blood pressure

Use in ACLS

1. Symptomatic sinus bradycardia, AV block at the nodal level, or organophosphate poisoning

Dose: 0.5 to 1 mg IV every 3 to 5 minutes for bradycardia to a total dose of 0.04 mg/kg or 3 mg

Adverse effects: Worsening of ischemia; rarely, VF, VT

ACLS DRUG LIST – AGENTS TO OPTIMIZE CARDIAC OUTPUT AND BP

Epinephrine

Action: α-adrenergic receptor-stimulating properties that increase myocardial and cerebral blood flow during CPR

Use in ACLS

1. Cardiac arrest
2. Symptomatic bradycardia after atropine, dopamine, and pacing, or pacing not available
3. Severe hypotension
4. Anaphylaxis associated with hemodynamic instability or respiratory distress

Dose in cardiac arrest: 1:10,000: 1 mg IV push every 3 to 5 minutes IV/IO

Dose for symptomatic bradycardia/anaphylaxis: 2 to 10 mcg/min infusion

Adverse effects: May cause myocardial ischemia, angina, and increased cardiac demand

Vasopressin

Action: Nonadrenergic peripheral vasoconstrictor

Use in ACLS

1. One-time alternative to epinephrine for vasoconstriction in cardiac arrest VFib/pulseless Vtach and asystole

Dose: 40 units IV × 1

Adverse effect: May provoke cardiac ischemia

Norepinephrine

Action: α- and β-receptor-stimulating actions; vasoconstrictor and inotropic agent

Use in ACLS

1. Severe hypotension (systolic <70 mmHg) and low total peripheral resistance

Dose: Initially, 0.5 to 1 mcg/min infusion titrated to effect

Adverse effects: Ischemic necrosis and sloughing of tissues with extravasation, possibly increased myocardial oxygen requirements

Dopamine

Action: Dopaminergic, α- and β-receptor-stimulating actions

Use in ACLS as BP Agent

1. Hypotension with symptomatic bradycardia
2. After return of spontaneous circulation for postresuscitation hypotension or shock

Dose: 5 to 20 mcg/kg/min infusion

Adverse effect: Tachycardia

Dobutamine

Action: Catecholamine and potent inotropic agent; predominant β-adrenergic receptor-stimulating effects that increase myocardial contractility and decrease left ventricular filling pressures

Use in ACLS

1. Treatment of severe systolic heart failure

Dose: 2 to 20 mcg/kg/min infusion

Adverse effect: Tachycardia

Nitroglycerin

Action: Relaxes vascular smooth muscle

Use in ACLS

1. Ischemic-type pain or discomfort, acute coronary syndromes, hypertensive emergencies, CHF

Dose

- For suspected angina 1 tablet (0.4 mg) sublingually and repeated at 3- to 5-minute intervals if not relieved
- Continuous infusion at 10 to 20 mcg/min and increased by 5 to 10 mcg/min until desired response occurs

Adverse effects: Hypotension (also, consider RV infarct; check R-sided leads), tachycardia, paradoxical bradycardia, hypoxemia, headache

Sodium Nitroprusside

Action: Potent, rapid-acting direct peripheral vasodilator

Use in ACLS

1. Severe heart failure and hypertensive emergencies

Dose: 0.1 to 5 mcg/kg/min infusion up to 10 mcg/kg/min

Adverse effects: Hypotension, headache, nausea, vomiting, abdominal cramps

Calcium

Action: Replenish calcium; cardioprotective effect

Use in ACLS

1. Hyperkalemia
2. Hypocalcemia
3. Calcium channel blocker toxicity

Dose: 10% solution of calcium chloride in a dose of 8 to 16 mg/kg (usually 5–10 ml and repeated as necessary at 10-minute intervals). Recheck ECG after calcium in hyperkalemia; if no decrease in peaked T waves or QRS width, give second dose

Sodium Bicarbonate

Use in ACLS

1. Preexisting metabolic acidosis
2. Hyperkalemia
3. Tricyclic antidepressant overdose (suspect of QRS >11 msec)

Dose: 1 mEq/kg initially; redose guided by blood gas and bicarbonate concentration

Adverse effects: Possibly extracellular alkalosis including shift of oxyhemoglobin curve, paradoxical intracellular acidosis, exacerbation of central venous acidosis, and inactivation of simultaneously administered catecholamines

Diuretics: Furosemide

Action: Inhibits reabsorption of sodium in the loop of Henle; direct venodilating effect in acute pulmonary edema

Use in ACLS
1. Acute pulmonary edema

Dose: 0.5 to 1 mg/kg slow IV

Adverse effects: Fluid and electrolyte abnormalities; hypotension

REFERENCES:

1. Adult Advanced Cardiovascular Life Support: 2010 American Heart Association Guidelines for Cardiopulmonary Resuscitation and Emergency Cardiovascular Care. *Circulation* 2010;122;S729-S767.
2. CPR Overview: 2010 American Heart Association Guidelines for Cardiopulmonary Resuscitation and Emergency Cardiovascular Care. *Circulation* 2010;122;S676-S684.

Pediatric pearls: High-yield facts from fever to drugs

Christopher Strother, MD

Normal Vital Signs by Age (Pediatric Advanced Life Support Guidelines)

Broselow-Luten tape is commonly used as a guide to weight and medication dosing. Using this system, medication doses and equipment sizing are color-coded based on the child's height.

Weight: (age × 3) + 6 = wt in kg (for school age only)

Systolic hypotension (numbers below are the 5th percentile, mean BP is higher)
- Newborn: <60 mmHg
- Infant: <70 mmHg
- > 1 year: <70 mmHg + (age in years × 2)

Heart rate
- Newborn to 3 months: 80 to 200
- 3 months to 2 years: 75 to 190
- 2 to 10 years: 60 to 140
- >10 years: 50 to 100

Respiratory rate
- Infant: 30 to 60
- Toddler: 24 to 40
- Preschool: 22 to 34
- School age: 18 to 30
- Teen: 12 to 16

Intubation

Endotracheal tube size and cuffs
- (age/4) + 4 OR (age + 16)/4
- About size of nares or pinky finger
- Use a cuffed tube down to 1 year of age
  - Infant size 3.5 to 4.0 at one year
  - Newborn size 3.0 to 3.5 tube
  - Premature neonate size 2.0 to 2.5 tube

Laryngoscope
- Miller blade to lift large floppy noncartilaginous epiglottis
- Miller 0 to 1 at birth, 1 to 2 for infants and toddlers

Fluids

- Fluid bolus: 20 ml/kg for crystalloid (blood often 10 ml/kg)
- Maintenance fluid rate:
  - 4 ml/kg/hr for 1st 10 kg of body weight
  - 2 ml/kg/hr for 2nd 10 kg
  - 1 ml/kg/hour for each kg over 20
    Example: 35 kg child maintenance fluid rate:

$$10\text{kg}(40\text{ml/hr})$$
$$+ 10\text{kg}(20\text{ml/hr})$$
$$\underline{\pm 15\text{kg}(15\text{ml/hr})}$$
$$= 35\text{kg}(75\text{ml/hr})$$

Burns

- Parkland Formula: weight (kg) × percentage body surface area (BSA) burn × 4 ml = fluids for 24 hours (in ml)
- Administer ½ over first 8 hours, ½ over next 16 hours
- Remember infant head is 18% body surface area (rule of 9s exception)
  Example: 40 kg child with 50% BSA burn:
  40 × 50 × 4 = 8000 ml
  4000 ml given over first 8 hours, remaining 4000 ml over the next 16 hours

Toxicology

What a toddler could have eaten is ALWAYS on your differential

Deadly in a dose

Drugs followed by severe symptoms (treatment listed if other than supportive)

- Tricyclic acids (TCAs): arrhythmia, hypotension, seizure
  - Treatment of wide QRS is $NaHCO_3$ bolus 1 to 2 mEq/kg, maintain serum pH 7.45 to 7.55
- Monoamine oxidase inhibitors (MAOIs): hypotension, bradycardia, seizures, severe hyperthermia, respiratory depression
- Chloroquine: seizures, coma, QRS widening, ventricular dysrhythmias, hypotension, shock, cardiac arrest, respiratory arrest
  - Diazepam may exert an antagonist action against chloroquine cardiotoxicity
- Phenothiazines: ventricular dysrhythmias, hypotension, coma
- Clonidine: hypotension, bradycarida, apnea
- Calcium channel blockers: dysrhythmias, acidosis, hypokalemia, hyperglycemia, CNS depression, acute renal failure, rhabdomyolysis

▶ Bradycardia: administer calcium chloride, glucagon, and pacemaker as necessary; atropine is usually not effective in this setting
▪ Sulfonylureas: protracted hypoglycemia
▶ Treat with glucose bolus then infusion, octreotide, bicarbonate for urine alkalinization (enhances elimination)
▪ Theophylline: seizures, hypotension, dysrhythmias, metabolic acidosis, hypokalemia
▶ Treatment: dialysis
▪ Opioids: respiratory depression, apnea
▶ Treatment: naloxone
▪ Iron: shock, acidosis, GI bleed, coagulopathy, hepatotoxicity, coma
▶ Decontamination, deferoxamine
▪ Salicylates (aspirin, oil of wintergreen, bepto-Pismol): respiratory alkalosis, metabolic acidosis, coma, seizures, hypotension, pulmonary edema, coagulopathy, cerebral edema, and dysrhythmias
▶ Treatment: hydrate, bicarbonate (for urine alkalinization), dialysis
▪ Camphor (mothballs): respiratory depression, seizures

Trauma Considerations

▪ Big head, little body compared to adults – C-spine injury more likely than L spine
▪ Large liver and spleen, weak abdominal muscles – tend to get liver or spleen lacerations before other bowel injuries; most can be managed nonoperatively (if patient is stable)
▪ Flexible rib cage – can get cardiac and lung contusions without rib fracture

Abuse (non-accidental trauma)

▪ Mandated reporter (you must report to authorities if there is any suspicion)
▪ Pattern injuries (Not ALWAYS intentional, but suspicious injuries)
▶ Retinal hemorrhage, subdural hematomas: shaken baby syndrome
▶ Spiral femur fracture (not toddler's fracture)
▶ Posterior rib fractures
▶ Sock/glove/diaper area submersion burns
▶ Belt/hand/cord mark patterns
▶ Story inconsistent with injury
▶ Story inconsistent with developmental milestones (ie, 2-month-old "rolled off the bed")
▪ Elbow, knee, and shin bruises are normal
▪ Mongolian spots often confused with back/buttock bruising

Rule out sepsis (fever without clear cause work-up)

▪ Younger than 28 days or toxic: antibiotics, CBC and culture, UA and culture, spinal fluid (cell count and culture), admission
▪ 29 days to 2 months: evaluation as aforementioned, consider discharge with next-day follow-up if well-appearing, labs negative, and reliable follow-up; consider antibiotics

■ 2 to 3 months: CBC and culture, UA and culture, consider discharge with next-day follow-up if well-appearing and reliable follow-up; consider antibiotics.

■ Remember to consider urine in all boys under 6 months, uncircumcised boys up to 1 year of age, and girls up to 2 years with significant fever and no other clear cause

Persistent crying

Consider corneal abrasion, hair tourniquet, urinary tract infection, meningitis, abuse

Limp – common causes

■ Septic joint versus transient synovitis
 ▶ Kocher criteria for hips
  ▷ Nonweight-bearing
  ▷ Erythrocyte sedimentation rate (ESR) >40
  ▷ Fever
  ▷ WBC >12,000
 ▶ 3 of 4 = 93% chance septic arthritis, 2 of 4 = 40%, 1 of 4 = 3%
■ Toddler's fracture: nondisplaced oblique distal tibial fracture from minor twist
■ Osgood–Schlatter: inflammation of the growth plate at the tibial tuberosity, teens,
 ▶ Overuse injury
■ Slipped capital femoral epiphysis: young teens, classically overweight, treat with urgent surgery
■ Avascular necrosis of the femoral head (Legg-Calvé-Perthes): idiopathic avascular osteonecrosis
■ Developmental dysplasia of the hip
 ▶ Congenital hip dislocation (diagnose with ultrasound in newborn)
 ▶ Ortolani and Barlow maneuvers (manipulation of the hip creates a clunk sound)

Newborn resuscitation

■ Warm, dry, stimulate, suction
■ Bag valve mask if HR <100, chest compressions if HR <60
■ Use umbilical line for critical access
■ Drugs which may be administered via endotracheal tube: lidocaine, epinephrine, atropine, narcan (LEAN) Note: ET meds are discouraged in recent guidelines, umbilical or intraosseous lines are preferred

Congenital heart lesions

■ Cyanotic heart disease (the Ts): Right to left shunts
 ▶ Tetrology of Fallot (ventricular septal defect, overriding aorta, pulmonary stenosis, right ventricular hypertrophy)
 ▶ Transposition of the great arteries (complete separation, need a shunt)
 ▶ Tricuspid atresia (no right atrium to right ventricle flow, need a shunt, often atrial septal defect)

▷ Total anomalous pulmonary venous return (pulmonary veins flow into systemic/right heart, need a shunt)

▷ Truncus arteriosus (single outflow artery straddling both ventricles)

▪ Prostaglandin E 1 should be considered for infants less than two weeks old presenting with cyanosis or shock as a shunt-dependent lesion may be the cause

▪ Noncyanotic heart disease (the Ds): left to right shunts

▷ Ventricular septal **D**efect

▷ Atrial septal **D**efect

▷ Patent **D**uctus arteriosis

▷ Atrioventricular **D**efect (also called AV canal or endocardial cushion defect)

▪ Obstructive disease

▷ Perivalvular or valvular stenosis (aortic, pulmonary, mitral)

▷ Coarctation (narrowing) of the aorta (remember increased upper extremity pulses and BP, decreased in the lower extremity)

▷ Hypoplastic left heart syndrome (severe mitral and aortic stenosis or atresia and aortic arch obstruction, inadequate LV)

Twenty common emergency medicine procedures: Indications, contraindications, technique, and complications

Reuben Strayer, MD

DEFIBRILLATION AND CARDIOVERSION

Indications
- Defibrillation
  - ► Ventricular fibrillation or pulseless ventricular tachycardia
- Cardioversion
  - ► Unstable ventricular tachycardia, supraventricular tachycardia, or atrial fibrillation/ flutter requires immediate synchronized cardioversion. Elective cardioversion may be used as an alternative to chemical cardioversion in stable patients with these rhythms. Note that pulseless ventricular tachycardia requires defibrillation, not synchronized cardioversion.

Contraindications
- No absolute contraindications exist for defibrillation or cardioversion except when the procedure poses an undue risk to healthcare providers (e.g., in a wet submersion victim).
- Defibrillation should not be performed on patients who have incompatible advanced directives for end-of-life care.
- Digoxin toxicity is considered a relative contraindication to cardioversion; however, therapeutic use of digoxin confers no additional risk for cardioversion. The treatment of choice in unstable patients with arrhythmia thought to be due to digoxin toxicity is digoxin antibody fragments (Digibind); if this therapy is unavailable or ineffective, the likelihood of benefit of cardioversion exceeds the likelihood of harm in most instances.
- Cardioversion of atrial fibrillation is relatively contraindicated unless the rhythm is known to be less than 48 hours old. In stable, low-risk patients with recent-onset atrial fibrillation, ED-based cardioversion (and discharge) has recently become a popular alternative to usual rate control and admission.
- Pregnancy at any stage is **not** a contraindication to defibrillation or cardioversion.

Equipment
- Monophasic or biphasic defibrillator with appropriately sized pads – infant paddles for patients less than 10 kg/1 year of age, adult paddles for all others
- Conductive gel, saline-soaked pads, or self-adhesive electrode pads

▨ Procedural sedation agents, if applicable

▨ Advanced airway equipment and ACLS medications in the event of complications

Technique

▨ Defibrillation

▷ Verify that the defibrillator is not in synchronous/cardioversion mode.

▨ Set the dose

▷ Adults: dose for monophasic defibrillators is 360 J. Dose for biphasic is unit-specific and should be indicated on face of unit; if unclear, use 200 J.

▷ Pediatrics: dose is 2 J/kg for the first shock, 4 J/kg for subsequent shocks in monophasic and biphasic machines.

▨ Apply conductive gel or alternative.

▨ Wipe away nitropaste or excessive secretions from patient's chest.

▨ Position paddles on chest. The "sternum" paddle is placed to the right of the sternum, below the clavicle; the "apex" paddle is placed left of the nipple in the midaxillary line, centered on the fifth intercostal space. Alternatively, anterior–posterior positioning is acceptable – the sternum paddle is placed over the precordium, and the apex paddle to the left of the spine, directly posterior to the heart. Twenty-five pounds of force are recommended to ensure appropriate contact between the paddle and the chest wall.

▨ Charge paddles.

▨ Verify that no personnel are in contact with the patient or stretcher "I'm clear, you're clear, we're all clear."

▨ Discharge defibrillatory shock. Immediately resume chest compressions after defibrillation; do not delay to check pulse or rhythm.

▨ Cardioversion – preferred when possible because shock is administered away from the vulnerable repolarization period in the cardiac cycle.

▷ Verify that the defibrillator is in synchronous/cardioversion mode.

▷ In stable patients, use analgesia/sedation. 10 mg etomidate in a normal size adult is a reasonable choice in most situations. Do not give propofol or midazolam to a hypotensive patient.

▷ Set the dose. Atrial fibrillation often requires a higher dose than ventricular and other supraventricular tachycardias, but the general recommendation is to start with 50 J, then 100 J, followed by 200 J for all rhythms, for both monophasic and biphasic machines. Pediatric dosing is 0.5 J/kg, followed by 1 J/kg, 2 J/kg, and 4 J/kg. Remember to verify that the machine is in synchronized mode before each shock – many units will revert to unsynchronized defibrillation after any discharge.

▷ Apply conductive gel or alternative, and position the paddles as described earlier.

▷ Charge the paddles and verify that personnel are clear, as described earlier.

▷ Discharge the synchronized shock. Note that a delay often occurs while the defibrillator evaluates the rhythm for synchronization.

▷ If no shock occurs, the R or S wave may be too small to sense. In that case, change the lead that the monitor is sensing or move the arm leads closer to the chest.

Complications

▨ Injury to skin and soft tissue – minimized by using conductive gel and wiping away excessive secretions (blood, perspiration, vomitus)

▦ Myocardial injury – minimized by using lowest effective energy dose and fewest number of shocks

▦ Cardiac dysrhythmias – any rhythm, including asystole, may follow defibrillation or cardioversion

▦ Injury to health-care providers – remember to verify that all providers are clear at time of shock

Notes

▦ If unwitnessed arrest, or if delay to defibrillation exceeds 5 minutes, some recommendations suggest five cycles of CPR (30 compressions and 2 breaths, five cycles = 2 minutes) before defibrillation. Best approach for the boards is to initiate chest compressions as soon as possible, while the defibrillator is being readied, then shock appropriate rhythms when possible.

▦ Before determining a rhythm to be asystole, increase the gain on the monitor and rotate the paddles 90 degrees or check another lead to rule out fine ventricular fibrillation masquerading as asystole.

▦ If patient has a pacemaker in situ, position paddle at least 1 inch away from pulse generator

CRICOTHYROTOMY

Indications

▦ Endotracheal intubation contraindicated

▦ Unable to intubate and unable to ventilate patient

▦ Anticipated inability to perform endotracheal intubation and ventilation of the patient

Contraindications

▦ Absolute

  ▶ Tracheal transection with retraction into the mediastinum

  ▶ Significant damage to larynx or cricoid cartilage

▦ Relative – may be overlooked when patient's oxygenation status is jeopardized

  ▶ Age <12 (transtracheal jet ventilation preferred)

  ▶ Bleeding diathesis

  ▶ Acute laryngeal disease

  ▶ Distortion of neck anatomy

Equipment

▦ Minimum: scalpel and an appropriately sized tracheostomy tube or an endotracheal tube

▦ Tracheal hook

▦ Tracheal (Trousseau) dilator

▦ Scissors

▦ Hemostats

▦ Tracheostomy tube (Shiley #5 in adults) or cuffed ETT (6–7 mm in adults)

▦ Needle and syringe with lidocaine for local anesthesia

▦ Suture or circumferential tie to secure tracheostomy tube in place

▨ Several prepacked percutaneous cricothyrotomy sets are available – these contain scalpel, needle, syringe, and guidewire and a specially designed tracheostomy tube fitted over a dilator to use with Seldinger technique.

Technique
▨ Hyperextend the neck if there are no contraindications.
▨ Identify the cricothyroid membrane below the thyroid cartilage and above the cricoid cartilage – one finger-breadth below the laryngeal prominence.
▨ Infiltrate the skin and subcutaneous tissue with local anesthetic if time permits.
▨ Sedate the patient if required (ketamine is a good choice if no contraindications).
▨ There are several accepted methods for performing cricothyrotomy, including the recently popular bougie-assisted procedure. The "Rapid four-step technique," is described here:
  ▷ Position yourself at the head of the bed, as if for endotracheal intubation.
  ▷ Reidentify the landmarks.
  ▷ Incise the skin and cricothyroid membrane with a single horizontal stab-like incision with a large (#20) scalpel. If the anatomy is ambiguous, make a vertical incision through the skin to identify the cricothyroid membrane and then a horizontal incision through the membrane.
  ▷ With the scalpel still in the trachea, insert the tracheal hook inferiorly to the scalpel blade and pull the cricoid ring anteriorly and inferiorly, as if performing laryngoscopy.
  ▷ Remove the scalpel, insert the tracheostomy tube or endotracheal tube, secure the device, ventilate, and confirm placement.

Complications
▨ Failure to successfully intubate the trachea
▨ Subcutaneous emphysema
▨ Bleeding
▨ Tube blockage/airway obstruction
▨ Infection (late complication)
▨ Subglottic stenosis (late complication)

Notes
▨ Mobilize airway consultants (anesthesia, ENT, general surgery) as early as possible in difficult airway situations.
▨ Difficult cricothyrotomy can be predicted using the mnemonic **SHORT** – neck **s**urgery, **h**ematoma, **o**besity, **r**adiation, and **t**umor.
▨ Failure to perform cricothyrotomy when indicated is an important airway pitfall. Do not hesitate to initiate this procedure in a can't intubate, can't ventilate/oxygenate situation.

TRANSCUTANEOUS PACING

Indications
▨ Hemodynamically significant bradycardia
▨ Bradyasystolic arrest (minimal benefit)

- Predicted or high risk for hemodynamically significant bradycardia, including second- and third-degree heart block, ingestion of negatively chronotropic drugs or toxins, and pacemaker malfunction
- Overdrive pacing of certain tachydysrhythmias, most commonly, torsades de pointes

Contraindications
- No absolute contraindications
- Warming the bradycardic and hypothermic patient is advised before pacing, as the cold heart is more susceptible to ventricular fibrillation.

Equipment
- Most EDs have combined defibrillator-transcutaneous pacemakers.
- The only other necessary equipment is a set of pacemaker pads to affix to the patient.

Technique
- Place the pads on the patient. The pads will be labeled front/back or anterior/posterior. The anterior pad is placed over the cardiac apex and the posterior pad is placed just medial to the left scapula.
- Verify that the defibrillator is in Pace Mode.
- For pacing bradycardic rhythms, set the rate to 70.
- For pacing bradyasystolic arrest, set the stimulating current to its maximum output and slowly decrease the output until loss of capture, then increase the output to above the needed current.
- For pacing hemodynamically significant but nonarrest bradycardias, start at the minimum current and slowly increase the current until capture is noted.
- For overdrive pacing of certain ventricular and supraventricular tachycardias, set rate at 40 bpm faster than the patient's heart rate and slowly increase the current until capture. Once capture is achieved, brief trains of 10 overdrive beats of asynchronous pacing are applied.
- If patient experiences significant discomfort from muscle contractions, provide analgesia/sedation.
- Prepare to initiate transvenous pacing.

Complications
- Failure to recognize an underlying dangerous rhythm (e.g., ventricular fibrillation) that is buried beneath pacer spikes is the most important potential complication. When in doubt, pause the pacemaker to assess the underlying rhythm.
- Induction of dysrhythmias is rare but possible. A defibrillator should always be available when pacing.
- Patient discomfort is common; skin burns are extremely rare but have been reported.

Notes
- Chest compressions can be administered directly over the pads while pacing. The power delivered during a typical pacing impulse is 1/1000th of defibrillation.

PERICARDIOCENTESIS

Indications
- The indication for emergency physician-performed pericardiocentesis is to relieve diagnosed pericardial tamponade in an unstable patient.
- In certain arrest or near-arrest situations, especially in the case of a pulseless electrical activity rhythm with jugular venous distension, pericardiocentesis is indicated as empiric treatment, before the diagnosis is made.

Contraindications
- There are no absolute contraindications to pericardiocentesis.
- Uremic patients with a pericardial effusion should be managed with dialysis, if circumstances permit, before pericardiocentesis, but only if hemodynamically stable.
- Hemorrhagic tamponade cannot be definitively managed by pericardiocentesis. In the case of traumatic pericardial effusion, pericardiocentesis may be performed on the arrested or near-arrested patient as preparations are made for thoracotomy, but should not delay thoracotomy.

Equipment
- The minimum equipment necessary is a syringe and a spinal needle (7.5–12.5 cm 18 gauge).
- Alternatives include larger-bore catheters and pigtail catheters, that may be left in the pericardial space for continuous drainage.
- ED pericardiocentesis is preferably performed under ultrasound guidance.
- In the absence of an ultrasound machine, electrocardiographic guidance may be achieved by attaching the clamp of one of the precordial leads on an ECG machine to the needle.

Technique
- Head of bed is elevated to 45 degrees, if possible, to bring the heart closer to the anterior chest wall.
- An NG or OG tube is placed if abdomen is distended.
- Lower xiphoid and epigastric area are prepped with sterile solution.
- Skin, route, and pericardium are infiltrated with local anesthetic in the awake patient.
- The classic technique is the subxiphoid approach. Needle is inserted between the xiphoid process and the left costal margin at a 30-degree angle to the skin and directed toward the left shoulder.
- The obturator/stylet is removed after the needle is through the skin.
- Ideally the needle is advanced toward the effusion under ultrasound guidance.
- Otherwise, the needle is advanced while aspirating until pericardial fluid enters the syringe. If using electrocardiographic guidance, the "current of injury" is seen on the ECG tracing – usually a wide-complex PVC with an elevated ST segment – when the needle is against the epicardium. If encountered, the needle should be withdrawn slightly.
- As much fluid as possible is aspirated from the pericardium.
- The needle is removed and a postprocedure x-ray is ordered to rule out pneumothorax.

Complications
- Dry tap
- Pneumothorax
- Dysrhythmia
- Myocardial or coronary vessel laceration
- Hemopericardium
- Air embolism

NEEDLE THORACOSTOMY

Indications
- Suspected or confirmed tension pneumothorax

Contraindications
- None

Equipment
- 10- to 14-gauge angiocatheter
- Syringe

Technique
- Locate the 2nd intercostal space (between the 2nd and 3rd rib) midclavicular line.
- The 2nd rib is the first rib palpable below the clavicle.
- Prepare the site with antiseptic solution, if time permits.
- Insert the needle just superior to the 3rd rib, perpendicular to the chest wall. A rush of air should be appreciated as the tension is relieved.
- Remove the needle, leaving the catheter in place.
- Immediately prepare to insert a chest tube.

Complications
- Cardiac injury/tamponade
- Chest vessel injury/hemorrhage
- Pneumonia
- Arterial air embolism

Notes
- The immediate placement of a chest tube is preferred to needle thoracostomy if possible – advancing a Kelly clamp through the pleura treats the tension pneumothorax.
- In obese patients, the usual chest tube insertion site (see below) may be preferred over the midclavicular line.

TUBE THORACOSTOMY

Indications
- Drainage of pneumothorax
- Drainage of hemothorax
- Drainage of empyema

Contraindications
- No absolute contraindications, especially in unstable patients
- Relative contraindications include coagulopathy and anatomic abnormalities (e.g., emphysematous blebs or pleural adhesions)

Equipment
- Sterile towels, antiseptic, local anesthetic, syringes, needles
- #10 scalpel
- Kelly clamp
- Thoracostomy tube
  - ▶ For pneumothorax, 22 to 24 Fr
  - ▶ For empyema or hemothorax, 36 to 40 Fr
- Scissors
- Petroleum and plain gauze
- Tape
- Suture
- Needle driver
- Chest drainage apparatus
- Clear, sterile plastic tubing
- Plastic serrated connectors

Technique
- A chest tube is placed fully sterile – gown, mask, and glove.
- Give patient supplemental oxygen and place the patient on a monitor.
- Elevate head of bed to 45 degrees, if possible.
- Restrain ipsilateral arm over patient's head.
- Sterilize the site. The conventional site is the 4th or 5th intercostal space, mid to anterior axillary line. This is roughly at the level of the nipple.
- Generously infiltrate local anesthetic into the skin, muscle, periosteum, and parietal pleura. Consider procedural sedation/analgesia if appropriate.
- Make at least a 3 to 4 cm transverse incision directly over the rib one intercostal space below the level to be entered.
- Using the Kelly clamp, tunnel and dissect a pathway immediately superior to the rib above the incision.
- Advancing through the dissected pathway, puncture the pleura with closed Kelly clamp. A rush of air or fluid is expected.
- Spread and withdraw the Kelly clamp to enlarge the rent in the pleura.
- Insert a gloved finger into the pleural rent to verify the track of entry and the absence of solid organs adjacent to the pleural rent.
- Leaving the finger inside the pleural space, guide the chest tube beside the finger into the pleural cavity.
- Advance the tube posteriorly and far enough that the last drainage hole is within the pleura.
- Attach tube to water seal device using plastic tubing and connector.
- Confirm placement with radiograph.
- Secure the tube by closing the skin and securing the chest tube to the skin with a stay suture.

▓ Apply petrolatum-impregnated gauze underneath plain gauze to the site where the chest tube enters the skin.

Complications
▓ Infection (pneumonia, empyema, local incision)
▓ Bleeding (skin, chest vessel laceration, solid organ injury)
▓ Malposition (subcutaneous, intraabdominal, inadequately advanced)
▓ Blocked drainage (tube kinking, clots within tube)
▓ Air leaks
▓ Reexpansion pulmonary edema

Notes
▓ Many patients with simple pneumothorax can be managed with observation or catheter-based drainage rather than a chest tube. The decision is based on the cause, size, and degree of symptomatology associated with the pneumothorax.

ED THORACOTOMY

Indications
Accepted indications
Penetrating thoracic injury

▓ Traumatic arrest with previously witnessed cardiac activity (pre-hospital or in-hospital)
▓ Unresponsive hypotension (BP < 70mmHg)

Blunt thoracic injury

▓ Unresponsive hypotension (BP < 70mmHg)
▓ Rapid exsanguination from chest tube (>1500 ml)

Relative indications
Penetrating thoracic injury

▓ Traumatic arrest without previously witnessed cardiac activity

Penetrating non-thoracic injury

▓ Traumatic arrest with previously witnessed cardiac activity (pre-hospital or in-hospital)

Blunt thoracic injuries

▓ Traumatic arrest with previously witnessed cardiac activity (pre-hospital or in-hospital)

Contraindications
▓ Blunt injuries
   ▶ Blunt thoracic injuries with no witnessed cardiac activity

▷ Multiple blunt trauma
▷ Severe head injury
▨ Lack of timely availability of surgical expertise to provide definitive repair after ED thoracotomy.

Equipment
▨ Antiseptic solution
▨ Scalpel with #20 blade
▨ Mayo scissors, curved
▨ Rib spreaders
▨ Vascular clamps
▨ Needle holder
▨ 10-inch tissue forceps
▨ Suture scissors
▨ Silk suture
▨ Foley catheter

Technique
▨ Patient should be intubated/ventilated.
▨ Prepare skin with antiseptic.
▨ Incise skin and subcutaneous tissue along 5th intercostal space from sternum to posterior axillary line – just below the nipple in males or the inframammary crease (with breast elevated) in females.
▨ Momentarily halt respirations and puncture the intercostal muscles at the anterior axillary line with Mayo scissors, then cut the intercostal muscles along the skin incision while separating the muscles from the pleura by following the path of the scissors with your second and third fingers of the nondominant hand.
▨ Insert rib spreader with ratchet pointed down and open the chest.
▨ Lift the lung to identify the pericardium; perform a pericardiotomy by incising and cutting the pericardial sac anterior to the phrenic nerve (pericardial incision is perpendicular to skin incision).
▨ Evacuate pericardial blood, tamponade any rents in the myocardium by inserting a Foley catheter, inflating the balloon, and performing a purse-string suture around the wound.
▨ Perform open-heart massage by compressing the ventricles in between two hands.
▨ Find the aorta by sweeping the hand along the posterior thoracic wall just superior to the diaphragm, separate from the esophagus, and cross-clamp using vascular clamp.
▨ If significant pulmonary hemorrhage, cross-clamp the affected pulmonary hilum.

Complications
▨ Trauma to phrenic nerve, coronary arteries, and solid organs
▨ Wound infection
▨ Provider blood exposure/needlestick

CENTRAL VENOUS ACCESS USING SELDINGER TECHNIQUE

Indications
▨ Inability to achieve adequate peripheral venous access
▨ Central venous pressure monitoring

▓ Volume loading, when large-bore peripheral access not available

▓ Central venous oxygenation saturation monitoring

▓ Frequent blood sampling requirement

▓ Infusion of agents that present an extravasation risk (dopamine, norepinephrine, calcium chloride), hyperosmolar solutions, and total parenteral nutrition

▓ Placement of transvenous pacemaker or pulmonary artery catheter

▓ Hemodialysis

Contraindications (all relative)

▓ Distorted local anatomy (including prior radiation therapy to the site, long-term venous cannula at that site)

▓ Coagulopathy, anticoagulation, or thrombolytic therapy (especially for noncompressible subclavian site)

▓ Suspected proximal vascular injury or vasculitis

▓ When pneumothorax presents a particular danger, subclavian site should be avoided

Equipment

▓ Sterile gown, gloves, mask, drapes/towels

▓ Lidocaine and antiseptic solution with corresponding needles and syringes

▓ Introducing needle

▓ Guidewire

▓ Dilator

▓ Catheter

▓ #11 Scalpel

▓ Suture

▓ Scissors

Technique (Seldinger/guidewire technique)

▓ Utilizing fully sterile technique, sterilize the area with antiseptic solution and infiltrate the skin overlying the access site with local anesthetic.

▓ Cannulate the vein with the introducing needle under ultrasound guidance if available. If unavailable, use anatomic landmarks as follows:

  ▶ The subclavian vein is most often cannulated by the infraclavicular approach, where the needle enters the skin at the costochondral junction (where the clavicle dives posteriorly) and is directed toward the suprasternal notch.

  ▶ The internal jugular vein is most often cannulated by the central approach, where the needle enters the skin at the apex of the triangle formed by the two heads of the sternocleidomastoid muscle and the clavicle and is directed toward the ipsilateral nipple at a 30-degree angle to the skin. The carotid artery is palpated with three fingers on the other hand; the needle is directed lateral to the lateral border of the carotid artery at all times.

  ▶ The femoral vein is cannulated by palpating the femoral artery at the inguinal crease and directing the needle cephalad at a 45-degree angle to the skin, 1 to 2 cm inferior and 0.5 to 1 cm medial to the femoral artery.

▓ Stabilize the needle in the vein and remove the syringe; flow of dark nonpulsatile blood should be appreciated.

▓ Introduce the flexible (usually J-shaped) end of the guidewire into the needle and advance the guidewire one quarter to one half its length. If increased ectopy noted on ECG monitor, withdraw wire.

▨ Remove the needle and stab the skin next to the wire with the scalpel.

▨ Place the dilator (or the dilator-in-catheter if using an 8.5 French introducer) over the wire and advance the dilator into the vessel using a twisting motion. The tip of the wire must protrude from the dilator before the dilator is advanced into the skin to prevent loss of the wire into the circulation.

▨ Remove the dilator and place the catheter over the wire into the vein.

▨ Remove guidewire.

▨ Confirm placement by aspirating blood from all catheter lumens.

▨ Sew the vein in place and confirm placement/rule out pneumothorax with a CXR if IJ or SC location.

Complications

▨ Vessel or thoracic duct injury

▨ Pneumothorax, hemothorax, hydrothorax (IJ and SC lines)

▨ Line infection

▨ Line thrombosis

▨ Catheter or wire embolism

▨ Air embolism

▨ Arrhythmia

▨ Myocardial perforation

Notes

▨ Rapid intravascular volume loading is ineffective in standard triple-lumen central lines. An 8.5 French introducer sheath should be placed in situations where aggressive volume expansion is necessary.

▨ In the event of difficulty threading the guidewire, the guidewire must never be retracted with force back through the needle – in this case, the needle and wire must be removed as a unit to prevent shearing of the wire with subsequent wire embolism.

INTRAOSSEOUS INFUSION

Indications

▨ Immediate vascular access is required and IV access is not available

Contraindications

▨ Fractured bone

▨ Recent IO cannula or multiple IO attempts on the same bone

▨ Overlying infection or burn

Equipment

▨ Any needle that has a stylet and is sturdy enough to penetrate bone may be used; a product designed specifically for IO access is preferable.

Technique

▨ The most commonly used site is the proximal tibia, on the antero-medial flat surface, two finger-breadths below the tibial tuberosity. The distal tibia (medial surface), distal femur (midline), proximal humerus, and sternum are alternative sites.

▓ The skin is scrubbed with antiseptic and, if the patient is awake, the site is infiltrated with local anesthetic.
▓ The needle is directed away from the nearest joint, at a 60- to 90-degree angle to the bone.
▓ Stabilize the bone with the nondominant hand while using the dominant hand to advance the needle through the cortex using a twisting motion (or drill, if this specialized equipment is available).
▓ Remove the stylet and aspirate marrow content using a syringe.
▓ If properly positioned, the needle should stand upright without support and fluids should infuse without extravasation.
▓ Secure and protect the infusion site.
▓ Remove when reliable IV access is achieved.

Complications
▓ Advancing the needle through the entire bone
▓ Lumen blockage
▓ Cellulitis or osteomyelitis at the insertion site (rare)
▓ Fat embolism (rare)

PARACENTESIS

Indications
▓ Therapeutic: to relieve symptoms from tense ascites, usually dyspnea
▓ Diagnostic: to characterize new ascites or rule out spontaneous bacterial peritonitis in patients with known ascites

Contraindications
▓ Overlying skin infection
▓ Underlying abdominal hematoma or engorged veins
▓ If gravid uterus or suspected distension of bowel or bladder, ultrasound-guided paracentesis is recommended

Equipment
▓ Sterile gown, gloves, mask, drapes/towels
▓ Lidocaine and antiseptic solution with corresponding needles and syringes
▓ 18- to 22-gauge needle; either standard 1.5 inch length or 3.5 inch for obese patients 20 to 60 cc syringe
▓ If performing therapeutic tap, tubing and vacuum bottles for collecting fluid

Technique
▓ The preferred site is the left lower quadrant of the abdomen, lateral to the rectus abdominis muscle, in the midclavicular line, inferior to the umbilicus.
▓ Utilizing fully sterile technique, sterilize the area with antiseptic solution and infiltrate the skin overlying the access site with local anesthetic.
▓ Insert the needle perpendicular to the skin and advance in 5 mm increments, aspirating at the end of each movement, until ascitic fluid is reached.
▓ For therapeutic taps, the needle may be left in the abdomen in cooperative patients.

Complications

▓ Perforation of vessels or abdominal solid/hollow organs

▓ Fluid and electrolyte shifts in large volume paracentesis – some advocate the administration of colloid such as albumin if >5 L of fluid is removed

▓ Local infection

▓ Abdominal wall hematoma

▓ Ascitic fluid leak – can be minimized by retracting the skin caudally before inserting the needle, using the "Z-tract" method

Notes

▓ Paracentesis may be performed without replacing either factors or platelets in the coagulopathic patient.

▓ The criteria for diagnosis of spontaneous bacterial peritonitis is 250 WBCs/μL with >50% PMNs.

▓ A serum-albumin gradient >1.1 g/dL rules in portal hypertension as the cause of ascites.

DIAGNOSTIC PERITONEAL LAVAGE

Indications

▓ Rapid diagnosis of intraperitoneal hemorrhage in the hemodynamically unstable trauma patient (ultrasound more commonly used for this purpose)

▓ Diagnosis of abdominal organ injury in the trauma patient, especially with the accuracy of abdominal examination compromised due to alteration of mental status or spinal cord injury (CT more commonly used for this purpose)

▓ Diagnosis of diaphragmatic injury

Contraindications

▓ Only absolute contraindication is when an urgent laparotomy is mandated

▓ Prior abdominal surgery/infections

▓ Obesity

▓ Coagulopathy

▓ Second- or third-trimester pregnancy (may still be performed – see later text)

Equipment

▓ Gown, gloves, mask, drapes, antiseptic, local anesthetic with appropriate syringes, and needles

▓ Seldinger introducer needle

▓ #11 scalpel

▓ Seldinger-type guidewire

▓ DPL catheter

▓ 1 L of warm standard normal saline or lactated Ringer's solution

▓ IV tubing

Technique

▓ More commonly used closed technique is described.

▓ Insert introducer needle attached to 10 ml syringe 1 cm inferior to umbilicus, at a 60-degree angle to the skin directed inferiorly.

▨ Advance the needle into the peritoneum past the linea alba and peritoneum (two pops should be felt).

▨ Advance 0.5 cm into the peritoneal cavity and aspirate for frank blood.

▨ If negative, place guidewire into the peritoneal cavity, directed toward the left or right pelvic gutter.

▨ Make a stab wound with the scalpel and advance the catheter over the guidewire, using a twisting motion. Aspirate for frank blood.

▨ If negative, infuse 1 L of warm, isotonic sterile saline solution into peritoneum.

▨ Agitate the abdomen to mix the fluid and any blood present.

▨ When 50 cc of fluid remains in bag, place bag on floor to siphon fluid out of the abdomen.

▨ Remove catheter and send fluid for analysis.

Complications

▨ Hollow viscous or solid organ injury

▨ Intraperitoneal vessel laceration

▨ Local skin infection at access site

▨ Lack of fluid return

Notes

▨ In penetrating trauma, DPL should not be conducted through the stab or missile entry site.

▨ An RBC count of >100,000/cc is considered positive with a blunt mechanism or a stab mechanism to the anterior abdomen, flank, or back.

▨ An RBC count of >5000/cc is considered positive with a gunshot mechanism or with a stab mechanism to the low chest when the indication is to exclude diaphragmatic injury.

▨ Elevated amylase and alkaline phosphatase levels in the lavage fluid suggest bowel injury.

▨ A supraumbilical, fully open technique is preferred in the context of pelvic fracture.

▨ A suprauterine, fully open technique is preferred in second- or third-trimester pregnancy.

LUMBAR PUNCTURE

Indications

▨ Suspicion of CNS infection, for example, meningitis/encephalitis

▨ Suspicion of subarachnoid hemorrhage

▨ Suspicion of certain CNS inflammatory conditions such as Guillain–Barré syndrome

▨ Therapy of idiopathic intracranial hypertension (aka pseudotumor cerebri)

Contraindications

▨ Infection of overlying skin or soft tissue (absolute)

▨ Unequal pressures between the supratentorial and infratentorial compartments, as evidenced by characteristic findings on CT scan (absolute)

▨ Indications for CT scan before performing lumbar puncture are as follows:

  ▷ Age >60

  ▷ Immunocompromise

▷ Seizure within 1 week
▷ Known CNS lesions
▷ Decreased level of consciousness
▷ Focal neurologic deficits
▷ Papilledema or suspected increased ICP
▨ Coagulopathy (relative)
▨ Brain abscess (relative)

Equipment
▨ Gown, gloves, mask, drapes, local anesthetic, and corresponding needles and syringes
▨ Spinal needle
▨ 4 specimen tubes
▨ 3-way stopcock and manometer

Technique
▨ Position the patient in either the lateral decubitus position with the knees drawn up to the chest (preferred) or the seated position with the back arched by the patient leaning forward onto a table.
▨ Identify the L3 to L4 interspace by using the imaginary line connecting the iliac crests.
▨ Scrub the area with antiseptic, infiltrate the skin overlying the site with local anesthetic, and drape the area.
▨ Infiltrate the deep tissues along the route the spinal needle will take with local anesthetic.
▨ Insert the spinal needle into the interspace and advance until in the subarachnoid space, usually 1/2 to 3/4 the length of the needle. Withdraw the stylet frequently as the needle is advanced to check for CSF return. A pop may be appreciated as the needle dissects the ligamentum flavum, immediately posterior to the subarachnoid space.
▨ If bone is encountered, adjust the angle of the needle. The adjacent interspaces may also be used.
▨ When CSF is expressed from the needle, attach the 3-way stopcock and manometer to measure the opening pressure. Normal pressure is 10 to 20 cm H_2O.
▨ Collect CSF for analysis.
▨ Replace the stylet and withdraw the needle, then cover the site with a bandage.

Complications
▨ Postlumbar puncture headache
▨ Backache and radicular symptoms
▨ Infection – skin and soft tissue infections as well as iatrogenic meningitis
▨ Herniation syndromes (see contraindications in the earlier text)

Notes
▨ Antibiotics must never be delayed for lumbar puncture or prelumbar puncture CT when meningitis is strongly suspected.
▨ Opening pressure cannot be measured when the patient is in the seated position.
▨ Prophylactic bed rest following lumbar puncture does not reduce the incidence of post-LP headache and is not recommended.

DORSAL SLIT OF PHIMOSIS

Indications
- Inability to urinate or pass a needed urinary catheter secondary to tight phimosis

Contraindications
- Dorsal slit should not be undertaken if the condition can wait for a formal circumcision, which is the definitive repair.

Equipment
- Antiseptic solution and gauze
- Lidocaine without epinephrine
- Syringe and small-bore needle (27 gauge preferred)
- Straight hemostat
- Straight scissors
- Needle holder
- 4–0 absorbable suture

Technique
- The incision runs along the dorsal midline aspect of the penis, from the coronal sulcus to the tip of the foreskin.
- Scrub the site with antiseptic and drape the area.
- Infiltrate the region, including the path of the incision, with local anesthesia.
- Advance closed straight hemostat between the glans and the foreskin, carefully avoiding the meatus and urethra. Gently open the hemostat to break up any adhesions.
- Remove the hemostat and reinsert a single jaw of the hemostat between the glans and the foreskin along the path of the foreskin, then close the hemostat, crushing the foreskin for 5 minutes.
- Remove the hemostat and cut the foreskin with scissors along the length of the crushed tissue.
- If the resulting flaps separate and bleed, they may be reapproximated with running absorbable suture.
- Refer the patient for formal circumcision.

Complications
- Bleeding
- Injury to urethra or glans penis

PARAPHIMOSIS REDUCTION

Indications
- All paraphimoses must be reduced to prevent tissue ischemia.

Contraindications
- None

Equipment
- 1% lidocaine jelly
- Crushed ice and water
- Size 8 latex glove

Technique
- Apply topical anesthetic to the paraphimotic foreskin and glans.
- A penile block and/or light sedation may be helpful.
- Compress the foreskin by encircling it with the hand and squeezing for 5 minutes.
- Applying slow, steady pressure, use both thumbs to push glans proximally while using both index and long fingers to pull foreskin distally over glans. Bring foreskin completely out over glans.
- If unsuccessful, fill glove with ice water and invert the thumb. Place penis into ice-water glove at the thumb slot and hold glove around penis for 10 minutes, then reattempt to pull foreskin over glans as described earlier.
- If still unsuccessful, a phimotic ring incision is generally performed by a urologist in the operating room.

Complications
- Injury to the underlying tissue is rare.

TESTICULAR DETORSION

Indications and contraindications
- Manual detorsion should be attempted on all cases of suspected testicular torsion; however, manual detorsion attempts should never delay operative intervention. All attempts at manual detorsion should occur simultaneously with preparations for immediate operative repair.

Technique
- Light sedation may facilitate the procedure. Some authors caution against the use of procedural sedation or spermatic cord anesthesia, as they obscure the endpoint of the procedure, namely, relief of pain.
- The procedure is more likely to be successful early in the course of the disease, before the onset of significant scrotal swelling.
- Position the patient in a reclining, supine, or, preferably, lithotomy position.
- The testicle usually torses from lateral to medial, and therefore is rotated from medial to lateral, as if opening a book.
- If difficult to perform or increased pain, attempt to rotate the testicle in the opposite direction.
- Simultaneous caudal-to-cranial rotation may be helpful in releasing the cremasteric muscle.
- If a single rotation improves pain or increases Doppler flow but significant pain remains, a further rotation may be attempted.
- In a successful detorsion, pain should subside and the position of the testicle should return to normal. Swelling and induration may take hours to resolve.
- Clinically successful detorsion does not interrupt the requirement for definitive operative scrotal exploration.

LATERAL CANTHOTOMY

Indications
- Retrobulbar hemorrhage (usually from trauma or recent ophthalmic procedure) resulting in decreased visual acuity, increased intraocular pressure, and proptosis

▓ In an unconscious patient with consistent findings, an IOP >40 also indicates lateral canthotomy.

Contraindications
▓ Suspected globe rupture

Equipment
▓ Sterile gloves, gown, mask, and drapes
▓ Local anesthetic with epinephrine, syringe, and needles
▓ Normal saline
▓ Straight hemostat
▓ Straight scissors
▓ Forceps

Technique
▓ Patient should be in a supine position.
▓ Infiltrate the lateral canthus with local anesthetic.
▓ Irrigate eye with saline to clear away debris.
▓ Crimp the lateral canthus with a straight hemostat for 2 minutes to exsanguinate the area and mark the incision line.
▓ Using scissors, cut the canthus along the crushed area to the orbital rim, taking care to avoid the globe.
▓ Expose the inferior crus of the lateral canthal tendon by grasping the lower lid with a hemostat and pulling it inferiorly and laterally.
▓ Cut the inferior crus and evaluate for relief of pressure and symptoms.
▓ If no improvement, lyse the superior crus.
▓ Arrange for immediate ophthalmologic evaluation.

Complications
▓ Mechanical injury to the globe and surrounding structures
▓ Bleeding
▓ Infection

PERIMORTEM C-SECTION

Indications
▓ Fetus is beyond the point of viability, usually considered 23 to 24 weeks' gestation. This corresponds to a uterine fundus 3 to 4 cm above the umbilicus.
▓ The decision to commence the procedure should occur after 3 to 4 minutes of aggressive resuscitation following a witnessed arrest, but may be considered up to 25 to 30 minutes postarrest.

Contraindications
▓ Previable fetus – all efforts should be directed at maternal resuscitation.
▓ A mother with anoxic injury but hemodynamically stable should not receive an emergency C-section.

Equipment
- Gown, glove, mask with face shield
- #10 scalpel
- Scissors
- Hemostats
- If available: bladder retractor, general retractors, forceps, gauze sponges, suction
- Standard obstetric pack: bulb syringe, 2 Kelly clamps, cord clamp, basin for placenta, towels, and blanket
- Neonatal resuscitation equipment: warmer, meconium aspirator, IO infusion needles, neonatal airway adjuncts

Technique
- CPR continues until the infant is delivered.
- If not already done, place a wedge underneath the right pelvis or manually displace the gravid uterus to the left.
- Incise the abdomen in the midline vertically from the symphysis pubis to the umbilicus.
- Cut through all layers of the abdominal wall to expose the uterus.
- If the bladder obstructs access to the uterus, it may be aspirated and reflected inferiorly.
- Make a 5 cm vertical incision to the lower uterine segment, taking care to avoid fetal injury.
- Insert the index and long fingers into the incision and lift the uterine wall away from the fetus.
- Use scissors to extend the incision to the fundus.
- Deliver the infant, suction the mouth and nose, cut and clamp the umbilical cord.
- Continue CPR for at least a brief period, as delivery sometimes facilitates successful maternal resuscitation.

Complications
- Fetal injury, especially by the scalpel

OROTRACHEAL INTUBATION

Indications
- Airway protection (intracranial catastrophe/trauma, compression of the airway by focal mass or angioedema, obstructing foreign body)
- Failure of oxygenation (pneumonia, COPD, asthma, CHF, ARDS)
- Failure of ventilation (sedative overdose, high spinal cord injury, ascending neuropathy, paralytic toxin)
- Reduce myocardial oxygen demand (sepsis)
- Patient must leave department and clinical course uncertain (e.g., for transfer to another hospital or the radiology department)
- Inability to control patient without profound sedation
- Need to perform procedures that involve the posterior oropharynx (charcoal, gastric lavage)
- Route to administer medications when IV access not available (intraosseous access preferred)

Contraindications
- Inability to open mouth
- Severe soft tissue swelling or distortion of airway anatomy
- Expected to be unable to visualize vocal cords with laryngoscopy, especially if expected difficult bag-valve-mask ventilation and/or difficult cricothyrotomy

Equipment
- Ambu bag connected to oxygen
- Laryngoscopy handles
- Laryngoscopy blades
- Suction
- Oral airways
- Nasal airways
- Colorimetric capnometer (if continuous capnography not available)
- Endotracheal tubes
- ETT stylet
- ETT securing device (tape if no device available)
- Gum elastic bougie
- Difficult airway equipment (e.g., laryngeal mask airway [LMA], combitube, cricothyrotomy supplies)
- Magill forceps if suspected foreign body

Technique
- Preoxygenate or bag the patient with 100% oxygen. Supplemental oxygen by high flow nasal cannula offers an additional oxygenation benefit and should be left on during intubation attempt.
- Position patient so that external auditory meatus is parallel to suprasternal notch.
- Adjust bed height so that patient's head is at operator's lower sternum.
- Administer pretreatment, induction, and paralytic agents, if applicable.
- Open the mouth as wide as possible, using finger-scissor technique.
- Insert the laryngoscopy blade into the mouth using the left hand and inch the blade posteriorly down the tongue until the epiglottis comes into view.
- Using the right hand, push the thyroid cartilage posteriorly (toward the bed) to increase the size of the vallecular space.
- While continuing to exert downward pressure on the thyroid cartilage, insert the laryngoscopy blade into the vallecula and lift the laryngoscope at a 45-degree angle to the horizontal – upward and toward the patient's feet.
- Identify the posterior notch and continue to lift the epiglottis to expose as much of the vocal cords as possible.
- Advance the endotracheal tube through the vocal cords, which has been molded straight to cuff with a 35-degree angle, from the side of the mouth, until the cuff is beyond the vocal cords.
- Inflate the cuff and confirm placement with end-tidal CO_2, breath sounds.
- Commence postintubation care.

Complications
- Failure to intubate the trachea with resultant hypoxia
- Unrecognized esophageal intubation

- Direct trauma to mouth, teeth, or larynx
- Vomiting with resultant aspiration
- Manipulation of the airway may cause increased intracranial pressure, bradycardia (especially in children), and laryngospasm

Notes
- If difficulty encountered when performing bag-valve-mask ventilation, insert oropharyngeal and nasopharyngeal airways, ensure proper mask size and reposition to improve seal, use jaw thrust and two-person technique, put in dentures, apply gel to bushy beard.
- If difficult airway suspected, do not attempt rapid sequence intubation (RSI). Call for help (ENT or anesthesia) and utilize alternate technique such as "awake" laryngoscopy without paralysis, fiber-optic or surgical airway (especially if anterior facial edema as in anaphylaxis) or, if anterior larynx/difficult view, use LMA, bougie, combitube, video laryngoscope.

The following topics do not lend themselves to the present format. There are a few important points in the management of dental trauma and joint reductions that are discussed subsequently.

DENTAL INJURY

- Ellis I fractures require routine dental follow-up.
- Ellis II and III fractures require a dressing (such as calcium hydroxide) if unable to see a dentist immediately, and prompt dental referral.
- Subluxed teeth require splinting with a cement if unable to see a dentist and prompt dental referral.
- Avulsed teeth require gentle cleaning and replantation, and if unable to see a dentist immediately, splinting with cement and prompt dental referral.

REDUCTION OF JOINT DISLOCATIONS

General principles
- Neurovascular status should be documented before and after all reduced dislocations.
- Unless urgent conditions contraindicate, prereduction films should be performed on all reduced dislocations.
- Postreduction films should be performed on all reduced dislocations.
- Sedation and analgesia are usually indicated to improve patient comfort and the chance of successful reduction.

Anterior shoulder dislocation
- Stimson maneuver: place the patient prone on a stretcher and hang 5 to 10 pounds weight from the patient's wrist. Apply gentle internal and external rotation with traction if needed; reduction should occur within 20 minutes.
- Scapular manipulation: position patient as for Stimson maneuver, with weights and slight external rotation of the humerus. Stabilize the superior aspect of the scapula with one hand while displacing the inferior tip of the scapula medially.

■ External rotation: in a supine patient, hold the arm in complete adduction with the elbow at 90 degrees of flexion. Placing the other hand on the patient's wrist, slowly and gently guide the arm into external rotation.

Posterior hip dislocation (Allis technique)
■ The patient is supine. An assistant applies direct pressure to both sides of the anterior pelvis, pushing it into the bed for countertraction.
■ The lower leg is grasped just distal to the knee and traction is applied in the direction of the deformity.
■ The hip is then brought to 90 degrees of flexion (perpendicular to the bed) and traction is applied in the anterior direction, toward the ceiling.
■ With continuous upward traction, the hip is gently internally and externally rotated until reduction is successful.

MCP/DIP/PIP dislocations
■ Exaggerate the deformity (usually hyperextension of the joint).
■ At the angle of maximal exaggeration, apply longitudinal traction.
■ While holding traction with one hand, use the other hand to reduce the joint by pressing the proximal aspect of the distal bone back into alignment.

Posterior elbow dislocation
■ An assistant grasps the proximal humerus in a supine patient to provide countertraction.
■ Grasp the wrist with one hand and apply steady traction with the elbow slightly flexed.
■ Grasp the distal humerus with the other hand and correct any lateral displacement.
■ Gently flex the elbow while maintaining in-line traction.

Knee
■ Traction–countertraction is usually sufficient to reduce femoral–tibial dislocation. If unsuccessful, direct displacement of the femur in the appropriate direction may be attempted while the leg is in full traction–countertraction.
■ Most knee dislocations reduce spontaneously; the injury and accompanying popliteal artery disruption must be suspected in cases of knee trauma where the ACL and PCL have been disrupted, that is, a "floppy" knee.

Radial head subluxation (nursemaid's elbow)
■ Place the child on the lap of the parent. Cup the elbow with one hand, placing the thumb over the radial head. With the other hand, grasp the wrist and supinate the forearm, followed by complete elbow flexion.
■ Hyperpronation of the forearm followed by elbow flexion may also be used.

Posterior ankle dislocation
■ The patient is supine; the knee is flexed.
■ Assistant applies cranially directed countertraction at the calf.
■ The foot is plantar flexed slightly and then traction applied longitudinally.
■ A second assistant pushes the distal tibia posteriorly (toward the bed) while the foot is reduced anteriorly while held in traction.

TMJ

▨ The practitioner must achieve leverage about the jaw; therefore the patient is either seated on the ground against a wall, in a chair against a wall with the practitioner standing on a stool, or upright in bed with the practitioner standing on the bed in front of the patient.

▨ Wrap both thumbs in gauze and place each thumb on the bottom row of teeth while grasping the mandible with the other fingers.

▨ Displace the mandible directly downward (toward the ground) with gradually increasing force, then reduce the mandible by pushing the chin posteriorly.

▨ The mandible may close forcefully as a result of masseter spasm; the thumbs may slide laterally into the space between the teeth and the buccal mucosa.

Further Reading

1. Roberts, JR, Hedges JR, eds. *Clinical Procedures in Emergency Medicine.* 5th ed. Elsevier; 2009.

2. Bailitz J, Bokhari F, Scaletta T, Schaider J. *Emergent Management of Trauma.* 3rd ed. New York, NY: McGraw-Hill; 2011.

3. Walls RM, Murphy MF, eds. *Manual of Emergency Airway Management.* 4th ed. Philadelphia, PA: Lippincott Williams and Wilkins; 2012.

Image answer key

Amish Shah, MD

Case	Figure	Modality	Answer
1	1.1	EKG	Normal sinus rhythm
1	1.2	x-ray	Normal chest x-ray
1	1.3A	x-ray	Nonspecific bowel gas pattern; no pills visible
1	1.3B	x-ray	Nonspecific bowel gas pattern; no pills visible
2	2.1	US	Pyloric hypertrophy
3	3.1	EKG	Sinus bradycardia with broad T wave inversions throughout
3	3.2	x-ray	ET tube in place; osteoporosis/degenerative joint disease
3	3.3	CT	Subarachnoid, intraparenchymal and intraventricular hemorrhage
4	4.1	EKG	Sinus tachycardia
4	4.2	x-ray	Right chest tube in place; no pneumothorax
5	5.1	EKG	Normal sinus rhythm
5	5.2	x-ray	Normal chest x-ray
5	5.3	US	Large gallstone and gallbladder wall thickening
6	6.1	x-ray	Normal chest x-ray
7	7.1	EKG	Normal sinus rhythm; occasional premature ventricular contractions
7	7.2	x-ray	Subcutaneous emphysema right shoulder and suspected pneumomediastinum
7	7.3A	CT1	Right pneumothorax
7	7.3B	CT2	Subcutaneous emphysema neck
8	8.1	MRI1	Epidural abscess near spinous process of L4
8	8.2	MRI2	Epidural abscess near spinous process of L4
9	9.1	EKG	Rapid atrial fibrillation
9	9.2A	x-ray	Normal chest x-ray
9	9.2B	x-ray	Normal chest x-ray
9	9.3A	x-ray	Normal knee x-ray
9	9.3B	x-ray2	No fractures; marked soft tissue swelling
10	10.1	EKG	Hyperacute T waves; sinus arrhythmia; Nonspecific IV conduction delay
10	10.2	x-ray	Median sternotomy wires and sutures suggest prior CABG; no focal infiltrate
12	12.1	EKG	Normal sinus rhythm
12	12.2A	x-ray	Normal chest x-ray
12	12.2B	x-ray	Normal chest x-ray
12	12.3A	x-ray	Dilated loops of small bowel
12	12.3B	x-ray	Air-fluid levels suggestive of small bowel obstruction; NGT in place
13	13.1	EKG	Normal sinus rhythm; minimal voltage criteria for LVH
13	13.2A	x-ray	Normal chest x-ray
13	13.2B	CXR2	Normal chest x-ray

Case	Figure	Modality	Answer
14	14.1	x-ray	Nonspecific bowel gas pattern
16	16.1	EKG	Normal sinus rhythm
16	16.2	CT	Normal head CT
17	17.1	EKG	Normal sinus rhythm; prolonged QT interval
17	17.2	EKG	Torsade de pointes
17	17.3	x-ray	Normal chest x-ray
18	18.1	x-ray	Markedly increased prevertebral space suggestive of retropharyngeal abscess
19	19.1	x-ray	L femoral head with growth plate widening
19	19.2	x-ray	L femoral head with growth plate widening
19	19.3	x-ray	Slippage of the capital femoral epiphysis
20	20.1	US	Testicular US showing limited arterial flow
20	20.2	US	Testicular US showing limited arterial flow
20	20.3	US	Testicular US showing limited arterial flow
21	21.1	EKG	Normal sinus rhythm
21	21.2	x-ray	Free air under the diaphragm
21	21.3	x-ray	Free air under the diaphragm with distended loops of small bowel
21	21.4	x-ray	Distended loops of small bowel
22	22.1A	x-ray	Normal chest x-ray
22	22.1B	x-ray	Normal chest x-ray
23	23.1	EKG	Normal sinus rhythm; biphasic T waves V5–6
23	23.2A	US	Enlarged aortic diameter
23	23.2B	US	Free fluid in Morison's pouch
23	23.2C	US	No free fluid in splenorenal recess
23	23.2D	US	No free fluid in pelvis
23	23.2E	US	No pericardial effusion
23	23.3	x-ray	Normal chest x-ray
24	24.1	EKG	Normal sinus rhythm
24	24.2	x-ray	Normal chest x-ray
24	24.3	CT	Normal head CT
25	25.1	x-ray	ET and NGT in place; no focal infiltrate
25	25.2	x-ray	Normal pelvis x-ray
25	25.3	CT	Normal head CT
26	26.1	EKG	Sinus tachycardia
26	26.2	x-ray	ET and NGT in place; no focal infiltrate
27	27.1	EKG	Sinus tachycardia; lateral T wave changes
27	27.2	x-ray	Normal chest x-ray
28	28.1	EKG	Sinus bradycardia
29	29.1	x-ray	Normal chest x-ray
29	29.2	EKG	Normal sinus rhythm
30	30.1	EKG	Normal sinus rhythm
30	30.2A	x-ray	Normal chest x-ray
30	30.2B	x-ray	Normal chest x-ray
31	31.1	EKG	Sinus tachycardia; prolonged QTc interval
31	31.2	x-ray	Hyperinflation suggestive of COPD; otherwise normal chest x-ray
32	32.1	EKG	Sinus bradycardia
32	32.2	x-ray	Normal chest x-ray
32	32.3	x-ray	Dilated loops of small bowel; clips in lower abdomen suggestive of prior surgery
32	32.4	AXR2	Air fluid levels suggestive of small bowel obstruction
33	33.1	EKG	Sinus rhythm; LVH; occasional PVC
33	33.2A	x-ray	Normal chest x-ray
33	33.2B	x-ray	Normal chest x-ray
35	35.1	EKG	Normal sinus rhythm; Right bundle branch block
35	35.2A	x-ray	Normal chest x-ray; small bilateral pleural effusions

(continued)

(continued)

Case	Figure	Modality	Answer
35	35.2B	x-ray	Normal chest x-ray; small bilateral pleural effusions
38	38.1	EKG	Normal sinus rhythm; biphasic T waves V5-6
38	38.2	x-ray	Normal chest x-ray
38	38.3	CT	Right acute subdural hematoma with slight midline shift
40	40.1	US	No intrauterine pregnancy; free fluid in pelvis
40	40.2	US	Free fluid in splenorenal recess
41	41.1	CT	Normal head CT
42	42.1	EKG	Sinus tachycardia; minimal voltage criteria for LVH
42	42.2	x-ray	Cardiomegaly
42	42.3A	x-ray	Stool noted in colon; Nonspecific bowel gas pattern
42	42.3B	x-ray	Stool noted in colon; Nonspecific bowel gas pattern
43	43.1	EKG	Sinus bradycardia; inferior ST elevations with lateral reciprocal suggest infarction
43	43.2	x-ray	Normal chest x-ray
44	44.1	US	Edematous R polycystic ovary with decreased flow
44	44.2	US	Edematous R polycystic ovary with decreased flow
44	44.3	US	Edematous R polycystic ovary with decreased flow
45	45.1	EKG	Normal sinus rhythm; inferior Q waves suggest old infarction
45	45.2	x-ray	Normal chest x-ray
47	47.1	EKG	Normal sinus rhythm
47	47.2	CT	Normal head CT
49	49.1	x-ray	ET and NGT in place; no focal infltrate
49	49.2A	US	No free fluid in morison's pouch
49	49.2B	US	No free fluid in splenorenal recess
49	49.2C	US	No free fluid in pelvis
49	49.2D	US	Pericardial free fluid present
51	51.1	US	Tubo-ovarian abscess near L ovary
52	52.1	EKG	Sinus tachycardia; minimal voltage criteria for LVH
52	52.2	CT	Normal head CT
53	53.1	x-ray	Normal chest x-ray
54	54.1A	x-ray	Normal lumbosacral spine film
54	54.1B	x-ray	Normal lumbosacral spine film
54	54.1C	x-ray	Normal lumbosacral spine film
56	56.1A	x-ray	Normal knee x-ray
56	56.1B	x-ray	Normal knee x-ray
57	57.1	x-ray	Normal chest x-ray
57	57.2A	x-ray	Stool noted in colon; Nonspecific bowel gas pattern
57	57.2B	x-ray	Stool noted in colon; Nonspecific bowel gas pattern
58	58.1	EKG	Sinus tachycardia; minimal voltage criteria for LVH
58	58.2A	x-ray	Cardiomegaly
58	58.2B	x-ray	Retrocardiac infltrate
59	59.1	CT	Normal head CT
59	59.2A	x-ray	Normal chest x-ray
59	59.2B	x-ray	Normal chest x-ray
60	60.1	EKG	Sinus tachycardia; diffuse ST elevations/PR depressions suggestive of pericarditis
60	60.2A	x-ray	Normal chest x-ray
60	60.2B	x-ray	Normal chest x-ray
61	61.1	EKG	Normal sinus rhythm
61	61.2A	CxR1	Normal chest x-ray
61	61.2B	CxR2	Normal chest x-ray
61	61.3	CT	Normal head CT
62	62.1	EKG	Sinus tachycardia

Case	Figure	Modality	Answer
62	62.2	CT	Normal head CT
62	62.3	x-ray	Normal chest x-ray
63	63.1	EKG	Sinus tachycardia; bigeminy
63	63.2	x-ray	Normal chest x-ray
63	63.3	EKG	Normal sinus rhythm
64	64.1	EKG	Sinus tachycardia; minimal voltage criteria for LVH
64	64.2	x-ray	Cardiomegaly; pulmonary vascular congestion suggestive of CHF
65	65.1	EKG	Sinus tachycardia; LVH; RVH
65	65.2	x-ray	Cardiomegaly
66	66.1A	CT	Left perinephric stranding and hydronephrosis
66	66.1B	CT	Left ureterovesicular junction calculus
67	67.1	EKG	Sinus tachycardia
67	67.2	CT	Normal head CT
68	68.1	EKG	Sinus tachycardia; minimal voltage criteria for LVH
68	68.2	x-ray	Normal chest x-ray
69	69.1	x-ray	Dilated loops of small bowel
69	69.2	US1	Telescoping of intestines suggesting intussusception
69	69.3	x-ray with barium	Contrast filling loops of bowel up to area of intussusception
70	70.1A	x-ray	Diffuse bilateral patchy infiltrates
70	70.1B	x-ray	Diffuse bilateral patchy infiltrates
71	71.1	EKG1	Superventricular tachycardia
71	71.2	EKG2	Normal sinus rhythm
72	72.1A	x-ray	Right lower lobe infltrate
72	72.1B	x-ray	Right lower lobe infltrate
73	73.1A	US1	No free fluid in morison's pouch
73	73.1B	US2	No free fluid in splenorenal recess
73	73.1C	US3	No free fluid in pelvis
73	73.1D	US4	No pericardial effusion
73	73.2	x-ray	Normal chest x-ray
73	73.3	x-ray	Normal pelvis x-ray
73	73.4A	CT1	C4 burst fracture involving body and posterior arches with subluxation
73	73.4B	CT2	C4 burst fracture involving body and posterior arches with subluxation
74	74.1	EKG	Sinus tachycardia; minimal voltage criteria for LVH
74	74.2A	CxR1	Normal chest x-ray
74	74.2B	CxR2	Normal chest x-ray
75	75.1	EKG	3:1 atrial flutter with ventricular rate of ~75, lateral T wave inversions
75	75.2	x-ray	Normal chest x-ray
75	75.3A	x-ray	Stool noted in colon; Nonspecific bowel gas pattern
75	75.3B	x-ray	Stool noted in colon; Nonspecific bowel gas pattern
76	76.1	EKG	Sinus tachycardia; minimal voltage criteria for LVH
76	76.2A	x-ray	Bilateral increased interstitial markings
76	76.2B	x-ray	Bilateral increased interstitial markings
77	77.1	EKG	Sinus tachycardia
77	77.2A	x-ray	Normal chest x-ray
77	77.2B	x-ray	Normal chest x-ray
77	77.3	CT	Normal head CT
78	78.1	EKG	Normal sinus rhythm; biphasic T waves V5–6
78	78.2A	CT	Normal head CT
78	78.2B	CT	Normal head CT
78	78.2C	CT	Hyperdense left middle cerebral artery suggesting thrombus
78	78.3	x-ray	Normal chest x-ray
79	79.1A	US	No free fluid in morison's pouch

(continued)

(continued)

Case	Figure	Modality	Answer
79	79.1B	US	No free fluid in splenorenal recess
79	79.1C	US	No free fluid in pelvis
79	79.1D	US	No pericardial effusion
79	79.2	EKG	Normal sinus rhythm
79	79.3	CT	Normal cervical spine x-ray
79	79.4	x-ray	Normal chest x-ray
79	79.5	x-ray	Bilateral pelvic rami fractures suggestive of open-book injury
80	80.1	x-ray	Normal chest x-ray
80	80.2	CT	Enlarged right kidney, no hydronephrosis
81	81.1	EKG	Sinus tachycardia; LVH with strain
81	81.2	x-ray	Small right lower lobe infltrate
81	81.3A	CT	Normal head CT
81	81.3B	CT	Normal head CT
82	82.1A	CT	Splenic laceration and hematoma
82	82.1B	CT	Splenic laceration and hematoma
82	82.1C	CT	Splenic laceration and hematoma
82	82.1D	CT	Splenic laceration and hematoma
83	83.1	EKG	Normal sinus rhythm
84	84.1	x-ray	Foreign body in pharynx; large stomach bubble noted
85	85.1	EKG	Normal sinus rhythm
85	85.2	x-ray	Normal chest x-ray
86	86.1	EKG	Anterior and lateral ST elevations with inferior depressions, likely acute anterolateral MI
87	87.1	EKG	Normal sinus rhythm
87	87.2A	x-ray	Large right lower lobe infltrate
87	87.2B	x-ray	Large right lower lobe infltrate
88	88.1	EKG	Sinus tachycardia
88	88.2A	CT	Normal head CT
88	88.2B	CT	Normal head CT
88	88.3	x-ray	Bilateral increased interstitial markings
89	89.1	EKG	Sinus tachycardia
89	89.2	US	Large pericardial effusion
89	89.3	x-ray	Cardiomegaly
90	90.1A	US	No free fluid in morrison's pouch
90	90.1B	US	No free fluid in splenorenal recess
90	90.1C	US	No free fluid in pelvis
90	90.1D	US	No pericardial effusion
90	90.2	x-ray	Right chest tube in place; no pneumothorax
91	91.1	CT	Sigmoid diverticulitis
91	91.2	CT	Sigmoid diverticulitis
91	91.3	CT	Sigmoid diverticulitis
91	91.4	CT	Sigmoid diverticulitis
92	92.1	CT	Normal head CT
93	93.1	Rhythm Strip	Rhythm strip with monomorphic ventricular tachycardia
93	93.2	EKG	monomorphic ventricular tachycardia
93	93.3	EKG	Normal sinus rhythm; lateral T wave changes
94	94.1	EKG1	Regular tachycardia; wide QRS with tall terminal R in avR suspicious for tricyclic overdose
94	94.2	EKG2	Normal sinus rhythm
95	95.1	EKG	Sinus tachycardia; minimal voltage criteria for LVH
95	95.2	x-ray	Hyperinflation suggestive of COPD; otherwise normal chest x-ray

Case	Figure	Modality	Answer
95	95.3	US	Hepatic abscess
96	96.1A	US	No free fluid in morison's pouch
96	96.1B	US	No free fluid in splenorenal recess
96	96.1C	US	No free fluid in pelvis
96	96.1D	US	No pericardial effusion
96	96.2	x-ray	Normal chest x-ray
96	96.3	x-ray	Normal pelvis x-ray
96	96.4	EKG	Sinus tachycardia; minimal voltage criteria for LVH
96	96.5	CT	Normal CT head
96	96.6	CT	Normal CT cervical spine
96	96.7	CT	Normal CT chest
96	96.8	CT	Splenic laceration with acute hemorrhage; perihepatic fluid suspicious for blood
97	97.1	x-ray	Dilated loops of small bowel wall with pneumatosis
98	98.1	EKG	Normal sinus rhythm
98	98.2A	US	Massive ascites
98	98.2B	US	Massive ascites
98	98.3	x-ray	Bilateral increased interstitial markings
99	99.1	EKG	Normal sinus rhythm
99	99.2	x-ray	Widened mediastinum; no focal infltrate
100	100.1	EKG	Normal sinus rhythm; biphasic T waves V5–6
100	100.2	x-ray	Normal chest x-ray
100	100.3	CT	Normal head CT
101	101.1	EKG	Sinus bradycardia; Osborn or J wave suggestive of hypothermia
101	101.2	x-ray	ET and NG tubes in place; Diffuse bilateral haziness suggestive of pulmonary
101	101.3	CT	Normal CT cervical spine
101	101.4	CT	Normal head CT
102	102.1	EKG	Sinus rhythm at approximately 130 bpm; LVH
102	102.2	x-ray	Severe cardiomegaly
104	104.1	EKG	Sinus tachycardia
104	104.2A	x-ray	Bilateral patchy infiltrates; hyperinflation
104	104.2B	x-ray	Lateral also reveals patchy infiltrates
105	105.1	EKG	Sinus tachycardia
105	105.2	x-ray	ET and NG tubes in place; no focal infltrate
105	105.3	x-ray	Mild pulmonary vascular congestion; no focal infltrate
105	105.4	CT	Normal head CT
106	106.1	EKG	Sinus tachycardia
106	106.2	x-ray	Mild pulmonary vascular congestion; no focal infltrate
107	107.1	x-ray	Normal L foot x-ray
108	108.1	EKG	Normal sinus rhythm; Nonspecific lateral and inferior T wave changes
108	108.2	CT	Normal head CT
108	108.3A	CT	Normal cervical spine series
108	108.3B	CT	Normal cervical spine series
108	108.3C	CT	Normal cervical spine series
109	109.1	EKG	Normal sinus rhythm; Nonspecific lateral and inferior T wave changes
109	109.2A	x-ray	Large bowel obstruction with massive dilation suggestive of volvulus
109	109.2B	x-ray	Large bowel obstruction with massive dilation suggestive of volvulus
110	110.1	EKG	RBBB with LAHB
110	110.2	CXR	Cardiomegaly, VAD, implantable device with single RV lead, interstitial edoma
111	111.1	x-ray	No acute fracture, radial head subluxation
112	112.1	CXR	Normal chest x-ray
112	112.2	EKG	Sinus tachycardia
113	113.1	Rhythm strip	Ventricular tachycardia

(continued)

(continued)

Case	Figure	Modality	Answer
113	113.2	EKG	Sinus tachycardia with incomplete RBBB
114	114.1	US	Color flow showing arterial flow on right side and absence of venous flow on left at rest. (Note the hyperechoic DVT in lumen of vessel on left.)
114	114.2	US	Vein during augmentation of venous return showing irregularity in vessel lumen indicative of DVT.
115	115.1	CXR	Widened mediastinum
116	116.1	Finger	Hydrofluoric acid burn of hand
118	118.1	EKG	Normal EKG
118	118.2	CXR	Normal chest x-ray with flattened diaphragms
118	118.3	CT	Normal head CT
119	119.1	EKG	EKG showing short QTc
119	119.2	CXR	Pulmonary mass and nodules
119	119.3	CT	Non contrast CT of abdomen with left renal calculus
120	120.1	Physical exam	Moon facies – rounding of the face , central fat deposit, striae
121	121.1	CXR	Normal chest x-ray
121	121.2	Bone marrow biopsy	Paucity of stem precursor cells with a predominance of fatty infiltrates
122	122.1	EKG	Sinus tachycardia
123	123.1	EKG	Normal sinus rhythm
124	124.1	EKG	Normal sinus rhythm
125	125.1	EKG	Normal sinus rhythm
125	125.2A	CXR	Normal chest x-ray
125	125.2B	CXR	Normal chest x-ray
125	125.3	CT	Normal head CT
126	126.1	EKG	Normal sinus rhythm
126	126.2	CT	Normal head CT

Index